SAVING THE PLANET: ONE BITE AT A TIME

Saving The Planet: One Bite At A Time

By Gary Null, Ph.D.

Foreword by Philip Wollen

GARY NULL
PUBLISHING

218 West 37th Street
New York, NY 10018
www.GaryNull.com
646-926-5422

ISBN 978-1-7328882-1-0

DISCLAIMER: THIS BOOK DOES NOT CONTAIN MEDICAL ADVICE. THE CONTENTS OF THIS BOOK, INCLUDING THE TREATMENTS AND MODALITIES MENTIONED AND REFERRED TO HEREIN ARE INTENDED FOR EDUCATIONAL AND INFORMATIONAL PURPOSES ONLY AND ARE NOT INTENDED TO SUBSTITUTE FOR PROFESSIONAL MEDICAL ADVICE, DIAGNOSIS AND TREATMENT.

The treatments and modalities mentioned or referred to in this book are intended to educate and inform viewers so as to enhance their ability to make their own nutritional and health choices. Always seek the advice of your physician or other qualified health care provider with any questions you may have regarding a medical condition. Never disregard professional advice or avoid seeking it because of something you read in this book.

Consult your health-care professional for individual guidance on specific health issues and before following this or any program. Persons with serious medical conditions should seek professional care. The author and publisher specifically disclaim any liability, loss or risk, personal or otherwise, which is incurred as a consequence, directly or indirectly, of the use and application of the contents of this book.

Any statements or claims about the possible health benefits of any foods or supplements have not been evaluated by the U.S. Food and Drug Administration (FDA) and are not intended to diagnose, treat, prevent or cure any disease.

To the insightful, courageous and outspoken individuals, past and present, who have illuminated the personal and global benefits of a healthy vegetarian lifestyle. May their wisdom and compassionate action direct and inspire many more of us to embrace this lifestyle as the preservation of life on Earth depends on it.

Acknowledgements

I'd like to acknowledge a dynamic and extraordinary creative team including Richard Gale, the Executive Producer of Progressive Radio Network and the Gary Null Program for the past 11 years, and Jay Graygor, my Art Director. Additionally, the quality of the manuscript with its structure, grammar and style, is due in no small measure to an outstanding team of editors; special thanks to Brian Connolly and his Editorial team of Lynn Komlenic, Michele Poff, Ruth Stuckey, Jennifer M. Holibaugh, and Zakira Karthiegeyan.

Table of Contents

Foreword

Tens of millions of Americans do not believe in global warming or deny that climate change is being driven by human activity. Others accept the consensus from the vast majority of scientists in the international community that anthropogenic climate change is real; however, most do not fully understand it. This lack of agreement and understanding is also true for the majority of elected officials and legislators who are expected to make wise decisions. As a result, virtually nothing constructive has been done in the past forty years to effectively mitigate the consequences of our lifestyles, habits, and addictions in order to slow global warming trends. Americans continue to demand more stuff: gas-guzzling SUVs and trucks; planes; meat, poultry, and fish; milk and cheese; genetically modified crops and all of the pesticides, herbicides, and fertilizers that accompany them; hardwood, sand for manufacturing concrete, coal-powered plants, hydrofracking, and oil drilling. All of this stuff is necessary to sustain the neoliberal myth of infinite progress that fuels booming and emerging economies. What is not being asked is: what are the consequences of the choices I make? Do I choose paper or plastic at the checkout counter? Shall I purchase water in a glass or plastic bottle? A hamburger or veggie burger? Will I make an effort to buy only organic produce or doesn't it matter? The outcome is that, during just the past two years, the increase in global warming has included some of the worst climate events and news in recorded history. Among the major climate and environmental news headlines that convey the severity of our planet's weakened immune system we read:

"Earth's Carbon Concentrations Have Soared to Levels Not Seen in 800,000 Years"

"Summers Are Getting Hotter Faster, Especially in North America's Farm Belt
New Study Shows Antarctic Melting Approaching 'Unstoppable' Tipping Point"

"Cut Carbon Now to Avoid Climate Tipping Points: The price to be paid for not cutting emissions of greenhouse gases could mean driving the planet across planetary boundaries, or "tipping points""

"Global Glaciers Melting up to Three Times Rate of 20th Century
Surge in Methane Emissions Threatens Efforts to Slow Climate Change
This Melting Glacier in Antarctica Could Raise Sea Levels By 11 Feet"

"Climate Change Could Flip Mediterranean Lands to Desert
Scientists Are Clear: Big Winter Storms Influenced by Warming Planet"

"NYC Can Expect More 9-Foot Floods"

"Almost Biblical: Amazing 3,000-ft high dust cloud shrouds Phoenix"

"Unprecedented Mass Die Offs as Pacific Ocean 'Turning into a Desert' Off California Coast"

"California Is Turning Back into a Desert and There Are No Contingency Plans"

"US Faces Floods of Climate Refugees"

"US Coastal Flooding Breaks Records as Sea Level Rises, NOAA Report Shows
'Unprecedented' Heat Wave Fueling Arctic Fires Made More Than Twice as Likely by Climate Change"

"Antarctica Ice Loss Tripled in 5 Years, and That's Raising Sea Level Risks Coastal Real Estate Worth Billions at Risk of Chronic Flooding as Sea Level Rises"

"Hottest July Ever Recorded in United States: California's Death Valley Busts Own Record - With 2018 on track to be one of the hottest years ever, the climate crisis is here. Now."

"NASA Scientists Say Ocean Circulation Is Slowing. Here's Why You Should Care."

"Europe's Extreme Summer Is So Hot It Melted the Highest Peak in Sweden, and Now It's Only the Second-Highest"

"State of the Climate Report Confirms Planet Has Entered 'New Neighborhood' of Global Temperatures"

"Human Activity Leaves Diminished Oceans: Humankind has already disturbed or degraded six-sevenths of the blue planet
Heatwave Deaths Will Rise Steadily by 2080 as Globe Warms Up"

"The Grotesque Truth about Florida's Red Tide Disaster: Lake O'Green Algae Dumps to Blame"

"Global Species Extinction: Humans Are Now the Asteroid Hitting the Earth"

"Methane Deathtrap Threatens Democracy"

"2016 was a year in the Arctic like we've never seen before."

"For the 37th consecutive year, alpine glaciers retreated across the globe."

"Global sea level was the highest on record"

"Humans Have Used a Year's Worth of Earth's Resources in Just Seven Months"

"Study Finds New Reason to Ban Plastic: It Emits Methane in the Sun"

Collectively, these headlines, among many others which could have been included, describe the new normal. We can reasonably expect Category 4 and 5 hurricanes annually. There is no evidence that wildfires across the American West and Northwest will abate. Prolonged droughts will persist. Extreme storms, floods, and hotter weather, which now threaten global food security, are also creating a new norm. These environmental trends and more should force us to concede that humanity is on course to exceed its capacity to sustain a quality life throughout much of the world, including half of the United States.

Yet, despite the lack of action in the US, there are nations and major cities around the world taking climate change seriously. Visionaries and scientists are creating unique and wonderful innovations in renewable energy to challenge America's hubris, denial, and complacency. Rather than descending into apathy, withdrawing into isolation and being unwilling to face these problems, this book intends to provide a deep and detailed strategy for how we can individually and collectively make a difference. And the foremost effort each of us can begin at this very moment is to adopt a healthy, plant-based diet. Not only is it affordable, but a vegan lifestyle will also strengthen our physical and mental health to face the challenges ahead. It is the single most important thing each of us can do to save the planet.

Introduction

What if I told you that going on the incredibly delicious, cost-effective plant-based diet would:

- Reduce your risk of *all* cancers by 50%,[1]
- Decrease your chance of developing diabetes by 50% and eliminate Type 2 diabetes,[2]
- Drop your chance of developing heart disease by 24%,[3] reduce your chance of dying from heart disease by 29%,[4] or if you have heart disease, reduce future cardiac events by 73%,[5]
- Lower your risk of colon cancer by 40%,
- Have an 80% chance of reducing arthritis symptoms in less than four weeks,
- Assist you in losing a minimum of one pound of body weight per week until you reach your goal, and without exercising[6] (although I recommend exercising too.),
- Significantly lower high blood pressure and unhealthy cholesterol levels,
- Double the number of natural "killer cells" in the body, thereby increasing the strength of your immune system,[7]
- Significantly lessen your likelihood of being obese,
- Help you have leaner, healthier children,
- Improve your sleep, your sex life, and your complexion,
- Give you more energy than you have ever had, and, most importantly, add quality years onto your life?

What if I also told you that in one year of eating this way, you would save the lives of approximately 400 animals (fish and shellfish included), plus, you would save 300,000 gallons of water,[8] nearly 90,000 pounds of grain[9] (which could go to feed humans), and more than 5,700 gallons of gasoline, all while generating 50% fewer carbon emissions[10]? You would also end your contribution through dietary choices to depleting rainforests, eroding topsoil, world hunger, and global warming, while standing for cleaner air, cleaner water in aquifers, rivers, lakes, and oceans, cleaner drinking water, the humane treatment of animals and humans, and the health of any number of species and the planet too.

Would you want to hear about it? Moreover, would you be interested in knowing that millions—and a growing number—of people in our country and around the world are choosing this diet and lifestyle right now, and for the very reasons I just pointed out?

A Brief Look at the Problem

Americans are sick; in fact, we are extremely sick. We are also tired, stressed, toxic, and confused. We work harder than most people, take fewer vacations, are sleep deprived, and our relationships are in frequent disrepair. We spend more on our healthcare than any other country in the world—$3.5 trillion, which is higher than any other segment of spending in America. Unfortunately, every year of increased spending translates into worsening health. We have more cancer, more heart disease, more mental illness, and more inflammatory conditions like arthritis. In addition, we have record-shattering numbers of people suffering from diabetes and obesity—in fact, America has more obese adults than any other developed nation; we also have the highest per capita rate of childhood diabetes in the world. So, our children are also now suffering from heart disease and diabetes. Shockingly, for the first time in modern history, many American children will now *die before their parents*—a disturbing reality, especially for a society that considers itself the greatest and most advanced country in the world. We are not only overeating; we are gorging. "Super-sized" is passé; we now have gigantic meals and frequently eat when we are not hungry. Many are experiencing a cognitive disconnect where "all you can eat," or "eat as much as you can" is the new norm. We are not eating to enliven, or eating for health, vitality, or restorative and regenerative purposes.

We are simultaneously approaching pandemic levels of brain conditions such as Alzheimer's, dementia, memory loss, and Parkinson's; and we are a nation that is depressed and anxious. Consider for a moment that 25% of all women between the ages of 25 and 45 (11 million women) are taking some form of antidepressant medication, selective serotonin re-uptake inhibitors such as Celexa, Lexapro, Prozac, Paxil or Pexeva, and Zoloft, while over ten million children are being medicated each day before they go to school with drugs such as Ritalin. Fatigue and pain are the two most common ailments for which people are seeking medical treatment. This is the picture of ill health that now shapes our nation.

We actually see women's lifespans shortening more so than any industrialized nation. Yet, we have more doctors, hospitals, nurses, research facilities, and federal agencies looking into more ways of treating the symptoms of these conditions. We've become so concerned, that our vernacular has changed. Our nation is at "war" with just about *everything* now: a war on cancer, a war on heart disease, and a war on obesity. But, unfortunately, like the wars on drugs, poverty, and terrorism, we are losing the war on health, too; and, frankly, cannot win with our modern approach of disease management.

One question we are not asking that actually could help us win is "*Why are we having all of these conditions?*" In short, we've confused the suffering and complexity of symptoms of these conditions with the *solution*—which is prevention; in this case, living healthfully. To prevent a disease is much easier than reversing it once it is in motion. Therefore, the purpose of this work, in part, is to describe a diet that is proven to prevent suffering and illness. So, we will take you step by step through these complex issues, while describing how the plant-based diet allows you to heal your body while easing pressures on our planet too.

Virtually all of the important statements herein have been scientifically verified, originating from quality, independent science published in peer review literature. It is no longer a mystery that the Mediterranean diet, the Okinawan diet, or the healthy vegan vegetarian diet are scientifically valid ways of reducing and eliminating key major medical conditions. Why? Because plant-based diets—or those founded on plant-based foods—have as their basis the living nutrients that maintain the integrity and health of our body's trillions of cells. These diets are anti-inflammatory and slightly alkaline; they are high in fiber but not excessive in protein. Most can be prepared with minimal to no heat and, hence, are easier to digest and safer and more effective for our biological processes.

But, until now we've only focused on our bodies. What about the planet?

When you stop and look around, you also see an environment that is imploding. We have a massive amount of land that is no longer able to sustain life. We are seeing the desertification of America's southwest, with dust storms similar to those of the 1930s and sand storms like those of the Arabian Peninsula. California is estimated to have one year's worth of drinking water left from its current reserves. The state is in perpetual drought and is now imposing mandatory restrictions. Last year, we had 12,000 unique weather events—the coldest day, the wettest day, the hottest day, the worst tornado, etc.—and this is the new norm.

It gets worse. There are 18 million children in America going to bed hungry each day, living with food insecurity, the state of being without reliable access to a sufficient quantity of affordable, nutritious food. One hundred million Americans are just at or above the poverty level, which is about one-third of our entire population, and nearly 29 million Americans, although not considered homeless, are living on couches in family and friends' homes. We now have students who are part of the teenage debt system. 50% of all college graduates today live at home with their parents because there's not a job for them in the area of their academic background, and graduate students can look forward to 20 years of paying off student loans. We also have the return of the debtors' prisons in 27 states, and in a minimum of 60 communities, we have made it illegal to feed the homeless.

Is there something wrong with this scenario? Clearly yes, but how do we change it? What is the good news?

The good news is that there are millions of Americans who are becoming increasingly conscious of the importance and value of the choices they make in every area of life, including food. You exercise that consciousness when you wake up in the morning and decide to have a nourishing smoothie or hot oatmeal with fresh berries and walnuts versus more standard American fare, such as bacon, sausage and eggs, toast, greasy hash browns with coffee, chemical creamers, and white sugar. And, as you will see, there's a substantial positive consequence when making these kinds of healthy choices.

Instead of sitting down to an unhealthy meal of steak and a "fully loaded" baked potato (butter, sour cream, and/or cheese) or burger and fries with a cola—a week's worth of protein, fat, and sugar in a single serving—members of this growing group are going to farmers markets, health food stores, their own backyards, and food co-ops and selecting functional health foods. They are also putting an end to overtaxing their kidneys and liver, thickening their blood, and putting blood sugar levels at risk.

The foods they are purchasing are fresh, organic, non-GMO grown whole foods, alive with nutrients—vegetables like kale, Swiss chard, kohlrabi, arugula, micro-greens, sprouts, tomatoes, spinach, garlic, and onions. And, as they're preparing these as part of a delicious meal—with red quinoa, organic brown rice, beans and legumes, or tubers—they're conscious that what they're putting in their bodies will make a difference to their health, not just in their sleep, digestion, and energy levels today, but in the long-term with disease prevention.

These people are also conscious that their health entails much more than just food or even exercise. The mental, emotional, and spiritual aspects of health are also critical and must be explored. Moreover, no conversation of health would be complete without speaking about the quality of the environmental resources that sustain us. So, we will be examining our water, air, land, and food-growing systems, as well as a host of other pressing ecological issues that are challenging humanity's very ability to heal and carry on with life as we are accustomed.

By considering the value of the information, principles, and guidelines that I am sharing here, my hope is that you will select what is reasonable to adopt and, in this process, enhance your natural, vital, and fulfilling existence. And, while there are numerous studies supporting the superior health benefits of a plant-based diet for warding off disease and reducing illness and for lessening environmental degradation, being a vegetarian does not guarantee health. Unfortunately, many well-intentioned individuals rightly choosing the vegetarian diet do not know how to be successful at it and end up reporting an overall lower level of health on average than those who are not vegetarian.[11]

Why is this? How is it possible? What does it take to be a healthy *vegetarian*? Moreover, what does it mean to be a healthy *human being*, and can we accomplish this in our fast-deteriorating world? As you will learn, these are not mutually exclusive questions. Becoming a healthy vegetarian does, in fact, lead to becoming a healthy human being, which I essentially define as someone with enduring health and vitality on all levels—*physical, mental, emotional,* and *spiritual.* And this vitality supports a person's full realization of their unique purpose in life and in service to others and the planet. But is a dietary change enough in this day and age to sustain health? As you will see, it is not.

So, why now with this message?

There have been numerous books on the link between dietary and planetary health—from *Diet for a Small Planet* by Frances Moore Lappé to *Diet for a New America* by John Robbins and many others; all of these have truths. But in America, our consciousness is what is on our mind today—especially since we are bombarded by so much information daily, and most people receive their information and education through the internet, which tends to be in the form of extremely brief news bytes. Hence, even good information from the past must be restated, updated, and presented within a current context. Furthermore, different stages in life bring different priorities. Those who were more active and interested in health at a young age may have married and become more involved in career, family, and education, with health taking a back seat. However, with increased responsibility comes increased stress—a key contributor to disease. When you couple the amplified financial and social stresses over the past 10 years—starting with the 2005 housing crisis, then the 2007–2009 recession, and the still-increasing costs related to living in America—with the fact that so many Americans turn to gravely, universally unhealthy "comfort" foods for relief from their pain, you can begin to understand why we are becoming a progressively heavier and sicker population. So, when people realize this—either through the deterioration of their own health or that of an aging parent or unwell child—they typically rekindle their interest in health.

Moreover, since our personal health is so inextricably linked to that of our environment, which is ever-changing, there is a need for ongoing discourse. But no matter where people are on their path, or their stage in life, my purpose is to help them find the health they are seeking. By supplying as much useful and practical information about the realities of health in *today's* world, you will have a better place from which to make important decisions. In addition, my hope is that by examining the information that is being presented here, readers can make healthier choices, and will find it easier to resist temptations and eliminate some of the negative feedback loops, such as emotional eating.

The idea that the only people who are capable of changing in America today are young, disillusioned, or idealistic kids is simply not true. I can tell you from my experience in the field for over 45 years that people of all ages, all walks of life, all ethnicities, and all educational backgrounds, when confronted with disaster will ask, "*What can I do to change the circumstances*?" So, we want to know what changes need to be made, and we think we want to change; but then comes the hard part—actually making the change. Most of us don't want to do it; we want to stay in our comfort zone. So we either don't make the changes, or we maintain our old habits while simply adding in a few very small modifications to appease ourselves but that do nothing to make much of a difference. What we really need is to start over; we need to write an entirely new story, with a whole new determination, and use the tools that are available for these changes.

We are living in a critical age, and if we don't make some major lifestyle changes and lightning fast, we're in for a "world of hurt." Most of you probably know that we are not living sustainably, and with a global population that has increased 7-fold in the last 60 years, we need to figure this out, and now. Can we grow enough food to supply for our current increasing population and future generations? The answer is "Yes," if we change our methods of farming and food distribution as well as the foods we consume.

If there has ever been a time to fully comprehend the breadth and depth of the individual and social ramifications of what we are putting into our bodies and how we are living our lives, it is right this minute. The human race is in trouble. As reported by NASA: "97% of climate scientists agree that climate-warming trends over the past century are very likely due to human activities, and most of the leading scientific organizations worldwide have issued public statements endorsing this position." While the corporate-owned media challenges science about the truth of this figure, and politicians and pundits debate over how much of climate change is actually caused by humans, my response is "*Who cares?*" Instead of debating who is right or wrong, we simply need to look at the science and address that.

So here's the science: Today, we are at 401.52 ppm (parts per million) of atmospheric CO_2, as measured from the Mauna Loa Observatory in Hawaii and reported on CO_2Now.org. (This is a combined total of a preliminary measured monthly average as of April 4, 2015 [Scripps Institution of Oceanography] and the preliminary monthly average as of April 6, 2015 [NOAA-ESRL].)

To put things into perspective, I turn to Bill McKibben, author, educator, and environmentalist. In a 2008 piece titled *The Tipping Point*, McKibben stated: "New evidence suggests that we have already passed a dangerous threshold for the amount of carbon dioxide in the atmosphere—and that the time for taking strong action is slipping away… If we are at 385 parts per million [now 401.52], and everything is melting, what does that tell you? What it tells you is: This is not a future problem. We're already past the line, out of the safe zone."

So, who are these people that I am speaking about—the ones who recognize what McKibben is saying and are changing their lives? They are the healthy vegetarians; people who support an organic plant-based movement because they want to be as healthy as possible throughout their hopefully long lives and are intelligent and responsible enough to recognize that the choices they make affect humankind and all life on our planet. They are acutely aware that every choice of a plant-based meal over an animal-based one markedly reduces animal suffering and environmental degradation; that switching to a meat, dairy, and egg-free diet does everything that I mentioned above and more.

If everyone went vegetarian *just for one day*, the US would save:

- 100 billion gallons of water, enough to supply all the homes in New England for almost 4 months;
- 1.5 billion pounds of crops otherwise fed to livestock, enough to feed the state of New Mexico for more than a year;
- 70 million gallons of gas—enough to fuel all the cars of Canada and Mexico combined with plenty to spare;

- 3 million acres of land, an area more than twice the size of Delaware; and
- 33 tons of antibiotics.

We would also prevent:

- Greenhouse gas emissions equivalent to 1.2 million tons of CO_2, as much as produced by all of France;
- 3 million tons of soil erosion and $70 million in resulting economic damages;
- 4.5 million tons of animal excrement; and
- Almost 7 tons of ammonia emissions, a major air pollutant.

This is the kind of significant impact that many are already realizing through the incredibly worthwhile and fulfilling choice of becoming a healthy vegetarian, and it is a choice that weighs on the consciousness of an ever-increasing group of Americans.

There is a growing group of people who are also fully cognizant that the Koch (pronounced 'Coke') brothers, Dow Chemical, BP, Exxon-Mobil, and other major polluters are not going to stop; they cannot stop because they've become addicted to their delusion of what real power is, as money is secondary to the influence they have gained. They have also bought the political system: They control the state legislators and the non-profit American Legislative Exchange Council (ALEC), which votes on "model bills" that change our rights and frequently benefit corporations' bottom lines at public expense. For 35 years, 20,000 laws have been enacted by a secret group representing 300 or so of the major corporations in America, like Coca Cola, McDonalds, Exxon-Mobil, Altria/Philip Morris, Humana, Bayer, GlaxoSmithKline, Wal-Mart, and Johnson and Johnson, all behind the backs of the American people.

But this doesn't mean that America's growing group of conscious individuals sits back and does nothing. No, we remain active participants in campaigns to raise awareness and to stop what can be stopped while also creating positive life-affirming organizations and initiatives, some of which you will read about here. The educated consumer also knows that the hundreds of thousands of lobbyists, contractors, and governmental agents are going to stay in Washington D.C. and look after the interests of the major food companies, agriculture companies, and energy companies, as well as the banking industry, insurance industry, and so-called "healthcare" and pharmaceutical industries; they're aware of that. The educated consumer also knows that the average person won't change, but for the individual that is aware of and working toward getting "off the grid" as much as possible, there's an enormous amount of opportunity *and* good—the type of good that occurs when you put your money in local nonprofit community banks or credit unions rather than in major banks (Bank of America, Chase, Wells Fargo, etc.), and refrain from purchasing cheaply made dresses made in sweat shops by disadvantaged women and children. Instead, you are buying "Green," consciously sourced goods that are "Made in America" by people paid a living or union wage. Getting off the grid has a lot to do with assuring your sustainability away from industry-structured energy sources, but it is also the process of intentionally disengaging from practices that are harmful—whether to humans, other living beings, or our planet.

As an example, when you're buying something that's locally grown, you are no longer contributing to the carbon footprint of something that was brought to your neighborhood from distant places. When you're eating an organic potato grown in the US, it might have taken 60 to 90 gallons of water to grow it instead of the hamburger you used to have that would have taken almost 3000 gallons of water.

You're conscious of that, and you're conscious of recycling in addition to using recycled materials and avoiding plastics as much as possible. You're also aware of how much you consume and whether you really "need" something or just want it; you challenge your relationship to "more." You feel better because you are no longer contributing to the floating "Trash Vortexes," the Western and Eastern Garbage Patches, which are harmful to aquatic life. (You may be interested to learn that the Pacific Trash Vortex now occupies an area equivalent in size to double that of the state of Texas.)

You're also mindful not to overeat or consume addictive, deficient foods. You're going to turn your yard, wherever possible, into an edible garden. If you cannot do that, you will consider Xeriscaping it—a term coined in 1985 to describe the idea of using landscaping that is water wise. You're going to be aware of the importance of honey bees and the dangers to them of Neonicotinoids, toxic pesticides that cause bee colony collapse, by supporting organic bee farmers. You're aware that if we do not stop this madness, one-third of all the food that we eat will disappear because it all requires pollination.

You're going to take a bag that is made out of natural fibers to the store to load up your produce; these little conscious acts make a significant difference when multiplied, and you will inspire more people to do the same. You're going to conserve water, even if you're not required to and, wherever possible, you're going to install solar panels on your roof to save the energy of cooling your house in hot weather. You will also consider collecting rainwater or participate in city planning to promote these same initiatives. Imagine how good it might feel to simplify and downsize your life, to trade your "stuff" for more free time, which could be used to craft a life that is viable, creative, *and* meaningful—one that promotes and "gives" life.

You could even join the millions of Americans as well as others around the world who are marching against Monsanto, DuPont, Syngenta, and Bayer, the GMO companies that are threatening life as we have known it for centuries. You might even feel the impulse to become a social activist, participating in closing down nuclear power plants and stopping gas hydro-fracking, thereby stopping the wanton destruction of nature, natural habitat, and species.

Can you also imagine a society where a large number of people earn their living from work and other initiatives that are non-destructive and that *cause* wide-ranging health and well-being—projects that are titillatingly efficient and effective in delivering ever-increasing levels of wellbeing to all that occupy this planet, while allowing it to heal? Imagine a growing number of people who are as concerned about others as they are about themselves, and who thrive on creating useful systems within which ALL are supported to thrive. These are people who know that joy comes from giving much more than they take; and they cultivate a mindset and practice of "enough," so that the less fortunate may have some, and, perhaps, even a bit more than just the basics. In this life, the rewards are immediate and real; one only need give it a try to see how enlivening and invigorating it can be.

Because once you open your mind to the truth of how we live, what and how much we consume, the unnecessariness of much of it, and the abuses to nature and animals that our current habits promote, you may find yourself too embarrassed and humiliated to ever think of living that way again. Instead, you will begin to look at all beings as sacred; you might even be the person who adopts an animal so that it won't have to be euthanized. For sure, though, you will never sit down to veal parmesan again, because you're now fully aware of how that little veal calf suffered—a torment that is unimaginable for a civilized society; and you become unwilling to consume this kind of "nourishment" ever again.

Instead, you will now be able to rejoice in the possibilities that your blood pressure is lower, your pulse rate lower, your cholesterol lower, and your inflammatory markers lower. You will also feel more confident knowing that you are less likely to have a heart attack or stroke, be overweight or obese, or suffer from cancer, diabetes or arthritis; and, you will rejoice in the fact that you are likely to live at least ten years longer. You will also celebrate a lightness of consciousness and greater peace and ease knowing that you aren't participating in the callous, insensible annihilation of sentient beings—animals, like us, that "cry out" for days, even weeks, when their babies are taken from them, never to be returned. No, once you see and know of the realities and take them deeply into your heart, you and your life will change for the better, and forever.

With the choice of becoming a healthy vegetarian, you are, in essence, becoming what I call a *vitalist*—someone who seeks the thoughts, actions, and deeds that energize the human spirit. Laudable vitalists include Voltaire, Michel de Montaigne, Maimonides, Socrates, Aristotle, Greek physicians Hippocrates and Galen of Pergamon, German biologist Hans Driesch, and French philosopher Henri Bergson.

As a vitalist, you will practically bounce out of bed in the morning. You will be burdened by few ailments; plus, no more dragging yourself through the day, artificially stimulating your energy with one cup of coffee or energy drink after the next. As your cells rebuild and replace themselves, you'll rebuild your adrenals, your skin, nails, hair, muscles, and bones; your body will start to transform for the better because you're flooding it with polyphenols, phytonutrients, chlorophyll, quality fibers, and plant-based proteins. Your thinking will also be clearer, your sleep more restful, and your spirit stronger.

We are the ones who are actively promoting a sustainable lifestyle, protecting animals from abuse and factory farming, respecting our fellow humans, and also engaging in being a model of this healthier way of living and aging for those who may be inspired by our example. We also respect the choices of others, as we are not here to be a kind of food or lifestyle police; we must acknowledge and preserve freedom of choice, even when we disagree. But when others are ready, we ask: what else can I do? We will be there to encourage them, to show them. Make no mistake; we are the future of sustainable living. And we are not a few; we are actually now numbering into the tens of millions.

The trouble is that our voices are not very loud or being heard enough yet on the global scene. There is yet to be a national and detailed survey of vegans: No one comes asking the many vegetarian teenagers or adults, "Are you eating a veggie burger instead of a hamburger, a hotdog, or fried chicken?" Or, "Why did you choose to become vegetarian?" Or, "What do you love about being vegetarian?" Or, "How has being a vegetarian helped you, your family, and your community?"

We do occasionally see it in the media from celebrities and other healthy vegetarian role models like Alicia Silverstone, Joaquin Phoenix, Ellen DeGeneres, Tobey Maguire, Anne Hathaway, and many more who have made these choices; as role models, they will continue to influence those that follow them. We also have more people, including celebrities, now than ever actively expanding their consciousness into body awareness through practices such as yoga, Pilates, and meditation. Then, there are those that take another step into social or political activism. They wouldn't automatically vote Democrat or Republican, but look for and support the independent candidate who has not been compromised nor will be compromised by the Washington industrial and lobbying machine. Instead, they will be there to protect the environment as well as animal and human rights and health. Once you become committed to the plant-based lifestyle, you're opening yourself up to an enormous new world of these wondrous, exciting possibilities.

Included here are recommendations from many studies, many people, and much learning and investigation into the foundations of health. Additionally, over my career, I've conducted more than 40 studies, with tens of thousands of participants in total. While these studies were all medically monitored and independently evaluated, their focus addressed changing lifestyle behaviors, including diet, exercise, and how to manage stress. They all had profound outcomes. Because protocols of scientific research were rigorously adhered to, these studies meet the criteria for establishing scientific evidence for living a longer, healthier life while overcoming or reducing diseases from arthritis to depression, from inflammatory conditions like Alzheimer's, Parkinson's, and dementia, to high blood pressure and elevated cholesterol. The people in my studies were real people with real symptoms, and my team and I typically worked with them for up to one year at a time. So, most of the comments are not simply anecdotal.

There is also growing support for the plant-based lifestyle, and not just from scientists: many physicians, including the ones noted in this book, are choosing to incorporate food and lifestyle protocols into their practices, and they are motivating and inspiring thousands of other physicians to take a step toward the prevention of conditions, not just treating the symptoms. Dieticians, with the support of the American Dietician Association, are now learning and supporting others on the vegetarian path, and even the US government is now recognizing the value of the vegetarian diet toward human health and sustainability.

From the time of my earlier books on vegetarianism 35 years ago, thousands upon thousands of studies and reports validate the health-promoting qualities of the plant-based diet, especially those including super foods such as pomegranate, blue-green algae, acai, grapes, wheatgrass, goji berries, and maca root, for example, which flood the body with phytonutrients, enzymes, probiotics, and prebiotics that are essential for optimal wellness. So, science (and good science) is supporting veganism. Meanwhile, there is no good independent science that supports being healthier by eating an animal-based diet.

We now have new understanding of food and its impact on the body, like resveratrol from grapes, and the anti-aging superstar carnosine, and how all these compounds stimulate the healing process. We know that the quality of fibers in grains, legumes, nuts, seeds, fruits, vegetables, and tubers help to keep our intestines clean, our cholesterol lower, and our intestines and colon free from polyps, pre-cancers, and cancerous tumors. We know that there are plant-based foods that will help our skin, eyes, and bones, and that our kidneys and liver need not be overwhelmed with the hazardous byproducts of fast-food processes. We will cover many of these and more.

As I noted earlier in this introduction, my *why* for creating this work at this time is twofold—to support *you* in your choice of health by providing new learning in the field of plant-based living and to support a shift that is desperately needed now for us to survive almost certain catastrophe. In reality, the solutions that we undertake now must be quick, and they must be impactful and effective. One qualifying solution is *to adopt the plant-based diet, now and completely,* never to look back. This is what I'm asking you to consider. And once you have done this, you will have joined the ranks of the millions serving as a living example of what is possible while beginning to enjoy the benefits of a life in harmony with the human spirit.

You do not have to make these changes quickly; they can be made gradually. What's most important is that you make them. Certainly, give yourself adequate time to sit with and reflect on the material I am presenting and to organize a new approach, but do not delay. We have already reached our crossroad; as confirmed by many, small changes will not be enough to reverse the current trend. We need big, bold, all-encompassing changes that are implemented with great love, care, and compassion.

Here is a brief outline of what we will be exploring, though I refer you to the detailed table of contents for a more finite presentation. We start section one with an exploration of the many pitfalls and challenges inherent in the Standard American Diet (S.A.D.) and what it takes to heal ourselves. We begin with the physical, as this is the easiest and most obvious place to make changes when we're talking about healthy vegetarianism. In this section, you will find: dedicated discussions on the vegetarian diet itself; our current food habits and where they come from; health reasons for adopting the vegetarian diet, including the toxic things that people put in your meat; reasons why vegetarian diets are better for you physically; what foods and vital nutrients comprise the vegetarian diet; and because it is still the number one nagging question by people considering vegetarianism as well as some long time vegetarians, I offer you an entire chapter dedicated to protein.

We then will take a look at the lifestyle of the healthy vegetarian, the religious and spiritual traditions that have fueled the practice of vegetarianism, the implications of taste as a healing mechanism, as well as what it takes to make and sustain change. This is, perhaps, the most important section of this book. Here we will explore what it is that causes people to choose a path and stay on it—to become so clear and resolute in service to their values and goals that they are living examples of actualized human beings. I will offer suggestions to get you in touch with your *why* in life and meaningful practices for keeping you on track with this. I will also give you a list of vegetarians, as well as an overview highlighting some important thoughts and accomplishments of its few most influential leaders, which may serve to inspire you on this journey.

In Section two, we focus on social responsibility from our local and national communities as well as the global community. You will begin to see firsthand how the entire world ties in and benefits from your choice of a healthy vegetarian lifestyle. This section includes discussions of morality as it relates to omnivorism and vegetarianism, along with everyday things you can do to promote a healthy vegetarian lifestyle; it also contains dialogue about the realities of our natural resources and global food resources and what is needed in terms of action there.

Section three turns the focus to what's next, as we consider what the healthy vegetarian lifestyle looks like in a broader social sense now and into the future. In this section, we will explore some of the initiatives—both local and global—currently being undertaken to address the sustainability issues that we bring attention to herein; we will also take a brief look at what it means to live sustainably. Finally, you will find appendices brimming with other helpful instructions and information that will help you along your healthy vegetarian path.

Do we know what is going to happen? No. But, as McKibben notes in his book *Eaarth*: "Our hope depends, on scaling back—on building the kind of societies and economies that can hunker down, concentrate on essentials, and create the type of community (in the neighborhood, but also on the Internet) that will allow us to weather trouble on an unprecedented scale. Change—fundamental change—is our best hope on a planet suddenly and violently reeling out of control and out of balance."

As this text is fundamentally about *healing*, it is obviously also about change; for something to be healed, we must discover it has been amiss and fix it. So, if we want to be a healthy vegetarian and expand from there into becoming a truly healthy human being, we must not only face our fear of change, we must embrace a different way of being and living in this world.

I leave you with the words of Paulo Coelho, a Brazilian lyricist and novelist of the widely acclaimed book *The Alchemist* (which has been translated into 80 languages and has sold over 65 million books worldwide), and who is considered one of the most influential writers of our time. This is an excerpt from his book, *The Devil and Miss Prym:*

> When we least expect it, life sets us a challenge to test our courage and willingness to change; at such a moment, there is no point in pretending that nothing has happened or in saying that we are not yet ready. The challenge will not wait. Life does not look back. A week is more than enough time for us to decide whether or not to accept our destiny.

My hope is that you accept this challenge, this call to a better life for you and the entire world.

Gary Null, Ph.D.

Part I:

Healing Yourself

> "What happens when people open their hearts? They get better."
>
> — *Haruki Murakami,* Norwegian Wood

What does it mean to *heal*? When you look up the word, you will get any variety of definitions: to make healthy, whole, or sound; to restore to health; to become free from ailment. It's a common word in medicine, in terms of healing wounds, bone breaks, or ulcerations and lacerations and such. It is also used when referring to breaks or chasms in relationships, such as healing a *broken heart*, which it turns out is both an emotional and physical experience.

In 1993, Harvard University began a nine-year study on "Broken Heart Syndrome,"—a phenomenon where a surviving spouse's death is linked to grief over the loss of a spouse. The highly publicized report[1] showed a stunning 66% increase in the rate of death of surviving spouses. Nicholas Christakis, M.D., Ph.D., professor in the Department of Healthcare Policy at the Harvard Medical School, had this to say about their findings: "Our study showed that people are connected in such a fashion that the health of one person is related to the health of another."

There are many reasons I bring up this study first, to illustrate that health is, in reality, inextricably linked to one's external environment, conditions, and situations;

second, to point out that *connection* is critical to animals, humans included; you will see this as a running theme throughout the book. Additionally, there is the premise that most of you have heard before and numerous other studies demonstrate: overall health is unequivocally tied to physical, emotional, mental, and spiritual health; they are dependent, and you cannot have health in one area without having it in the others.

Furthermore, health is much more than just the absence of disease, as we have tended to think of it here in the US. The definition of health by the World Health Organization is: "As a complete state of physical, mental, and social well-being, not merely the absence of disease and infirmity."[2] So, we will need to take a look at social factors too.

How any one person defines and achieves health is different; however, the foundational components of health (exercise, rest/sleep, pure water, nourishment, recreation, purpose, community, consciousness development, etc.) that we will explore in this section are largely similar across cultures and disciplines and arouse general agreement from a majority of health practitioners and philosophers for some time now.

In our country, particularly, we tend to look at things as separate components. What is required, then, for healing to occur, is to first correct our thinking along these lines. We need to start thinking holistically. Then, we need to take it upon ourselves to recognize when we are out of balance and bring wholeness to these areas. The world (as we know it) will heal itself as each of us takes responsibility to heal our self.

This holistic approach that I'm speaking about is, in fact, the essence of traditional medicine practices, such as Chinese Medicine or Ayurveda. While these systems and the healing practices associated with them have been largely dismissed by Western medicine, there is growing acceptance of them—one-third of Americans now partake[3]—along with plenty of scientific evidence backing their efficacy in healing.

The following discussion of Native American ancestors' philosophy about health and healing encapsulates my thinking and, in essence, summarizes the great task we have in not only defining the components of health but also what is required for healing.

> With more than 2,000 tribes of indigenous people in North America, the healing practices varied widely from tribe to tribe, involving various rituals, ceremonies, and a diverse wealth of healing knowledge. While there were no absolute standards of healing, most tribes believed that health was an expression of the spirit and a continual process of staying strong spiritually, mentally, and physically. This strength, as well as keeping in harmony with themselves, those around them, their natural environment, and Creator, would keep away illness and harm. Each person was responsible for his or her own health and all thoughts and actions had consequences, including illness, disability, bad luck, or trauma. Only when harmony was set right, could their health be restored.[4]

Let's take a look now at what all of this might entail for us in modern society today, addressing the question: what does it take to become truly healthy?

Chapter 1

Getting Started on the Vegetarian Diet – An Overview

"Find me someone who is eager to live, so far as is possible, in accordance with intellect… and let him demonstrate that meat eating is easier to provide than dishes of fruits and vegetables; that meat is cheaper to prepare than inanimate [vegetarian] food for which chefs are not needed at all; that compared with inanimate [vegetarian] food it is… lighter on the digestion, and more quickly assimilated by the body than vegetables; that it is less… conducive to obesity… than a diet of inanimate [vegetarian] food. But if [as I believe will happen] no doctor, no philosopher, no [athletic] trainer, no laymen ventures to say this, why do we not voluntarily detach ourselves from this bodily burden [of eating meat]?"

— *Porphyry,* On Abstinence from Killing Animals *(written about 275 CE)*

Where Do We Begin?

There are no two people reading this page right now who are starting at the same place. You may be a person that has been a vegetarian at some point in your life but found that you couldn't follow through with it at that time, for whatever reason.

Maybe you are still a vegetarian but recognize you aren't as healthy as you would like to be. For example, there are a lot of young people who will not eat meat because of ethical reasons—they don't want to see an animal sacrificed for a hotdog or hamburger—but they might be consuming a lot of foods high in refined carbohydrates (bread, pastas, pizzas), or partaking of foods that taste and smell like animal products like soy bacon. They may be doing this without awareness of the challenges associated with them, such as they often contain gluten and flavor enhancers like MSG.

Or, perhaps you have become aware of the benefits of a plant-based diet and are looking for some healthy parameters within which to launch your exploration; you're an athlete who's concerned about adopting a plant-based diet because you were told that you'll lose your muscle mass, your strength, your endurance, or speed; or, you're a connoisseur of fine foods who goes out to eat a lot and are afraid that you will miss the variety of foods that you are accustomed to or worse have not yet been exposed to the amazing world of gourmet plant-based cuisine.

Whatever your reasons for reading this book, know that being a healthy vegetarian means so much more than just eating vegetables; it is a state of mind, a consciousness, a way of life. But let's just say you're that person who wants to make positive, healthy choices, and you simply do not know where to begin. You know that you want to look better, feel better, sleep better, have more energy, enjoy clearer thinking, and wake up feeling excited about the day. Or, maybe you're tired of the indigestion, the constipation, the headaches, the insomnia, the high blood pressure, the elevated blood sugar, the excess weight, foggy brain, poor memory and the pains; you don't want this anymore. Okay, but where do you actually begin? Let's start with the actual diet because that is the most obvious, and physical health has a huge impact on other areas of life.

Getting Rid of What's Harmful

In terms of the diet, we always begin with *elimination*.

Step one in becoming a healthy vegetarian is to eliminate anything that may be causing a lower energy state. Go into your refrigerator, go into your storage pantries, and look to see: Is the food that you are eating a living food? Is it a vital food? Does it really represent health at its highest level? If not, throw it away. Throw it away because you don't want it in your body.

Here's the short list: all dairy; eggs; meat in any form, including fish, chicken, beef, pork, venison, nothing with eyes or a head; no artificial sweeteners; no processed foods (chips, TV dinners, etc.); no refined carbohydrates or sugary foods, meaning bagels, most breads and cereals, pastries, cookies, cakes and most crackers; no deep-fried foods; no artificial flavors, sweeteners, coloring agents; no sodas or coffee—nothing that triggers an inflammatory reaction. Inflammation is one of the bedrocks of most diseases—cancer, diabetes, heart disease, arteriosclerosis, arthritis, Alzheimer's, Parkinson's, osteoporosis, ALS, fibromyalgia, macular degeneration, cataracts, glaucoma; all of these disorders exist because of inflammatory agents. If you want to be healthy—or become a healthy vegetarian for that matter—you've got to get rid of these items. Instead, you will be consuming food from the delectable, health-giving world of plant-based foods and, as you will see, it is a vast and wondrous one.

A vegetarian diet free from animal products is alkalinizing to the body, which is in harmony with the body's natural slightly alkaline state; it rejuvenates the body and promotes health and healing. Whereas, the foods that I mentioned just above are acidic; they throw off the body's natural pH balance and promote inflammation and disease. Even though we like them and they taste good, even though they comfort us on many levels—we like the salty, crunchy, soft, and sweet and sugary—these are the foods that are proven to negatively impact our well-being and cause our diseases. So, we're going to eliminate them all. Now, you may feel deprived for a period of time, but that will completely resolve itself once you start eating healthily. For some people, it's not possible to get rid of everything unhealthy. In this case, I would then suggest that you get rid of one unhealthy item per week, like beef in any form in week one; chicken, week two; fish, week three; pork, week four; alcohol, week five; caffeine, week six; sugars, week seven; artificial sweeteners, soft drinks, colas, week eight; French fries, pizzas, week nine; and dairy, week ten. What's nice is there are natural vegan alternatives that are healthy and vital for all of these. As soon as you take this important step, you are starting to become healthier. Congratulations, you are now on your way!

What's So Bad about Inflammation?

Inflammation is a natural and complex biological process initiated by the body in response to harmful stimuli, the aim of which is to protect the body so that damaged cells, irritants, pathogens, etc., can be removed, and the body can begin the healing process. Inflammation, specifically acute inflammation, shows that the body is trying to heal itself. Take the example of a sprained ankle: inflammation prevents us from "walking on it" until we have given the inflammation sufficient time to subside. Inflammation, however, does not mean *infection*, even though infection causes inflammation. Infection is caused by a bacterium, virus, or fungus, while inflammation is the body's response to it. In and of itself, inflammation is an incredibly helpful and healthy reaction; the problem occurs when inflammation becomes chronic, as is typically the case in people consuming the Standard American Diet.

I've noted in previous works that it is a complete myth that an inflammatory attack is tissue-specific when, in fact, the contents of your blood are reaching every cell in your body. Inflammation in the body from any source extends throughout the entire body, negatively impacting all cells. For example, the pro-inflammatory cytokines produced in the body after eating a well-done hamburger may cause a person's knees to swell. Even though it appears that the knees are the only affected part, the cytokines are also, for instance, contributing to the buildup of toxic amyloid plaque in the brain and impairing normal liver function. By the same token, a lack of knee swelling after eating the hamburger doesn't mean that someone isn't being affected by inflammation on the fundamental level. This is the dangerous thing about inflammation. Let's say every time you eat a hamburger, your knees don't swell. Does this mean that your joints and other organs are not being affected or that your brain or liver are fine? The answer is "no." Chronic inflammation is problematic for everyone, and it affects everybody; it just may take years or even decades until the damage is so severe that you've reached your tipping point.

Unfortunately, by this time you have a verifiable, diagnosable condition, and you are long past the moderate response stage—you are, in reality, at the end stage, which is different, but your doctor cannot tell you so. What we do know is that one person may end up with arthritis or fibromyalgia, and someone else with diabetes or cancer, all of which are diseases of inflammation. This is what the healthy vegetarian diet will help you avoid.

Here is a list of acidic foods, which are to be avoided on a healthy diet:

- Refined sugar (basically all conventionally prepared baked goods)
- Refined flour
- Dairy (milk, egg and cheese products)
- Meats of all kind especially ham, bacon, and foods cooked with lard
- Seafood
- Soft drinks
- Alcohol
- Coffee
- Deep-fried foods
- Overcooked foods
- Processed foods
- Trans fats (partially hydrogenated oils)
- Synthetic sweeteners (Splenda®, NutraSweet®, and Equal®)
- Artificial colors
- Food additives
- Food preservatives
- Genetically Modified (GM) foods, or foods containing GMOs (Genetically Modified Organisms)

Dangers Lurking in Processed Foods

Why must we eliminate the foods I've just mentioned if we want to be healthy? The short answer is because they are toxic to the body. They can create chronic states of inflammation and disrupt our pH balance, and significantly, many of these foods are highly processed. This means, among other things, that they are full of chemicals in the form of harmful additives and preservatives. There are essentially two types of processing—mechanical and chemical. What I am speaking about mostly here is chemical processing. However, even with mechanical processing, where you think chemicals are not being added, this is likely not the case. In 2004, the FDA approved the "Modified Atmosphere Packaging" (MAP) system[1] (reportedly used in up to 70% of packaged meats[2]), which is the process of treating meat by sucking oxygen out of a package and pumping in carbon monoxide (CO), which preserves the red color of meat just after processing. The practice, which saves meat processors billions of dollars a year[3]—in that consumers do not want to purchase unappealing-looking meat—is just one of the tricks that food processors use to increase the appeal or shelf life of foods. One report noted that to enhance the meat's color and freshness and to mask any discoloration from spoilage, the carbon monoxide is combined with myoglobin, a globular protein of 153 amino acids, to form carboxymyoglobin—a bright cherry red pigment that is injected into most red meats, including pork.

And it's not as if "fresh foods" are safe, either. Non-organic apples, for example, which are typically harvested in September and October in the US, are picked when they are slightly unripe and then treated with the chemical 1-methylcyclopropene (also known as "SmartFresh,") waxed, boxed, and then stacked on pallets, where they are kept in cold storage warehouses for an average of 9-12 months.[4] In fact, according to the USDA's Agricultural Research Service, "On average, treated apples stayed firm for 3 to 6 months longer than untreated controls when placed in controlled-atmosphere storage conditions. Red Delicious apples, for example, stayed crunchier 2 to 3 weeks longer than untreated controls after removal from storage."[5]

But let's get back to chemical processing. In reality, nothing but harm can come to the body from bombarding it with endless chemicals. Here are just a few of the noxious substances used in the processing of foods[6]: Nitrites and Nitrates, which have been implicated in cancer; Sulfites and Sulphur Dioxide, which are known allergens for many asthmatics; and Aspartame, a popular additive in many beverages and athletic supplements today, which accounts for over 75% of the adverse reactions to food additives reported to the FDA.[7] including seizures and death. The FDA even denied approval for aspartame for 20 years because of brain tumor findings in animals.[8] Other noxious substances include BHA (Butylated Hydroxyanisole) and BHT (Butylated Hydroxytoluene), which is considered a possible human carcinogen by The World Health Organization's International Agency for Research on Cancer[9]; Benzoic Acid/Sodium Benzoate, a preservative often added to milk and meat products, fruits juices and soft drinks, low-sugar products, and cereals that temporarily inhibit the proper functioning of digestive enzymes and cause headaches, stomach upset, asthma attacks, and hyperactivity in children; Potassium bromate, used to increase volume in white flour, breads, and rolls, is linked to increased cancer risk for humans; High-Fructose Corn Syrup has been noted as a causative factor in heart disease, as it raises blood levels of cholesterol and triglyceride fats while making blood cells more prone to clotting; the more well-known Monosodium Glutamate (MSG), the world's most utilized and controversial flavor enhancer, has been implicated in tightening of the chest, headaches, and a burning sensation in the neck and forearms as well as obesity. Since the public does not want to consume MSG, the food processing companies have become wise to this and instead now disguise it in many forms: hydrolyzed vegetable protein, autolyzed vegetable protein, textured vegetable protein, hydrolyzed yeast extract, autolyzed yeast extract, plant protein extract, sodium caseinate, calcium caseinate, yeast extract, textured whey protein, and textured soy protein; even the innocuous terms spice and natural flavor can designate the presence of MSG[10]; and, we'll stop at Olestra, a fake fat commonly known to cause "anal leakage" and other gastrointestinal problems, forcing the FDA to require foods containing it to carry a warning label.

Do you get the idea? Processed foods, which comprise most of the food sold in supermarkets, convenience stores, fast food restaurants, many restaurant chains, and gas stations across America, are not health-promoting in the very least. Most processed foods also contain sugar, excess salt, and fats; they are also low in nutrients and fiber[11] and easy to consume quickly. Food manufacturers go out of their way to combine chemicals for the sole purpose of creating "foods" that are highly intoxicating and addictive, which leads to overeating. If you cannot pronounce the ingredients on a label or know what something is, don't eat it; it's not going to help you, no matter how "good" it tastes.

As if this weren't enough, we have two additional topics to discuss here related to the heating of some of the foods I talked about previously. First, let's look at the browning of carbohydrates—the bagels, toast, pizza crust, buns, and potatoes, in particular—and the link to cancer. The National Cancer Institute notes research pertaining to the heating of certain foods, including vegetables, to a temperature above 120 degrees Celsius (248 degrees Fahrenheit), which causes the chemical acrylamide to occur. Potato chips and French fries were found to contain higher levels of acrylamide compared with other tested foods, and foods prepared below this temperature did not contain acrylamide.[12]

The International Agency for Research on Cancer considers acrylamide a "probable human carcinogen."[13] "Acrylamide has also been linked to nerve damage and other neurotoxic effects, including neurological problems in workers handling the substance. While the EPA regulates acrylamide in drinking water, and the FDA regulates the amount of acrylamide residue in materials that may come in contact with food, they do not currently have any guidelines limiting the chemical in food itself."

In 2003, Swedish researchers analyzed the acrylamide levels of some common foods such as processed potato products, bread, breakfast cereals, biscuits, cookies, snacks, and coffee. They estimated the average daily intake of the chemical to be high enough to be associated with potential health risks according to US Environmental Protection Agency (EPA) and World Health Organization (WHO) data.[14]

Let's now turn our attention to the chemical that occurs during the cooking of muscle meats such as beef, pork, fowl, and fish products—the Heterocyclic Amines (HCAs) and how they are carcinogenic and also mutagenic[15], meaning they can change DNA. One study conducted by researchers from the National Cancer Institute's Division of Cancer Epidemiology and Genetics found a link between individuals with stomach cancer and the consumption of cooked meats. They also found that people who ate beef four or more times a week had more than twice the risk of stomach cancer than those consuming beef less frequently, and additional studies demonstrate an increased risk of colorectal, pancreatic, and breast cancer associated with high intakes of well-done, fried, or barbequed meats.[16] Moreover, HCAs are not present in significant amounts in foods other than meat cooked at high temperatures.[17]

So, in summary, we're eliminating two known cancer-causing items in the diet, but also a large number of pro-inflammatory agents that result in any of the numerous lifestyle diseases that our nation is plagued by today. There is enough evidence on both of these fronts, however, to demonstrate the value of replacing all of these foods with healthier plant-based alternatives. But, before we discuss what to eat, I want to take a moment to address portion sizes and America's appetite for food, both of which tend to be large, and the negative effects associated with this.

America's Need to Super-Size

Let's talk about portions and learning to control our appetite. Also, let's examine why we also must eliminate super-sizing as a way of eating and living. We have become accustomed to eating way more than the body needs and can possibly handle. For example, the body cannot store protein. So when we consume more protein than the body can use, it's stored as fat, which adds a host of additional problems. We need, therefore, to eat smaller quantities of protein—which a plant-based diet inherently provides—three times a day in order to stay trim. In doing this, not only will we drop unnecessary weight, we will be protecting our kidneys, our heart, our liver, and in reality, our overall health.

Meat isn't the only problem as it pertains to super-sizing. As a population, we are obsessed with sugar; in fact, according to the USDA, the average American consumes 150 lbs. of added sugar a year[18]; by "added," we are not speaking about naturally occurring sugars in fruits, such as fructose, or glucose and sucrose in vegetables. Added sugars include agave syrup, brown sugar, corn sweetener, corn syrup, sugar molecules ending in "ose" (dextrose, fructose, glucose, lactose, maltose, sucrose), high-fructose corn syrup, fruit juice concentrate, honey, invert sugar, malt sugar, molasses, raw sugar, sugar, syrup.[19] The problem has gotten so bad that the World Health Organization issued a plea early in 2014 for a significant reduction in the consumption of added sugar, saying: "There is increasing concern that consumption of free sugars, particularly in the form of sugar-sweetened beverages, may result in... an increase in total caloric intake, leading to an unhealthy diet, weight gain, and increased risk of noncommunicable diseases."[20]

Too much sugar consumption is linked to everything from metabolic syndrome to depression, obesity, diabetes, and cancer. One example of a disorder related to a diet that is high in processed sugars, is non-alcoholic fatty liver disease (NAFLD), which affects 40% of the adult population. As the name suggests, NAFLD isn't from alcohol; it's from sugar in the diet. In fact, the American Liver Foundation notes that NAFLD tends to develop in people who are overweight or obese or have diabetes, high cholesterol, or high triglycerides.[21] They specifically say that rapid weight loss and poor eating habits also may contribute to the disease. NAFLD may cause the liver to swell (steatohepatitis), which, over time, can cause scarring (cirrhosis) to the tissues, and may even lead to liver cancer or liver failure.

This is why we must let go of all the foods I'm discussing. In reality, a diet full of meat, dairy, and processed foods is a harmful diet that leads to disease. And, as you read on, you will learn even more about the toxins in these foods that are preventing you from experiencing the health that you desire. From pesticide-ridden foods to environmental pollution to negative thinking, literally everything needs to be examined and evaluated for its effectiveness in helping you create a joyous, happy life. Before we get into a more in-depth look at these, however, I want to spend a little time speaking about what it takes to create health in the physical body related to what we eat.

What Can We Eat, Then?

You say, "Okay, I've got rid of all or most of this unhealthy stuff, so what do I eat now?!" And this is where we go to the healthy vegetarian diet. The healthy diet, which we will speak more about in Chapter 5, includes:

VEGETABLES of all kinds, including tubers (yams, potatoes, Jerusalem artichokes, etc.), root vegetables (carrots, parsnip, daikon, etc.), stalk vegetables (celery, asparagus, kohlrabi, etc.), leafy vegetables, including dark green leafy vegetables (kale, lettuces, cabbage, etc.), inflorescent vegetables, meaning we eat the *flower* of the vegetable (broccoli, cauliflower, artichokes, etc.), and fruit-like vegetables, meaning foods that we call vegetables but that are botanically considered fruits (a seed-bearing structure that develops from the ovary of a flowering plant such as olives, tomatoes, avocados, peppers, cucumbers, peas and beans, etc.), and sea vegetables (arame, kombu, wakami, etc.).

FRUITS, the best being apples, pears, peaches, nectarines, plums, grapes, or citrus fruits. Although the sugar content of these fruits is fairly high, it is diluted with water and released relatively slowly into your system as you chew and digest the cellulose-encased cells of the pulp. Bananas and other tropical fruits should be eaten in moderation by those sensitive to sugar, since their sugar content is higher. Similarly, dried fruits, including figs, prunes, raisins, dates, dried apricots, pears, and apples contain three times the sugar dose of the fresh fruit, and as such, they should be eaten sparingly.

Basic WHOLE GRAINS, for example, are a good source. These include whole wheat, rye, triticale (a cross between rye and wheat you may be able to tolerate if you are allergic to real whole wheat), corn, barley, brown rice, oats, millet, and buckwheat.

BEANS and LEGUMES such as soybeans and soy products such as tofu, tempeh, and miso, as well as mung beans, lentils, azduki beans, split peas, black-eyed peas, kidney beans, navy beans, red beans, pink beans, pinto beans, black beans, turtle beans, fava beans, chick-peas (garbanzos), and peanuts.

NUTS and SEEDS such as sunflower, pumpkin, chia, sesame, alfalfa, chia, and flax seeds, as well as almonds, cashews, walnuts, pistachios, and pine nuts.

Let's look at what a typical day of eating might look like. Starting the day with a healthy smoothie is one of the best ways to get the nutrition you need at the beginning of the day. Take your favorite liquidapple juice (if you do not have sugar sensitivities like in the case of diabetes), rice milk, almond milkthen add some chia seeds, perhaps some blueberries and pomegranate seeds, a little bit of almond, cashew, walnut, or pistachio butter, a teaspoon of organic coconut or flaxseed oil, and a tablespoon (of about 20 to 30 grams) of high-quality plant-based protein, from hemp, split pea, rice, or organic soy. Now you've got a full spectrum of what you need to start your day: protein, fats, and carbohydrates. Add a little bit of non-dairy yogurt (for probiotics) or some powdered probiotic for intestinal health and a teaspoon of vitamin C, and you are good to go—all the fiber, polyphenols, phytonutrients, and antioxidants needed for one meal. It's a great way to start the day, and you can vary the fruits and the nut butters for variety; you can even get vanilla and chocolate flavored proteins or just add raw cacao powder, or if you are in the mood for banana flavor, just add a banana.

When you're thirsty during the day, have coconut water with lemon juice (two ounces of lemon juice and 16 ounces of coconut water), instead of soft drinks, sweetened fruit juices, or teas. This concoction will quench your appetite, give you electrolytes and potassium, and doesn't spike your blood sugar. If you don't want coconut water, then some purified water with some citrus or some decaffeinated green tea will do the trick.

Have your major meal in the afternoon: try to include a little bit of sea vegetable (those from the Atlantic coast are best because some from the Pacific Ocean have tested positive for radioisotopes as a result of the Fukushima disaster), a little bit of fermented vegetables, and some starchy vegetables such as parsnips, kohlrabi, squash. Have beans or legumes as an entrée dish, served over brown rice or quinoa pasta, or as toppings to a big green salad. Then, in the evening, have your smallest meal, such as a bowl of soup or some salad. If you're hungry at night, you don't want to ingest anything that will keep the metabolism going, such as fruit or sugary snacks which will spike your blood sugar, or even a heavier snack. Instead, have organic popcorn, which will satisfy the appetite but doesn't add calories and doesn't affect your blood sugar. Eating before bed is not a good idea, as the food will sit in your stomach, which could cause restless sleep. If you don't want food, then have iced lemon water; it will kill your appetite. This is even better for your body, especially if you want to reduce your weight.

The world of plant-based eating is so vast and astounding; you could spend years experimenting with the diet and not exhaust the possibilities. If you live in a multicultural area, which many of you do, visit different food markets to get a sense for what I am saying. Go to a Korean market, a Japanese market, a Chinese market, an Indian market, a Spanish market, a Caribbean market; you will find interesting and amazing foods that will expand your foray into plant-based eating. These cultures all have healthy foods; they also all have unhealthy foods. If you go to an Indian market, for example, in New York City around 27th Street and Lexington Avenue, there are several. I can guarantee that if you go in there, you've never experienced those particular kinds of smells and wonderful aromas. They might have 30 different types of lentils, and you're used to one. Along the same lines, Chinatown will have 25 different types of dried mushrooms, and mushrooms are very important—shiitake mushrooms and maitake mushrooms in particular. Americans usually eat white cap mushrooms, and we don't eat the medicinal nutritionally rich mushrooms, so go to the specialty markets to find those.

You can start by incorporating some into soups, or mix them into grains with other vegetables. I also encourage you to experiment; get creative and blend things that you know you enjoy the taste of separately (or in other dishes), and mix them together—that is how we expand our food experience. As an example, take some fresh tomatoes and blend them in a blender with a little ginger, garlic, fresh basil, raw spring onion, and a pinch of cayenne—that's a phenomenal gazpacho! Add some chunks of cucumber and avocado for a heartier meal. Not only does this taste great, but it fills you up, and it's healing—kills viruses and bacteria. Purchase a number of vegetarian cookbooks that help build your excitement to the delectable world of plant-based foods. Vegetarian recipe books not only provide valuable information on plant-based foods, but they can give you hundreds of tips and ideas while helping you plan meals in advance.

A lot of these items can be cooked in advance. You can even make smoothies and juices in advance—make them all on Sunday, for example, and then freeze them into containers. The night before, place what you want to consume for the next day in the refrigerator; the next morning your juice or smoothie is thawed and ready to go. The same principle can be applied to grains, soups, legumes, or stews: cook them all one day a week and freeze them, thawing the night or day before as you go along; this way you don't have to do a lot of cooking. Salad prep is so much easier today with our modern air-tight storage containers. Cleaned salad greens that are either blotted or spun dry with a salad spinner, with chopped vegetables (ones that do not decay quickly) such as carrots, cabbage, celery, onion, grated beets, turnips, rutabaga, etc., can easily be stored for a week in air-tight containers. If you want to add other fruits like apples, pears, pomegranate seeds, etc., or vegetables like cucumber, pepper, and fennel that spoil more easily, simply chop and add those throughout the week.

So it's joyful, it's fun; it's exciting. You do all your food prep on one day; you do your food selection on the previous day, and you have meals for a week! The vegetarian diet offers a far greater range of tastes and dishes than you've ever experienced in your life. But in order to gain the full benefit of it, you've got to break the habit of just eating the same foods and especially the ones that are highly addictive and highly allergenic, such as dairy and processed wheat.

But when you do, you'll find weight drops off easily and quickly. You're also going to have more energy because plant-based foods are far more easily digested and assimilated by the body. Plus, it will not be constantly stressed by having to digest such massive amounts of food. Most people don't realize they've eaten so much (in terms of quantity and calories) for breakfast that by the time lunch comes round, they still have breakfast in their stomach; then, by the time dinner comes round, they haven't fully digested lunch; by the time bedtime comes, they have dinner, or a late-night snack, in their stomach—that's why we have so much insomnia and indigestion. Eat vegetarian, lighter; eat less; eat living foods.

It really is simple on one hand: the diet should be 70–75% raw, uncooked foods, and 25–30% lightly cooked, so the nutrients are actually liberated—I will explain this next—and we can enjoy the experience of warm food. When you heat broccoli, asparagus, Brussels sprouts, and cauliflower, for example, you're actually breaking down the vegetable slightly so that more phytonutrients are available to you. You can break down a vegetable or fruit for that matter in a couple of ways; I recommend juicing or blending and steaming or sautéing for a short period of time.

Juicing is important. Start with one fresh 16-ounce glass of vegetable juice or combination vegetable and fruit juice (with emphasis on the vegetables) per day for one week. The next week, add a second one, and so on and so forth up to six weeks; at the end of the six weeks, you will be drinking six glasses of juices a day, which will be flushing toxins, cleansing and purifying your blood, your kidneys, and your liver. During this process, your blood will become thinner, lessening your likelihood of having a stroke or heart attack; you will also become energized as your tissues become oxygenated, healthy, and thriving. So within three months, you will have lost weight, cleaned up your complexion, experienced more energy and better sleep, as well as improved digestion and elimination, to name a few. You will also have a new and exciting diet that you love.

Plus, in the ever-expanding world of plant-based cuisine, we now, of course, have younger, creative people getting into the field. With their youth and vitality, they're bringing new passion to the field and helping to form new opinions about vegetarian living. They're actually opening up vegan restaurants that have chefs trained in plant-based food preparation who are creating inspiring dishes with a wide range of tastes, appealing to both the eye and to the palate. We also have more raw foods being introduced to the health market that are assisting those on the health journey, and we have more gourmet frozen vegan dishes than ever before. So, today it has never been easier to find foods to support you in the vegetarian diet. At the back of this book, you will find some helpful resources.

The Importance of an Alkaline Diet

The internal environment of our bodies is maintained at a slightly alkaline pH range of 7.35–7.55 (anything below 7 is considered acid). According to Russell Jaffe, M.D., PhD., "When an alkaline environment is maintained in the body, metabolic, enzymatic, immunologic, and repair mechanisms function at their best. Maintenance of this state is a dynamic, not static, process mediated moment to moment by numerous reactions that produce acid products... For necessary reactions and functions to occur, our body must maintain a proper pH." Jaffe goes on to say that "the acid-forming metabolics of stress and inflammation and of high fat and high protein foods are adequately and effectively neutralized only when sufficient mineral-buffering reserves are present. Mineral-buffering reserves are the gift that alkaline-forming foods give to our body. A diet that is predominantly alkaline forming is essential to the maintenance of sustained health. Most vegetables and fruits contain higher proportions of alkaline-forming elements than other foods... In foods containing large amounts of protein and fat, the acid-forming elements predominate over the alkaline-forming elements."[22]

So, the foods that I suggested that you part with earlier in the chapter cause both inflammation and an imbalance in pH, both of which lead to disease in the body that over time leads to diagnosable conditions, some of which can shorten one's life by a wide margin. The health situation of our nation's people is so out of hand that the CDC has gone on record to say that for the first time in recent history, today's newest generations are expected to die at a younger age than their parents.[23] This, indeed, should tell us that something is very wrong with the way we are thinking about health and how we are going about establishing and maintaining it.

This is what we are taking on in this book—to provide you with the important information you need in a straightforward format so that you too can create a truly healthy existence for you and our planet. To do this, we need to reconnect to what is natural for our bodies, which, as I said, begins with the elimination of what is not natural. Let's continue this conversation with a discussion on food processing, and then we will move to portions and how we learn to eat in rhythm and harmony with our body, thus controlling our appetite.

Alkaline-Forming Foods

To optimize prevention and healing of chronic diseases such as arthritis, the diet should consist of 80% alkaline-forming foods. In addition to most vegetables, some common alkaline-forming foods are:

Vegetables

Alfalfa sprouts, artichokes, asparagus, bamboo shoots, green, lima, wax, string beans, beets, broccoli, cabbages, carrots, celery, cauliflower, chard, chicory, corn, cucumber, dill, dulse, eggplant, endive, escarole, garlic, horseradish, Jerusalem artichokes, kale, leeks, lettuce, mushrooms, okra, onions, parsley, parsnips, peas, bell peppers, potatoes, pumpkin, radish, romaine lettuce, rutabagas, sauerkraut, spinach, sprouts, squash, sweet potatoes, turnips, watercress, and yams

Beans/Legumes

Green beans, lima beans, peas, soybeans, sprouted beans, tempeh (fermented), and tofu (fermented)

Nuts and Seeds

Alfalfa, almonds, Brazil nuts, chestnuts, chia, coconuts, radish, and sesame

Whole Grains

Amaranth, buckwheat, millet, quinoa, and teff

Fruits

Apples, apricots, avocados, bananas, berries, currants, dates, figs, grapefruit, grapes, kiwis, lemons, limes, mangoes, melons, nectarines, olives, oranges, papayas, peaches, pears, persimmons, pineapple, quince, raisins, raspberries, strawberries, tangerines, and watermelon

The most alkaline-forming foods are lemons and melons.

Dietary Vegetarianism Defined

The Various Names for Vegetarianism

To most people, being vegetarian means nothing more than abstaining from the flesh of anything with eyes or a face, but people partake of this abstaining by drawing the line on what they will eat at different points. Some vegetarians eat dairy; some eat eggs; some eat fish; some eat varying combinations of these. Here are a few examples:

- Total vegetarians or ethical vegans live on plant foods alone, eating vegetables (including greens, sprouts, and juice of grasses), fruits, nuts, seeds, grains, and legumes. This regimen rigorously eliminates all animal foods, including meat, poultry, fish, eggs, dairy products, and honey (because it is made by insects), and abstains from using products *derived* from animals, such as leather, wool, and silk, to name just a few. See page 268 for a list of popular products that utilize animal-based components.
- Vegans abstain from eating all animal foods and dairy products, including honey, and live on the same plant-foods listed above; and depending on where they are on the spectrum, they also may not use products derived from animals, such as leather, wool, or silk.
- Lacto-vegetarians include dairy products in their diet in addition to vegetables.
- Lacto-ovo-vegetarians consume eggs along with dairy products and vegetables.
- Pesco-vegetarians add fish to their diet. Such a diet is common in Asia where hundreds of millions live on rice, fish, and vegetables.
- Pollo-vegetarians eat poultry (chicken, duck, game, and birds) but omit red meat.

The term vegetarianism has evolved to connote diet alone, whereas, originally, it was used to describe the lifestyle of someone who lived naturally, in harmony with their surroundings, and acted in ways that did not harm fellow humans or the animals with which they co-existed. The word vegetarian hails from the word *vegetare*, meaning "to enliven." So, a vegetarian not only was thought to make something more exciting and vital, but to honor life through their every action. In its essence, vegetarianism is a spiritual undertaking, which we shall see by examining a brief history of the vegetarian movement.

Further, the term vegan was coined by Donald Watson in 1944, who defined it as follows: "Veganism is a way of living which excludes all forms of exploitation of, and cruelty to, the animal kingdom, and includes a reverence for life. It applies to the practice of living on the products of the plant kingdom to the exclusion of flesh, fish, fowl, eggs, honey, animal milk and its derivatives, and encourages the use of alternatives for all commodities derived wholly or in part from animals."[24]

A Brief History of Vegetarianism

Vegetarianism has been around for a long, long time. In fact, in the book of Genesis in the Bible, Adam and Eve were vegetarians. And they were living in the Garden of Eden. What better recommendation is there than that?

More seriously, this first book of the Christian religion does advocate a decidedly vegetarian diet of fruits, seeds, and nuts. Genesis (the first book in the Bible) chapter 1, verse 29, says, "Then God said, 'I give you every seed-bearing plant on the face of the whole earth and every tree that has fruit with seed in it. They will be yours for food.'"[25]

While the Bible is one place to find ancient references to vegetarianism, other roots of vegetarianism are found elsewhere in the early history of the East. A number of ancient religions believe that a soul could "transmigrate" back and forth between animals and humans. A man may come back in the next life as a cow while, vice versa, a cow may in the next life be reborn as a person. This led followers of these religions to maintain a vegetarian diet out of respect for the animal life that might be housing human souls. Buddha later commanded, "Do not butcher the ox that plows thy field," for, after all, that ox may contain the soul of an ancestor. Buddhism quickly spread eastward from India, becoming the state religion of China around 500 A.D. and arriving in Japan a century later. For Japanese Buddhists, vegetarianism included the belief that eating animal flesh polluted the body for a hundred days.[26]

While not every Eastern religion believes in transmigration – I will give a fuller exposition of this doctrine later in the book—vegetarianism is a hallmark of many of these faiths. In the Hindu religion of India, vegetarianism is founded on health standards that go back to the epic poem *The Mahabharata,* which states:

> Those who desire to possess good memory, beauty, long life with perfect health, and physical, moral, and spiritual strength, should abstain from animal foods.

Jainism, another religion that started out in India, preaches nonviolence and abhors the killing of animals for food. Believers strive to move toward a greater purity, resembling that of higher beings, and they find vegetarianism is part of the life of these angelic entities.

Yoga, not so much a religion as a set of practices to help achieve a more integrated body and mind, arose in India and draws on the vegetarian beliefs of the Hindus and Buddhists, teaching that all life is formed and sustained through prana, the "life force." One gains and sustains one's life energy by eating foods rich in it, including vegetables, fruits, nuts, legumes, and grains. It follows that the meat of dead animals, which have lost their prana along with their life, is useless for true nourishment and should be avoided.[27]

Moving to the Near East and looking at ancient Egypt, where the state religion did not promulgate vegetarianism, it is interesting to find that analysis of the intestinal contents of mummies has shown that some Egyptians were also vegetarian. This group in Egyptian society has been named by students of the society "the eaters of bread."[28] Much later in the Middle East, Mohammed's holy book of Islam, the Koran, prohibited the eating of "dead animals, blood and flesh," although, like the injunctions against meat-eating in the Bible, this prohibition was seldom strictly practiced by followers.[29]

Of the ancient civilizations that have been customarily (though perhaps not correctly) put as the direct forbears of Western culture, one, Greece, was named a place of thinkers, and the other, Rome, the land of warriors. Both these types of humans had a penchant for vegetarianism. Among Greek thinkers, Pythagoras pioneered and Plato and Socrates followed. What began as a green-eating policy coming out of religious and ethical concerns moved on to become in classical

Greek society a full-spectrum belief that saw vegetarianism as natural, hygienic, and necessary for healthy living.[30]

Perhaps more surprisingly, the Romans, who were considered the warriors among the ancient societies, carried out their conquest of the known world with an army fed in large part on bread and porridge, vegetables, wine, and occasional fish. "The Roman army conquered the world on a vegetarian diet," writes historian Will Durant. "Caesar's troops complained when corn ran out and they had to eat meat."[31]

While a vegetarian philosophy continued in the East, after the fall of the Roman Empire, it was no longer on the front burner in the West for the next 1,200 years since the Catholic church, which promulgated what was the dominant world view, did not emphasize plant-based diets outside of those eaten by a few cloistered orders of monks or nuns, such as those belonging to the Benedictine and the Cistercian orders.

However, the ancient teachings were revived during the Renaissance, which went in the direction of "back to the future." In other words, the Renaissance thinkers and artists made major innovations, inspired by new translations of Greek and other old, forgotten writings. In this period, modern vegetarianism was born. This humanist movement of the Renaissance, which put the emphasis on humans rather than on god as the Middle Ages had, is the world view which still prevails today.

Along the way, some of the world's greatest humanists, whether scientists or artists, were vegetarians, including such people as Frances Bacon, Shakespeare, Voltaire, and Benjamin Franklin.[32]

Moving closer to the present, while there was a general increase in meat-eating in the nineteenth century, partly because a growing fraction of the lower classes could now afford to add meat to their diets, there was also the growth of organized vegetarian movements. These differed from earlier moves toward vegetarianism, which had either been connected to religious belief, in the case where green eating had many adherents, or were the chosen paths of intelligent but quirky individuals such as Franklin. While the 19th century movement did have many religious adherents, such as William Metcalf, the minister who was mentioned at the head of this section, it now also had many secular spokespeople.

One of these was Anna Kingsford, a medical practitioner who devoted much of her scientific writing to the subject of vegetarianism. She emphasized, against meat-eaters' propaganda, the physically empowering effects of a green diet. She reported, for instance, that the strongest animals in the world, including the horse, elephant, hippo, and rhinoceros, were herbivorous, eating only plant foods, and she drew parallels to the amazing athletic prowess of the ancient Greeks.[33] With powerful boosters such as Kingsford, in the US in 1850, the American Vegetarian Society was established. This remained a small but vocal movement in the 19th century.

In World War I, meat scarcity prompted scientists in the US to re-evaluate the national diet.[34] Forced to find alternative sources of protein, they worked to persuade people to switch to a green diet and began to discover the health benefits of non-meat-eating at the same time. Other countries that were similarly war-wracked followed suit. In 1917, Denmark, for example, asked its citizens to adopt a simple, meatless wartime diet based on whole grains, vegetables, and dairy products. The result was overall improved health and lowered mortality rates in the country.[35,36]

The need for restricting meat consumption also arose in many countries during World War II. In Norway, the public drastically cut its meat consumption, turning instead to cereals, potatoes, and other vegetables. As it turned out, this new diet improved the country's health and lowered mortality rates. As you might have predicted, these health statistics were reversed when the war ended and "normal" meat consumption resumed.[37]

Even though vegetarianism began to take root within the society throughout the 1960s, it was still closely identified with a countercultural lifestyle. Nowadays, it is more mainstream, attracting anyone who is sophisticated about health and social/spiritual issues, and aware of the potential dangers of meat-based diets.

Still, meat eaters are the bulk of the population, and vegetarianism has a long way to go to once again become the dominant choice. To my mind, meat eaters are in a situation that can be characterized as "ignorance is bliss." They continue blithely along consuming animals because they have not learned about the practice's negative health (and ethical) effects nor tasted the joys of vegetarianism. I'm guessing that if a confirmed meat eater picked up a book such as this or heard a persuasive vegetarian speaker, that individual *would think twice about loading up their fork with toxic and acidic meats*. One thing that could possibly shift them in this direction is finding out that their favored meat myths, such as that about the necessity of getting protein from meat, have been completely shattered.

Vegetarianism Today

I've said that in the last 20 years there has been an upsurge in vegetarianism in the US. In this instance, our country is getting in touch with the rest of the world, where a plant-based diet is often the norm. There are a whole lot of people out there who do not eat animal flesh and therefore are technically vegetarians, but they don't live anything resembling a healthy vegetarian lifestyle. If you live on breads, pasta, French fries, and ketchup, then yes, you're technically a vegetarian—one who will certainly develop a host of health issues as you age. To eat a vegetarian diet does NOT automatically mean that your diet is a healthy one, and that is NOT the brand of vegetarianism we are promoting in this book.

Healthy vegetarian eating means getting the host of nutrients that your body needs into your body. This is the first step, after elimination. To do this, you need to eat the full range of fruits, vegetables, grains, legumes, seeds, and nuts available to you. Some might eschew peanuts and pistachios, for example, because of their acidic pH, but that is another discussion. And as long as these people are eating other nuts, they're fine.

As an example of a population of people that eats a vegetarian diet that is primarily an unhealthy one, take India, which contains over 1.2 billion people (roughly 17% of the world's population).[38] The number of Indians who are thought to be vegetarian ranges from 20 to 42%.[39] The Indian society is, perhaps, the largest collective of vegetarians on the planet today because of their native religion of Hinduism, which deems the cow as a holy animal and therefore not to be eaten.

While these numbers and ones we would find in other less developed nations dwarf those in industrialized nations, even in the latter the number of vegetarians is growing. A 2000 Zogby poll found that 2.5% of Americans were vegetarian, while a 2003 Harris poll put the figure at 2.8%.[40] Today, a reported 16 million Americans are vegetarians or vegans, which is about 5% of the population. You will see studies later on in the book that speak about the number of "vegetarians" who do consume meat from time to time. However, my optimism about the growth of this movement is hardly dampened by this. Americans are now starting to get the message: If you want to decrease your risk of developing any one of the so-called "lifestyle" diseases (heart disease, cancer, diabetes, obesity, etc.), eat a plant-based diet; you will begin reaping the benefits almost instantly.

As the number of vegetarians grows in the West, so does a vegetarian support system, including restaurants offering gourmet vegetarian entrees, meatless cookbooks, even radio shows and magazines produced specifically for vegetarians. Plus, dieticians across the nation are now increasing their support in rising numbers. From these facts alone, we can glean that eating a plant-based diet will only continue to increase in popularity. We've even invented other names for people partially on the path, such as "flexitarian." This, indeed, is a sign that our population is becoming more aware of the benefit of a plant-based lifestyle and desiring to be a part of it. Still, there is a lot of confusion about what it means to be a healthy vegetarian, let alone what it means to lead a healthy lifestyle, all of which will be addressed within the pages of this book.

First, we will take a look at the physical component. It is, perhaps, the easiest and quickest way to become healthier and more vital. I have seen this first-hand in coaching people for decades. When you give the body the essential nutrients it needs to function well, through foods that it can readily assimilate, you will be surprised and maybe even shocked about what is possible for you, in terms of healing symptoms, improving sleep, gaining vital energy, promoting positive thinking and emotional balance, and feeling alive and well in general. The body is incredibly resourceful and responds rapidly to good, properly applied nutrition. Some people realize significant benefits in their body in as little as three weeks.

After we address the physical aspect of health and healing, I will be spending time in the last two chapters of this section addressing the mental, emotional, and spiritual components of wellness. The American Psychological Association reported that studies show that your mind and your body are strongly linked. As your mental health declines, your physical health can wear down, and if your physical health can wear down, it can make you feel mentally "down."[41]

Along the same lines, Professor David Goldberg of the Institute of Psychiatry, London, UK, reported that the rate of depression in patients with a chronic disease is almost three times higher than normal. He explains, "Depression and chronic physical illness are in reciprocal relationship with one another: not only do many chronic illnesses cause higher rates of depression, but depression has been shown to antedate some chronic physical illnesses."[42]

To support the importance of this aspect of health, I turn to the APA, once again. This time, the study, led by author Sonja Lyubomirsky, Ph.D., of the University of California, Riverside, upended assumptions that success *makes* people happy. Instead, the study found that happiness *leads to success* via positive emotions. The report notes:

> ...happiness does lead to behaviors that often produce further success in work, relationships and health, and these successes result in part from a person's positive affect. Furthermore... a person's well-being is associated with positive perceptions of self and others, sociability, creativity, prosocial behavior, a strong immune system, and effective coping skills, and... that happy people are capable of experiencing sadness and negative emotions in response to negative events, which is a healthy and appropriate response.
>
> Much of the previous research on happiness presupposed that happiness followed from success and accomplishments in life, said the authors. "We found that this isn't always true." Positive affect is one attribute among several that can lead to success-oriented behaviors. Other resources, such as intelligence, family, expertise and physical fitness, can also play a role in people's successes... and happy individuals are more likely than their less happy peers to have fulfilling marriages and relationships, high incomes, superior work performance, community involvement, robust health and even a long life.[43]

It is important to note from the above studies that all of them speak about some aspect of physical health. So, as we bring wholeness to our personal experience, we build on our opportunity to affect the health of those closest to us, perhaps others around the globe, and the planet at large. To this end, we will start first by asking ourselves: how do we heal the physical body? Once we detail the answers to this, we will discuss emotional, mental, and spiritual well-being within the context of the vegetarian lifestyle, and how to put that to work in your life for the greater good of humanity and the planet.

Chapter 2

What We Eat Now... and Why

"I cannot teach anybody anything. I can only make them think."

— *Socrates, Philosopher*

How We Learn Anything... Including What to Eat

Let us think for a moment about the concept of *epistemology*. *Epistemology* is a two-dollar word that essentially means *knowledge*. But it's a little more than that: epistemology considers *how we know what we know*. This is an idea that Ancient Greek scholars deliberated thoroughly, and like many of their musings, it remains as viable a question today as it was then.

How do we know what we know?

The Ancient Greeks determined that knowledge essentially comes from one of two sources. Either you experience something yourself or someone told you. This sounds simple enough, but it's actually quite complex. Let's briefly consider these ideas, starting with the *someone told you* piece.

When we learn from others, we are receiving *their* interpretation of information they've received. This is true when we read journalists' accounts of events in the newspaper, when we attend to a religious speech or sermon, when we face the judge in a courtroom, when we read a textbook, and in every other life circumstance. There's no getting around this. Whenever you speak, it reflects your understanding of whatever it is you're talking about. Your perspective of the topic comes from the sources you've read and/or listened to. This might be news reports, political speeches, TED talks, movies and/or documentaries, and the internet, to name a few, and of course your coworkers, friends, and neighbors.

We take this base information we receive and most of us tend to add our own thoughts and ideas to it. This is absolutely normal. Now, in effect, we're interpreting someone else's interpretation. ("The preacher said *this*, and I think he was talking about *that*, so *this* and *that* must be related.") We then share our perspective with others. They add their own layer of interpretation and share the message further. It soon begins to look like the childhood game "telephone," but the difference is that it's not a game, and it's not meant for amusement.

This is how we get our information. This is how we gain knowledge. Sure, we might occasionally check sources, but if most people generally believe something to be true, it's much easier for us to accept it as true. Also, it's very easy to believe something if "all of the authority figures" promote a certain perspective. If I do a web search for a certain thing and get 2 million hits that reinforce a certain perspective, and among that list are powerful and credible sources, that's a much easier position for me to accept than if my web search yields 10 reinforcing hits from entities I've never heard of.

You can start to see how this is becoming more complex. Not only are we subject to greater influence when information comes from sources we consider authoritative, such as the preacher speaking on religious tenets or the farmer speaking about crops, but we also tend to gauge the quality of information by *how many sources back it up*. Most of us are more willing to believe something that 2 million people agree on than a position that only 10 people agree with. If enough people believe a certain way, this position becomes the status quo.

It gets better (or actually, worse). Research in marketing shows that people prefer to purchase from sellers they're familiar with. Since human nature finds uncertainty uncomfortable, we seek to reduce it; so it makes sense that as consumers, we're more likely to purchase from someone we're more familiar with. Big Business spends billions of dollars on creating familiarity with their company and their products for just this reason. Over time, we as consumers become familiar with companies through their extensive advertising. As we become familiar, we are reducing uncertainty and developing trust. So this familiarity means that as a consumer, I'll more likely purchase from the company I'm familiar with and that I (therefore) trust. This is one reason advertising works to increase sales and profits.

The same can be said of ideas rather than products. When a message is consistent over time, it builds familiarity, which reduces uncertainty and builds trust in the information—whether the information presented deserves that trust or not. Further, when a particular idea is promoted by an authority figure or authoritative institution, such as our government, it's harder for us to justify dismissing it as patently untrue. Our leaders know this and rely on it. Consider George W. Bush's admission of selling propaganda as truth in his comment, "See, in my line of work you got to keep repeating things over and over and over again for the truth to sink in, to kind of catapult the propaganda."[1] If a powerful public figure says the same thing enough times, people will begin to accept it as truth. Also, when the status quo latches onto a perspective, it becomes increasingly difficult to swim against that powerful social stream, which by definition will label you a nonconformist and maybe even worse. This is why many say that "change takes time"—a statement rooted in the knowledge that change is an initiation of new ways of thinking and being in the world, which goes against our strong human need for comfort and stability. As Arthur Schopenhauer, the great German philosopher (1788–1860) said, "All truth passes through three stages. First, it is ridiculed. Second, it is violently opposed. Third, it is accepted as being self-evident."

So getting back to the question of *how do we know what we know?* As you can see, there are a lot of cooks adding to that soup we call our knowledge.

As for the other component of that question, the *personal experience* prong, that's not straightforward either. We interpret our experiences based on our current knowledge. But remember that our knowledge is subject to the slant of whatever source we're adhering to. So even when we experience something personally and learn from it, there's a good chance that what we learn from that experience is also tainted by the information we've received from others in how we interpret what we're experiencing. So even when we learn by directly experiencing something ourselves, that knowledge is deeply influenced by what we know from others. Take the example of divorce: if your closest friend experienced a nasty divorce, where neither they nor their former spouse could agree on terms and both experienced tremendous pain and anguish through the proceedings, chances are your idea of divorce, whether you have experienced it or not, would be affected, possibly jaded. Then, in the event that you divorce, some of your friend's experience would be in the back of your mind—no matter how amicable the situation; and it will likely influence your actions.

Now, let's consider these ideas within the US capitalistic milieu of today. To provide focus to this discussion and because this is a book about healthy living, including food, we'll start with the food industry.

The *authoritative sources* in the US for information about what's good for us to eat are the Food and Drug Administration (FDA), the Surgeon General, the United States Department of Agriculture (USDA), and maybe the Centers for Disease Control (CDC). These are governmental institutions, funded and operated by the federal government—paid for by you and me.

In making their recommendations about what's healthy for us, we like to believe, indeed we *need* to believe, that these institutions have our best interests at heart. Why would a governmental institution make recommendations that would harm the population it serves?

Yet, as soon as we utter this question, there's another voice in our heads that laughs at the idea that the government has our best interests at heart. Some of us need to believe this, but most of us know that this is a utopic illusion and not our present day reality.

If you don't live under a rock, you know that today's political parties and the way they legislate is a mess. The left and the right fight just for the sake of it. Whatever party is not in the oval office blocks the president's agenda because they can. Rather than working together—unifying—to best serve our nation's people, our politicians are busy taking sides and remaining intractable—separating—and protecting themselves and their ideological tenets. Politicians are subject to huge donations from special interest groups that result in those same politicians voting a certain way on a certain issue, one that conveniently advances the special interest group's agenda, and swaying colleagues to do the same. In fact, recent research has determined that the US is no longer a democracy but rather an oligarchy, run by those with the most money. Those who actually run this country aren't "the people," as democracy promises, but rather the huge corporations that purchase profit-enhancing rights and privileges via political contributions, and to heck with the people! Why else would billions be spent in campaigning for a job that takes home less than $200,000 per year?

This is relevant to our discussion because the FDA, Surgeon General, USDA, and CDC are governmental bodies—and are just as riddled with politics and corruption as Capitol Hill. To prove my point, let's look at one recent example—the occurrence of senior CDC vaccine safety scientist, Dr. William Thompson. In a blog dated February 12, 2015, Robert F. Kennedy, Jr.—one of the nation's most prominent environmental attorneys—said that Dr. Thompson, who invoked the protection of the Federal Whistleblower Statute following the release of his taped conversations disclosing pervasive corruption within CDC's Vaccine Safety Division, is maintaining that his bosses forced him and other researchers to lie about the safety of mercury-based vaccines,[2] when the research clearly showed otherwise. Indeed, Dr. Thompson said: "Thimerosal (a controversial mercury based preservative) from vaccines causes tics… I can say tics are four times more prevalent in kids with autism. There is biologic plausibility right now to say that Thimerosal causes autism-like features."

The worst aspect of this, perhaps, is the latent corruption between the CDC and pharmaceutical concerns as noted in Dr. Thompson's account of what occurred when bringing this indiscretion to the attention of his superiors: In 2004, he sent a letter to CDC Director, Julie Gerberding, alerting her that CDC scientists were breaking research protocols to conceal the links between Thimerosal and brain damage in children. Gerberding never responded to Thompson's allegations, but her deputy, Robert Chen, then head of CDC's Immunization Safety Office and Thompson's direct boss, confronted Thompson in an agency parking lot threatening him and screaming, "I would fire you if I could." In 2009, Gerberding matriculated to Merck as Chief of the company's Vaccine Division. Two years prior to the move, she approved Merck's HPV vaccine for pre-adolescent girls—an estimated billion dollar value to the company. Following Thompson's revelations, Merck transferred Gerberding from its Vaccine Division to Executive Vice President for Strategic Communications, Global Public Policy and Population Health.[3]

Special interest groups have tremendous influence over the information that these governmental bodies—which we trust to decide in our best interests on what is safe for us to consume—disseminate. It is well publicized that these governmental bodies and the large corporations affected by their decisions are run by the same people, as I just noted above. Decision-makers once employed by Monsanto and Pfizer now make decisions within these governmental institutions that affect these corporations, and vice versa, back and forth, and there are numerous examples of this revolving door relationship between government and industry and the conflict of interest that results. It is not only unethical; it needs to be made illegal in order for the public's best interest to be protected.

What this means for the American people is that the information that our governmental institutions give us about what is healthy for us to consume is deeply influenced by corporations standing to profit immensely from the release of some information and the withholding of other information. For example, Marion Nestle reports that in her then-new job as manager of the editorial production of the first ever *Surgeon General's Report on Nutrition and Health* in 1986, she was given these rules on her first day of work:

> No matter what the research indicated, the report could not recommend 'eat less meat' as a way to reduce intake of saturated fat, nor could it suggest restrictions on intake of any other category of food. In the industry-friendly climate of the Reagan administration, the producers of foods that might be affected by such advice would complain to their beneficiaries in Congress, and the report would never be published.[4]

This was a very real concern, as federal health officials had suffered nearly constant congressional interference with their dietary recommendations for nearly a decade.

Getting back to epistemology and how we know what we know, we rely on our leaders for our information about what is healthy for us to consume. The FDA, Surgeon General, USDA, and CDC steer public health in this nation. They are our most accepted and largest authoritative sources for our personal health. These institutions and the news reports and governmental agendas generated from their reports, are our primary sources for how we know what we know about food, nutrition, and health in the US. Yet, the information they give us is highly tainted with the agendas of the profit-seeking corporations these bodies are in bed with. In other words, our government will tell us what it is told to tell us *by* corporations like Monsanto and Pfizer so *that* they will keep increasing their profits. Yes, this happens at the expense of our health and in spite of the fact that our tax dollars are paying their salaries.

In fact, the entire medical industry, including the pharmaceutical and hospital businesses, relies on our being ill or they don't make any money. People with this agenda in mind are the same people telling us what to eat.

So now that we know a bit more about *how we know what we know* regarding what is healthy to consume, let's set everything aside for a moment that we've ever been taught about what is healthy for us to eat. Set aside your beliefs and your current knowledge on this topic. And think about it. Think about what it means to rely on animal flesh and other animal products for our livelihood, to sustain life through the process of killing other living, breathing beings. Think about what our dependence on animal products means to the very large and powerful meat, dairy, and poultry industries, and to the numerous other industries connected to them. In short, our ill health is their wealth. I also ask you to think about the health risks of continuing a meat-based diet—as we'll see in this book, there are many—and the conditions in which these animals are raised, their only purpose in life to be made fat and then slaughtered and sold for hamburgers or chicken nuggets. With this as their sole life purpose, no care is given to their living conditions, which are riddled with disease, overcrowding, and, immense suffering from the beginning of their miserable lives to the end. Is this what it means to be human, to bring living creatures onto this planet for the sole purpose of serving our wishes, without any thought to the suffering involved with this? In a humane world, how can we actually believe that the suffering of others doesn't matter as long as we get what we want?

In considering our consumption of animal flesh, think also about our fellow human beings and the jobs they endure in these factory farms and the slaughterhouses, and consider their working conditions and abuses. Consider what it would be like to do this work for a week or even an hour. Imagine walking around on the kill floor, ankle deep in blood, air thick with the stench of death and decay, howling animals' last cries of fear and suffering ringing in your ears and echoing in your soul—50 hours a week. Think about *how many animals* we need as a growing global population to feed the world's people over time, how many resources we need to feed these animals, and whether, as a responsible people, this actually makes sense. Think about the culture of violence that murdering for our food contributes to.

Then think about why you eat meat. I mean really, why? Once you remove yourself from everything you've ever learned about the benefits of meat consumption, why do you eat it? The *it's healthy* argument is out, because it's not healthy, so there are really only two reasons remaining: *because everyone else does* and *because I want to*. Well, I won't go into the dangers of leading an unhealthy lifestyle *because everyone else does*. As a kid, didn't your caregiver ask you "If everyone else jumped off the bridge would you jump too?" You make a conscious choice whether or not to 'drink that dangerous Kool-Aid.' So let's talk about the *because I want to* argument. In a hedonistic society, that's reason enough. But in a responsible society, that just doesn't cut it.

The Almighty Food Industry

Let's turn for a moment to the very large and powerful meat, dairy, and poultry industries, and consider whether their profit-seeking agenda might have influenced what we've been taught about these food sources. I'm going to cut you a little slack here and present some information that demonstrates that, as much as we want to believe our choices are our very own, our food choices are in truth so deeply influenced by the food industry that we, as individuals living busy lives, simply can't fight that powerful tide. In many cases, it's a tidal wave we don't even know about or see because, unsurprisingly, it's not addressed with the public directly by the government or the food industry. Consider animal cloning as one example. Cloning typically involves removing genetic information (DNA) from a cell taken from one animal and placing it into an unfertilized egg that has had its own DNA removed. This egg is then artificially stimulated to start developing into an embryo and placed into a surrogate mother. Most people are completely unaware of this practice or that they absolutely may be consuming cloned meat or dairy products from cloned animals.

Why is this? Well, in 2008, the FDA "concluded that meat and milk from cow, pig, and goat clones and the offspring of any animal clones are as safe as food we eat every day."[5] This is even after acknowledging the existence of health risks for clones and their progeny. And, because the agency is not requiring food from clones or their offspring to be labeled, consumers are purchasing these novel foods without knowledge or consent. Think about that: the government requires ingredients like food additives to be labeled, but it does not require labeling of foods from or of cloned animals. This is an atrocity, especially because there are a number of serious health issues with cloned animals.

According to the Center for Food Safety, "These animals tend to have difficulty delivering live young and develop lameness. These illnesses may lead them to be heavily treated with hormones and antibiotics, which can enter the food supply and put human health at risk."[6] Additionally, the Royal Society for the Prevention of Cruelty to Animals (RSPCA) notes: "Where animals are born alive, they often have breathing problems, tumors, liver defects or other abnormalities, and have a reduced lifespan."[7] As an important side note, according to the Humane Society of the United States, cloning involves invasive and painful procedures to the animals. The egg 'donors' and/or surrogate mothers are subjected to painful hormone treatments to manipulate their reproductive cycles as well as invasive surgeries to harvest eggs or implant embryos. Also, surrogate mothers endure an additional surgery to deliver the baby.[8]

Some additional insight from academic nutritionist Dr. Marion Nestle, from her acclaimed book *Food Politics,* helps us to better understand these dynamics and illustrate how powerless we are in deciding what we put into our mouths.

Nestle astutely points out that unlike other animals, humans don't have an innate sense of nutrition or of how to provide our bodies with the essential nutrients they need. So, we have to be *taught* what to eat. A hundred years ago, food was in short supply. Much of the population wasn't getting the nutrition it needed. In efforts to guide the American people into better health, the US government promoted "eat more" campaigns. Then we moved into relative prosperity, where food became abundant, yet we still retained the "eat more" mentality of days gone by. Facing epidemics caused from overeating, such as obesity and heart disease, the US government switched its public message to "eat less." Not everyone got that message.

We now live in an age where there is an overabundance of food produced. We produce more than we can eat. This overabundance keeps food costs low—and also creates pressure on food manufacturers to add value through processing. With processing, marketers can convert potatoes (cheap) to potato chips (expensive), or even to those fried in certain fats or coated with certain things (even more expensive). This is an example of how marketers add value to basic food commodities. Fruits and vegetables can be processed as frozen, canned, or precut, which makes a lot more money for these food preparation companies than consuming produce in its fresh state. The market for processed food is driven by economics and convenience. Today, nearly one-half of all meals are consumed outside the home.

Salt is an essential ingredient in processed food. It binds water and thus increases the food's weight at a very low cost. With salt, processed foods become palatable, and people become thirsty. It promotes "eat more." Although diets high in salt can increase blood pressure levels and contribute to heart disease,[9] there is some controversy as to the benefit of following a low-salt diet. For example, a study by scientists from the Albert Einstein College of Medicine reported an inverse association between salt intake and mortality from cardiovascular disease, and suggest "a survival advantage accompanying a lower sodium diet."[10] On the contrary, the WHO recommends we decrease our daily salt intake from 10 grams to 5 grams, and suggests that by doing so, we could help reduce global rates of cardiovascular disease by 17%,[11] and the American Heart Association (AHA) suggests cutting salt intake even more drastically to less than 1.5 grams daily.[12] Nevertheless, governmental efforts to restrict salt intake through public messaging have been vehemently opposed by the salt industry, who aims to raise doubt that salt intake and high blood pressure are at all related.

The various food industries (salt, sugar, beef, poultry, dairy, etc.) assert a great deal of pressure on governmental agencies and individual representatives to influence public messaging in favor of their product. "Food companies use every means at their disposal to promote their product," Nestle explains.[13] Many governmental executives, tempted by larger salaries, become industry executives. Many industry executives also take positions within governmental institutions. Corporations and industry executives have been known to give elaborate gifts, such as luxury vacations, to lawmakers. Corporations fund research projects both within academia and privately, all aimed to provide scientific support that their food is healthy. They work continually and methodically to blur the lines between food advertising and dietary advice. These are just some of the efforts by food companies to influence the dietary advice that is disseminated to the public.

Nestle explains, "dietary advice affects food sales, and companies demand a favorable regulatory environment."[14] So, companies assert immense pressure on regulatory agencies to issue information favorable, and at the very least not unfavorable, to their industry. *Food companies want to make money. They don't care about your health.* For example, in 1991 the USDA was manipulated into blocking the publication of the Eating Right Pyramid due to industry pressure. The proposed pyramid did not promote certain food groups, such as beef and dairy, enough to satisfy those industries, so those affected industries threw a fit and the USDA had to respond by altering the Eating Right Pyramid to satisfy these industries. Just to be sure that last part isn't lost on you, *the beef, dairy, poultry, salt, sugar, and other food industries made the government change its public message so they could sell more of their products, even though eating too much of their products cause disease and in some cases even death.* I hope it's clear that the government and its agencies created and sustained with our tax dollars do not have the general public's best interest at heart when offering dietary recommendations.

Follow the Money Trail

The various food industries have no shortage of funds to develop advertising that works to sell their products. Campaigns are carefully researched within target markets, marketed carefully, and repeated frequently. These companies have far more money to put into advertising than the government does, and, it's not hard for them to upset the government's central message of "eat more fruits and vegetables and less fat, sugar, and salt." That's not novel or exciting information. Food corporation marketers promote highly processed, elaborately packaged, and fast foods. Their advertising works below the consciousness of everyone, including nutritionists and the general public. They are a Goliath that no individual or entity can put down.

It may interest you to know that many of today's largest food companies are owned by tobacco companies. These are presented in the figure below.

Table of food companies owned by tobacco companies and dates of acquisition

COMPANY	DATE ACQUIRED
Philip Morris	
Miller Brewing Co	1969-1970
7-up (97%)	1978
General Foods	1985
Sells 7-up to Pepsico	1986
Kraft Foods (combines with General Foods)	1986
Jacobs Sachard, a Swiss coffee and confection company	1990
Kraft (Philip Morris) buys **Taco Bell**	1996
Philadelphia Cream Cheese	1999
Kraft (Philip Morris) buys **Nabisco**	1999-2000
RJ Reynolds	
Nabisco	1985
Sells Nabisco to Philip Morris	1999-2000

You know the tobacco companies, right? They helped kill millions of people by denying that cigarette smoke was bad for you. Now, guess what? These very same people and companies are now preparing your food and telling you what's healthy to eat. I hope you find this as alarming as I do. Then of course there's the "food" giant Monsanto, which actually made a name for itself as a vicious chemical company that created such humanly devastating chemical substances as napalm. They now own most of the global market on genetically modified seeds, which form the basis of our daily diets.

As if it weren't enough that corporations spend billions of dollars to convince otherwise competent adults to purchase their products, we're not their only targets. Your children are often the targets of insidious food advertising that uses entertaining animation to capture young children's attention and then provides enough information on the health benefits of the product to give the child the necessary arguments to nag their parents into purchasing it.[15] Our nation's children are also exploited by food companies that push their high fat, salt, and sugar items into school cafeteria vending machines, and through "social programs" carried out using taxpayer dollars, such as utilizing the police force to provide McDonald's coupons promoting bicycle safety to children wearing helmets. Corporations will go to any length to hook a young customer because they know it generally means a customer for life.

The aim of processed food manufacturers is to create confusion within the American public, for the food industry reaps the greatest benefits of a confused public because this confusion makes people more subject to the effects of advertising. Food manufacturers focus on a single nutrient to amplify the perception of the food's unique nutritional value, regardless of its overall deleterious impact. Take milk as an example. Dairy producers fortify milk with vitamin D to promote milk as a healthy food for bones, which it is not. These products are not only acidifying, they are mucous-forming and loaded with hormones, antibiotics, pus, and other undesirable contents. Further, dairy consumption is directly correlated with osteoporosis. But in reality, *all* foods have *some* nutritional value—they're food! Moreover, researchers contribute to this confusion by constantly focusing and reinforcing their studies on single nutrients. This allows the food industry to give the impression that they are merely reflecting and promoting scientific findings for greater nutrition.

GMOs and Your Right to Know

No discussion on food or health would be complete without a conversation about GM (Genetically Modified) crops, GMOs (Genetically Modified Organisms), and pesticide use. With the passing of every month and year, new discoveries and findings reveal further scientific evidence that the promises of GM crops are fraudulent if not downright heretical. Anti-GMO advocates have been warning of a global food, health, and environmental catastrophe for over two decades. Now, the evidence is in—independent science, outside the halls of Monsanto's and the USDA's control, are vindicating these voices. As one example, an article in the February 2014 issue of *The Ecologist* "GM Crops Are Driving Genocide and Ecocide: Keep Them Out of the EU,"[16] summarizes the dramatic consequences nations who bought into the GMO mythology face with growing poverty, epidemic levels of still births and birth defects from glyphosate spraying, unstoppable destruction of habitats and biodiversity, the rapid decline in essential pollinators to sustain other food crops, and GMO's mounting failures with reduced crop yields and more resilient pesticide-resistant weeds and pests.

The most recent alarming finding has been a recent critical review of published studies associated with the 47 GM crops now approved for human consumption. The survey found only 21 total studies in the scientific literature supporting these crops, and among these 21 studies, only 9 of that 47 plants are represented. Is there something seriously wrong with this picture—that 38 GM foods are scheduled for approval and not a single peer-reviewed study supports their health safety?

While there are an increasing number of studies in the scientific literature identifying the health risks associated with GMO consumption and glyphosate independently, no research has yet been conducted to assess the combined synergistic adverse effects of GMOs and pesticides in animal models and humans. The original foundation of agricultural biotechnology was to advance sales of pesticides by engineering crops to become immune to toxic spraying. While weeds and insect pests would be eradicated, targeted crop would be spared, thereby allowing farmers to spray massive amounts of chemicals on soy, corn, cotton, sugar beets, and other agricultural foods without injury. This was the assumption that led to the agro-genetic revolution. Only during the past decade, with more and more GM products in our diets and more and more farm acreage being sprayed with glyphosate and other toxic pesticides and herbicides, are the long term health risks to animals, humans, and the environment being more fully recognized within the scientific community. Annual runoffs of pesticides into rivers, streams, and reservoirs have complicated the extent to which humans are being exposed to life threatening chemicals on a daily basis.

In a major paper published by Earth Open Source, "GMO Myths and Truths: An Evidence-Based Examination of the Claims Made for the Safety and Efficacy of Genetically Modified Crops," Kings College molecular geneticist Michael Antoniou, molecular biologist John Fagan, and GM Watch's Claire Robinson outline the known health risks now shown to be associated with glyphosate:

- DNA damage
- Premature births and miscarriages
- Birth defects including neural tube defects and anencephaly (absence of large parts of the brain and skull)
- Multiple myeloma
- Non-Hodgkin's lymphoma
- Disruption of neurobehavioral development in children, including attention deficit disorder and attention deficit hyperactivity disorder.[17]

Since the release of the study in the journal *Entropy*, a researcher at MIT and a member of the Union of Concerned Scientists have discovered that glyphosate is in fact taken up by plants from the soil and found in our food—an accusation Monsanto continues to deny. The study says that the negative impact of glyphosate accumulation "is insidious and manifests slowly over time as inflammation damages cellular systems throughout the body. "In addition to being linked with problems ranging from cancer to infertility, a connection may also be made to the rising number of adults acquiring Parkinson's Disease.[18] A couple of earlier studies on individual cases found a correspondence between glyphosate exposure and the onset of Parkinson's.[19] There are now growing concerns that glyphosate consumed by mothers and infants in GM tainted foods might be giving rise to the autism epidemic that continues to worsen each year and now stands at almost 1 in 50 children.

With each passing year, the body of scientific data challenging the safety of glyphosate expands. In several peer-reviewed studies conducted by researcher Andres Carrasco of the University of Buenos Aires, glyphosate was observed to cause teratogenic impairment of neural signaling and microcephaly, leading to craniofacial malformations.[20]

In early 2014, the *International Journal of Environmental Research and Public* Health published a study linking glyphosate runoff in Sri Lanka's water systems to an epidemic rise in a fatal unknown chronic kidney disease or CKDu. Until recently, scientists were unable to offer up evidence of what has been causing this new form of illness affecting the kidneys. Similar observations have been made in El Salvador and Nicaragua, where more men die of CKDu than AIDS, diabetes, and leukemia. However, in each regional population studied, Roundup exposure is rampant. Sri Lankan scientists hypothesize that glyphosate, originally discovered to act as a chelating chemical in 1964, takes up toxic heavy metals and binds them in the kidney without the body's detection. According to the researchers, the buildup of these heavy metals ultimately leads to kidney failure and death.[21]

In early 2014, the Ministry of Health in Cordoba, Argentina noted a dramatic rise in deaths from cancerous tumors– twice the national average. It just so happens that the elevated rates of malignancies were being reported in those regions where GM crops and toxic agrochemicals are most readily used.[22]

What do the studies say about GM crops specifically? Studies cannot be conducted directly on humans because of moral and ethical reasons; however, in another sense, we are all test subjects, since so many of our major crops are now GM crops. Nonetheless, some studies suggest that glyphosate, for example, may be altering human reproduction. The rate of male fertility in the US has been dropping steadily since GM foods started to saturate the average American diet. Today, according to the American Pregnancy Association, 1 out of every 6 men in couples is infertile.[23]

The American Academy of Environmental Medicine (AAEM) stated, "several animal studies indicate serious health risks associated with GM food consumption including infertility, immune dysregulation, accelerated aging, dysregulation of genes associated with cholesterol synthesis, insulin regulation, cell signaling, and protein formation, and changes in the liver, kidney, spleen, and gastrointestinal system."[24] The AAEM went on to consider the possible role of GM foods in the disease processes and to advise patients to avoid GM foods until their safety is proven.

The Institute for Responsible Technology further notes: "Before the FDA decided to allow GMOs into food without labeling, FDA scientists had repeatedly warned that GM foods can create unpredictable, hard-to-detect side effects, including allergies, toxins, new diseases, and nutritional problems. They urged long-term safety studies but were ignored."[25] They also reported findings including:

- Thousands of sheep, buffalo, and goats in India died after grazing on Bt cotton plants.
- Mice eating GM corn for the long term had fewer and smaller babies.
- More than half the babies of mother rats fed GM soy died within three weeks and were smaller.
- Testicle cells of mice and rats on a GM soy changed significantly.
- By the third generation, most GM soy-fed hamsters lost the ability to have babies.
- Rodents fed GM corn and soy showed immune system responses and signs of toxicity.
- Cooked GM soy contains as much as 7-times the amount of a known soy allergen.
- Soy allergies skyrocketed by 50% in the UK, soon after GM soy was introduced.
- The stomach lining of rats fed GM potatoes showed excessive cell growth, a condition that may lead to cancer.
- Studies showed organ lesions, altered liver and pancreas cells, changed enzyme levels, etc.

Another major blow against Monsanto has been the republication of Dr. Seralini's paper showing a correlation between severe kidney and liver damage, advanced tumors, and pre-mature death in rats fed Monsanto's NK603 maize in the peer-reviewed journal *Environmental Sciences Europe*. Seralini's paper has undergone more scientific review and scrutiny than any other study either proving or disproving GMO safety. With its republication, the paper should officially replace Monsanto's flawed safety study purporting the health safety of its NK603 corn.[26]

Who Controls Your Health Choices?

For now, in terms of health, the only prudent choice is *USDA certified* organic foods; only these are guaranteed to be GMO-free, which brings me to my next point. With the rise in popularity of organic foods, many of the organic food brands that you see in health food stores today are, in fact, now owned by large multinational food conglomerates that have little to no interest in consumer or environmental health. Here are just a few examples of the many natural and organic brands now owned by major multinational corporations: Boca Burgers, Green & Blacks & Back to Nature (owned by Mondelez, formerly known as Kraft), Kashi (owned by Kellogg), Dagoba (Hershey Foods), Seeds of Change (M&M Mars), White Wave/Silk and Horizon Dairy (Dean), Kettle (Diamond Foods), Stonyfield & Brown Cow (Dannon), Lara Bar, Cascadian Farm, Food Should Taste Good, and Muir Glen (General Mills).[27] See Appendix E for a complete list of corporate acquisitions of health food companies.

Dr. Philip H. Howard of Michigan State University, creator of the popular *Organic Industry Structure: Acquisitions and Alliances, Top 100 Food Producers in America chart notes*: "Frequently the acquisition of an organic brand by a larger company often means the watering down of a company's standards."[28] Moreover, when an organic brand is controlled by a corporation, not only can product quality suffer, but worse, your dollars spent on these products benefit the parent corporation—most of whom don't think GMOs are a problem and likely even donated money to prevent GMO labeling. Here is just a brief rundown of anti-GMO labeling contributions by major food companies who, along with GMO makers like Monsanto, Dow and Bayer, and other GMO-proponents, defeated GMO labeling laws in California's Proposition 37:

- Pepsico, Inc. - $2,485,400 (Naked Juice)
- Kraft Foods Global, Inc. - $2,000,500 (Back to Nature, Boca Burger)
- Coca-Cola North America - $1,690,500
- Nestlé USA, Inc. - $1,461,600 (Gerber Organic Baby Food, Powerbar)
- General Mills, Inc. - $1,230,300 (Cascadian Farm ["organic"], Good Earth, Food Should Taste Good ["organic"], Lärabar ["organic"], Muir Glen ["organic"], and Nature Valley)
- Kellogg Company - $790,700 (Kashi)

- Campbell Soup Company - $598,000 (Bolthouse Farms)
- The J.M. Smucker Company - $555,000 (Natural Brew, R.W. Knudsen Family, Santa Cruz Organic)
- Hershey Company - $518,900 (Dagoba)
- Mars Food North America - $498,350 (Seeds Of Change)
- Unilever - $467,100 (Ben and Jerry's Ice Cream)
- Dean Foods Company - $253,950 (Horizon Organic milk products, Silk organic and natural plant-based products, Brown's Dairy dairy products etc.[29]

GM seed companies and the Grocery Manufacturers Association are dumping millions into propaganda campaigns to defeat the popular civil demand to label GM foods and products, in part with the message that labeling would substantially increase the cost of food. Ironically, the October 2014 issue of *Consumer Reports*, which reaches over 7 million readers, has determined that the cost to consumers for labeling GMO products would be at most a meager $2.30 per person annually,[30] less than a penny a day. The Consumer Union has fully endorsed GMO labeling and also noted that its survey found that three quarters of Americans try to avoid GMO consumption as a vital issue for having a healthy diet.

The importance of these labeling laws cannot be understated.They would go a long way to bring an end to the misinformation associated with the wording of "natural," which currently does not exclude GMO ingredients and other deleterious substances such as synthetic and non-synthetic substances including cellulose—which is wood pulp—used as an anti-caking agent and filtering aid; chlorine materials, used for disinfecting and sanitizing food contact surfaces; non-synthetic waxes such as Carnauba wax and wood resin; and animal enzymes, such as rennet, catalase (from bovine liver), and animal lipase.[31] In short, because there are few regulations governing the labeling of "natural" foods, food manufacturers can include ingredients that may not be considered natural by some consumers. In reality, the only way to ensure that you are eating a truly plant-based food is if the words "suitable for vegans" or a symbol like this Ⓥ (meaning a food is completely animal-free—in terms of both ingredients and processing) appears on the label. Read more about the dangers lurking in your foods on p. 271.

Whenever possible, it is best to support independent, family-owned certified organic companies. Because they continue to operate independently, they can uphold product integrity and their commitment to their customers' health equal to that of their business, as well as freedom in educating about GMOs.[32] These companies are also free to spend their money in the fight for GMO labeling, unlike organic brands owned by major food corporations.

Here is a list of companies with organic products that you can support knowing that they are presently free from corporate influence and that purely organic products are free from GMOs[33]:

Amy's Kitchen	Late July	R.W. Garcia Tortilla chips
Apple and Eve	Let's Do Organic	Raw Revolution
Artisana Nut Butters	Lotus Foods	Road's End Organic
Bearded Brothers	Lundberg Family Farms /	Rudi's Bakery
Betty Lou's Bars	Wehah Farms	Sambazon
Bionaturae	My Grandpa's Farm	SOL Cuisine
Bob's Red Mill	Native Forest	SquareBar
Bueno Foods	Nature Factor	Sunshine Burger
CB's Nuts	Nature's Legacy / VitaSpelt	Teddie Peanut Butter
Clif Bar	/ Purity Foods	Theo's Chocolates
Core Foods	Nature's Path	Uncle Matt's Organic
Crofter's Organic Fruit	Newman's Own Organics	Shiloh Farms
Spreads	NuGo Nutrition bars	Sweet Creek Foods
Dave's Killer Bread	Nutiva	Tasty Brand
Eden Organic	Once Again Nut Butter	Two Moms in the Raw
Edward & Sons Brands	One Degree Organic	Vermont Village Applesauce
Feridies Peanuts	Organic Food Bar	VitaSpelt
Fiordifrutta Organic Fruit	Organic Valley	Vivapura
Spread	Pacific Beach Peanut Butter	Wild Friends Foods
Grindstone Bakery	Pascha Chocolates	Yogi Tea
Grown Right	Pure Bar	YummyEarth / YumEarth
Healthy Times	Que Pasa	Zulka

Furthermore, here is a short list of brands that *currently use Monsanto GMOs*. If you want to make an impact, stop purchasing these products or supporting these companies; and consider letting them know why. If enough of us do this, these companies will be forced to change their ways.[34]

Aunt Jemima	Hosum	Ore-Ida
Aurora Foods	Hormel	Ocean Spray
Banquet	Hungry Jack	Orville Redenbacher
Best Foods	Hunts	Pasta-Roni
Betty Crocker	Interstate Bakeries	Pepperidge Farms
Bisquick	Jiffy	Pepsi
Cadbury	KC Masterpiece	Pillsbury
Campbells	Keebler/Flower Industries	Pop Secret
Capri Sun	Kellogg's	Post Cereals
Carnation	Kid Cuisine	Power Bar Brand
Chef Boyardee	Knorr	Prego Pasta Sauce
Coca Cola	Kool-Aid	Pringles
ConAgra	Kraft/Philip Morris	Procter & Gamble
Delicious Brand Cookies	Lean Cuisine	Quaker
Duncan Hines	Lipton	Ragu Sauce
Famous Amos	Loma Linda	Rice-A-Roni
Frito Lay	Marie Callenders	Smart Ones
General Mills	Minute Maid	Stouffers
Green Giant	Morningstar	Schweppes
Healthy Choice	Mrs. Butterworth's	Tombstone Pizza
Heinz	Nabisco	Uncle Ben's
Hellman's	Nature Valley	Unilever
Hershey's	Nestlé	V8

The "Basic Four"

In their efforts to promote a healthy society, the USDA developed a diagram of what foods should be consumed in what quantities. It showed certain quantities of grains, meats, dairy, fruits and vegetables, and sugars, salts, and fats that should be consumed for a healthy diet. This diagram was introduced in 1956 and purported to be a way to simplify the complexities of nutrition for the public. But, the truth is, the only thing this really simplified was the process of lining the pockets of agribusiness, since this grouping did little to ensure proper nutrition.

What isn't reflected on the food pyramid's surface recommendations is the intense politics behind these decisions. If an industry felt it was not being adequately promoted for its own tastes, it came down hard on the USDA with lobbying pressure, getting thousands of mothers (many of whose families were employed by the industry) to bombard the regulatory agencies with effective phone campaigns until the USDA made the requested changes to the pyramid.

Let me digress for a moment into a bit of social theory that I believe will help explain what's happening here. Picking up the argument of *epistemology* and how we know what we know, we see that we receive our knowledge almost exclusively from other people. In other words, we learn what they teach us as being the truth of our reality. If the USDA food pyramid suggests 12 servings of wheat a day, then that is the truth of the reality of what our bodies need.

But we have to keep in mind that our reality, our "truth" as we perceive it, comes from other people. Thus, it's really hard to get at the actual "truth" of something—anything—because it's all always reflective of others' realities. This is the essence of the theory of social constructivism or social constructionism as it's also called. Reality, truth, are constructed by people—socially constructed.

We are wise to keep this in mind when evaluating information disseminated as "truth" or "reality." Indeed, what we are receiving is someone else's truth and reality, which may or may not be good for us.

In fact, the USDA food pyramid, and the categories of foods it reflects, are purely a social construction. It is constructed by people. Those people have their own agendas to meet. In this case, the USDA has an agenda of some degree of pandering to food industries. This pandering is reflected in the final chart of food recommendations—which is disseminated to the general public.

Of course the meat and dairy groups take a lot of space on the food pyramid—these are exceptionally powerful industries in the US, and it's not hard for them to pressure the USDA into promoting their products.

At its core, even the USDA food pyramid is about generating profit for the industries it most promotes.

Notwithstanding, in their 2015 report, the USDA recognizes America's health problems and recognizes them as stemming from our standard diet (the very same unhealthy diet they have been promoting for decades). Simultaneously, despite what's happening on Capitol Hill, the USDA acknowledges the challenges to sustainable food sources if we continue on our current path:

> Consistent evidence indicates that, in general, a dietary pattern that is higher in plant-based foods, such as vegetables, fruits, whole grains, legumes, nuts, and seeds, and lower in animal-based foods is more health promoting and is associated with lesser environmental impact (GHG emissions and energy, land, and water use) than is the current average US diet.[35]

The same USDA report actually recommends the *Healthy Vegetarian* diet as a way to reduce disease and environmental impact. Media reports indicate that the current recommendations of vegetarian dietary patterns are the strongest to date.[36] Some complain, however, that the inclusion of meat and low-fat dairy remains part of the USDA's general recommendations because all meat and low-fat dairy products cause disease, according to Dr. Neal Barnard.[37]

The High Cost of Meat and Dairy: It Must Be Good for Someone

If you're envisioning images of the beef industry consisting of small ranches working together to accomplish their ends, it would probably be because you are still caught up in a vision of yesteryear, when meat and dairy foods were handled by rugged, hard-working farmers toiling on small plots in scenic valleys, walking their herds over picturesque pastures, carefully selecting their best products for the marketplace. That was before the advent of monopolies, those business behemoths like Monsanto that arose in the late 1800s in the US and gradually crushed and swallowed up most small competitors. Today, over half of all US farm sales come from only 3% of the farms—mega corporations owned by non-farming businessmen who hire foreman and women (rather than farmers) to supervise the low paid help who do the raising, drugging, and slaughtering. As it stands, four corporations take care of at least half of all food industry sales.[38] Swift and Pillsbury, for example, control an estimated 90% of the chicken market.

These mega-conglomerates usually working through their associations, such as the National Egg Board, the American Egg Board, the United Dairy Industry Association, the National Livestock and Meat Board, and the National Pork Producer Council, to pour on the advertising when their food is under attack, or simply in order to shape public perception about the health benefits of eating their commodities. Of course, these advertising costs are eventually passed on to the consumer, who pays not only for the product, but also for the so called "privilege" of being persuaded to buy it.

Unlike the sassier or more frivolous-seeming ads that might be used to sell toys or shoes, a great deal of this food advertising puts on a serious air, so as to "inform" the viewer or reader with a *scientific sounding* communication concerning the fact that a glass of milk or a pat of butter or a lean cut of pork is essential to a well-balanced diet. You might almost mistake it for a public-service announcement. Indeed, that's why it was crafted the way it was by the advertisers, to make you believe that the information is coming from a health book or other credible source. This type of advertising has become a major focus of the meat and dairy industries in recent years as they struggle to combat falling sales resulting from their own inflated prices, the greater availability of vegetarian alternatives, and, especially, from the rising public awareness of the severe health hazards of meat and dairy foods.

King Cattle

I want to emphasize how powerful the influence of these meat and dairy interests are, with cattle raisers usually in the lead in promoting their agenda—an understandable situation if one looks at the history of cattle raising.

In the early part of the 19th century, cotton was king. It was the chief cash crop of the US, benefiting farmers who grew it and industrialists who made finished products from it. Cotton production also relied on a large slave population.

History moved on, slavery ended, King Cotton was dethroned, and the vast plantations were laid to waste. Soon enough, King Cattle saw an opportunity and moved in. Like its former ruler, King Cattle provided wealth for the few at the top, impoverishment for those in the lower ranks, and devastation of the land. The battle to drive up meat consumption began.

Between 1938 and 1956, the American Meat Institute sponsored educational and promotional programs to drive up meat sales, investing more than $30 million in consumer advertising within that period to convince Americans that meat is a fine food. Today, the US government alone spends $550 million on USDA-managed programs.[39] The industry spends in the billions of dollars with Cargill, JBS (Brazil's largest meat-processing company) and Tyson alone, counting for close to $4 billion.[40] They touted meat as offering "magical results"—it was a cure-all that reversed everything from pernicious anemia to pellagra, warded off bad habits, and was "a nutritional necessity for the steady drinker and smoker" because it could reduce the ill effects of overindulging in drinking and smoking. Meat was advertised as a "health guardian for man, woman, and child."[41] They worked at our core American values arguing that, along with voting and possibly serving in the military, the third thing a patriotic American could do to show love for his or her country was to dig into a good helping of T-bone steak or other meat, aiming to increase meat consumption to "a pound per day or even more."[42]

Apparently their efforts worked. We are now a full-blooded animal killing and eating culture. As recently as 1950, Americans were annually consuming an average of 60 pounds of beef, 60 pounds of pork, and 25 pounds of poultry.[43] By the 1970s, though, per capita beef and poultry consumption had doubled. By 2006, Americans' per capita beef consumption was 96.56 pounds. America is second in beef consumption only to Argentina, where cattle raising is a leading industry and the culture is steeped in the gaucho machismo of beef eating. The European Union lags far behind in these grotesque figures, recording only 39.46 pounds per person of beef consumption in 2006.[44]

According to the National Chicken Council, annual consumption rates of meat for 2015 are 54.1 pounds of beef, 50 pounds of pork, 89.6 pounds of chicken, and 16.3 pounds of turkey for a total of 211.1 pounds of meat a year per American.[45]

The last estimates of fish and shellfish were in 2013, where the average consumption was at 14.5 pounds per person.[46] The amount of dairy products—all sources—consumed by Americans in 2012 was 275.9 pounds.[47] According to the United Egg Producers, the average number of eggs consumed by Americans in 2014 was 263 eggs.[48] The report also noted that the USDA's Per Capita Consumption figures show egg consumption at the highest in 30 years.[49]

Deceptive Dairy

Meanwhile, the dairy industry was not being left behind. Don't forget that back in the 1930s when our cattle saga began, many more mothers nursed their babies or had them tended by professional wet nurses. Giving infants cow's milk was considered a decided second best. Indeed, many Americans shunned dairy products, in part because they recognized milk caused mucus and allergic reactions.

In stepped the National Dairy Council, the largest provider of nutrition-education materials for our school systems, vigorously promoting the merits of milk and cheese, sponsoring self-serving research, and ultimately winning the hearts of American consumers. Infants were pulled from their mothers' breasts and introduced to the milk bottle, and for decades now, cheeses and milk (including chocolate milk) in the school cafeteria have been as common as beer in a bar.

Dieticians and school teachers were enlisted in the campaign to get people to eat what the meat purveyors claimed were complete (meat and dairy) as opposed to incomplete (vegetables and fruits) proteins.

Also, milk is far from a beneficial source of calcium as its advocates claim—given that much of the calcium it contains cannot be absorbed by the human body. That's why, surprising as it may be to holders of the status quo, "Most research shows that dairy products are not beneficial to bone health" at any age.[50] Milk also contributes to the excess protein many Americans are getting, which can be as ruinous to their health as a lack of protein and is discussed in greater detail in Chapter 6. Plus, the antibiotics and other pharmaceuticals given to cows make milk less a pure drink than a drug cocktail. It doesn't promote weight loss though, as the dairy industry asserts; rather, the Physicians Committee for Responsible Medicine won a lawsuit against the dairy industry in 2005 for touting dairy's benefits as important for affecting and maintaining weight loss. In fact, milk and dairy products do just the opposite; they add to the obesity epidemic.

Certainly, on the face of it, there is something rather unreasonable in imagining that the milk of one species—the cow—crafted by evolution over thousands of years to properly nourish its own young, could be simply hijacked and given to the young (and even the adults) of another species, humans, and be expected to provide the same nutrition without any difficulties. The milk of one species is not formulated to fully support the health of another species, period. And this is without exception. There are, for example, natural hormones in cows' milk for the mother cow to pass on to her calf. When humans drink that milk, we ingest these hormones that are programmed specifically to regulate the biochemistry of the cow's system, not ours.

One of the major proteins of milk, casein, constitutes some 80% of milk's proteins and is often frequently included in processed foods as an ingredient. As the body digests casein, casomorphins—natural morphin-like substances—enter the bloodstream. One study demonstrated that autistic children had higher levels of casomorphins in their urine,[51] hinting at a link between autism and milk consumption.

Increasing numbers of people seem to have an intolerance to casein, suffering from constipation, gas, bloating, and diarrhea, and studies have linked casein consumption to an increased production of mucus[52] and increased wheezing in children with asthma.[53]

It is important to note that the beef, dairy, poultry, and related industries have a LOT to gain from convincing us to eat their products. They will stretch the truth in any direction necessary to get us to give them our money.

Your Consumer Rights: Who Will Uphold Them?

Some state legislators bend over backwards to help the embattled beef industry, which should give you some idea about how good such lawmakers are at protecting your interests. That is, they know who's filling their campaign coffers: meat and dairy producers, and who's not: the public. Those that gain the most from friendly meat and dairy agribusiness owners tend to become boosters of their contributors' industries, even following a wild line of argument the industry has recently unveiled that holds that we should put less emphasis on raising grain for humans and more on growing it to feed livestock, because, as one pro-meat industry observer puts it, "It's cheaper to ship a pound of beef than it is to ship eight or ten pounds of grain."[54]

I don't mean to imply that our politicians cannot ever be reached. While even a hardened meat company executive, for example, will withdraw an ad if the public is outraged by some claim made in a particularly offensive way, he or she is still not as dependent on public good will as a politician who periodically needs to be re-elected. That's why I say you and I *can* make our voices heard to some extent, just as the special interests do. I believe your senator and congressman will listen when you write or call concerning specific legislation that upholds your rights as a consumer. So let them know how you feel. Use your influence. Those who have no interest in your welfare are certainly using theirs! Also, please check out the list of resource organizations in the back of this book.

Cooperation in Getting Food Alternatives

But what about reaching the meat and dairy industries? It would be a bit quixotic to expect them to alter their ads to make them more honest if this would be undercutting their sales. The better strategy is just to stop buying their products and go green. It's equivalent to a boycott that never ends.

That means shopping at health food stores, for one, but if you are more adventurous, you can start or join a food cooperative and bypass the middleman retailer. All you need is a group of like-minded people that can place bulk orders large enough to be able to buy directly from wholesalers and producers at a wholesale price. This will give you access to the quality food you want at savings of up to 40-60%. The shelves in your coop will be stocked only with food you want; not, for instance, with overpriced, over-sugared breakfast cereals or piles of the meat of dead animals.

Also, in uniting with people who share common interests, the cooperative system of buying establishes a network that can serve as a model for further group action in various directions, such as food, housing, medical supplies and care, and much more. It gives members a sense of the power they have as a group, and they begin to realize that they, too, can exert influence in the political realm, which should never have been left to the pernicious lobbying of the large monopolies and agribusinesses.

You can get even more actively involved in providing yourself with the kinds of foods that promote health and prevent disease by growing them yourself, assuring your very own supply of fresh organic produce. You don't need much space, just a small plot in your yard or city roof top or community garden. You can learn the basics from the internet, books, or magazines such as the popular *Organic Gardening* and *Farming*.

The Vegetarian Alternative

For a moment, let's imagine that you had to construct a pyramid that had application not only for the US but for the world. Immediately, you would have to slice off the meat layer. Why? The vast majority of the world's people can't afford to eat meat, so even if they wanted it they would have no means of obtaining it. So let's imagine a transcultural food grouping with five categories. These would be the three principal dietary staples—grains, legumes, and vegetables—and two smaller groups consisting of raw foods like fruits, and possibly nuts, and foods containing vitamin B12.[55] Our new pyramid contains every food needed by people in any socio-economic or cultural group in order to maintain a healthy, active life.

While most people in underdeveloped countries already eat exclusively from this global pyramid, if Americans started making the shift to using it, what a boon it could be, not only to them but to their neighbors across the globe. Agricultural expert Lester R. Brown argues that if Americans were to cut their annual meat consumption by a mere 10%, it would save roughly 12 million tons of grain, which alone could negate an entire year's nutritional deficit in India.

Social Norms

The Influence of Mass Media

Part of the reason for our widespread confusion about health and the defeatist attitude it breeds is that most of us simply are not scientists or nutritionist or chefs for that matter. As such, we don't have easy access to the technical literature or, perhaps, the know-how and skill set involved in succeeding in a healthy lifestyle, including preparing wholesome meals.

And we cannot count on the mass media for help. Decision-makers in the news business often bypass less flashy but ultimately more significant research findings in favor of those that are more dramatic, even ones that may seem contradictory. Such is the nature of the media industry. After all, from their point of view, confusion and conflict arouse interest, which generates increased viewer ratings and therefore more advertising dollars and profit. Hence, dramatic reversals and controversies are often times considered the "best" stories.

Moreover, as our look at history has suggested, when the meat and dairy industry was able to flood the media with glowing scientific reports about the benefits of their products, these stories seemed to find their way into print and over the airways with much less ease than did findings on the health hazards of what they were selling. But with scientific reports that back the claims of animal-based agribusiness becoming few and far between and new facts about the health dangers of meat- and dairy-centered diets becoming almost daily occurrences, the media turns to controversy and confusion. Why? Because it is uncomfortable and calls their credibility into question. They'd rather broadcast stories that promote dietary confusion than ones about the abuses and health risks associated with agribusiness or the "boring" findings on the health benefits of vegetables and whole grains—which (they say) won't command any attention—even though such reaffirmations would be life-saving for many right now.

In fact, media provides an extremely powerful force in shaping and guiding public opinion, so what they report matters. Most vegetarianism press is negative, including the recent (December 2014) scourge of reporting on The Humane Resource Council's report that demonstrated a large number of vegetarians return to meat eating within a year of adopting a vegetarian lifestyle. Consider the headlines: *Almost All Vegetarians End Up Going Back to Meat Eventually*; *84% of Vegetarians Become Meat Eaters Again*; *Vegetarian Statistics: How Many Will Fail?*

While the HRC report also mentions that a full 37% of the former vegetarians and vegans surveyed said they would consider adopting the diet again, the finding was buried in most reports. This perhaps is the most important news, for it allows us to see that the growing number of people are actually positively moving away from eating meat, at the least, and see and/or know the benefits associated with *becoming more of a vegetarian*, even if they still consume animal products. I believe that the increased level of awareness these people have as a result of their attempt at the diet will keep them closely related to fruits, vegetables, and grains for a long time. And those that do return to meat, fish, or poultry will most likely eat less than they had consumed previously and will almost always consume, as much as possible, organic, free range meats and poultry from local farms and wild caught fish. I also think that it demonstrates that our level of consciousness (at least around physical health) is, indeed, rising. With proper focus and support, in my estimation, more people could and would sustain a plant-based diet.

As humans, we are social animals, hard wired to seek each other's company for cooperation and compassion. Further, humans have a high need for comfort, physically and emotionally. So, when we find out some news that is disquieting to our nature—how sickeningly harsh and unimaginably inhumane the treatment of a chicken or steer is prior to making its way to our plate, for example—very few will act readily upon the information. Instead, most of us cover up that discomfort by ignoring the facts. One way of doing this is to make excuses, to distract ourselves or even go so far as to refute the evidence (without any hard data), or to take a headline from a piece of news and use it to strengthen investment in the status quo. These are favorite ways for humans because, in reality, we not only *dislike* change, but most of us get really upset when our beliefs and ideas are challenged. This certainly gives more meaning to the word "comfort food," doesn't it?

Identifying incongruent behavior is one of the most difficult things for us to do. Even if we know it and we know what's good for us, Americans' diets are largely harmful and not in the best interest of personal or planetary health. But we don't think that. One study of 1,234 US adults conducted for consumer reports noted that 89.7% of Americans described their diet as "somewhat" (52.6%), "very" (31.5%), or "extremely" (5.6%) healthy.[56] Shockingly, 9 out of 10 Americans think their diet is actually on the health spectrum, when close to 7 out of 10 adults are now overweight, with 35% of these adults obese. Something is clearly askew in the minds of Americans.

Food runs our lives, literally, as it provides the necessary fuel for us to live our lives. So, it makes sense that food is at the forefront of many people's thoughts and concerns. What should be on people's minds is just making sure they actually get enough fruits and vegetables and enough variety of these items. But there are plenty of forces outside of media working against this intelligent and life-affirming thought process.

Time and Health…*What the Science Says*

The Value of the Slow Food Movement

Today, people rarely take their time eating at home, and often or not, they're standing on one leg at a kitchen counter, picking at food, and they've got their cell phone up to their ear, a television on in the background, and a radio playing. People are jumping around, running in and out, and to them, that is normal. When was the last time you saw a movie where everyone sat down, took their time, and there was no rushing? You can't remember because those scenes are rarely filmed. Instead, it's dashing here or there, and no one has any time.

This is also now common in restaurants, even in the so-called more up-scale restaurants. The environment is noisy, and the place is over-cramped; even some vegan restaurants in New York are packed, and the food is poorly prepared and displayed and, at times, uneventful in terms of taste. I won't even eat at one of the most popular restaurants in America because the service is abominable, the food is boring, and it's noisy. But younger people frequent it and they're happy because they're not used to slow cooking, slow conversation, and slow living. Not only this; they don't look at each other, they're twittering while at a table, they couldn't care less about the service or the taste of the food because they don't know what anything really natural tastes like because they were raised on fast, processed foods.

When I go to Europe, I see just the opposite. When you watch people shopping and eating there, whether it's in India with their huge food bazaars, or in Romania—they take their time. Food is very important to them. They know something has to be fresh to taste good so they want their bread fresh that day. They don't buy a week's worth of bread or vegetables; they go to the market every day. If you go into most of their kitchens, their cupboards are largely empty. They either like making things themselves or buying fresh food that day. Fresh is the key. I remember visiting a restaurant in a small village in Italy one summer. When we asked for some food, they were very happy to prepare it from scratch. We enjoyed the bucolic setting from the front patio while the food was being prepared in the kitchen. This gave my travel companions and I the opportunity to visit with the owners of the restaurant and other guests, while enjoying a rest in the middle of the day. We must have been there for nearly three hours, but the experience was so rich and the food so incredibly delicious and fresh.

In certain more traditional parts of Europe, the main meal is almost always in the early afternoon, and it's very common for people to take two to three hours away from work to enjoy it. Watch how they prepare food and visit and talk with one another; it's a joyful celebration of life. Nothing is rushed or deep-fried; everything is slow—because eating is an integral part of life. And so they're living longer lives, exhibiting less disease—certainly less heart disease, stroke, and cancer, whether colorectal, prostate, or breast cancer—and we wonder why.

In the US, every day we have multiple stopwatches that we click on: click on to get up, click on to commute, click on to get our exercise in, click on to catch ten minutes of the news. We live by regimented, ritualized time restraints and hence, we're always stressed. We find it really hard to relax, we find it hard to unwind, even when we go on vacation, we attempt to fit everything in: "Okay, well we paid 1500 dollars to be here for the week, so we've got to do everything," and then we come back exhausted and unrested for the next stretch of our automaton-like existence.

So more than ever, we need a complete break from our overstressed, fast-forward society: the slow food movement came about to address these concerns as well as to help us shift our habit toward valuing quality over quantity and long-term over short. According to Carlo Petrini, the Slow Food founder and president, "Slow Food unites the pleasure of food with responsibility, sustainability, and harmony with nature."[57]

Slow Food was founded in 1989 to counter fast food and defend a slower pace of life. It is now a global organization involving millions of people and is active in over 150 countries. The movement's motto is good, clean, and fair food, meaning high quality, healthy food whose production does not harm the environment, sold at accessible prices for consumers, and with the producers receiving fair pay.

Following on from the Slow Food Movement, the Slow Movement has extended to almost all aspects of life, including Slow Education, Slow Parenting, Slow Travel, and Slow Money, in an effort to promote our own and others' wellbeing by reconnecting with the natural world and its natural rhythms. Carl Honoré, author of *In Praise of Slowness*, describes this as "a cultural revolution against the notion that faster is always better. The Slow philosophy is not about doing everything at a snail's pace. It's about seeking to do everything at the right speed; savoring the hours and minutes rather than just counting them; doing everything as well as possible instead of as fast as possible."[58]

The Slow Movement and particularly Slow Food, encourages many of the issues we've discussed previously, such as buying whole, ethical, organic, local produce; growing some of our own food, even if it's in pots on the windowsill; in addition to joining community schemes and lobbying against the use of genetic engineering, factory farms, and pesticides. See the resources section in the back of this book for more information on the organizations promoting this way of living.[59]

Food and Time in America

One of the challenges to eating a healthy vegetarian diet for many Americans is the time factor involved in meal preparation. A 2014 report in the *American Journal of Preventive Medicine* indicated that Americans only currently spend an estimated 33 minutes per day on food preparation and cleanup. Also, limited time available for cooking may be one of the barriers to the adoption of more healthy diets. Social class also plays a role. In fact, time scarcity was prevalent among working parents earning low wages in the US. Even those parents who valued healthy family meals often served their children foods that were fast and easy to prepare, including hot dogs, pizza, and macaroni and cheese. Research on low- and middle-income working parents showed that they coped with time pressures by relying more on takeout and restaurant meals and basing family meals on prepared entrees and other quick options.[60]

It may very well be that time may end up not being on our side when it comes to health. A study conducted at Ohio State University reported that American adults who prepare their own meals and exercise on the same day are likely spending more time on one of those activities at the expense of the other. The research showed that a 10-minute increase in food preparation time was associated with a lower probability of exercising for 10 more minutes for both men and women, and applied to single and married adults as well as parents and those who have no children. Dmitry Tumin, one of the co-authors of the study summarized: "There's only so much time in a day. As people try to meet their health goals, there's a possibility that spending time on one healthy behavior is going to come at the expense of the other. I think this highlights the need to always consider the trade-off between ideal and feasible time use for positive health behaviors."[61]

While I understand the time constraints that many face, I do believe that part of being a healthy vegetarian means doing all we can do to incorporate daily exercise and healthy vegetarian eating, with as much home cooking as possible. With home cooking, you can control the amount of fat, sugar, and salt in your foods, and studies do indicate that it indeed improves health. The same study I noted two paragraphs before, published in the *American Journal of Preventive Medicine,* concluded that greater amounts of time spent on home food preparation were associated with indicators of higher diet quality, including significantly more frequent intake of vegetables, salads, fruits, and fruit juices.[62]

Furthermore, consider the quality of life and positive interaction with one's self, family, and friends when preparing and enjoying a meal together. Also, home cooking need not be a chore. In a blog dated October 9, 2014, Mark Bittman, American food journalist, author, and columnist for *The New York Times* writes, "When I talk about cooking, something I've been doing for the better part of five decades, I'm not talking about creating elaborate dinner parties or three-day science projects. I'm talking about simple, easy, everyday meals. My mission is to encourage novices and the time- and cash-strapped to feed themselves… we need modest, realistic expectations, and we need to teach people to cook food that's good enough to share with family, friends…"[63]

Bittman also touches on a topic related to food that I see as a key motivator for the vegetarian movement: "Shouldn't preparing—and consuming—food be a source of comfort, pride, health, well-being, relaxation, sociability? Something that connects us to other humans? Why would we want to outsource this basic task, especially when outsourcing it is so harmful? Sure, there are challenges to cooking; there are challenges to fixing income inequality too. Our goal should be to make things better, not to accept such a dismal status quo. Because not cooking is a big mistake—and it's one that's costing us money, good times, control, serenity, and, yes, vastly better health."

Think about it: Food is our primary source of life, and we have fundamentally lost touch with this when we eat convenience foods. In reality, the basics in life (whole foods, clean water, proper amounts of sleep, as well as rest and play) support us to do our most rewarding work in the world, which is to serve humanity. Why, then, do we literally relegate food to the shelves, while substantially elevating other activities such as shopping, watching television, and playing computer or video games? If we know the answer to this question, we have an opportunity to reverse this devastating trend and make a real impact on our own health and the health of our entire culture.

Food Availability

The truth is, not everyone has access to the necessary foods to comprise a healthy diet; it's as simple as that. The people of impoverished nations suffer from malnutrition, be they vegetarians or not. Impoverished US residents also suffer from malnutrition. If you don't live in an area with a variety of healthy foods that fit your budget, it's extremely difficult, perhaps nearly impossible, to live a healthy vegetarian lifestyle.

In fact, several elements contribute to the difficulty of accessing healthy affordable foods in low-income US neighborhoods. The Food Research and Action Center (FRAC) in Washington DC cites relevant research on this topic. For one thing, they report, full-service grocery stores and farmer's markets are often lacking in low-income neighborhoods, while corner markets and convenience stores abound. This means that a variety of fresh fruits and vegetables and whole grains are difficult to come by. Research has demonstrated that area residents with better access to supermarkets and more limited access to convenience stores tend to enjoy both healthier diets and reduced obesity risk.

Secondly, even when it is available, healthy food is usually more expensive than the refined grains with added sugars and fats. One way to stretch a household food budget is to buy cheap, energy-dense, filling foods to stave off hunger. Unfortunately, energy-dense foods tend to have lower nutritional value, and because of caloric overconsumption, are linked to obesity.

Thirdly, even when it is available in lower income neighborhood markets, the quality of the produce offered is generally poor, diminishing the appeal of these items. Additionally, the wide availability of fast food restaurants in lower-income neighborhoods, especially near schools, contributes to obesity. Fast foods are toxic, denatured, energy-dense, nutrient-poor, cheap foods. Frequent consumption, of course, typically leads to weight gain.

This "grocery gap" is a reason why our school cafeterias are so important. Schools are where our community learns and grows. They are considered to be safe spaces, particularly for younger children, with positive influences. Nutritional information is mostly being "taught" via the foods the children are fed. Also, school is where we, as a society, learn not only the three R's, but also how to be members of this society. We learn social codes, norms, and values. School lunches aren't only supposed to be giving our children proper nutrition for the day, but are also about teaching our nation's children about proper nutrition for a lifetime. If the school serves unhealthy food out of bags and boxes, it's difficult to later argue that we shouldn't be eating out of bags and boxes; it is confusing to demonstrate one way and then ask them to act differently. The school provides a role model to our children and our community and shapes the future of our children's diets. We, as a society, need to pay more attention and, more importantly, get involved with what our school children are being fed. It affects all of us, because it affects our nation's health and the future of our nation's health.

There is a new movement afoot to combat food scarcity, and it is a movement that will continue to grow in prominence and importance; let's call it "Friends who farm." Let's say you live in a food desert, but there are a few families who are willing to farm; or, perhaps, you live in the suburbs or city, and work in the city, but have never been to a farm. Now, and moving into the future, you will have the opportunity to buy into a farm, thereby securing your opportunity for fresh produce. The way this typically works is that you invest money that you earn in another profession, such as an engineer, an accountant, a construction worker, or a seamstress to purchase a "share" of a farm's produce. The farm is worked by others and supplies food for its own workers as well as its investors. Within this structure, there is also room for the creative possibility of trading services, such as the ones noted above, for shares as well. This is a wonderfully creative solution to improve food availability in a way that preserves natural resources.

Food and Culture

Scholars of culture have defined a culture as a *learned, shared meaning system of symbols, values, norms, and language*. Food fits into most of these categories, underscoring the importance of food and food behaviors in any culture. Certain foods *symbolize* certain things. For example, when you see turkey, stuffing, mashed potatoes, gravy, and pumpkin pie on the table, you know it is Thanksgiving or Christmas. Our foods also express our *values*. For example, those who place a high value on health don't put junk into their bodies, and you're much more likely to find them speaking about the values of vegetarianism or veganism in their local health food stores or farmer's markets than cruising through the fast food drive–thru. The food we eat is also definitely guided by cultural *norms* or regular ways of being. For example, a typical US breakfast might be bacon and eggs, French toast, oatmeal, or cold cereal with milk. However, a typical German breakfast might be bread, butter, sausage, and possibly beer, while a typical Costa Rican breakfast has its own name: *gallo pinto* is mixed beans and rice served with eggs, tortillas, and cheese. Italian dinners consist of the pasta course first, followed by the meat course, and the salad at the end of the meal to cleanse the palate. Salad is followed by cheese perhaps, or fresh fruit. In the US, dinner is followed by a sugary dessert—pie, cake, ice cream, torte.

Our celebrations in the US are marked by sugary desserts. At birthdays, graduation parties, and especially weddings, cake is the most honored guest. It is often elaborately decorated—and rich in refined sugars and saturated fats. It is ceremoniously cut, passed around, and enjoyed together as part of the celebration. Indeed, cake is integral to these celebrations. Zucchini fritters in its place would be a harsh surprise for everyone.

But just because we can't topple the important role of sugary desserts in US culture doesn't mean we have to comply with that expectation either. Animal milk ice cream can easily be replaced by coconut milk ice cream. The desire for sweets can be met with imaginative renditions of sugary fruits such as ripe mangoes, pineapples, berries, and melons. If that's not sweet enough, sweet natural syrups such as maple and cane should do the trick. Particularly for these events, it is important to hunt recipe boards and cookbooks for innovative natural dessert delights that will satisfy both your guests' cultural need for sweetness and your own desire to make a healthy change.

Cultural Influences

As I mentioned a few sections ago, close to 70% (more than two-thirds) of all Americans are overweight and about 35% are now obese.[64] Since obesity—all by itself—poses such a major health hazard, a great many Americans are constantly dieting and otherwise trying to avoid or stop being overweight. But they are drawing the line at what would really help them: becoming inspired and enthusiastic plant-based eaters. The result can even be that when a person is on a fad diet, he or she becomes undernourished. And what people don't realize is that being a healthy vegetarian is NOT a fad or a "diet" in the sense that diets are spoken about in America; it's a lifestyle—a way of eating (and living) in harmony with nature, including the nature of human biology.

When we think of a person not getting enough to eat, we usually think of malnutrition, something found in abundance in the underdeveloped world. However, according to the USDA, in 2013, 14.3% (17.5 million) of US households were food insecure at some time during the year. It also revealed that an astounding 50 million Americans, including almost 9 million children, experienced food insecurity.[65] With the exception of one year since then, it has continued to increase. They are too poor to get enough to eat. This is the new reality in America reflected in a 2013 statistic that reported 45.3 million people in poverty, which is the largest number in the 52 years for which poverty statistics have been published, incidentally up from 37.3 million in 2007.[66] Also it seems that poorer people often have large families in the belief that every new member will be another hand to contribute to the household economy.[67] But nowadays—because of our country's shift away from a family-based agrarian society—a new member in a family is oftentimes an economic hardship, another mouth to feed rather than a helping hand. Agri-business has displaced farmers, taking their land to graze cattle or to raise export crops, and farmers are forced to leave their lands (where new hands were needed) to relocate to overpopulated cities where malnutrition is endemic.

If poverty and displacement breed malnutrition for lack of food, wealth and dieting can lead to undernourishment, fueled by dietary programs that do not carefully weigh the components of the foods they recommend. This is the kind of leanness—lean on nutrition—that we can do without. But it is endemic to the dieting culture, which seems to follow what I call the "boom and bust cycle." One example of this cycle is meat eaters who fatten up on high protein, high cholesterol foods, and then reverse gears and try to slim down with drastic and even health-endangering weight-loss programs. Another example is the group that undertakes unhealthy low-fat diets, where the main staples of the program are chemical-laden, processed foods. These diets are harmful to the human body and cannot be sustained for the long run. Moreover, once these people revert back to "normal" eating, the weight inevitably goes back on and, in many instances, increases.

In fact, to end this section on an extremely tentative positive note, both the health dangers and, to an even greater degree, the vast expenses of meat eating have been getting to the public in small streams. This is registered in the fact that per capita beef consumption dropped from 76.4 pounds in 1980 to 65.4 pounds in 2005, a healthy reduction of just over 14%, with a further reduction to 57.1 in 2012, for a total reduction of about 25% over 32 years.[68] However, total poultry consumption has increased radically in the US from 47.4 in 1980 to 86.4 in 2005. While poultry consumption dropped to 80.8 in 2012, this is still an overall increase of 70%! Even with its hot-air-filled leanness campaign, pork, too, has been taking a hit (just over 20% reduction since 1980), as American consumers turn from it and beef to favor chicken and turkey.

While overall meat consumption has decreased steadily since 2007, the US still ranks among the top in total meat per person consumption. According to one 2009 report, we only rank behind Luxembourg and Hong Kong.[69] In reality, according to one 2012 report, meat consumption in China is now double that in the United States.[70] While the Chinese do have 1.35 billion people to the US's 319 million, I raise this point in support of the data that as countries increase their wealth, meat consumption rises, which ultimately affects all of us. There is no doubt that meatless meals are catching on in the US, but the demand for meat in emerging economies is growing. As an example, Brazilians ate 43% more meat in 2009 than 2 decades earlier, and the Chinese consume 58% more, according to the most recent UN figures.[71]

We can only hope that many American consumers are soon drawn away from poultry and dairy products, and, in search of more economical alternatives, begin dining on leafy green vegetables, root and other vegetables, whole grains, beans, and fruits. It would also be a blessing if we could somehow, through our transition to eating more plant foods and the resulting health effects, assume a greater leadership role in the restoration of sanity to the rest of the world.

Chapter 3

Why Adopt the Vegetarian Diet

> "The medical literature on the causes of food poisoning is full of euphemisms and dry scientific terms: coliform levels, aerobic plate counts, sorbitol, MacConkey agar, and so on. Behind them lies a simple explanation for why eating a hamburger can now make you seriously ill: There is shit in the meat."
>
> — *Eric Schlosser,* Fast Food Nation: The Dark Side of the All-American Meal

One of the first exercises that someone may take on in order to bring healing and balance to the physical body is to detoxify and cleanse the body of accumulated toxins. There are two key principles that are simultaneously at work in health-based detoxification programs and are the reasons for its great success. First, you remove the foods and substances that are the cause of the problem, then you nourish the body with radically healthy foods and substances such as vegetables and fruits–fresh squeezed juices and purified water, for example. Detoxification works quickly because of these two forces working in combination with the body's natural healing tendencies.

We begin this discussion with an overview of additives in meat, poultry, and fish. In effect, in order to heal, you've got to know first what could be causing your body to be out of balance so you are inspired to remove the food substances that are at the heart of a low functioning, low-energy body. As such, I will be speaking a bit about the deleterious substances in the animal products that you may be eating and the diseases you can get from eating meat. I will also speak about bad meat, our culture's unnecessary obsession with protein, and the dangerous fad diets that are high in protein and low in carbs.

The Dangers Lurking in Animal-Based Foods

Additives

Meat Additives

For lack of a better word, the meat sold in this country's grocery stores and restaurants is from animals so "shot up" with hormones, antibiotics, tranquilizers, preservatives, additives, and pesticides that it is almost *more pharmaceutical than nutritional.* These added toxins have been linked to negative long-term effects on health. Here's just one example: the highly toxic organophosphates and brain damage.[1] Human electro encephalograms showed that *a single exposure* could alter the electrical activity of an infant's brain for years and possibly cause abnormal behavior and learning patterns. The study, conducted by Harvard Medical School concluded that "there is a dangerous possibility that organophosphate pesticides have the potential for causing long term brain damage." As a side note, organophosphates also decrease sex drive, impair concentration, and cause memory loss, schizophrenia, depression, irritability and more; plus, the US Environmental Protection Agency has taken steps to limit their availability to the public.[2]

One group—the most egregious in some ways—is colored dyes used to beautify meat. I guess their use is implicit acknowledgment by the industry that they would lose flocks of consumers if they tried to sell their meat in its untouched-up state, as slimy, brownish green, rotting flesh. Like morticians, meat packers artificially treat this organic material to give it the colors of life. Red and violet dyes are added to beef and pork, while yellow dyes are put into chicken feed to enhance the color of the chickens' flesh. Even pet food is cosmetically treated in this manner.

The majority of synthetic colorings used by the food industry are coal-tar derivatives. Some of them, such as the infamous Red Dye No. 2, banned by the

FDA as a carcinogen, have been kept out of our food. Others, even when labeled "US Certified," meaning they meet minimum government standards, have not been sufficiently tested to prove they are safe, and some of these have been correlated with increased incidence of cancer and reproductive damage leading to birth defects, stillbirths, and infertility in animals.

A much more necessary group of chemicals from the meat industry's standpoint, is preservatives such as two petroleum derivatives: butylated hydroxytoluene (BHT) and butylated hydroxyanisole (BRA). They prevent the fat in meat from becoming rancid. You'll find them everywhere –from lard, chicken fat, butter, cream, bacon, sausage, cold cuts, milk, vegetable oils, potato chips, peanut butter, shortening, raisins, breakfast cereals, and chewing gum. Though the industry depends on them to prolong their products' shelf life, they are hardly safe, with their toxicity being associated with skin blisters, fatigue, eye hemorrhaging, and respiratory problems.

I've previously gone into nitrosamines and a few other additives, so let me end this section by more briefly noting three of the more potentially problematic and common of those that remain:

- Artificial flavorings, some which have proven to be carcinogenic
- EDTA, used to prevent the oxidation of fats and oils, in large enough amounts will kill cells
- Monosodium glutamate (MSG): a flavor enhancer that can cause the popularly titled "Chinese restaurant syndrome" (taken from the fact that far too many restaurants overuse this additive), which is characterized by headache, tightness in the chest, prickling skin sensations, impaired concentration, and fatigue; there is also evidence that MSG, in any form, exacerbates cancer,[3] and when manufactured using acid hydrolysis contains cancer-causing substances.[4]

Antibiotics

Overuse of antibiotics (from the Greek word *anti*, meaning against, and *bios*, life) is prevalent in human society. While most of us think of antibiotics as "good" in that they can save our lives from threatening harmful bacteria, we erroneously don't think of them as dangerous to our bodies when, in fact, they are if used in excess.

Those who pay attention to the news will know that the overuse of antibiotics in both animals (cattle, pigs, chickens, etc.) and people has helped to generate new, more resolute strains of bacteria that put up massive and severe resistance to drugs meant to cope with them. Why and how does this happen? Well, first, adaptation is a rule of nature, which, in biology, is the process by which an animal or plant species becomes fitted to its environment.[5] Adaptation is a continuous and ongoing activity, which is why much of science is regularly organizing itself around a new "bug" or "pest" (think pesticides) to fight. This is how drug-resistant bacteria and "superbugs" come into existence in our foods.

Because antibiotics are prevalent in animal-raising today, if you consume these products three times a day, as the typical American does, there is an accumulation of these toxins in your blood stream and tissues over time. A person eating such a contaminated animal may also be consuming the antibiotic-resistant bacteria that developed in the animal, increasing a person's risk for illness.

In one study, grocery store products in Minnesota were tested and showed resistant bacteria in meat samples, especially turkey. In fact, I'm sure that consumers would be devastated to learn that their "food" is infected with *Listeria, E coli, and Salmonella,* three of the most serious contaminants in inexpensive meat products over the past ten years. Not only do these bacteria withstand the antibiotics meant to suppress them, but they often escape lax quality control processes at some of these farms. Thus, the presence of *Salmonella, norovirus, botulism, and E.coli* have been reported in meat products across the country in such trusted brands as Safeway, McDonalds, Walmart, and Arby's. As a side note, sadly, children and the elderly—many of whom have struggles with nutritional deficiencies, unhealthy living environments, and heavy dosages of medications, including vaccines—are especially susceptible to these bacteria-infected meats.

Let's take a look at what could happen when you become ill. Typically, you would take an antibiotic, which means you are bombarding your system directly while adding to the antibiotics already accumulated in your tissues. At the same time, you are weakening your body's ability to fight-off other pathogens that require increasingly more powerful antibiotics to handle. In time, through ongoing assault, the body's system fails—it could be a heart attack, a stroke, cancer, or bacterial infection or virus that cannot be contained, any of which can lead to rapid death.

Take the case where a person, let's say it is a man who is a heavy meat and dairy eater, is prescribed antibiotics for an illness. He may find he is suffering antibiotic overload, due to the combination of the prescription he received from the doctor and the ingested antibiotics he receives from the foods he consumes. Too many antibiotics in the system end up indiscriminately eliminating friendly bacteria, such as those necessary for proper digestion, and ultimately health. Will the body of this antibiotic-surfeited man now serve as a harem for the creation of new strains of drug-resistant germs just as, we noted earlier, factory farmed animals are?

A report in the *New England Journal of Medicine* linked 18 cases of food poisoning, which claimed one life and hospitalized 11 people, to hamburger meat riddled with a *drug-resistant* form of Salmonella. The contaminated beef was traced to a cattle farm in South Dakota where the livestock were consuming grain that had been over treated with the antibiotic tetracycline.

Let's continue with our example of the meat and dairy-eating man. Suppose he were taking penicillin for a throat infection, and that he also had in his system the drug-resistant Salmonella, which, as the *New England Journal of Medicine* article indicates, is present in our food. The penicillin he takes will wipe out the bacteria causing the sore throat while the antibiotic-resistant Salmonella bacteria will multiply, and rapidly. Holmberg of the Centers for Disease Control, whose thoughts on Salmonella were noted before, estimated that in 1984 alone, 1,500 humans died from exactly this toxic effect. Further studies on food-borne diseases have shown that human death is more common in food-poisoning cases involving consumption of these resistant strains of bacteria.[6]

So believe me when I tell you that the price of utilizing these antibiotics in animals to the extent that they are today in the US is extremely high—and I'm not just referring to the cost of the drugs alone, which exceeds $300 million dollars annually in the US; globally, antibiotics given to livestock and poultry account for $800 million in annual sales, increasing each year.

Let's just glance at a few more figures to round out this picture. Since these drugs were first introduced into animal feed in 1949, the annual use of antibiotics has grown from 490,000 pounds in 1954, to 1.2 million in 1960, to approximately 16 million in the 1980s, to over 30 million pounds today.[7] This is in stark contrast to the 6 million pounds of antibiotics used annually on men, women, and children combined in the US. Currently, over half of our nation's annual antibiotic production goes into livestock and poultry.

Is there a problem with this vast tonnage of antibiotics used in food animals? You bet there is. Maybe this is why the FDA is being sued over their refusal to release data on antibiotic use in animals. The alarms have been sounded because the saturation of our food supply and human population with antibiotics is the primary cause for the staggering explosion in cases of methicillin-resistant staphylococcus Aureus (MRSA) infection. MRSA is blamed for more than 94,000 infections and 18,000 deaths each year in the US.[8]

As the numbers suggest, the hard-nosed business people that run these factory farms do not administer antibiotics to their livestock lightly, or in a careful and controlled manner. They have become beholden to these drugs for the survival of their businesses. The antibiotics are given as a regular course to stave off the disease that would otherwise be rampant in the close, unsanitary, injurious conditions in which meat and dairy animals are forced to live. If they did not dose these animals with a bumper load of pharmaceuticals, these owners would have far fewer "healthy" animals for slaughter. In the case of young cattle, however, there is a second reason for the dosing. Some animals are deprived of iron and rendered anemic in order to yield the white, pale meat preferred by those who prepare and eat veal. Being sickly, the calves are prey to all sorts of infection, which the antibiotics help to stave off.

I don't mean to imply that every single animal gets the antibiotic treatment, but estimates suggest that 70-80% of the antibiotics used in the US go to farm animals and fully three-fifths to four-fifths of American animals receive antibiotics. That's 4 out of 5, or 80%, of all animals, resulting in extremely high odds that most Americans are consuming antibiotics through their food multiple times daily. (By the way, this percentage is much higher than that found in Europe where control on drug use in animals is tighter.)

In addition to being using prophylactically, antibiotic drugs are also supplied when an animal comes down with a specific disease, such as, leprospirosis, parvovirus, erysipelas, *E.coli infection*, atropic rhinitis, gastroenteritis, *C. perfringens,* and pseudorabies.

As we've discussed previously, this over-reliance on antibiotics is helping birth a new generation of pathogens that can withstand the power of our strongest drugs. It is remarkable and frightening that not only can some of these hardier bacterial strains resist a drug to which they have been exposed, they can also ward off the effects of a similar drug. Thus an animal's pathogen may simultaneously have a wide and dangerous immunity to many drugs on the market.

One of the more notorious of the new resistant agents is *Enterococci*. In one study, a high percentage of *Enterococci* bacteria found in food products, including meat, dairy and poultry, were resistant to such common antibacterials as tetracycline (over 30% of the strains were resistant), erythromycin (over 20% resistant), and streptomycin (over 10% resistant). Even more shocking, a small 0.7%, were resistant to ciproflaxin, one of the strongest antibiotics on the market. Of course, at this point that percentage is very low, but it is quite possible that in a host such a strain will live on, gathering strength until even the strongest antibiotics cannot weaken it.

Things are getting so bad with the growth of antibiotic-resistant pathogens that the World Health Organization has issued a warning directive claiming that infectious diseases will soon outstrip our ability to contain them with any existing medicines. Antibiotic resistance is one big contributor to this trend, and feeding antibiotics to farm animals, which then gets into meat-eaters' diets, plays no small part in this tendency toward developing super-resistant pathogens.

Let's quickly note some other grim results of the overuse of drugs—antibiotic and otherwise—in animals. For one, many additives given to animals are not tested for their safety to people, since it is (I believe, erroneously) assumed that *if* the administration of the antibiotics is discontinued well before the animal is slaughtered, *then* traces of it will not remain in the meat. Take the hormone Carbadox, used to enlarge market-bound pigs, and removed from their diet a month or so before the animals are killed; or the drug Paylean, which is given to pigs to shift their biochemistry from fat production to meat production. Neither has been evaluated for its effect on humans, which is beneficial, of course, for enterprising drug companies and the governmental regularity bodies they control through "contributions" of sorts, but it is completely deleterious for consumers.

Antibiotics also have the effect of helping animals add weight. Moreover, additional additives, including colorings and preservatives of sorts are added to the meat during processing. So people who are allergic to antibiotics like penicillin or sensitive to food dyes and any other chemical enhancements may unknowingly aggravate their allergies by eating meat with traces of such drugs.

Most shocking of all considerations, if these antibiotics and other drugs don't reach meat eaters through land-animal flesh, they may unknowingly be getting them from the sea. Industrial runoff and dumping are allowing drugs to drain into the oceans, and, due to this, catches of sea life are more toxic than ever before. So fish and other seafood may be contributing to the current antibiotic resistance we are experiencing since they can be contacting traces of antibiotics in the water that they breathe.

Unfortunately, the meat and dairy industries are not required to inform consumers which products have been treated with antibiotics and other pharmaceuticals, and which have not.[9] (For that matter, they don't even have to inform us if the meat comes from factory manufactured cloning.)

The first question you might ask about all this is: why is it that the government agencies that are charged with protecting our health don't do something about this?

Believe it or not, they actually have tried. In 1977, the FDA tried to ban antibiotics in the animal industry, but their efforts were shot down by the successful lobbying of the powerful livestock and drug companies, such as the largest manufacturer of livestock antibiotics, American Cyanamid.[10] It's a sorry story of the government lying down to wealthy, free-spending companies, who used the same argument then as they do now, which is—as the pro-industry American Farm Bureau Federation puts it—curtailing the widespread use of antibiotics will cause a jump in the cost of meat. And we know they are not figuring in the gigantic tally of health bills run up by those suffering unnecessarily from *additional* illnesses attributable to the widespread use of these chemicals. Of course they are not, because it is not in their interest to do so; and I've spoken for decades in my books and on my radio program about our nation's investment in sickness and illness as being a core reason for the lack of real and durable change.

In any case, slow to change as it is, the meat industry has made innovations in relation to antibiotics. Don't get your hopes up. They are not thinking of eliminating them; they are simply trying out less commonly used antibiotics as way to possibly curtail the human health hazards of the more popular ones. One new candidate is barnbermycin, recently adopted and widely used in chicken feed. The National Broiler Council says this item poses no health risk. By the way, this is the typical response you get from industry advocates who know little about human health and how the body works. However, when they are introduced, no one knows with certainty the short or long-term health risks of these drugs. A biochemist at the National Resources Defense Council believes "all antibiotics [even the newer ones] can cause resistance to occur eventually."[11] And one of the newer ones, chloramphenicol, even in low doses has already been shown to induce aplastic anemia in humans, a deadly disease that prevents the production of red blood cells in the bone marrow.[12]

You can see how the meat industry could actually boast: *You no longer need to go to the doctor when you have an infection. Just take a bite of one of our products and you'll get a full spectrum of antibiotics.*

Hormones

No discussion of meat safety would be complete without mentioning that the FDA allowed DES (diethystilbestrol), a synthetic hormone in meat. It was used to rapidly increase the size and weight of cattle. On average, a calf weighs about 80 pounds and needs to grow to anywhere from 700-1,200 pounds for sale in just 14-16 months! According to John Robbins, author of *The Food Revolution*, "That kind of unnaturally fast weight gain takes enormous quantities of corn, soy-based protein supplements, antibiotics, and other drugs, including growth hormones."[13] In contrast, according to Homestead Organics, it takes 2-4 years for natural grass-fed cattle to go to market.[14] As an important side note, shifting a cow from its natural diet of grasses and hay to corn and soy can be fatal if it's not done gradually and with a constant supply of antibiotics. Okay, back to hormones. You may recall that it was not long ago that the FDA allowed DES to be prescribed to women to reduce the risk of miscarriage and premature births. There was a 40 fold increase in rare vaginal tumors in women and girls that were exposed to this drug in utero. There was also a significant rise in breast cancer in women exposed to this drug. The FDA banned the use of DES in women in 1971, but it was permitted to remain in cattle feed until 1980. However, today, they still allow the use of synthetic steroid hormones in cattle like estrogen, progesterone, and testosterone to name a few. We now know after many human trials that these very same hormones, which are prescribed to millions of women for the treatment of their menopausal symptoms, have been proven to increase the risk of certain cancers, cardiovascular disease, and dementia. And to think that the FDA is the anointed watchdog for both food and drugs in the United States is mind boggling; it strains credulity to say the least.

Hormones are one of the main additives used in the US for regulating breeding, and to tranquilize and promote weight gain. The downside for us, if not for the meat sellers, is that synthetic hormones can cause cancer in the recipient animals. This is not a down side for the business side of animal agriculture since it usually doesn't affect the marketability of the meat.

But what we know at this time is that estrogen, one of the hormones commonly fed to these animals, may increase women's chances of contracting uterine and breast cancer, and may cause children to enter puberty prematurely. Add Raigro to this list, an estrogen-like compound; Synovex, a naturally occurring hormone, which has been seen as affecting weight gain; Lutalyse, a prostaglandin (often given to an entire herd so that they will all ovulate at the same time), which may disrupt women's menstrual cycles and cause pregnant women to miscarry; and, finally, the hormone androgen, which may cause liver cancer.

DDT and Other Additives

By cooking meat, a chef creates chemicals (HCAs) that are health hazards. This could be avoided by, for instance, eating beef raw, as is done in some cultures. But it is a terrible and potentially deadly idea due to worms, parasites, and life-threatening bacteria. Furthermore, there is nothing that can be done (short of abstention from eating meat) to guard against the chemicals that are put into it, such as food coloring, antibiotics, and hormones as well as add-ins that are introduced into livestock at the breeding phase. Throughout their existence, livestock and dairy cows are fed large amounts of chemically treated feed. To judge whether a particular meat has traces of these additives would be difficult, not only because meat is difficult to analyze, but because the government offers little help, allowing the use of over 500 chemical additives while very lightly monitoring how these chemicals are administered.

As an example of the noxious chemicals that contaminate meat, let's look at DDT. This pesticide is so dangerous it was banned in 1972, following on the heels of Rachel Carson's *Silent Spring*, which brought to public notice the cancer-causing properties and other dangers associated with this pesticide. The chemical became popular in the '40s, and was used extensively for nearly three decades. Many people don't know that the DDT that got into plants came not through what had been sprayed on them to kill bugs but through the soil. After plants were dosed with it every year for decades, our soil became saturated with DDT. That means that even when farmers stopped spraying the plants, its presence would remain, and for up to 2 to 15 years.[15] Next step, livestock eat the crops and concentrate the chemical; then we eat the livestock, DDT and all. DDT is extremely persistent and can still be present in crops and soil in the US today, largely through our atmosphere: other parts of the world still use DDT in agricultural practices and in disease-control programs, so the deadly toxin makes its way here via wind patterns.[16] This is also something to be mindful of when purchasing non-organic products outside of the US.

I'm not talking about super-miniscule amounts either. Livestock consume roughly 16 pounds of food to produce one pound of flesh. And because DDT gets stored whole in body fat, a pound of beefsteak, say, may contain significant quantities of DDT residues. The DDT we then ingest in our burgers is stored in our body fat, where it sits idle until we diet or come under stress. When we begin to burn fat, the stored DDT is catapulted into the bloodstream. It can even be passed on to babies through mother's milk. While every hazard to the health brought on by DDT has not been assessed, we do know that DDT plays a part in causing anorexia, tremors, and fever.

As we see, DDT is a substance that inadvertently gets into animals through the food chain, but many other unfriendly chemicals are purposely given to livestock. The food additive sodium nitrate, used as a color fixative in most processed meats, including hot dogs, bologna, cured meats, bacon, meat spreads, sausage, and ham, is terribly detrimental to health. When ingested, nitrates form potentially cancer-causing substances called nitrosamines. While vitamin C has been found to block the formation of some nitrosamines, and some bacon producers have added vitamin C to their products to make them less of a cancer threat, about two-thirds of C's power is lost during cooking.

Because the cattle pens are not only filled with germs but insects, the animals are commonly and frequently sprayed with pesticides such as Vapona, which is in the same family as nerve gas. This is the chemical used on "No Pest Strips," ones so toxic that the World Health Organization set the daily allowable limit at .004 milligram per kilogram. You could exceed this limit by merely staying indoors with one of these strips for nine hours.[17] But that's another story. The danger is that somehow these pesticides will get into our meat.

And meat is not the only animal product that shows the effect of these pharmaceuticals. The chemicals fed to and sprayed on milk cows pass into their milk while those given to chickens appear in their eggs. So, with any animal product you eat, you can't help getting *a side order of drugs.*

Tranquilizers and Other Miscellaneous Additives

Other apparently innocuous meat additives like tranquilizers have also been shown to be responsible for many ailments. Tranquilizers have been added to livestock feed for the last 30 years, but this is not to help animals calm down in their harsh living conditions. The reason, rather, is that tranquilizers slow down an animal's metabolism so that it plumps up more quickly.

It's dangerous to think you can escape these additives by eating eggs. Hens are often fed a combination of antibiotics, sodium bicarbonate, and terephthalic acid, a "three-niter mash," which assures a hard eggshell. Yolks are also manipulated through chicken-feed additives to correct any pigmentation abnormalities. Many of these chemicals are toxic, so when you buy, for instance, "jumbo" eggs, they should realize the adjective does not only apply to the size but to the jumbo dose of additives found in the food.

Rather than go further down the list of health-weakening additives that go into animal products, it will be enough here to simply underline the idea that the effects of the toxins in animal products are not quickly evident. One doesn't eat a slab of bacon and get sick the next day. The toxins work slowly but insidiously as Rudolph Ballentine, M.D. explains. He writes that illness begins with toxicity at the cellular level. Cellular toxicity and death progresses from the organelle stage, to the cell stage, to the organ stage. "When a great enough number of the cells that constitute an organ die, then the organ becomes diseased."[18]

Pesticides… and the Link to Our Water Supply

Previously in this book, I examined the way DDT, a long-banned pesticide substance, is still finding its way into meats and milk through our soil and air and the foods raised to feed cattle. Pesticides are no small health problem either. It is estimated that over 100,000 people in the United States are subjected to pesticide poisoning annually—and not only farmers and farm workers, but a countless number of other individuals who unknowingly ingest pesticides in their daily diet. After DDT, among the most common pesticides contaminating meat are cadmium, carbon tetrachloride, and hexachlorobenzene.

So how many of these pesticides are we getting and where are they coming from?

For the average American's intake, the total is approximately 40 mg of pesticide residue every year. Of this, about 4 mg are stored in fat tissue and can lead to toxicity symptoms such as headaches, fatigue, muscle aches, and fever. The meat advocate might object here, since even vegetarians may be getting these deadly residues through plant foods. Consider, however, that when a cow consumes soybeans containing pesticide traces, much of the poison permanently settles in the animal's fat tissue. The person who comes after and devours a T-bone from this cow is getting *concentrated* amounts of toxic residues. By contrast, if the pesticide-treated soybeans were eaten directly, the toxins would be much less concentrated.

As to where these pesticides in our foods are coming from, a government report estimates that one-sixth of all meat and poultry eaten in the US contains "potentially harmful residues of animal drugs, *pesticides* or environmental contaminants." The report goes on to note that of the nearly 150 known drugs and pesticides found in meat and poultry products, "42 (nearly $1/3^{rd}$) are known to cause or are suspected of causing cancer, 20 of causing birth defects, 6 of causing mutations, 6 of causing adverse effects on the fetus, and others of causing similar toxic effects."

I might highlight in the roster of pesticide infamy, a particularly toxic one, Monsanto's Roundup® weed killer, which is commonly used by farmers in the production of grains or grasses like alfalfa, a common food staple for meat cattle and dairy cows. "The active ingredient in Roundup®, glyphosate, is linked to non-Hodgkin's lymphoma—a cancer—and the inhibition of steroidogenesis—the obstruction of steroid creation in the body," according to the research of Paul Goettlich.[19] So it's both a carcinogen and an endocrine disruptor.

To move for a moment off our current focus on how full our food and drink supply is with these pesticides, let me also emphasize that these poisons pollute the water supply through runoffs into lakes, streams, and rivers. This enormous leakage infiltrates "63% of rural America, [home to] some 39 million people, who are drinking water that may be unsafe," according to *The New Farm* magazine. This same water is given to the animals being readied for slaughter and consumption.

Moreover, further studies reveal that the beleaguered, pesticide-tainted, water-drinking population is spread across our country. Three-quarters of rural Western populations are quaffing this excessively contaminated beverage; 65% in the Southern and North-Central states; and 45% in the Northeast. To make matters worse, along with these pesticides are several other health-destabilizing substances such as the following:

- Lindane: a noxious insecticide that affects the central nervous system
- Mercury: known to cause kidney and neurological damage
- Cadmium: a toxic metal associated with high blood pressure and kidney damage

- Lead: known to damage the nervous system and kidneys
- Nitrates: the chemical precursor of cancer-causing nitrosamines

Any and all of these substances can and are likely to be in your water supply. For now, let's return to our main topic of meat and dairy's inclusion of pesticide traces; let me not forget to mention milk. A few sections ago I indicted it for being tainted with hormones, pus, and antibiotics. Now let me add that it is often high in pesticide residues, and so may be associated with higher breast cancer risk.

I suppose after perusing the last few sections, you might join me in suggesting to the meat and dairy industries that they create a replacement food pyramid, upon which they highlight the "features" of the products they are selling. Instead of such categories as meats and dairy, they would have to add pesticides, dyes, antibiotics, and preservatives, too!

"Natural" Toxins

But let's ignore the possibility of bacteria getting in the meat and think of other contaminants.

Animals, like humans, continuously eliminate waste products from their tissues and cells to the surrounding blood. This natural process comes to an abrupt halt when the animal is slaughtered; the waste material then present remains intact, and we ingest it when eating its flesh. You might say that our bodies' various organs of elimination—lungs, bladder, kidneys, sweat glands, and liver—should be adept at disposing of such wastes, but do you really want to add to their workload, which is already consumed with ridding our bodies of worn-out cells and the by-products of digestion? Asking them to take on the additional task of dealing with the animal wastes is hazardous at best. Our organs may well respond, if overloaded, by developing any of several degenerative diseases.[20]

I talked earlier about the dangers of meat staying for too long in the digestive tract; it begins to putrefy, which can cause noxious gas, headache and lethargy, among other symptoms. However, I neglected to mention that meat can also putrefy outside before we even consume it. Unlike fruits and vegetables, meat starts to degrade the moment the animal dies, and continues to degenerate during processing, packaging, and transportation to the market or butcher. After slaughter, a steer is sectioned and moved into cold storage. Some cuts may then be aged for a time to increase tenderness. The meat may be stored in a warehouse before finally being sent to a butcher or supermarket for packaging. Of course when it is refrigerated degeneration is slowed, but for parts of its processing time it is not kept cool.

It is important to note that for any of the time that the meat was left out of refrigeration, the bacteria were proliferating like mad. Each gram of sausage stored at room temperature for 20 hours has its live bacteria count increase by 70 million, each gram of beef by 650 million, and each gram of smoked ham by a whopping 700 million.[21] While no one would, except by accident, let meat sit out for such a long time, you really can't be sure how the meat was handled before you bought it.

If you are a meat consumer, you are unlikely to leave meat sitting out for extended periods but you may well reheat the food one or more times. The Michigan State University Department of Human Ecology came out with a warning against the practice, noting that reheated food could contain the toxins of bacteria previously in the food, and it warns that though the bacteria may have been killed by the original cooking, the toxins might still be present.[22]

And even worse, some bacteria form spores that are not killed by cooking. Then, once the leftovers are set aside, the spores germinate and grow. The new bacteria may be strong enough to survive a second heating. Moreover, even if new bacteria do not grow, the toxins they release may stay around to inflict damage. Dr. Al B. Wagner, Jr., of the Texas Agricultural Extension Service backs this notion by saying of certain bacteria, that "although cooking destroys the bacteria, the toxin produced is heat stable and may not be destroyed."[23] A February 2008 article in *Science Daily News* details the debilitating effects of bacterial toxins that may be left in meats after the bacteria are killed. They can shut down the body's immune response by affecting a cell mechanism essential to attacking threats such as viruses and bacteria.[24] In other words, they are what in military terms used to be called "sappers," soldiers who undermined the walls of the fortress so the enemy (bacteria) would find it easy to invade when they came on the scene.

I'm not saying, by the way, that the toxins in reheated meat wouldn't also be in the meat (if it contained bacteria) the first time around—that is, when it is first cooked. They certainly would be. In any case, this whole issue of remaining toxins is not one that seems to have been learned by agribusiness directors, who think nothing of taking *bacterially contaminated* meat and cooking it in order to "purify" it, as has been the practice of companies looking to cut their losses from sick slaughterhouse cattle.[25] A 2002 Knight Ridder Tribune News Service article describes how ConAgra Foods was planning to recycle beef contaminated with *E. coli* into cooked canned foods for either human consumption—such as chili, beef ravioli or meat spaghetti sauce—or for pet consumption. The article reports:

> Consumers might buy a meal containing recalled meat [and this is perfectly] legal—and wholesome—according to the US Department of Agriculture. The federal agency must OK the company's plans for recalled meat. [But this is hardly unusual in that,] cooking recalled meat is common practice in the food industry. "I think we can say any product that is cooked per the guidelines established by the USDA and recommended by the Colorado Department of Health is perfectly safe for human consumption and to indicate otherwise is irresponsible," ConAgra spokesman Jim Herlihy said.[26]

Even though the USDA seems to find this procedure safe when done by meat companies, on the USDA's *own* website, they take time to warn consumers, not meatpackers, that "if raw products are left out at warmer temperatures, pathogens can produce a heat-stable toxin that might not be destroyed by cooking."[27]

Given what to most will seem like a reckless procedure in terms of meat safety—all to save a few bucks—by selling meat that is known to be contaminated, you can now see why I have little confidence in the meat industry. After mulling over these latest findings, I have even less. Would you knowingly eat meat, or any food for that matter, that was recalled for containing *E.coli* or other harmful bacteria? Of course not. But big food companies have decided that it's okay for you, and they've got the FDA's blessing.

More than the dangers that face us through ingestion of these animal products is an even greater danger—*our inaction* toward a healthier vegetarian lifestyle that does *not* include a diet of animal products. How is it that we can stand by—when we know the suffering of these innocent, sentient creatures—and allow this insanity to continue? Have we lost all connection to our humanity and our sensibilities? It appears so, as many can still seemingly justify this means to an end. Yes, there are very practical health reasons for putting an end to factory farming as we know it today, but there are even more compelling reasons for putting an end to the human behavior that is causing suffering—not just in these animals—but to ourselves. In truth, we cannot be truly healthy when we are actively engaged and participating in the suffering of others—be it animals or humans.

Dairy Additives

At this point in history, however, the presence of natural hormones in cow's milk and their effect on us seems almost minor compared to the dangers now associated with the product due to the industrialization of animal-raising today. I've already highlighted the main issues in speaking about meat production—the over-crowding, disease-causing conditions of factory farms, and the onslaught of drugs, especially antibiotics, to which these animals are subject—all to forestall diseases that are created by the system itself.

Now we must turn quickly to another pollutant of milk and dairy products that accompanies the raising of livestock industrially: the additives given to animals to kill disease that also hasten their growth, and add "value," say these business persons. I want to get right to this because, so far, I have not handled the most controversial of all the drugs given to cattle, recombinant bovine growth hormone (rBGH), which is routinely injected in dairy cattle to increase milk production.

For years, Monsanto—perhaps the world's wealthiest and largest agro-developer and food industry lobbyist—had been marketing rBGH under the trade name Posilac, and it created a global monopoly on the manufacture and sale of this dairy additive. The company was earning $270 million every year on this single product.[28] With such a "cash cow" on its hands, Monsanto lobbied aggressively with the FDA and the National Dairy Council to sustain its freedom to sell Posilac to dairy farmers. Why it had to make this argument will be explained more fully in a moment, but suffice it to say that many were voicing health concerns about the use of the hormone. There became such an outcry that, in 1999, the United Nations Food Safety Agency, representing 101 nations, ruled unanimously on a moratorium against Monsanto's genetically engineered hormonal milk.[29] Nevertheless, the United States, which of late has been frequently standing alone in international discussions—for example, in refusing to sign the Kyoto Protocols, an agreement to address global warming through reduced greenhouse gas emissions, signed by 187 nations—didn't adopt the ban, and rBGH remains a standard fare in the raising of dairy cows.

If the shortsighted politicians in our country ignored health concerns, Monsanto itself seemed to get the message and ducked the controversy that was building by selling its rights to the product. In August 2008, the company divested its stakes in the controversial growth hormone, which was later purchased by Eli Lilly's agriculture division, Elanco. That, though, has not stopped the hormone from flowing into cows and then their milk. The only difference now is it comes through a new spigot. As of today, you can only drink milk certified as organic with any degree of confidence that it's free from rBGH.

Why is there such alarm over rBGH's use? For one, before we get to the possible health effects, it is possible that the hormone is addictive. Some evidence of this appears in the stockyards where "in some cases [there is seen] an inability to successfully wean treated cows off the drug BGH."[30] While so far there is no research into whether humans can become "hooked" on this milk additive, it is certainly not encouraging that certain hormones, such as estrogen, have addictive properties for humans. One more thoroughly investigated health concern is that a comparison between milk of cows with or without the hormone has shown that rBGH leaves more bacteria in final milk products. It also aides in preserving traces of antibiotics if any were used to treat infections that appeared following injection of the hormone.

But that's not the main fear over the hormone's health threats. The primary reason for the United Nation's decision against Posilac use is that it has been linked to colon, breast, and prostate cancers. One agent that may well take part in the development of cancer and other diseases is IGF-1, a biomolecule associated with severe inflammatory illnesses, which is found in milk from rBGH treated cows. IGF-1 levels can be as much as ten times higher in this milk than in untreated milk. Also, it appears that the IGF-1 in treated milk is more potent, because it binds more strenuously to human proteins than that in milk of cows who didn't receive the hormone."[31] There is evidence that this IGF-1 molecule, and hence the rBGH that carries it, plays a major role in diabetic complications and during the early stages of diabetic nephropathy—kidney damage resulting from high protein in the urine.[32]

Samuel Epstein, M.D., author of *What's in Your Milk*, has done extensive research on how the health threats of rBGH occur. He writes that traces of rBGH "are absorbed through the gut… supercharged with high levels of… IGF-1, which is [also] readily absorbed through the gut," where "excess levels of IGF-I have been incriminated as a cause of… colon cancer." The molecule weakens the body's defenses since "IGF-1 blocks natural defense mechanisms against early submicroscopic cancers." And not only does IGF-1 appear to allow for the emergence of colon cancer from its stronghold in the gut, Epstein warns that IGF-1 can also cause breast and prostate cancers.[33]

When a cow is administered rBGH, it is followed by administration of a sulfur-based drug to prevent infection due to injection of the growth hormone. I mentioned above that traces of these antibiotics are found in the milk, and these sulfur drugs may be cancer causing.

On top of that, as mentioned previously in relation to antibiotic administration to animals in general, it tends to make bacteria drug resistant, and these bacteria often make their way into the milk. Moreover, in fighting the bacteria, which either came into the cow in connection with the hormone injection or in relation to the unhealthy conditions of the animal's living quarters, pus forms in the cow as its body fights against the pathogenic intruders. This is par for the course and accepted by the FDA, *which labels pus in milk as an accepted "additive."* After all, the FDA reasons, it is a natural by-product. With this in mind, the FDA permits 750 million pus cells to be present in every liter of milk.[34] And if you think that's overly generous, consider this: Since the ratio of milk to cheese is 10:1, a pound of cheese can (while meeting FDA "health" stipulations) contain 7.5 billion pus cells!

I mentioned how many antibiotics go into cattle but haven't noted in particular how this affects our milk. As the Toronto Vegetarian Association notes, "Antibiotics, mostly penicillin, are given to cows for treatment of mastitis [an inflammation of the mammary gland]. Cows are not supposed to be milked for 48 hours after receiving penicillin. When this precaution is not followed [which is not an uncommon occurrence], the penicillin appears in the milk."[35] We know by now that antibiotics, which in other writings I have noted are overprescribed for humans, also seem to be given too freely to animals. "Fifteen million pounds of antibiotics are used in animal production every year which end up in dairy products and meat."[36] What I'm stressing here is that these drugs end up in the dairy products you may be consuming. "Consumers Union and the *Wall Street Journal* tested milk samples in the New York metropolitan area and found the presence of 52 different antibiotics. Eat ice cream, yogurt, and cheese toppings, and you're also consuming antibiotics."[37]

Fish Additives

It may seem that while there may be negative health consequences to eating fish, at least a portion of these animals are not suffering the intolerable living conditions that land beasts raised for meat are forced to endure. But consider this: fish live in oceans and lakes that are so polluted that no person in their right mind would dare drink from them.

Because fish are floating in seas of pollutants, every time we eat them, we are ingesting, along with their meat, noxious chemicals, heavy metals, and disease-bearing organisms.[38] That's a fact that has been noted by leading physicians, such as Neal Barnard, M.D., Director of the Physicians Committee for Responsible Medicine (PCRM), who has explained, "As a result of human pollution of aquatic environments, eating fish flesh has become a major health hazard."[39]

In more striking terms, as Richard Schwartz points out in his article, "Troubled Waters," the fish we eat today are little more than "a mixture of fat and protein, seasoned with toxic chemicals."[40] And, they are "seasoned" with other unwanted additives as well. During the course of a six-month investigation, the Consumers Union brought this out when it found that nearly half of all fish tested from markets in New York City, Chicago, and Santa Cruz were contaminated by bacteria from human or nonhuman feces, pathogenic worms, and parasites.[41]

I've said that fish oils contain the valuable omega-3 fatty acids and other important nutrients, but looking at the way fish pick up so many toxins from our polluted waters causes me to ask: what if the widespread, deep contamination of fish neutralizes the positive effects that eating them might otherwise have?

A number of health watch groups are coming to the conclusion that now the risks of fish consumption outweigh the practice's upsides. For one, The National Academy of Science's Institute of Medicine presented a report on October 17, 2006, which reviewed "the scientific evidence on seafood's benefits and risks, [being led to this step] because seafood is the major source of human exposure to methylmercury,"[42] a potent neurotoxin known to cause cognitive impairment, memory loss, and coordination difficulties. The report's conclusions were not ones the seafood industry is likely to boast about. An examination of the study noted, "Evidence suggesting that people who have suffered heart attacks can reduce their risk of future heart attacks by eating seafood is weaker than previously thought, the committee concluded. It is also not clear whether consuming seafood might reduce people's risks for diabetes, cancer, Alzheimer's disease, or other ailments."[43]

Such hesitant words from a respected scientific group, which argue that the evidence for the health claims of fish eating is inconclusive at best, do not go over well with the often outlandish claims of fish-eating promoters. Dr. Hope Ferdowsian and PCRM nutritionist Susan Levin have written about these inflated ideas in scathing terms, saying, "It's a whopper of a fish story. And, unfortunately, some consumers are swallowing it—hook, line, and sinker." This is to say, to continue with a metaphorical way of expressing things, the fishing industry has caught the public in what amounts to a net of propaganda. "For years," Ferdowsian and Levin say, "The fishing industry has worked overtime to persuade Americans to ignore well-founded concerns about mercury and other pollutants in fish."[44]

In many tuna fish, for example, which is a favorite American food, there are traces of methylmercury. Vas Aposhian, a toxicologist and professor of molecular and cell biology and pharmacology at the University of Arizona, who served as a key "scientific" advisor on mercury issues to the FDA and EPA, reported (as noted in Lanou and Sullivan) that mercury levels in albacore tuna are so high [all] consumers should avoid the fish completely. "[Even] eating small amounts of some fish may be unsafe."[45]

And unlike the agribusiness-sponsored scientists whose research always seems to discover good things about meat and dairy consumption, which says little about these scientists' integrity, Aposhian stands by his guns. He resigned his advisory position in protest when the FDA and the EPA issued "a national health advisory warning that children and women of childbearing age should limit mercury intake by eating no more than six ounces [one can] of albacore tuna a week,"[46] a warning that Dr. Aposhian criticized as "dangerously lax." As he saw it, the food industry had exerted influence to weaken the agencies' mercury warnings.

Having just mentioned tuna, let me turn to another of America's favorite (and riskiest) fish, salmon. Salmon's popularity has grown rapidly in recent years, mainly for being high in omega fatty acids. Currently, though, it should also be gaining not fame, but notoriety for being one of the most polluted fish in the sea. This is due to the high burden of PCB contamination, which is infiltrating the animals via the PCB-containing agricultural runoff, human and livestock sewage, and industrial wastes.[47] PCBs, known carcinogens, are used as coolants, in waterproofing compounds, in paints, and for many other industrial purposes. They are now all-pervasive in factory and factory farm environments.

I talked of fish ingesting the poisons from polluted seas and other free waters, but those are not the only place from which we draw fish. Many are raised in fish farms, living their lives in tanks or other enclosed areas, which poses the same issues of feedlots, which I will discuss in a few minutes. In fact the majority of fish sold in restaurants today come from unhealthy fish farms. This is not only done for the industry's convenience and financial gain, but because wild fish stocks are being greatly depleted, down as much as 50% in some species. At the current rate of wild-catch exploitation, the United Nations Food and Agriculture Organization (FAO) estimates that the world's fish supply will be completely depleted by 2048.[48] Fish in the depleted category are so few it is no longer feasible to try and catch them.

Adding to the problem of depletion is that much of the fresh fish caught in the world today are fed as fishmeal to pigs, chickens, and farm-raised animals—some 37%,[49] actually. The fishmeal fed to livestock is usually produced from small forage fish, including anchovies and sardines, which are near the bottom of the ocean food chain and are a food source for larger fish, ocean mammals, and seabirds. Thus, the excessive removal of these small fish from the ocean are hurting the species that feed on them. There are other concerns, of course: I spoke earlier about food inefficiency; these small fish could easily be consumed directly by humans as a source of nutrition, rather than shipped to manufacturing facilities and then to farms to feed livestock. This is especially true for areas of the world where people rely on fish for survival. Further, when you are consuming land animals, you are also now consuming the accumulated toxins from the fish stores.

Indeed, this is another example of the insanity of raising animals for food. A full 90% of the forage fish caught each year—some 31.5 million tons[50]—are dried and ground into fishmeal. To put this amount into perspective, pigs and poultry worldwide consume more than six times the amount of seafood consumed by the (human) US market.

There are obvious concerns about fish stocks collapsing, and alternative livestock feed would be an enormous help for struggling fish populations. "Plus," states Daniel Pauly, co-author of the study Forage Fish: From Ecosystems to Markets, "it is not what pigs or chickens naturally eat. When is the last time you saw a chicken fishing?"

The problem is worse than we suspect. In 2013, the Scientific Journal *Nature* reported that only 10% of all large fish—both open ocean species including tuna, swordfish, marlin as well as the large groundfish such as cod, halibut, skates and flounder—were left in the sea.[51] You've got to wonder about the implications of such a large depletion. One thing is for sure, fewer of today's children will have the opportunity to experience fish as we boomers have—in their natural environments, abundant, lively, and healthy.

Because the future of ocean fish is so bleak, there has been a swelling of funding and industrial development in aquaculture fish farming with participation from just about every developed and many developing nations with borders on a seacoast. According to a 2007 report in *Time*, 40% of seafood eaten today derives from aquaculture, which is the "fastest growing food group" earning $78 billion for the fishing industry.[52] These commercial fish "farms" not only alter the natural conditions by which fish spawn and thrive; they are hauntingly similar to the agricultural factory farms we have been discussing.

The fish raised in aquaculture's tanks are facing the same situations, such as being overdosed with antibiotics, which we saw were affecting factory-farmed livestock. Due to the environmental conditions created for aquaculture, farmed fish are far more susceptible to a variety of diseases, such as bacterial infection and attacks by a host of different parasites. To protect and preserve the financially lucrative aquaculture, fish raisers use vast amounts of antibiotics.

As in the case of raising land animals, the use of antibiotics in aquaculture is largely unregulated. According to one study, these antibiotics are not biodegradable and remain in the fishery waters for long periods of time, thereby generating the perfect conditions for new forms of pathogenic, drug-resistant organisms to emerge.[53]

The antibiotics, along with any infectious organisms and bacteria that remain in the fish, are ultimately ingested by consumers. To take one additional example of these drugs' presence, let me mention the fungicide known as malachite green. It was banned in the 1990s because of its association with varied cancers, genetic mutations, and endocrinal disorders. Nevertheless, it has been documented that this fungicide is still used illegally in fish factories.[54] To make matters worse, the preparers of farmed fish use a variety of artificial dyes to make fish more appealing to buyers. The use of these dyes has increased three-fold and one in particular, canthaxanthin, is linked to ocular and retinal damage and defects.[55]

The fact that these farmed fish have to be treated with antibiotics and other drugs to keep down disease is not unexpected given that, like livestock, these fish are kept in ridiculously cramped quarters. You can expect to find about 50,000 fish in two acres of water. They are packed in so close that they bump into each other, suffering damage from the collisions and becoming sickened with various diseases and infections. Given this situation, farmed fish's toxicity is at much higher levels than that of wild varieties. This is why, according to Dr. J.G. Dorea, the infusion of the fish with drugs as well as the toxicity of the water in which they are swimming is giving rise to high levels of toxic chemicals in the fish flesh we buy and eat.[56]

In three separate independent studies, conducted between 1999 and 2002 of 37 fish pellet samples (animal feed made from fish) used in six countries, each sample was found to have PCB contamination.[57] While this may seem a trifle less threatening than other studies since the fish pellets were given to animals, don't forget that the animals were usually being raised for meat. More than likely, these fish will store the PCBs in their fat to ultimately be passed to humans. Closer to home, a study of fish filets sold to humans found that many had unwanted chemical additives and noted the two fish with the highest level of health-threatening chemicals, including PCBs, are bluefish and rockfish.[58] Besides PCB contamination, dangerous pesticides such as DDT and dieltrin as well as flame retardants have also been found at risk levels in studies of salmon samples, especially in farmed fish.

The resemblance of fish farming to livestock raising has already been noted in terms of the need the growers have to maintain their yields by dosing the animals with drugs. Another similarity is in how these businesses sap so many vital resources.

In order to raise cattle, as we saw, huge amounts of land and feed crops are required. The same, as I noted previously, is true for aquaculture.

What has evolved, then, is an absurdly paradoxical cycle. Fish purveyors turn to aquaculture because they realize the ocean fish stocks are running out, but in doing so, they rely on fish taken from the seas to feed their in-house creatures—a practice that not only ads to further depletion of free stocks, but that is putting the American public at greater health risk.

Animal Foods: You Get Far More than You Bargained For

Let's turn back to something I said in passing in the last section, namely, the costs that are passed on to the unwary American who is consuming these products. As mentioned previously, millions are spent by food companies to convince us of the need to eat in abundance meat, dairy, fish, and the processed foods that contain them. Besides advertising, there is the cost of lobbying and contributions to politicians. According to the Center for Responsive Politics, annual lobbying on agriculture for 2014 was nearly $127 million,[59] while total campaign contributions amounted to almost $77 million[60]—all to ensure that their products continue to be seen in a positive light. This, of course, means that any health risks are underplayed and out of the way of hostile legislation that might better protect citizens from the dangers of such health destroyers as mad cow disease.

You probably remember the headlines about this illness, which first emerged during Christmas in 1994. In Great Britain, 180,000 animals were infected with the illness that can be transmitted to humans who eat meat from sickened animals and resulted in 165 deaths in the United Kingdom. When this outbreak occurred overseas, the beef lobby here rushed to assure Americans that its beef was fine.

Mad cow was attributed in part to "rendering," where parts of animals sent to the slaughter were added back into animal feed; a disgusting practice that turns peaceful grass eating cows into unsuspecting cannibals as well as turning herbivore animals into carnivores. The same feeding method was going great guns in the US. Thankfully, after the panic and deaths in England, the process was banned in the US in 1997. But this didn't mean that if a cow looked sick, it couldn't be led to the slaughterhouse and sold. As long as it was checked and didn't have mad cow, it was good to go. And some state politicians were so much in the pockets (literally and figuratively) of the meat industry that they passed laws to stop activists from publicly talking about their fears of eating tainted meat when it hadn't been "proved" to be unsafe. Is it a surprise that reports indicate politicians with ties to the meat lobby defended cattle owners' rights to sell meat from sick cattle?

Eventually, because of continual threats of mad cow disease (whose outbreaks didn't end in 1994) and the rousing efforts of activists, a December 2004 ban became reality. Even though these sick or "downer" cattle are federally banned from our food supply, there are two major problems currently: some companies do not heed the ban, and a loophole exists that still allows young downer veal calves to be sent to slaughter. On the first issue, in 2013, the Humane Society of the United States (HSUS) exposed the Westland Meat Co., in Riverside, California, one of the nation's leading suppliers of the school lunch program, for the illegal slaughter and sale of sick and downer cattle. This was in spite of the fact of a reported eight on-site USDA inspectors.[61] The regulations forwarded by the USDA in the Spring of 2014 "permit such calves to proceed to slaughter if they are able to rise and walk after being warmed or rested."[62] Sadly, this has led to food manufacturers using cruel and inhumane methods including beating, kicking, and the use of electric prods to get these sick animals to the kill room.[63]

The *L.A. Weekly* cynically stated that the meat lobby may have caved in on this issue because its members felt that they could still get around the industry-friendly regulatory boards that were set up to enforce the laws dealing with these sales.

The propaganda from the meat industry doesn't stop at downplaying the possible health hazards that are associated with its products, but extends to making rather unmerited claims. For instance, The National Pork Producers' Council recently has been running ads to reassure us that "pork has been on a diet," and that "America is leaning on pork."[64] Lean, according to meat industry definitions, means less than 10% fat. And, of course, as the industry will go on to tell you, many cuts of pork are lean, *once you trim off all the fat.*

However, as you've learned already, the question of whether meat has a lot or a little fat, while important, is hardly the only or even the primary consideration that should occupy someone thinking about eating pork or any meat for this matter.

Illnesses from Improper Meat Handling

Animal Flesh

The contribution of animal products to domestically-acquired Illnesses and deaths between 1998 and 2008 is estimated at 48.1% to illness and 50.4% to deaths.[65] Poultry, in particular, accounted for the most deaths (19%); many of those were caused by *Listeria* and *Salmonella* infections. While the CDC did not say why meat accounts for a greater number of deaths, I speculate that it is linked to immune function. The bacteria linked to meat and dairy products are extremely dangerous to those with weakened immune systems—which is just about anyone consuming the Standard American Diet. Some of the bacteria linked to meat contamination are quite virulent. *Listeria* bacteria, for example, can survive refrigeration and even freezing.

One additional note: this report indicates that 5% of illnesses and 2% of deaths were attributed to other commodities, and additional 1% of illness and a full 25% of deaths were not attributed to commodities but rather pathogens, such as the toxoplasma parasite, not in the outbreak database. I was about to say, "Remember that the health effects of food poisoning can be long lasting." But that wouldn't be quite correct since *readers can't remember what they have never been told.*

Even when the media mentions the latest cases of toxicity, they, at best, name the number killed or sickened, usually reporting the story as if those who are ill will soon recover and be back on their feet. Trouble is, once someone has experienced food poisoning, there are recurrent physical experiences after the initial bout. The University of Maryland Medical Center made a partial list of them:

- After shigellosis, white blood cell problems and kidney problems
- After *E. coli* infection, renal and bleeding problems
- After botulism, long hospital stays (1 to 10 months) with fatigue and difficulty breathing for 1 to 2 years or, if worse, respiratory failure
- After salmonellosis, Reiter syndrome (an arthritis-like discase) and inflammation of the heart lining
- After campylobacteriosis, Guillain-Barré syndrome (a nerve disease).[66]

A 2008 Associated Press article takes up the same theme, noting another seldom presented danger of food poisoning—that physical effects often don't manifest till years down the road:

> It's a dirty little secret of food poisoning: *E. coli* and certain other food-borne illnesses can sometimes trigger serious health problems months or years after patients survived that initial bout. Scientists only now are unraveling a legacy that has largely gone unnoticed. What they've spotted so far is troubling. In interviews with The Associated Press, they described high blood pressure, kidney damage, even full kidney failure striking 10 to 20 years later in people who survived severe *E. coli* infection as children, arthritis [coming] after a bout of salmonella or shigella, and a mysterious paralysis that can attack people who just had mild symptoms of campylobacter… For now, some of the best evidence comes from the University of Utah, which has long tracked children with *E. coli*. About 10% of *E. coli* sufferers develop a life-threatening complication called hemolytic uremic syndrome, or HUS, where their kidneys and other organs fail.[67]

Because knowledge of these lingering effects is so little known, people have not yet faced some of the most troubling consequences of contaminated food. Further, they may not even be aware that legal rights are suspended upon initial settlement. This means that should diseases present themselves down the road, the patient could have no additional legal recourse. As Marler says, "Most people who get a food-borne illness never figure out what it is that made them sick. Others who have their suspicions often fail to act. The only way to change bad food-service behavior is to catch it. It's the only way to loop back to the company and say, 'You did a bad thing.'"

Dairy

To take this one step further, we know that, as with all animal products, milk—raw and pasteurized—is a potential breeding ground for harmful bacteria. The list of bacteria contaminating milk and dairy products is similar to those associated with meat: S*almonella, E. coli, Listeri*a (frequently in cheese), *Campylobacter*, and *Staphylcoccus.*[68]

Faulty Inspection Regimes

But why is all this bad meat, as testified by the recalls racked up in the last few years, showing up? Are our livestock now more contaminated than they used to be? It certainly seems so.

Several theories have been suggested as to why so much bacteria-infected meat has been appearing of late. One is that rising oil prices have encouraged greater production of ethanol, which creates a corn byproduct that increasingly is being used as cattle feed. This feed appears to make the animals' digestive tracts even more hospitable breeding grounds for the toxic strain of *E. coli* bacteria. This opinion comes from Kenneth Petersen, an assistant administrator in the Office of Field Operations at the US Department of Agriculture.

Droughts in some regions might also have contributed to the survival of more virulent forms of the bacteria, and better investigation methods can now link far-flung cases of beef contamination to a single cause.

But, putting all that aside, it seems the main obstacle to preventing the spread, in particular, of toxic *E. coli* are inadequate government inspection and meat-handling practices, particularly in slaughterhouses, where contamination is most likely to occur. "Slaughter plants are the primary source of *E. coli* contamination, so the USDA should be putting more resources toward recording and tracing back the original source of contaminated meat detected in test samplings at smaller down-line processing facilities," stated John Munsell, former owner of a Montana-based meat packing and slaughter company who has testified about beef contamination at congressional hearings.

Once you know his story, you'll see where he is coming from with this charge.

Munsell owned a company, Montana Quality Foods, which got in trouble when the USDA discovered his firm's hamburger was contaminated with *E coli*. But, he protested, the meat was contaminated when it came to his plant, and he even identified the source, none other than ConAgra where it had passed inspection by the same USDA before it came to his facility. This experience soured him on meatpacking and turned him into an activist.

Other shortfalls in the safety system identified by experts include:

- Carcasses can move through slaughterhouses at a rate of up to 390 per hour, making inspection difficult.
- If meat tests positive for the bacteria, companies are allowed to cook it for sale (as we've seen) in other products such as pizza or tacos. While thorough cooking should kill E.coli, diverting tainted meat creates an opening for cross-contamination; that is, the transfer of the germs to other meats before it has been cooked.
- It should be underlined that consumer illnesses, not government or industry testing, triggered recalls for the majority of the 61.8 million pounds of beef subject to E.coli-related recalls over the past five years, according to the US Food Safety and Inspection Service.[69]

Of course, and with good reason, fears of meat contamination peaked with the appearance of Mad Cow Disease. As we saw earlier, in reaction to its outbreak in England, the US meat industry spent a lot of money combating the danger of... bad publicity. It's such a terrifying disease because there is no known treatment for this neurodegenerative affliction that can and usually does result in death. Moreover, it may be decades after contraction of the germs for the disease's symptoms to appear.

America has hardly been untouched by this startling disease. In February 2008, the Hallmark meat packing company slaughtered large numbers of cattle that were suspected of having Mad Cow disease. What was the telltale sign that alerted the overworked inspectors? One reason to suspect an animal might be infected is its inability to stand or walk. Apparently, Hallmark's plant workers manually held up unstable cattle for USDA inspectors before being given the green light to slaughter the animals. Then the cattle were carried to the killing floor on forklifts.

In the largest call back in US history, 143 million pounds of meat were recalled. The vexing problem was not that the weak cattle had Mad Cow disease, which was never learned, but that the USDA had not detected the likelihood that these animals were carriers, even in their enfeebled condition.[70] It was an animal rights group that made known the conditions, not the USDA inspectors. The Hallmark plant was subsequently shut down, but that is not much comfort to those who know they ate possibly tainted meat from this plant before it was recalled or those who have put faith in the government's workers to detect such diseased meats.

In January of 2015, Food Safety reported that in 2014 a total of 2.5 million pounds of meat and poultry were recalled for pathogen contamination. The report noted a total of 94 recalls, and nearly half were because of undeclared allergens, while 16 were due to *E. coli, Listeria*, or Salmonella contamination.[71] Just last year, a Petaluma, California slaughterhouse had voluntarily halted operations, as it attempted to track down beef shipments from Jan. 1, 2013 through Jan. 7, 2014 to distribution centers and retail stores in California, Florida, Illinois, and Texas. The US Department of Agriculture announced that the company was recalling more than 8.7 million pounds of beef products.[72]

We mentioned that another element that hampers inspection of livestock is the speed of the "disassembly line," which keeps being boosted by companies seeking any means to increase productivity. As Farmed Animal Watch recently reported regarding the poultry being processed at one plant: "The US Department of Agriculture (USDA)'s Streamline Inspection System for slaughter was designed for 70 birds per minute. The New Line Speed inspection system is designed for 90 birds per minute... [The company] Meyn has since received approval from the USDA to process chickens at unbelievable speeds of 140 birds per minute."[73] Even at the lower rate of 90 birds a minute, 6,300 birds an hour pass through this slaughterhouse, an amount which would seem to severely challenge the inspectors, that is, if we had enough inspectors. Yet, at an average of only 1.25 inspectors per slaughterhouse, the sheer volume of animals being slaughtered daily threatens to overwhelm the inspection regime. The USDA work force hardly seems adequate, and as the *Los Angeles Times* reported, "The [USDA] has 7,800 pairs of eyes scrutinizing 6,200 slaughterhouses and food processors across the nation."[74] And the problem is not just a recent one and it's not just poultry. In 1990, the USDA reported that "large meat plants slaughter from 200 to 400 cattle per hour or 3,000-5,000 cattle per plant per day."[75]

Even more mind-boggling is that some firms find the US meat inspection system, lax as it is, to be too rigorous, and they look for ways to get around it. This was addressed in 1993 by meat inspector William Lehman, who said this in testimony before congress:

> I came here today to tell you that food poisoning deaths, like the Jack-in-the-Box tragedy [over 700 became ill and four died], are certain to multiply under USDA's import inspection procedures. The US-Canada Free Trade Agreement has taken the "meat" out of the meat inspection program. Australian beef is being shipped into the United States through Canada to escape both strict inspection and the payment of duties owed to the taxpayers. Add to this the fact that USDA has recently decided to allow the importation of ground meat. Together, you have the recipe for more public health disasters.[76]

Lehman went on to give vivid details about the incredulous way Canadian importers skirted the rules, which were already very relaxed to begin with. As the Free Trade Agreement was put in place, our northern neighbor adopted the Canadian Streamlined Inspection System. As Lehman outlined:

> Streamlined inspection reduced inspection rates over 90%. Instead of inspecting all of the meat imported to the US from Canada, only approximately one in 10 trucks was stopped for Inspection. Streamlined inspection also notified the Canadian packers which of their trucks would be inspected before those trucks ever left the Canadian packing plant. To make matters worse, the Canadians were allowed to select the very cartons or carcasses to be inspected by USDA. Furthermore, the General Accounting Office discovered that many times trucks designated for inspection failed to even stop at the border.[77]

In other words, it would seem one way this streamlined system saves time is simply by making sure it doesn't find anything amiss with the cattle coming into the US. And, while the USDA's Streamlined Inspection System for Cattle (SIS-C) is less flagrant, one might question how much better it is than the negligent Canadian system. A Committee on Evaluation was established within the Food and Nutrition Board of the Institute of Medicine of the National Academy of Sciences to evaluate SIS-C. Their report blandly notes that the inspection system cannot be expected to weed out diseased meat, although it's good for maintaining quality control. This is to be expected since it relies on the Cumulative Sum method for its inspection. Using this method, random samples are taken from the mass of animals being slaughtered and judgment is made based solely on those samples. The reader might think this may offer some hope that contaminated livestock will be excluded from the food chain since, maybe, if one is sick, then most are sick, and this will show up in the random assessment. The report, however, shoots down this thought. I have italicized the most striking parts of this passage.

> The Cumulative Sum (CUSUM) [method] … is a good choice to help control the process and ensure uniformity of processing. *However, many people erroneously believe CUSUM as used in SIS-C is intended to ensure that no contaminated or otherwise defective meat reaches the consumer. That is not its purpose*, and it is inadequate to provide that assurance in cattle slaughtering operations.
>
> Therefore, *CUSUM in SIS-C will not directly ensure a* pleasing, clean, wholesome, and *toxin- or pathogen-free product.*[78]

Let's look at a number of pathogens in the meat supply in order to give more specificity to our understanding of how well the inspection system works. In this quote from the Centers for Disease Control (CDC), again I have italicized the most damning parts. "Although commercial 'ready to eat' pork products are required by law to be cooked, frozen, or otherwise treated to kill *T. Spiralis* larvae [which cause trichinosis], federal or state inspection procedures do not actually include examination of pork for the presence of larvae at the time of slaughter. *The burden of responsibility lies with the consumer.*"[79]

Admittedly, there are fewer cases of trichinosis today than we saw in the past due to widespread use of freezers and the discontinued practice of feeding garbage to hogs, yet given the low inspection standards here, whose notoriety means many other countries are reluctant to import our pork, the disease will continue to occur.

It is brought on by undercooked pork products that carry the larvae of the nematode worm. This is where the comment about the "responsibility" of the consumer comes in. If the consumer had cooked the pork properly, he or she wouldn't have gotten the dread disease, we are told. That's overlooking the fact that if the inspectors had been warier and the pork seller in less of a hurry to get the meat sold, pork with the larvae would never have been in the marketplace.

I called trichinosis a dread disease with good reason. The larvae are first ingested in the intestinal tract, then later in active muscles—the calves, diaphragm, and tongue—which are weakened until the victim can barely move. Even non-pork eaters can pick up the illness, as this organism can get into other meats by the intentional or inadvertent mixing of pork with chopped beef in supermarkets, butcher shops, and restaurants.

While the effects on humans of trichinosis are well known and much feared, another disease found in animals, foot-and-mouth disease, which stems from the aphthovirus, has been ignored because it is believed it cannot pass over to humans even if they do ingest its causative virus. It's not that hard for this disease-causer to be found in meat that gets to the stores, given that, depending on the stage of infection at the time of slaughter, the virus may go undetected. Initial signs of infection may not appear until after a two-to-eight day incubation period, and it's possible they may never become apparent. This highly infectious virus is biochemically active during the decaying process. However, when the action of enzymes and acids are halted by quick freezing of meat, the virus can remain intact and dormant to become active again when the meat is thawed. There are studies investigating whether the presence of this pathogen in meat raises health issues for humans with at least hints that those suffering from chronic degenerative diseases or individuals using immunosuppressant drugs for cancer and other illnesses that affect the immune system may be affected by this agent.

A couple of other deadly bacteria that have been detected in meats that made their way to the supermarket shelves or restaurant tables are *listeria* and *salmonella*. *Listeria* contamination was responsible for five of the eight large recalls listed at the beginning of this chapter. It only rarely infects humans, but when it does, it is quite lethal, with a 25% fatality rate. It acts by getting into the cell and then propagating by moving cell to cell, avoiding reentering the bloodstream where it might be detected by antibodies. Those most at risk are newborns, the elderly, pregnant mothers, and AIDS patients.[80] Given its lethality, special biochemical detection assays have been developed to determine its presence in commercial food products.

Salmonella is an enterobacteria that is often associated with food-poisoning and food-borne illnesses. It is responsible for causing typhoid and paratyphoid fevers. There is no realistic hope of wiping out the possibility of *Salmonell*a infection as long as we continue to eat animal foods. As the National Academy of Sciences says, "Reluctantly, we are forced to recognize the unfeasibility of eradicating salmonellosis at this time." Dr. Scott Holmberg of the Centers for Disease Control says that *Salmonella* poisoning affects "two to four million humans each year, and one of every thousand [30,000 every decade] will die,"[81] many of them elderly or infants. The symptoms of *Salmonella* poisoning might appear less than life-threatening: nausea, vomiting, and diarrhea, but this infection is much more hazardous than the common flu or other soon-passing infections.

It should also be stressed that the presence of one bacteria in a meat product does not preclude in the same cut of beef, a second, third, or even more pathogenic intruders. Laboratory studies have indicated that contaminated meat likely contains more than one disease-causing microbe. *E. coli* in cultures taken from animals, for example, is often backed up by brother germs, such as Enterbacteriaceae, and *Salmonella*.

And remember, even if meat leaves the factory farms pure, it will not necessarily reach your plate that way. Let's say for a moment that meat did come untainted from the slaughterhouses and meat-packing plants. There is still a second line of hazards for someone eating in a restaurant or institution (such as a hospital or school cafeteria). According to the CDC, mishandling of food in such places is the major factor in outbreaks of botulism, a serious nerve toxin and form of food poisoning. The agency identifies, among other factors that lead to food-borne illnesses, improper storage temperatures, inadequate cooking time, and poor personal hygiene of food handlers.[82]

What has been discussed in the last few pages—from the overworked and (seemingly) often negligent inspectors, to the way one recall after another has rocked the meat industry, to the long-term, health-undermining effects of seemingly mild bouts of food poisoning—should have made you aware that you take your life in your hands or, rather, on your fork, every time you dine on prime rib, chicken, or any other meat.

Meat-related illness costs Americans billions of dollars a year, to echo a point I've been making throughout this book. The Senate Select Committee on Nutrition and Human Needs found that an increase in the rate of malnutrition and obesity had a direct correlation to a decrease in the quality, not quantity, of food consumed.[83] At the same time, meat consumption results in a direct increase in the rate of heart disease, cancer, hypertension, arthritis, and other degenerative diseases. I believe much of this illness results from *incorrect eating*.

Unhealthy Meat-Based Diets

The Paleo Diet

One of the more recent popular diets to sweep the nation is the Paleo Diet. The Paleo Diet operates on the principle that before the agricultural revolution, people didn't eat grains, rice, or legumes. Rather, as the argument goes, they hunted and foraged, living—and evolving—on animal and plant protein, and the nutrients derived from the range of fruits, vegetables, nuts, and seeds at their disposal. So, if they didn't eat it, neither can you.

Robb Wolf, author of best-selling book *The Paleo Solution*, claims to be a research biochemist (though his credentials aren't easy to come by), and argues for the health benefits of the Paleo Diet. On his website, Wolf claims, "The "Paleo diet" is the healthiest way you can eat because it is the ONLY nutritional approach that works with your genetics to help you stay lean, strong, and energetic!" Well, there are a lot of people who would disagree with that bold statement, including for example, all vegetarians through time and a whole lot of nutrition and genetics experts. Wolf goes on to argue that our modern US diet is leading to a plethora of disease, which is not disputed—but that still doesn't mean that the Paleo Diet is a good idea.

A second website promoting the Paleo Diet argues, "Paleo" is based on the idea that this mismatch between our bodies and our diet might be the reason for modern health problems like diabetes, obesity, and heart disease. Just like any other animal, humans suffer when we stray from our natural diet, but when we return to it, everything changes. Food stops making us sick, and starts making us strong, energetic, and vibrant with health."[84]

Here is the diet plan for the Paleo Diet, according to Wolf:

Okay To Eat	Avoid
Fruits	Dairy
Vegetables	Grains
Lean Meats	Processed Food and Sugars
Seafood	Legumes
Nuts and Seeds	Starches
Healthy Fats	Alcohol

Paleo Leap goes on to label those foods Wolf has placed in the "avoid" column as *toxic!* In actuality, the only way grains, legumes, and starches such as potatoes are toxic to the human body is when they're loaded with chemicals.

As you see, fruits, vegetables, nuts and seeds, and healthy fats are in the "okay to eat" column—and that is a good place for those items in order for the human being to achieve optimal health. Similarly, dairy, processed foods, sugars, and alcohol are in the "avoid" column—which is another excellent idea. So, I agree that some of the recommendations of the Paleo Diet are healthy. *But*, that doesn't mean that the Paleo Diet is a good idea in general.

There are two essential problems with the Paleo Diet. The first is, obviously, that animal proteins are in the "Okay to Eat" column, and the second are the grains, legumes, and starches in the "avoid" column. Animal proteins are not okay to eat, in fact. A 2014 study published in the *International Journal of Exercise Science* noted that the "Paleo" diet worsens cholesterol levels. Forty-four adults were placed on the diet as well as on a circuit training program. After ten weeks, LDL ("bad") cholesterol increased by 12.5 mg/dL and total cholesterol by 10.1 mg/dL; triglycerides also increased slightly. The authors also stated that any improvements from an exercise program may be negated by the "Paleo" diet.[85]

Michael Pollan, author of a number of best-selling books on food and agriculture, including *Cooked: A Natural History of Transformation* explained, in a 2014 podcast, that the trouble with the Paleo message is that it asserts that the diet is akin to what our ancient ancestors ate when it is probably nothing like the diet of hunter-gatherers. "I don't think we really understand… well the proportions in the ancient diet," argues Pollan. "Most people who tell you with great confidence that this is what our ancestors ate—I think they're kind of blowing smoke."[86] Meanwhile, in an article appearing in *Scientific American*, Rob Dunn, a science writer and biologist in the Department of Biology at North Carolina State University, states "If you want a justification for eating a meaty 'paleodiet,'… the search should be for evidence that some aspect of our bodies evolved in such a way as to be better able to deal with extra meat or other elements of our stone age diets that differed from the primate norm. It could be there, as of yet undetected."[87] In other words, our guts have evolved from and are most like that of our nearest cousins the great Apes, who eat a predominantly vegetarian diet. This also happens to be Dunn's conclusion about humans and our ancestors.

Further, an article titled *Neanderthal medics? Evidence for food, cooking, and medicinal plants entrapped in dental calculus* published in the journal *The Science of Nature* reports "Our results provide the first molecular evidence for… ingestion of a range of cooked plant foods. We also offer the first evidence for the use of medicinal plants by a Neanderthal individual. The varied use of plants that we have identified suggests that the Neanderthal occupants of El Sidrón had a sophisticated knowledge of their natural surroundings which included the ability to select and use certain plants."[88]

The second problem with the Paleo Diet is its prohibition of grains, legumes, and starches. Now, I'm not saying you should overdo these in the diet, but I'm also not going to suggest that these things aren't good for you or that they don't have vital nutritional value, when in fact they do. Further, legumes are the primary source of protein that I am recommending, but grains and starchy vegetables also contain essential amino acids and plenty of nutrients. As you will read in Chapter 5, I am suggesting 9-11 servings of vegetables a day, including starches, tubers, and root and stalk vegetables; there, you will see studies noted about their nutritional value. I am also recommending fruits, as well as nuts and seeds, which is covered thoroughly in Chapter 5.

The last point that I wish to make about the Paleo Diet, which is often ignored by proponents, is that the diet is environmentally destructive and unsustainable. Much of this is covered in this text, so I will leave you with a few points raised in *Earth Island Journal's* article *Can Seven Billion Humans Go Paleo?*[89]:

- The United Nations Environmental Program cites meat production as one of the top three causes of ecological problems and one of the main drivers of climate change.
- According to the United Nations Food & Agriculture Organization, 53% of the world's fisheries are fully exploited, and 32% are overexploited, depleted, or recovering from depletion. More to the point, "The global fishing fleet is 2-3 times larger than what the oceans can sustainably support." Most of the developed world now relies heavily on aquaculture, but farmed fish still requires feed made with wild fish.[89]

I will leave you with a quote from Yale researchers Dr. David Katz and Stephanie Meller, who in their 2014 report concluded that: "A diet of minimally processed foods close to nature, predominantly plants, is decisively associated with health promotion and disease prevention."[90]

High Protein/Low-Carb Diets

Another popular weight-loss diet promotes heavy meat consumption and extremely low carbohydrates. Promoters of these diets claim animal protein is low in calories and so helpful in weight-loss plans, while carbs, on the other hand, add the pounds. What they don't tell you is that eating this way can be lethal. It increases your risk of a heart attack by as much as 86%. Further, increasing the daily intake of fruit alone—high in carbs—can reduce your chances of a heart attack by 40%.[91-94] In fact, the American Heart Association tracked over 4,000 people who had had a heart attack, and found that those who followed a diet high in animal protein and low in carbs were 51% more likely to die from heart disease.[95] Add to this that consumption of red meat is linked to a 22% increased likelihood of developing breast cancer,[96] and this diet makes less and less sense.

It is true that carbohydrate deficiency generates a condition known as ketosis, which is a state where your body does burn fat. But this comes with ghastly side effects including gastrointestinal issues, fatigue, organ damage, and bad breath, among other symptoms.[97]

Further, while animal protein, if it was isolated in foods, might be low-cal, it doesn't arrive that way. Even in "lean" meats, the protein is normally accompanied by a large amount of fat. An average 16-ounce steak, for example, has about 1,250 calories, and about 80 grams of fat.[98] One of the things, in addition to simple or refined carbohydrates, contributing to the US's astonishing levels of obesity is excess meat consumption. Carbohydrates, except for those found in refined carbohydrates and sugars, are much lower in calories than animal products. Sixteen ounces of long-grain brown rice, for example, contains just 503 calories—one-third that of a steak, and only 4.8 grams of fat.

As if that weren't enough, a diet high in animal protein leads to an earlier death. A study of more than 6,000 Americans over the age of 50 showed that those who ate the most animal protein had a 5-fold increase in the risk of diabetes-related death. Those under 65 who ate the most animal protein had a 74% increase in the risk of death from any cause and a 4-fold increase in cancer-related death. Critical to note is that these risks of death were diminished or even entirely absent with plant-based protein diets.

In fact, carbohydrates—not protein—are the body's primary energy source and should make up the majority of what you eat. A high fiber/high complex carbohydrate and low fat/low protein/low dairy diet may actually prevent prostate cancer.[99] Carbohydrates can be found in grains, fruits, vegetables, and beans.

One thing about this high protein diet is certain: you could die from it.[100]

Chapter 4

The Good News about Vegetarian Diets

> "Few of us are aware that the act of eating can be a powerful statement of commitment to our own well-being, and at the same time the creation of a healthier habitat. Your health, happiness, and the future of life on earth are rarely so much in your own hands as when you sit down to eat."
>
> —*John Robbins, Author of* Diet for a New America *and* Food Revolution

Now that we've seen plenty of evidence that the perils associated with an animal-based diet are real and true, we will spend some time speaking about the good news related to vegetarian diets, including the host of diseases and disorders you will avoid, or significantly reduce your chances of developing in your lifetime by adopting this diet.

Following a vegetarian diet has been demonstrated to offer more associated health benefits than a meat-based diet. These include increased protection for a host of chronic conditions: from heart disease and cancer to obesity and diabetes 2.[1]

No doubt health is the concern that leads many people to opt for and stay with vegetarianism, or a predominantly plant-based life. It boils down to the fact that replacing fatty meats with lighter plant proteins radically shifts what is nourishing your body in a way that boosts general health and lowers the risk of contracting many diseases. By eliminating the saturated fats and cholesterol found in meats in abundance, for example, one depresses one's chance of coming down with breast and colon cancer, which have been linked to consumption of these substances. Meats' fats and cholesterol also contribute to hardening of the arteries and heart disease. Eating too much animal protein, coincidentally, has been tied to a long list of diseases, including stroke, osteoporosis, liver and kidney disorders, and arthritis. Let's take a look at some of the correlations between the vegetarian diet and health as it exists today.

Fiber, Disease and Vegetarianism

We Need More Fiber

Those that turned to vegetarianism because they wanted enhanced physical well-being did so not only to avoid the toxins and cholesterol in meat and dairy, but because of the positive nutritional benefits of a diet of vegetables, fruits, grains, and seeds. Important among these benefits is that vegetables and grains are rich in fiber. A diet high in fiber improves the functioning of the digestive tract, resulting in less constipation and gas as well as helping ward off gastrointestinal diseases.

There are two different types of fiber, soluble and insoluble; soluble fiber dissolves in water and insoluble fiber does not. Both are important in the diet, and to some degree these differences determine how each fiber functions in the body and benefits your health. Soluble fiber attracts water and forms a gel, which slows digestion. It is incredibly helpful in controlling weight because it delays the emptying of your stomach and promotes a "full" feeling. Slower stomach emptying may also affect blood sugar levels, which can be helpful in controlling diabetes and symptoms like lethargy and moodiness linked to shifting blood sugar levels. Soluble fiber can also help lower harmful LDL blood cholesterol levels by interfering with the absorption of dietary cholesterol. Examples of soluble fiber are oatmeal, lentils, apples, oranges, pears, oat bran, strawberries, nuts, flaxseeds, beans, dried peas, blueberries, cucumbers, celery, and carrots.[2] Insoluble fiber provides roughage. I brought this up before when I put down a few bullet points about the benefits of fiber found in plant foods, not meats. As I said previously, fiber "scours the intestinal walls, removing some potentially toxic agents, which would otherwise accumulate." It is the considered gut-healthy fiber because it has a laxative effect and adds bulk to the diet, helping prevent constipation. Since this fiber does not dissolve in water, it passes through the gastrointestinal tract relatively intact, and speeds up the passage of food and waste through your gut. Insoluble fiber is mainly found in whole grains and vegetables. Sources include whole grains, wheat bran, corn bran, seeds, nuts, barley, couscous, brown rice, bulgur, zucchini, celery, broccoli, cabbage, onions, tomatoes, carrots, cucumbers, green beans, dark leafy vegetables, raisins, grapes, fruit, and root vegetable skins.[3]

Let's look at why a few years ago the role of fiber came as such a revelation to many in the medical world. Dr. Denis Burkitt, one of the foremost researchers in the field of dietary fiber and disease, explains that fiber has been "neglected because it contributes little nutritionally despite its important role in maintaining normal gastrointestinal function."[4] Because it is not a "nutrient," in the sense that fiber itself doesn't supply vitamins or minerals, it wasn't getting much respect. The important role of fiber was all but dismissed or ignored until, that is, the absence of its "services" begun to come to light.

This may be why American eaters acquiesced in the changeover to a low-fiber diet, which began in the 1870s, when new milling techniques replaced stone mills. White bread suddenly became readily available to everyone, replacing the healthier, hearty brown and black breads previously eaten as a staple by the less-than-wealthy. Overall consumption of whole, unrefined grains has decreased since the late 1800s, where there has been a prolific increase in refined grains, breads, cereals, etc., as well as more treacherous foods such as meat, dairy, and both sugar and salt in the form of various confections, potato chips, and other hazardous "treats" in the American diet. Between 1890 and 1960, the national intake of sugar more than doubled, and fat intake also rose.

While the majority of the US public continues heedlessly to eschew fiber, Dr. Burkitt's work substantiates the wisdom of the common vegetarian practice of including "whole foods" in the diet—whole grains, whole-wheat breads and pastas, and skin left on fruits and vegetables, all filled with fiber. Before these green eaters had the scientific backing that Burkitt and others provided about the value of fiber, they were eating something in abundance that we now know is invaluable.

"Many diseases common in modern western civilization have been related to the amount of time it takes food to pass through the alimentary tract, as well as to the bulk and consistency of stools," Burkitt writes. He adds, "These factors are influenced by fiber in the diet, especially cereal fiber," which speeds the flow. His research shows that *lack of fiber* leads to "changes in gastrointestinal behavior" that is suspect in such ailments as appendicitis, diverticulitis, gall bladder disease, cardiovascular disease, diabetes, hemorrhoids, varicose veins, hiatus hernia, and certain forms of cancer.[5] Benign and malignant tumors and ulcerative colitis are "more dependent on environmental than on genetic factors," Dr. Burkitt reported in the *Journal of the American Medical Association*.[6] The colon's "environment" is predominantly determined by the quality of the food that passes through it and the speed of its transit.

With a low-fiber diet, there is generally not enough weight and bulk in the fecal waste to move it quickly through the intestinal tract. The waste then becomes concentrated and sluggish, as it makes its slow progress. Prolonged bowel transit time is suspect in appendicitis as well as in colon and rectal cancer. Not only do low-fiber diets slow digestion, they may lead to changes for the worse in the type and number of fecal bacteria, which has been linked to increased incidence and severity of bowel disease.

A very slowed-down movement of waste through the intestines is another name for constipation, which typically leads to more serious ailments over time. As Dr. Burkitt writes, consuming the right amount of indigestible fiber can both prevent and cure constipation.

A diet lacking it [fiber]—that is, one made up chiefly of meat, peeled potato, white bread, and concentrated sweets—is a common cause of atonic constipation (when the colon is not responding to normal signals to evacuate waste), because the food mass moves sluggishly through the digestive tract and the lack of moisture-holding bulk makes the stool dry and difficult to pass. Constipation is a factor in health problems; because of the straining, it can cause varicose veins, which affect some 10% of the American adult population. In this, the intra-abdominal pressure is abnormally increased, which may lead to the damaging of the proximal valves in our legs. This mechanism seems to lead to the onset of hemorrhoids and hiatus hernia. Almost half of our over-50 age group suffers from this preventable and often extremely painful condition.

Constipation is uncommon among people who live largely on unrefined plant foods from which the cellulose (as in the bran of grains) has not been removed. We digest the digestible parts of what we eat and the rest remains as bulk for bowel hygiene. Cellulose residue absorbs and holds moisture and so gives bulk to the bowel contents. This stimulated peristalsis prevents stagnation of materials in the colon, and keeps the fecal matter soft and easy to evacuate.[7]

Alas, this clear and informative message, written more than 30 years ago, remains hidden in a periodical stashed on a back shelf in most medical libraries, seldom consulted except by those who want to look beyond the alleged common sense of today's meat extollers. Indeed, a recent study conducted at the University of New Hampshire indicates quite clearly that it is those who cling to the meat gospel who are most likely to suffer constipation problems.

The findings showed that there were five distinct eating groups, of which the largest, the "meat and potatoes" crowd, tended to be overweight, lower middle-class, conservative, small-town residents. Chronic constipation was rampant in this group; many believed a weekly bowel movement was normal. On the other end of the spectrum, representing some 15% of those surveyed, was the "naturalist" group. These people tended to be younger, more affluent, interested in creative cooking, and—this is key—more conversant on health matters in relation to diet, as well as more conscious of food additives and preservatives. Notably, constipation was far less of a problem among them.[8]

Diabetes and Lack of Fiber

The connection of fiber consumption to intestinal health is easy to understand in contrast to the links between a lack of fiber and diabetes, which are far from obvious. And this difficulty in grasping the relationship, which translates into a general lack of awareness, is not helped by the fact that important medical groups also ignore the connection. The diet condoned by both the American Diabetic Association and the American Dietetic Association is an example of this ignorance, in that the diet is high in saturated fat, cholesterol, and refined carbohydrates and deficient in complex carbohydrates and dietary fiber.

Dietary fats decrease the utilization of what little insulin the diabetic may still be able to produce, while fiber, on the other hand, is needed to regulate blood-sugar fluxes. (As most readers know, diabetes arises when a person's body has trouble either producing insulin (type-1 diabetes) or utilizing insulin (type-2 diabetes), which regulates the amount of sugar in the blood.) While the recommended diet causes trouble to the diabetic, studies suggest a low-fat, high-complex-carbohydrate diet can reverse both diabetes mellitus (type-2 diabetes) and hypoglycemia. At this point, I'm now not talking simply of fiber, but of a broader dietary program that draws from the whole panoply of green foods.

Those who advocate this plant-based program for people suffering from diabetes, recommend total consumption of carbohydrates be increased, with emphasis on complex carbohydrates. Concurrently, the consumption of refined sugars should be significantly decreased or altogether eliminated. These goals can best be accomplished by substituting grains, legumes, vegetables, and fresh fruits (all high in fiber *and* nutrients), for meat, dairy products, and refined and processed foods.

Moreover, all the physical problems I've mentioned so far have to do with eating properly cooked meat. Health disaster after disaster has appeared in the news where people were hospitalized when they undercooked, for instance, a pile of ground beef that was contaminated with E coli or other bacteria. Each time such an outbreak occurs, the government tells meat consumers to make sure they prepare and cook their food properly, implicitly acknowledging that the government itself cannot adequately prevent poultry and mammalian food contamination.

Let me add that the government's admission that it can't protect consumers from diseased meat does not mean those few who hunt game in the wild are safer than the majority who get their meat from a butcher. It's been discovered that a large population of deer and elk in the West are afflicted with prion, which causes severe neural degeneration.[9] Although there have been no proven cases of direct transmission, potential infection should cause concern for any wild game hunter.

So whether you shoot it yourself or pick it up at the nearby food mart, meat is unhealthy, either in the short-run, if the meat is contaminated, or in the long run, since years of meat consumption typically end in sickness.

In a 2011 analysis of the scientific literature on vegetarianism and vegan diets entitled *Health Implications of a Vegetarian Diet: A Review*, researchers confirmed a wealth of evidence demonstrating the health-promoting effects of vegetarianism and veganism. The scientific data convincingly establishes that a plant-based diet reduces many of the leading causes of morbidity and mortality such as obesity, diabetes, cancer, and heart disease as well as some types of cancer. Furthermore, the vegetarian diet increases life expectancy.[10]

General Muscle Health

One additional area is muscle strength, which is a good area for us to begin with since most bodybuilders argue that meat is essential for strength. In general, muscle strength is of vital importance in maintaining one's capacity for physical activity and mobility. And protein is required for the repair and creation of muscle tissue. In a revealing study, researchers looked at the incidence of sarcopenia in the elderly. Sarcopenia is characterized by the loss of skeletal muscle tissue and an increase in muscle fat. Often times, we are not aware that this process is occurring, and typically osteoporosis is blamed for falls and hip fractures when researchers have found that the real culprit is a loss of muscle strength that *increases* the risk of falling. Their conclusions support the fact that it is a decrease in the synthesis of muscle protein and poor nutritional status in the elderly that is the primary cause of sarcopenia. This is highly relevant because animal-based proteins require more energy for digestion and assimilation than plant-based proteins. Further, because humans lack the necessary enzymes to digest animal products completely, a certain amount of these foods remain undigested, cheating the body of nutrients. Poorly assimilated protein would naturally lead to a corresponding decrease in muscle protein synthesis.[11]

On a similar but related topic, new research shows a correlation between lack of exercise and free radical damage to intramuscular mitochondrial DNA as contributors to loss of muscle strength. Mitochondria are the power plants for every cell in our body, and as mitochondria die, there is a corresponding decline in muscle function.

In addition, muscle quality is negatively affected by protein cross linking—a process whereby two proteins link together to form strong chemical bridges—which further damages the mitochondria and resultant tissues. An example of this effect, which you may be familiar with already, is related to skin aging. In this case, glucose molecules link themselves to the amino groups of tissue proteins such as collagen, and slowly rearrange their youthful structure into culprits that end up causing wrinkles, discoloration, and loss of elasticity to name a few. Consequently, protein that is derived from foods high in saturated fat accelerates this cross-linking process.

Throughout this book, it will become transparently clear that a vegetarian diet provides *more than enough protein* to support a healthy physiology, but it also does far more; it preserves the natural state of the body. The vegetarian diet packs an overwhelming advantage with an antioxidant counterpunch that helps to neutralize the free radical and cross-linkage damage that naturally occurs from protein metabolism.

Critics and skeptics abound regarding the protein adequacy of a vegetarian and vegan based diet. One such critic was the American Dietetic Association. They have retracted their former position and now acknowledged the fact that protein requirements are met on a plant-based diet. Importantly, the ADA has also acknowledged the undeniable health benefits derived from vegetarianism, including vegan diets, in their updated position paper. They stated that "appropriately planned vegetarian diets, including total vegetarian or vegan diets, are healthful, nutritionally adequate and may provide health benefits in the prevention and treatment of certain diseases. Well-planned vegetarian diets are appropriate for individuals during all stages of the life cycle including pregnancy, lactation, infancy, childhood and adolescence and for athletes."[12]

In another important study published in the peer-reviewed journal *American Journal of Clinical Nutrition,* investigators found that a variety of "plant proteins can serve as a complete and well-balanced source of amino acids for meeting human physiological requirements."[13]

While no studies to date have analyzed muscle quality between vegetarians and omnivores, there are studies that prove that vegetarians weigh less and have a lower body mass index. BMI is one way to calibrate the fat content in the body relative to a person's height and weight. Even though the quality of one's diet is closely linked to body composition, be mindful of the fact that exercise, too, can significantly impact the strength and quality of muscle tissue, which affects BMI, since muscle is denser and weighs more than fat.

Still, one quick search on the Internet will reveal any number of powerful looking vegan bodybuilders. In fact, one Romanian Olympic athlete study found those who took 1.5 grams of Supro soy protein daily for two months experienced greater increases in body mass, strength, serum proteins, and calcium, as well as dips in post-training fatigue, compared to athletes who didn't take soy protein.[14] The key to all of this is to get away from monotheistic thinking about diets and purposes for certain diets—for example, the unfounded and harmful myth that "I'm going to be a meat eater because that will get me better muscle development." This will only lead to health problems down the road, as we've discussed a bit so far and will see in more detail later.

Bone Health and Vegetarianism

Bones are far more complex than they are given credit for. They are the solitary source of many important minerals—like calcium and phosphorus—and furnish these minerals to all of the other organs in the body. Every nerve and muscle cell requires calcium to send chemical signals; the bones provide the calcium. Every cell requires phosphorus, and the bones supply that as well. Calcium and phosphorus are so vital to the health of the body that the proper amounts of each must be properly sustained for tissues to function properly. The bones serve as the body's sole repository for each of these precious minerals.

One major affliction related to bones is osteoporosis, which is linked to the loss of calcium. According to a report issued in June of 2014 by the National Osteoporosis Foundation, 54 million Americans are living with or at-risk of *osteoporosis* and low bone mass, which causes two million bone breaks every year.[15] The number is speculated to increase to 71.2 million by the year 2030. Amy Porter, executive director and CEO of NOF, notes the burden to our nation by stating that Medicare (our tax dollars) pays the cost for repair in 80% of these bone breaks.

A common error that many make when speaking about warding off bone loss is to recommend dairy products. In fact, a 12-year Harvard study of 78,000 women reported that those who drank milk three times a day actually broke more bones than women who rarely drank milk. A similar study in Sydney, Australia, showed that higher dairy product consumption was associated with *increased* fracture risk.[16] Furthermore, one UK study sponsored by the Government's Food Standards Agency (FSA) found that only 43% of the mean intake of calcium in adults came from milk and milk products.[17] This demonstrates that a large share of the calcium in our diets is derived from sources other than dairy foods, which is not surprising as most people in the world (around 70%) obtain their calcium from plant-based sources rather than dairy products.[18]

As I wrote in my book *Get Healthy Now!: A Complete Guide to Prevention, Treatment, and Healthy Living*, registered nurse and acupuncturist Abigail Rist-Podrecca noted, "When I was in China, we noticed that no dairy was used. We expected to see a high incidence of osteoporosis, rickets, and other bone problems. In fact, we saw the lowest incidence. In the West, dairy is used a lot and osteoporosis is rampant. Something is not quite right here."

While the NOF misses the boat by recommending dairy and "plenty" of it, they also extol the benefits of a wide variety of fruits and vegetables. They also note that recent research has found olive oil, soy beans, blueberries, and foods rich in omega-3s like flaxseed oil may also have bone boosting benefits.[19] Additionally, adequate levels of vitamin D are required for calcium absorption.

In reality, the value of the vegetarian diet for bone health is superior. Plant foods promote bone growth and repair. Green, leafy vegetables contain vitamin K, beta carotene, vitamin C, fiber, calcium, and magnesium, which enhance the bones. Other calcium-rich foods include broccoli, nuts, and seeds.

Sesame seeds have high calcium content. The Chinese, who as mentioned earlier have low rates of osteoporosis, use sesame often in their foods and cook with sesame seed oil.

Foods to avoid include sugar, caffeine, carbonated sodas, and alcohol, as these contribute to bone loss. Chicken, fish, eggs, and meat are also contraindicated. These are high in the amino acid methionine, which the body converts into homocysteine, a substance that causes both osteoporosis and atherosclerosis.

Other Health Issues Benefited by a Vegetarian Diet

Vegetarianism and Health: What the Studies Show

The plain fact is that reliable, undivided science does support the benefits of adopting a properly balanced vegetarian way of eating. In an almost symbolic acknowledgement of this fact, on January 2, 1996, for the first time the US Secretary of Health and Human Services endorsed the healthfulness of a vegetarian diet. In fact, for the first time ever, *in 2015 the USDA acknowledged that a plant-based diet is sufficient for good health.* The data has been in for decades now, and they demonstrate one thing: Vegetarianism offers significant health benefits. The studies are there—hundreds of them—in peer-reviewed scientific journals. I know because I have numerous reprints in my office.

But remember what I said earlier in the book when speaking about how we learn (the field of *epistemology*). By the time we have learned something and it becomes social norm (an agreed upon set of social behavior), we must go through a similar process of *un*learning something when this formerly agreed up on set of behavior proves invaluable for the society at large. My primary purpose in presenting this material is to fortify efforts toward creating a new social norm when it comes to health, including the foods we find acceptable to consume in our society.

So far in this book, I have thrown in a number of passages that speak to the value of green eating, noting, for instance, the importance of having a lot of fiber in your diet. But I admit a lot of what we've covered health wise are the disastrous consequences of meat and dairy consumption. Such discussions may have frightened you. When you read the following pages and find out more about the health-improving and disease-curtailing effects of a vegetarian diet, you will shed your fear and boost your spirits.

Vegetarianism and the Heart

Let's stay with this broader perspective as we further investigate disease and diet, first taking a look at cardiovascular disease, the leading cause of death in America. We should note that a major risk factor in heart disease is hypertension, or high blood pressure. The symptoms, such as fatigue and poor circulation in the extremities, are frequently ignored because people consider them normal parts of aging. But they're not. In heart disease, the blood vessels are narrowed, typically because they are coated with cholesterol and plaque, and the heart has to pump harder to get blood through these ever-narrowing channels. Extra exertion in the form of exercise or stress can put the body in jeopardy. Because the heart is working harder, and the actual amount of blood getting through the vessels is reduced, there may be insufficient oxygen supply to the muscles and the brain with these extra demands. Heart attack and stroke are possible consequences.

As established previously, meat, dairy, and refined foods bear major responsibility for the cholesterol overlay in the blood circulation channels. What I haven't noted yet is that a vegetarian diet has a blood-pressure lowering effect, which has been documented numerous times. In fact, if many of the claims for the value of vegetarianism are based on research done in the last few decades, as noted in one recent study,[20] scientific interest in this beneficial effect of a meat-free diet goes back to the early decades of the 20th century, when it was shown that hypertension was worsened by meat intake. In studies done at that time, vegetarian college students who added meat to their diets saw their blood pressure increase significantly within two weeks.

Since those early days, research about the connection between diet and blood pressure has not ended, nor have the results been much different from those found at the beginning of the last century. You can know this simply by glancing at a recent article in *The American Journal of Clinical Nutrition,* whose conclusion reads, "There is now strong evidence for a blood-pressure lowering effect of a lacto-ovo vegetarian diet… The effect is independent of sodium and energy intake and of other aspects of lifestyle that tend to characterize vegetarian populations." Furthermore, the report points out that "cardiovascular risk in general is low in people adhering to a lacto-ovo vegetarian diet, not only because their blood pressures are lower and tend to rise less with age, but also because they carry less excess fat and tend to have healthier blood lipid profiles than do meat eaters."[21]

You might have noted in the last but one quote the use of the words "independent of," which is to say, the effects of lower blood pressure were found even after discounting for other factors. I've brought up this point before, as have adversaries of research pertaining to vegetarians: In studies of the health of vegetarians, it can be hard to pin down exactly how much a benefit is tied to green eating and how much might be the product of other good habits vegetarians typically cultivate, such as exercising regularly, consuming less alcohol, not smoking, yoga and meditation, regular sleep, and so on.

Ischemia, or coronary heart disease (IHD), is the most common cause of death in the West[22], with no sign of it being dethroned in the foreseeable future. While the role of diet in IHD has been controversial over the years, new research is surfacing to prove the effectiveness of a plant-based diet in the prevention and significant reduction in cardiac events.

In his book, *Prevent and Reverse Heart Disease: The Revolutionary, Scientific, Nutrition-Based Cure*, Caldwell Esselstyn, Jr. M.D. asserts “Coronary heart disease is a benign food-borne illness which need never exist or progress,” and presents the results of a 20-year study—the longest study of its kind ever conducted—proving changes in diet and nutrition can actually cure heart disease. Dr. Esselstyn, a former internationally known surgeon, researcher, and clinician at the Cleveland Clinic, argues that conventional cardiology has failed patients by developing treatments that focus only on the symptoms of heart disease, not the cause.[23]

The study included 17 patients with advanced coronary artery disease who had a total of 49 cardiac episodes and had undergone aggressive treatment procedures, including multiple bypass operations. Five of them were given *less than a year to live*. Participants’ cholesterol levels, angina symptoms, and blood flow improved dramatically after a few months. After 5 years, their average cholesterol dropped from 246 mg/dL to 137. (Above 240 mg/dL is considered “high risk,” below 150 mg/dL is the total cholesterol level seen in cultures where heart disease is essentially nonexistent.) This is the most profound drop in cholesterol ever documented in the medical literature in a study of this type. Twelve years later, these participants had no further cardiac events. Those who adhered strictly to the diet, eliminating meat, dairy, fish, and added oil, survived beyond 20 years symptom free.

Their angiograms showed a widening of the coronary arteries, and thus a reversal of the disease. Dr. Esselstyn notes:

> "The dietary changes that have helped my patients over the past twenty years can help you, too. They can actually make you immune to heart attacks. And there is considerable evidence that they have benefits far beyond coronary artery disease. If you eat to save your heart, you eat to save yourself from other diseases of nutritional extravagance: from strokes, hypertension, obesity, osteoporosis, adult-onset diabetes, and possibly senile mental impairment, as well. You gain protection from a host of other ailments that have been linked to dietary factors, including impotence and cancers of the breast, prostate, colon, rectum, uterus, and ovaries."[24]

While, as noted, this is the longest study on the subject to date, there are other studies demonstrating the positive relationship between a plant-based diet and the reversal of IHD.

Research on Seventh-day Adventists, acknowledging that their overall health may also be the result of their refusal to drink alcohol or smoke, compared a group of Adventists with a group of meat-eating Mormons, similar in their religious commitment and abstinence from caffeine, alcohol, and tobacco. The Adventists had significantly lower blood pressure, obesity, and cholesterol levels than the Mormons.[25] Similar results have been found in other studies involving comparisons between vegetarian Adventists and other groups that have similar profiles except that the other groups are not green eaters.[26] Even more telling are studies that compare these meat-eating Adventists and their vegetarian counterparts; they showed, with the exception of those under 25 years of age that the meat eaters had higher serum cholesterol levels than the vegetarians.[27]

A similar study comparing cholesterol levels of vegetarian and non-vegetarian Seventh-day Adventist teenagers (aged 12-17) found that the vegetarians had significantly lower cholesterol levels.[28] While heart disease is not typically a concern for adolescents, patterns established early in life tend to continue on into later years, when risks of heart disease increase.

In addition to higher cholesterol in meat-eaters, levels of triglycerides—substances found in animal fats, which, when found to be in elevated levels in the blood, are connected to the occurrence of heart problems—are also higher in meat eaters.[29] Perhaps most telling of all is what we find when we look at death rates from heart problems. Again, looking at Adventists, a study in *The American Journal of Clinical Nutrition* found that "the risk of fatal coronary heart disease among non-vegetarian Seventh-day Adventist males, ages 35 to 64, is three times greater than [that for] vegetarian Seventh-day Adventist males of comparable age."[30] The report cites lower total or saturated fat intake and higher intake of dietary fiber as probable factors in the better statistics for the vegetarian group.

But the evidence doesn't stop there; recently, more and more information is coming to the fore regarding the value of a proper vegetarian diet in the reduction of heart disease. One study, published in January 2013 in *The American Journal of Clinical Nutrition*, reported that going meatless reduces the risk of heart disease by 32%. The study involved 44,561 men and women (34% of whom consumed a vegetarian diet) living in England and Scotland who were taking part in the European Prospective Investigation into Cancer and Nutrition (EPIC)-Oxford study.[31] The EPIC study—the largest detailed study of diet and health ever undertaken—commenced in 1992 and included 500,000 people in 10 European countries. Oxford was one of two United Kingdom "cohorts" (a large group of people who have joined a study and whose health is being followed). The strategy for establishing the EPIC-Oxford cohort was to recruit participants with a *wide range of diets* by targeting vegetarians as well as participants from the general UK population. Researchers praise the EPIC-Oxford for its great scientific value because the diets of vegetarians, and especially vegans, differ substantially from those of meat-eaters and this range in diets made it easier to detect relationships between nutrition and health.[32]

Another eye-opening study published in April of 2013 in the journal *Nature Medicine* by a research team led by Stanley Hazen, M.D, Ph.D., of Cleveland Clinic, unequivocally demonstrated the cardiovascular health benefits of vegan and vegetarian diets.[33] This time the study was not about saturated fat or cholesterol—two leading factors contributing to atherosclerosis (the hardening or clogging of the arteries)—it was for *carnitine*, a compound abundant in red meat and regularly added as a supplement to popular energy drinks.

In this case, the results of this study are significant in that they demonstrate the positive effects of a plant-based diet toward the prevention of heart disease, unrelated to lifestyle factors OTHER than the diet itself. Therefore, the results do not fall into the trap I noted above, where the value of the diet could be in question because of the health-enhancing effects of the vegetarian lifestyle.

Specifically, the study showed that bacteria living in the human digestive tract metabolize the compound carnitine, turning it into trimethylamine-N-oxide (TMAO), a metabolite—which simply means a product of metabolism—the researchers previously linked in a 2011 study to the promotion of atherosclerosis in humans. The research further found that a diet high in carnitine *promotes* the growth of the bacteria that metabolize carnitine, thereby compounding the problem by producing even more of the artery-clogging TMAO.

The study tested the carnitine and TMAO levels of omnivores, vegans, and vegetarians, and examined the clinical data of 2,595 patients undergoing elective cardiac evaluations. The researchers found that increased carnitine levels in patients predicted increased risks for cardiovascular disease and major cardiac events like heart attack, stroke, and death, *but only in subjects with concurrently high TMAO levels*. Additionally, they found that baseline TMAO levels were *significantly lower among vegans and vegetarians* than omnivores. Remarkably, vegans and vegetarians, even after consuming a large amount of carnitine, did not produce significant levels of the microbe product TMAO, whereas omnivores consuming the same amount of carnitine did.

"The bacteria living in our digestive tracts are dictated by our long-term dietary patterns," Hazen said. "A diet high in carnitine actually shifts our gut microbe composition to those that like carnitine, making meat eaters even more susceptible to forming TMAO and its artery-clogging effects. Meanwhile, vegans and vegetarians have a significantly reduced capacity to synthesize TMAO from carnitine, which may explain the cardiovascular health benefits of these diets."

Not that this holds more weight than studies by major hospitals like Cleveland Clinic, but even the American Heart Association now endorses various forms of vegetarian diets saying: "They're also usually lower than non-vegetarian diets in total fat, saturated fat and cholesterol. Many studies have shown that vegetarians seem to have a lower risk of obesity, coronary heart disease (which causes heart attack), high blood pressure, diabetes mellitus, and some forms of cancer."[34]

It is certainly advisable to reduce or eliminate as many risk factors to this disease as possible by introducing stress-reduction programs such as regular exercise, meditation, and yoga. In fact, *Mindfulness Based Stress Reduction (MBSR)*, a program created by Dr. Jon Kabat-Zinn at the University of Massachusetts Medical Center, has proven effective in reducing symptoms of anxiety and depression, perceived stress, blood pressure, and Body Mass Index (BMI) in patients with Coronary Heart Disease.[35] Over 18,000 patients with all manner of diagnoses have successfully completed the eight-week course, and 1,400 physicians have referred patients to the program. Published evaluations of the medical outcomes resulting from patient participation have shown a 35% reduction in the number of medical symptoms and a 40% reduction in psychological symptoms (stable over four years).[36, 37]

Further, the addition of meditation training to standard cardiac rehabilitation regimens has been shown to reduce mortality (41% decrease during the first two years following, and 46% reduction in recurrence rates) morbidity, psychological distress, and some biological risk factors (plasma lipids, weight, blood pressure, and blood glucose).[38, 39] Meditation practice alone has been shown to reduce exercise-induced myocardial ischemia in patients with coronary artery disease.[40, 41] We will speak more about the importance of mindfulness practices later in the book. Suffice it to say that learning how to live in the present moment has tremendous benefit, beyond improving physical health conditions.

Now back to our conversation on the effects of a plant-based diet on coronary heart disease. The 2015 USDA report recognizes the connection between lowering heart disease and eating a healthy diet, including a vegetarian diet. One study, comparing mortality in vegetarians and non-vegetarians, analyzed the combined data from five prospective studies to conclude that "mortality from ischemic heart disease was 24% lower in vegetarians than in non-vegetarians."[42] Another study from Loma Linda regarding Adventists found that vegetarians of African-American decent are at a lower risk for heart disease.[43] The study compared the cardiovascular risk factors between black vegetarians and non-vegetarians among more than 26,000 black Seventh-day Adventists from the Adventist Health Study-2 (AHS-2). Those who are vegetarians are at lower risk for heart disease, compared with their meat-eating counterparts. Black vegetarian Adventists were at less risk for hypertension, diabetes, high blood pressure, total cholesterol, and high blood-LDL cholesterol. Vegans and vegetarians who consume eggs and dairy were the least at risk for cardiovascular disease, followed by vegetarians who infrequently eat meat, vegetarians who eat fish, and non-vegetarians.

Another meta-study, on the possible relationship between fruit and vegetable consumption and strokes, the third leading cause of death in America[44], analyzed the data from eight studies on 257,551 people, with an average follow-up of 13 years. Also, as reported in *The Lancet*, researchers found that those who ate more than five servings of fruits and vegetables a day were 26% less likely to suffer a stroke over the course of the study than those who ate less than three daily helpings.[45]

An examination of hypertension among four diet groups—meat eaters, fish eaters, vegetarians, and vegans—found "significant" differences in both rates of hypertension (self-reported) and mean blood pressure across the groups, with meat eaters at the high end of the measures and vegans at the low end. The authors of the study concluded, "Non-meat eaters, especially vegans, have a lower prevalence of hypertension, and lower systolic and diastolic blood pressures than meat eaters, largely because of differences in body mass index."[46]

The ability of vegetarian eating to lower a person's chances of suffering certain health problems may be because a healthy organic diet of whole plant foods contains a proper balance of fruits, vegetables, nuts, seeds, legumes, and healthy oils—walnuts, walnut butter, olive oil, olives, black cumin seed oil, flaxseed oil, the omega–3 fatty acids—all of which have been shown to lessen the degree of heart disease and stroke. Multiple studies from Loma Linda University in California studying Seventh-day Adventists have shown that the group that adheres to a vegetarian diet has less heart disease, and they're able to obtain the essential nutrients, including calcium, for their bones.[47] Their intake of iron and vitamins A, B, and C is higher than average as well. Vitamin B1 is more plentiful in the vegetarian diet because it's found in wheat germ, buckwheat, and legumes.[48] In fact, the vegetarian diet closely resembles the Dietary Goals for the United States developed by the Senate Select Committee on Nutrition and Human Needs.

Having seen such investigations and statistics on vegetarian eating, an increasing number of doctors are speaking out about the health benefits of a plant-based diet. Dr. Neal Barnard, M.D., president of the Physicians Committee for Responsible Medicine, has mustered an impressive army of studies and sources to support his contention that non-meat-eaters have a lower prevalence of such cardiac risk factors as elevated cholesterol, obesity, and high blood pressure and consequently lower levels of IHD and of heart disease mortality. "The prevalence of ischemic heart disease is markedly reduced in populations which avoid meat… Those who avoid meat products also have a reduced risk of heart disease mortality."[49]

Indeed, Dr. Barnard is quite a booster of vegetarianism. He believes the literature demonstrates that "cancer risk is elevated by foods that are high in animal fat," and that "those who avoid fatty meat products… have a much lower incidence of non-insulin-dependent diabetes, compared to non-vegetarians."[50]

Lowering Cancer Risk

Cancer comes in many varieties. In looking at factors that may reduce its incidence, as researchers did with heart disease, scientists have turned to examining the health patterns of Adventists. The results have been encouraging indeed.

First off, let us note that broadly speaking the consumption of animal products in numerous studies, as summarized in a piece in the *International Journal of Cancer,* has been correlated with the appearance of cancers of the colon, rectum, pancreas, breast, ovary, uterine corpus, and prostate.[51] By contrast, those who rely on plants for their nutrition, such as the vegetarian Seventh-day Adventists, fare much better. It's been reported that "the risk of fatal cancer among Seventh-day Adventist males is 53% of the risk among all US white males of comparable age. For Seventh-day Adventist females, the risk is 68% of that in all US white females."[52] Furthermore, a recent study shows that vegetarians are 22% less likely to develop colorectal cancers[53], which is the second-leading cause of cancer death in the United States after lung cancer. The risk was reduced by 16% for vegans, although the least at risk were vegetarians who ate fish compared to non-vegetarians. Data from food questionnaires and medical records was analyzed for over 77,000 subjects from the Adventist Health Study-2 over seven years. "The main message is to avoid all meats, as the main result was that all vegetarians as a group did better than the non-vegetarians," said Dr. Gary Fraser, principal investigator for Adventist Health Studies-2 and study co-author, in an e-mail interview. He continued by saying that "replacing meats with vegetables, nuts, legumes, and fruits will most likely decrease risk of colorectal cancer."[54]

A writer in the *Journal of Environmental Pathology and Toxicology* speculates that such positive outcomes may be the product of certain chemicals, either present or lacking, in the vegetarian diet. According to the writer:

> Perhaps as a result of their vegetarian diet, Adventists have a lower intake of benzopyrene and nitrosamines and a higher intake of flavones, which are strong inducers of the enzyme systems responsible for detoxifying such carcinogens. In addition, they may have a higher intake of vitamins A and C, recently suggested as possible protective agents against certain chemical carcinogens. Thus, it seems reasonable to suggest that the typical Adventist diet may protect against many of the major sites of cancer.[55]

Let's continue for a moment with this theme of the possible cancer-preventive ingredients in a vegetarian diet. Two studies found anti-cancer properties for phytosterols in humans, reporting that "total phytosterols were associated with a strong inverse relationship with stomach cancer,"[56] although the other did not find such an effect.[57]

Aside from phytochemicals, another component of a vegetarian diet that may be playing a system-protective role in cancer prevention is fiber. I shared its properties, including speeding of digestion, earlier in this book. Here let me simply emphasize (with my own italicization) some conclusions found in a piece on dietary links to colon cancer in *Annals of Surgery*:

> Current epidemiologic data have shown that there are striking differences in the incidence of colon cancer in various parts of the world. It has been demonstrated that the occurrence of cancer of the colon is much lower in East Africa, India and Japan than in Western Europe or North America... Nutritional substances such as *fiber*, refined carbohydrate, animal fat and protein have all been advanced as being the significant factor responsible for the variance in incidence rates of colonic cancer... [The article, then shifts from the components of a vegetarian diet that may reduce cancer risk, and notes one important action of these components.] Further studies have shown that the levels of bile acids, as well as the degradation products and enzymes responsible for the degradation of bile acids in the colonic lumen, are decreased in this group of vegetarians.[58]

The bile acids referred to are associated with colon cancer risk, and they have been shown to be lower in vegetarians.[59] It's noteworthy that the vegetarian-oriented Adventists have a colon cancer mortality rate only 61% that of the general US population for males, and 70% for females.[60]

Again and again diet comes up as an important factor in colon cancer. From *The American Journal of Clinical Nutrition*:

> Recent epidemiological studies associate colon cancer with specific types of diet. In general, highly developed countries have a high incidence of colon cancer, and less well developed countries have a low incidence. Japan represents an exception in that it is highly developed but has a low incidence of large bowel cancer. Japanese who adopt a Western diet, however, develop colon cancer with increased frequency; among Japanese immigrants, the frequency approaches that of Native Americans.[61]

From another report: "Cholesterol and its metabolites, together with bile acids, are implicated as risk factors in the genesis and progression of colon cancer…"[62] As we know, a high-meat regimen increases levels of these harmful substances.

Let's turn to a second widely occurring cancer, that of the prostate, which for American men follows only lung cancer in malignancy.[63] Vegetarians seem less prone to be brought down by this killer. One study noted that green-eating Seventh-day Adventist men aged 45 to 70 have a prostate cancer mortality rate only 30% that of men in the general California population. (Many Adventists live in that state.) This suggests that vegetarianism may be a protective factor against the disease, and researchers who have studied this conclude, "Implications include the possible modification of prostate cancer risk through dietary intervention."[64]

As has already been suggested, across the board Adventist vegetarians have reduced cancer risk. A 1994 article in The *American Journal of Clinical Nutrition* titled, "Cancer Incidence Among California Seventh-day Adventists, 1976-1982," found:

- For prostate cancer, a high consumption pattern of beans, lentils, peas, tomatoes, raisins, dates, and other dried fruits was associated with lower cancer risk in this analysis.

- High consumption of fruits was significantly associated with lower lung cancer risk even after adjusting for smoking. Higher risk of colon cancer was associated with higher consumption of saturated fats. Lower risk of colon cancer was associated with higher fiber and legume consumption.
- Higher consumption of soy-based products was associated with markedly lower risk of pancreas cancer in this population. Consumption of dried fruits, beans, lentils, and peas was also significantly associated with lower risk. … Risk of bladder cancer increased twofold in association with high meat intake.[65]

I wanted to stress how broadly their vegetarian diet appears to protect Adventists from cancer, and so diverted my attention from the last specific cancer we were discussing, that of the prostate.

There are other studies relevant to the link between prostate health and a vegetarian diet. In a sign of the times, even The American Cancer Society website notes, "Another study found that men who choose not to have treatment for their localized prostate cancer may be able to slow its growth with intensive lifestyle changes." They continue on to note a study conducted by University of California, San Francisco, researchers. The men in the study ate a vegan diet and exercised frequently; they also took part in support groups and yoga. After one year the men saw, on average, a slight drop in their PSA level.[66] Another study conducted by Doctors at the University of Massachusetts Medical School in Worcester reported similar findings: Men that had been diagnosed with prostate cancer slowed the disease's progression by switching to a low-fat, vegetarian diet.[67]

Furthermore, in 2005, University of California researchers determined that men who have been treated for prostate cancer are less likely to have a recurrence if they maintain a healthy weight. The study specifically reported that obese men, defined as those with a body mass index (BMI) greater than 30, were found to have a 30% increased risk of cancer recurrence, compared with those with lower body weights. Very obese patients (BMI greater than 35) had the greatest risk of recurrence—about 70% higher than thinner men. Results emphasize the importance of maintaining a healthy weight.[68]

Even though the purpose of this section is to inform you of the health-protective features of green eating as it relates to cancer, there are too large a number of studies espousing the values of a plant-based diet to run through them here. Let me merely end the section by mentioning, as a final contrast, two other notable findings—one attributing cancer-avoiding properties to a plant-based regimen, the other pointing the finger at a meat-based eating plan in relation to another cancer. An article on pancreatic cancer risk in the journal *Cancer* reported, "Increasing consumption of vegetarian protein products, beans, lentils, and peas, as well as dried fruit, was associated with highly significant protective relationships to pancreas cancer risk."[69]

Finally, research on brain tumors reported in the journal *Neuroepidemiology* found that "increasing use of meat, poultry or fish… was associated with increased risk estimates for gliomas [tumors]. This increase in risk was especially apparent for consumption of pork products." The report went on to explain that "since many pork products are cured with sodium nitrite, this may be consistent with the hypothesis that foods containing high concentrations of N-nitroso compounds may increase brain cancer risk."[70]

I have given you some information on how vegetarianism offers relief from two of the major killer diseases. These topics were mentioned in passing in the book, but one other pressing matter I want to get to has not yet been addressed. This is the particular value to women of going green.

Women's Health Concerns

As talked about in our general remarks on Seventh-day Adventist vegetarians, women from this group have lower cancer mortality rates than women in the general population, including from breast and endometrial cancers. One reason for this may be that diet affects hormonal patterns, and these patterns are critically important factors in women's disease risk.[71]

One way hormones are linked to disease relates to the age of a young woman's first menstruation. An early onset of this physical change has been seen as contributing to greater breast cancer risk. The increasing appearance of breast cancer in the West, then, may be tied to the fact that the age of menarche, or first menstruation, has been decreasing. Such a speeding up of puberty seems to be the product of our changing diet, with more fat, simple carbohydrates, and hormone-laden meat.

How much of an issue is it? [72] Let's say that the statistics are curious. In an article appearing in the Women's Health Activist Newsletter in the fall of 2009, Kathleen O'Grady reports that, "the average age of first menstruation in White US girls has declined by several years, from an average of 13 to 17 years of age… White girls in the US now menstruate at an average age of 12.6 years; African American girls at 12.1 years; and Latinas at 12.2 years." It is believed that these differences result from continuous exposure "to low-level endocrine disruptors in their diets, drinking water and air supply" which mimic hormones in the body.

It stands to reason, then, that living as *naturally* as possible—from the food and water we consume to the products we use—is essential for a balanced physiology, and psychology for this matter. We used to be able to say living "close to nature" was the way to go, and it would be if we weren't currently experiencing the level of toxicity that we do in our water, soil, and air.

Even still, researchers have proven experimentally that this "trend toward early menarche can be reversed when a balanced vegetarian diet is selected in place of the ordinary American diet."[73] Other researchers, again turning to the valued subject of Adventists, have found that the maturation delay of vegetarian Adventist teenage girls, compared with meat-eating schoolgirls, "may carry potential health benefits in adult life. A later age of menarche has been consistently associated with decreased risk for several cancers, particularly of the breast."[74]

Turning our look now from early on in a woman's life cycle to much later, it is agreed that maintaining necessary mineral content in bones is a primary concern for older women. Here, too, vegetarians have an advantage, as green eating has been shown to contribute to strong bones in post-menopausal women. As researchers explain, "The primary dietary characteristics of a lacto-ovo vegetarian diet that may be of benefit to bone tissue are the sources of protein and quantities of calcium and phosphorus in the diet. Investigators [further]… suggest that vegetable protein produces a lower-acid ash than animal protein when metabolized and thus helps to conserve calcium."[75] Statistics reported in the *Journal of the American Dietetic Association* back up this contention: "Lacto-ovo vegetarian women 50 to 59 years of age lost 18% bone mineral mass while omnivorous women lost 35%."[76]

However, take caution in interpreting this, as you can eat all the dairy products that you wish. Amy Lanou Ph.D., author of *Building Bone Vitality, and c*hair and associate professor of health and wellness for the University of North Carolina, Asheville, states that, "The countries with the highest rates of osteoporosis are the ones where people drink the most milk and have the most calcium in their diets. The connection between calcium consumption and bone health is actually very weak, and the connection between dairy consumption and bone health is almost nonexistent." She continues: "Vegetarian diets can help people build strong bones, and plant-based diets reduce the risk of heart disease, diabetes, and cancer. To build strong bones and healthy bodies, people need weight-bearing exercise and low-acid, plant-based diets rich in fruits and vegetables."

Moreover, the 12-year-long Harvard Nurses' Health Study found that those who consumed the most calcium from dairy foods broke more bones than those who rarely drank milk. By the way, this is a broad study based on 77,761 women aged 34 through 59 years of age. In the authors' own words, "These data do not support the hypothesis that higher consumption of milk or other food sources of calcium by adult women protects against hip or forearm fractures."[77]

In an article on SaveOurBones.com, Vivian Goldschmidt, MA writes, "Even drinking milk from a young age does not protect against future fracture risk but actually increases it."[78] Shattering the '"savings account"' calcium theory, Cumming and Klineberg report their study findings as follows: "Consumption of dairy products, particularly at age 20 years, was associated with an increased risk of hip fracture in old age."[79]

What does the research currently say about vegan diets and their effect on bone health? Two things: One study reports that vegetarian diets, particularly vegan diets, are associated with lower BMD (Bone Mineral Deficiency), but that the magnitude of the association is clinically insignificant.[80] A second study by the same authors reported that a vegan diet did not have adverse effect on bone loss and fracture. The report further notes that corticosteroid use and high intakes of animal protein and animal lipid were negatively associated with bone loss.[81]

Here are some lifestyle topics and suggestions from Harvard School of Public Health for being the healthiest possible vegetarian:

- Getting regular exercise, especially weight-bearing and muscle strengthening exercise.
- Getting adequate vitamin D, whether through diet, exposure to sunshine, or supplements.
- Consuming enough calcium to reduce the amount the body has to borrow from bone.
- Consuming adequate vitamin K, found in green, leafy vegetables.
- Not getting too much preformed vitamin A.[82]

Again, the effect of vegetarianism on women's health is too large a topic to cover in one section, but enough has been said to make clear that balanced green eating offers a cornucopia of health benefits to women.

From Dental Health to Diabetes: The Benefits of Vegetarianism Abound

We've talked about a number of important areas in which green eating has proved to be remarkable in fending off disease and lowering the risk of physiological factors that are a prelude to ill health, such as the presence of unhealthy cholesterol. I don't want to try to cover all the regions in which there have been studies testifying to the worth of vegetarianism, because there's far too much out there. The evidence on the health-enhancing effects of green eating has been piling up for years. Still, rather than neglecting this other material totally, it might be of value to give you a sample of the range of information that has been accumulating regarding the health enrichment and protection that follows from green eating.

Beginning in this section, I will call attention to a few articles by quoting them in sample form and continuing. Then I will give more details when I get to the topic of plant nutrients in the next chapter, so as to convey a sense of the scope and depth of the available research, which has been replicated repeatedly. Yes, it will be something of a grab-bag, but one from which I don't doubt you will pull some facts that are significant for you. Here are some conclusions drawn by various scientists following scientific investigations into the value of vegetarianism:

- ...[It was found that] the dental and periodontal status of the Seventh-day Adventist group was significantly better than that of the controls, suggesting that vegetarianism is beneficial to oral health.[83]

- … when healthy elderly vegetarian women are compared with closely matched non-vegetarian peers, the vegetarian diet is associated with several benefits, primarily lower blood glucose and lipid levels.[84]
- After controlling for height, boys and girls in the Seventh-day Adventist schools were found to be leaner than their public school peers… These results suggest that a health oriented lifestyle in childhood and adolescence, such as the one followed by Seventh-day Adventists, is compatible with adequate growth and associated with a lower weight for height.[85]
- During 21 years [of study and follow-up], the rate of diabetes as an underlying cause of death in Adventists was only 45% of the rate for all US whites.[86]
- All-cause mortality showed a significant negative association with green salad consumption and a significant positive association with consumption of eggs and meat. For green salad and eggs, the association was stronger for women; for meat, the association was stronger for men. All the observed associations were adjusted for age, sex, smoking history, history of major chronic disease, and age at initial exposure to the Adventist Church.[87]
- Systolic [maximum] blood pressure in Adventists was lower in early adult life and rose less with aging than in the other two groups [from the general population]. This pattern also occurred with diastolic [minimum] blood pressure. [Maximum and minimum rates depend on when the heart has acted, the flow being stronger right after the heart pumps.]… The differences in plasma lipid levels between Adventists and other population groups can be explained by a vegetarian diet, and this may have contributed also to the blood pressure levels.[88]
- [In a study] vegetarian students consumed significantly higher amounts of calcium and phosphorus than did omnivore students, suggesting that… the vegetarian students were making superior food pattern selections.[89]

Having given you a lot of detail quickly in that spate of citations, let me now finish up by enlarging a little on the ideas presented in the last note—that vegetarians tend to have superior nutritional status as shown by measures of important nutrients. This idea has been seconded by numerous studies, such as one presented in the *Journal of the American Dietetic Association*, whose method was to first match groups of vegetarian and non-vegetarian elderly women for a variety of non-dietary factors, and then ask them to keep records of what they ate over a week-long period. Looking at the results they provided, it was seen that vegetarians consumed significantly less cholesterol, saturated fatty acids, and caffeine, but more carbohydrates, dietary fiber, magnesium, vitamins E and A, thiamin, pantothenic acid, copper, and manganese. "In summary," said the report, "when healthy elderly women were compared with closely matched non-vegetarian peers, the vegetarian diet was associated with improved nutrient intake and associated reductions in blood glucose and lipid levels."[90]

You see in this study that the vegetarian diet was providing not only more nutrients, but a better internal environment with less cholesterol in the blood. These results were backed up by another study pairing vegetarian and omnivorous postmenopausal women, with the diets of the vegetarian being found to provide:

- Higher nutrient density for folate, thiamin, vitamin C, and vitamin A
- Lower total fat, saturated fatty acids, and cholesterol
- Higher dietary fiber.[91]

Other studies further emphasize the nutrient- and fiber-rich nature of vegetarian eating.[92-94]

Still, you will want to take note here that there are consistent vitamin deficiencies (vitamin D, iron, B12, etc.) that vegetarians are susceptible to and need to guard against. These will be addressed in the next chapter on the diet of the healthy vegetarian. Before this, we will finish our conversation on the good news about vegetarianism.

Aging Gracefully

In one recent, six-month, in-depth holistic lifestyle study, incorporating vegetarianism and extensive supplementation, our aim was to show that vegetarians can not only reap the benefits of living healthier, longer lives, but can also look better and younger while aging gracefully.

As I've discussed in other books, when I talk about looking better and aging gracefully, I'm not speaking about images promulgated by Madison Avenue—ultra-thinness for women and chiseled jaws for men—but rather the glow of loveliness that almost always accompanies a fit person free from disease and distress that honors themselves, others, and the natural world by living purposefully into a peaceful existence.

Conventional medicine focuses on treating symptoms of diseases after healthy functioning has broken down, rather than on creating health. Our goal in this study was to maintain and improve already existing healthy functioning as well as to bolster areas in which optimal functioning had lapsed. Specifically, we wanted to improve the condition of the subjects' hair and skin, which are observable indicators of the aging process, and of some weakening of metabolic processes. Many participants had experienced balding, thinning, or graying hair for at least seven years. While the general public explains such changes in older people as the inevitable and unavoidable expression of their years, my perception before starting the study was that many, not all, of these effects were the result of a breakdown that was *reversible*.

To see how to accomplish a shift in these typical aging patterns, we studied the effects of changes in five lifestyle components: nutrition, physical activity, stress management, attitude, and personal environment. This study was part of a larger, ongoing study that measured levels of function in participants, using such parameters as weight, blood pressure, cholesterol levels, hormone levels, and overall wellness. For this particular six-month component of the examination, we focused in on measuring the quality of the subjects' hair and skin.

Our study, focused on people who had the type of hair change and loss that most people consider a "natural" part of aging. We were aiming at the seemingly impossible goals of inducing new hair growth in bald areas, slowing thinning, and reversing graying. For skin, our second concern, the goal was to reverse the effects of sun damage and premature aging.

Participants aged 55 and older did well with the protocols, scoring improvements in hair, skin, and functioning; but the mean scores of younger participants were significantly better in 11 of the 42 measures. Also, the mean scores of women were significantly better in 12 of the 42 measures. Please see Appendix A for further details on this study.

The Bottom Line—a Longer, Healthier Life

My last point in this discussion is more holistic. I frequently noted that the adoption of a vegetarian diet is often, and should be, linked to a particular worldview, one that emphasizes harmony with nature—an environmentalist ethic, per se. While the scientists who have studied vegetarians are looking at them simply as green eaters and not delving into their philosophies, they have found one holistic relationship: that the many health benefits seen so far all add up to green eaters living longer and healthier lives.

Here is one finding from a book on plant proteins: "Compared to Adventists who heavily use meat, the vegetarian Adventists have a substantially lower risk of fatal coronary disease, fatal diabetes and death from any cause, especially among men. Among men who use few animal products... the risk of fatal prostate cancer is one third that of Adventist men who heavily use such products."[95]

Studies conducted at Loma Linda University revealed that Seventh-day Adventists (aged 45-54) who eat meat six or more times per week are three times as likely to die of heart disease as vegetarian Seventh-day Adventists... [and] have twice the incidence of obesity (30% overweight or above), which is related to increased death rate from diabetes... Vegetarian Seventh-day Adventist women aged 55 and above have significantly less osteoporosis than the meat-eating non-Seventh-day Adventists.[96]

Remember my earlier mention of the European Prospective Investigation into Cancer and Nutrition (EPIC)-Oxford study, which showed that vegetarians had a 32% lower risk of hospitalization or dying from cardiovascular disease.[97] Researchers owe these results to the improved cholesterol profiles and lower blood pressure in the vegetarian population.[98,99]

Good health in your later years is intimately tied to your quality of life, throughout life. While the effects of smoking and heavy drinking can be largely reversed, this must be done with a radical change of lifestyle and early enough in life to result in a longer, healthy lifespan. Those who are in poor health, who consistently rely on pharmaceuticals throughout life, and who make frequent visits to the hospital don't have the chance to reap the rewards of their long experience or of the greater free time they may have received at retirement.

The same point made in the last-cited study is repeated in an examination of lifestyle and the use of health services described in a 1994 issue of *The American Journal of Clinical Nutrition*. Close to 30,000 Seventh-day Adventists were divided into four groups: vegetarian and non-vegetarian, men and women. They were then tracked for a year to see how much health care they required.

The results? Non-vegetarians reported more overnight hospitalizations, surgeries, and X-rays than their vegetarian counterparts. Medication use by non-vegetarian males was double that of their peers, while the rate for non-vegetarian females ranged from 70 to 115% higher. In short, the vegetarians were simply healthier. "We conclude that a vegetarian diet may decrease the prevalence of chronic disease, medication use, and health services use, and thus, potentially, health care costs," said the study.[100]

I myself have been convinced of these conclusions and have been for a long time. One has only to examine the vast body of scientific literature to see why. Though I want to continue looking at health benefits in the next chapter, these last two studies are ones to always bear in mind. It's not only that green eating helps you prevent and/or avoid disease, but that it is a foundation for overall well-being. When 17th-century English poet and Anglican priest George Herbert wrote, "Living well is the best revenge," I believe he was not talking about having tons of money, but rather was referring to something much better in the long run—keeping throughout your long life the full bloom of health. This is what we will explore next: What is the diet and lifestyle of the healthy vegetarian?

Chapter 5

The Diet of a Healthy Vegetarian

> "When I was 88 years old, I gave up meat entirely and switched to a plant foods diet following a slight stroke. During the following months, I not only lost 50 pounds, but gained strength in my legs and picked up stamina. Now, at age 93, I'm on the same plant-based diet, and I still don't eat any meat or dairy products. I either swim, walk, or paddle a canoe daily and I feel the best I've felt since my heart problems began."
>
> *—Benjamin Spock, M.D., The famous Dr. Spock pediatrician and author (1903-1998)*

We've just discussed many of the health reasons to turn to a vegetarian diet. Now we will take a look at what the diet of a healthy vegetarian looks like and how to actually make this transition.

Making any changes in one's life requires three basic things: *knowing what you want and visualizing the outcome, getting enough education and support to make the change*, and then *finding joyful ways of engaging in the new pattern that you desire.* Before you know it, you will have accomplished your new reality. Life is meant to be a fun and joyful exploration; this can also be said about adopting a vegetarian lifestyle… at any age!

Making the Shift to Vegetarianism

It's Getting a Little Easier Now…

Our lifestyle study, mentioned in the *Aging Gracefully* section in the previous chapter, was not a boot camp in the traditional sense, because participants were still living their normal lives, going to work, relaxing, and socializing. Nor was it an environment where hostile authorities forced participants to follow the rules. But it did resemble such a training camp in one way. People who fully participated had to throw much of their old way of living out the window.

Our study is not the only one that supports the benefit of an entire lifestyle reversal. Even the 2015 USDA report recommends a lifestyle overhaul. In fact, some practitioners argue for an even more abrupt immersion in change. Dr. McDougall, whose work we discussed earlier, feels that people can turn around "chronic" diseases of aging, such as high levels of blood-serum lipids, obesity, and hypertension, *in two weeks or less*. Though mainstream scientists discount Dr. McDougall's claims about re-growing hair and improving joint and skin conditions through nutritional efforts, our study suggest that his claims have merit.

McDougall was alerted to this direction for his vegetarian program when he was living in Hawaii and noted that seniors who ate a mostly plant-based diet lived longer, healthier lives than their offspring, whose diets were more typically American, bursting with animal protein and fats.

Some researchers, such as doctors W.S. Collens and G.B. Dobkins, continuing a point made earlier, say the green diet is far better health-wise because our bodies aren't suited for meat. They argue, "While designed to subsist on vegetarian foods, [modern man] has perverted his dietary habits to accept the food of the carnivore… Herein may lie the basis for the high incidence of human atherosclerotic disease."[1]

The basis of their claim resides among such facts as our flat teeth are not sharp enough to tear through hide, flesh, or bones. Earlier, I noted the inadequate length of our digestive systems for processing animal flesh, which cannot, like that of omnivores, quickly dispose of the meat they eat before it putrefies. Our long digestive system (which can be up to 30 feet in an adult male) is closer to those found in herbivores, and the enzyme we secrete in our mouth, amylase, (one that carnivores don't have) breaks down complex plant cells. Further, carnivores have an enzyme (called uricase) that humans don't have to break down the uric acid in meat. Excess amounts of uric acid are a strain on the human body. As we learned previously, the kidneys, in an attempt to neutralize the toxic effects of meat, can be overstrained, resulting in such unwanted results as the formation of calcium urate crystals, which are responsible for many painful conditions like gout, bursitis, rheumatism, and lower back pain.

Having come this far in the book, you won't likely need to compare herbivore and carnivore physiology to be struck by the numerous health advantage of vegetarianism. Still, there is plenty of writing on this in other publications, like the bestselling book *The China Study* by T. Collin Campbell, Ph.D. or *Food for Life: How the New Four Food Groups Can Save Your Life* by Neal Barnard, M.D. if you require more convincing. Moreover, it is important to note that plant-based eating is adopted not only by green eaters, but by individuals arriving at higher levels of consciousness on any number of issues—spiritual, environmental, and social, to name a few.

Medical Professionals Are Catching On

Modern health professionals, who have been diligently and patiently educating their colleagues and the public about the health benefits of vegetarianism, did not just come on the scene. Greek physician Hippocrates, born around 400 BC and known as the father of modern medicine, used a plant-based diet to help people heal from a host of illnesses. He is famous for having said "Let thy food be thy medicine, and thy medicine be thy food." There are a number of physicians throughout the centuries since then who recommended green eating. More recently, in the 1700s, a vegetarian diet was prescribed, not unreasonably, for dissolving kidney stones and curing gout. In the 1800s, medical journals described flesh-free diets for treating tumors and cancerous ulcers. Bringing these historical references closer to today, in 1945, celebrated physician Antone Cocchi gained attention by proclaiming the preventive and healing benefits of the vegetarian diet.

However, most doctors, like the average American green eater, become interested in vegetarianism, not after looking at cultural studies of more vegetarian societies or even spiritual viewpoints, but because of its undeniable health aspects. Dr. Philip White, a director of the Department of Foods and Nutrition of the American Medical Association (AMA), brings up this component of the vegetarian outlook in these remarks: "Several studies have shown that vegans have lower serum cholesterol levels than their non-vegan counterparts, undoubtedly due to the substitution of vegetable oils for animal fats… There have also been studies suggesting that a diet high in fiber can bring about a decrease in serum cholesterol."[2] Like many enlightened doctors, White is focused on prevention. In this case, he is forestalling the difficulties associated with high cholesterol and the impact of vegetarianism on the problem.

Dr. Mark Hegsted, former chief nutritionist for the federal government, editor of *Nutrition Review,* and member of the National Academy of Sciences, also has placed a major focus in his own educational work on stopping disease as opposed to fighting it after it has already cropped up. This is why he finds fault with a meat-heavy diet. "The risks associated with eating this diet are demonstrably large. The question to be asked, therefore, is not why we should change our diet, but why not? What are the risks associated with eating less meat, less fat, less saturated fat, less cholesterol, less sugar, less salt, and more fruits, vegetables, unsaturated fat, and cereal products, especially whole grain cereals? There are none that can be identified and important benefits can be expected."[3] These thoughts are mature reflections on a study Hegsted and his Harvard co-workers published in 1955, in which they defended vegetarianism against detractors who argue such eating leads quickly to ill health. In the study they state that, on the contrary, "It is difficult to obtain a mixed vegetable diet, which will produce an appreciable loss of body protein." In their eyes, a vegetarian diet is quite healthy or, metaphorically said, "A step in the right direction."[4]

More recently, The Nutrition Institute of Mexico echoed these ideas by asserting, "The Western habit of eating meat is not necessarily healthy. It is a false assumption that only a diet based on animal products helps you stay in good health."[5] In a report, this institution went on to say that the traditional diet eaten by many in the developing world, based largely on grains and vegetables, is actually ideal for everyone.

Around the same time as the Mexican report was published, back in the 1980s, the AMA countered such pro-green eating assertions with the blunt statement, "A strictly vegetarian diet may lead to deformities and even death."[6] Alex Hershaft, president of the Vegetarian Information Service, didn't take this jibe lying down. The comment, to his mind, simply reflected the level of consciousness of the institution issuing it, so he said: "The AMA has experienced a loss of credibility." Even more unfortunate, as he reflected on the situation, was that many who still believed in the AMA would shun green eating on its flawed advice. These are his poignant words:

> The biggest losers are those who… deferred their turn to vegetarianism and a healthier, more ethical life, because they believe in the competence and honesty of AMA news releases. Each year, nearly 500,000 people in this country die of heart disease, 200,000 of stroke and over 80,000 of cancer of the colon and breast... an overwhelming fraction of these deaths are linked to the consumption of animal fat and meat, cholesterol, salt and sugar. Any individual or organization that deters the American people from embracing a meatless diet… must bear the responsibility for some of these deaths.[7]

Taking a broader view, the *Vegetarian Times* said at the time, "The handling of this story by the press and the AMA shows that we still have a long way to go in clearing up the misinformation and confusion that exists when it comes to vegetarianism."[8]

I don't bring up this argument to hark back to ancient history. Rather, I am trying to make clear that in the US some of the same stones are being cast at vegetarianism today as were being hurled 30 years ago. But there is a difference. Today, with more scientific evidence demonstrating the adequacy—even the superiority—of the vegetarian diet, and now the US Department of Agriculture acknowledging the diet as superior for both health and the sustainability of our species, the attacks on vegetarianism are becoming easier to repel.

The 18th-century French economist and politician Brillat-Savarin said, "The destiny of a people depends on the nature of its diet." I say, a country can change its direction if it changes its diet. I've been, perhaps idealistically, steadfastly harkening for several decades now that if the more affluent part of the world's population shifted toward vegetarian eating and settled on a new value set—a more modest, less consumption-obsessed existence where creative service to humanity and the sustainability of the planet were the priority—there would most certainly be more to go around. Hence, we would see a significant drop-off in the violence and wars so characteristic of our "modern" world, most often stemming from fights over possessions and the oppression of others. This, of course, flies in the face of what humans most want, which is a cooperative, loving, creative experience on the human plane. The vegetarian diet most certainly supports this… and more.

What a Healthy Vegetarian Diet Looks Like

The Basics

Eating a healthy vegetarian diet isn't difficult. You have to be sure of two things: 1) You're eating a full variety of fruits, vegetables, legumes, grains, nuts, and seeds and 2) You're getting the essential nutrients you were used to getting from animal flesh, including vitamin B12, iron, Omega-3s, and protein.

I will take up the discussion of protein in the next chapter because it is a discussion unto itself, in particular because there are far too many false ideas related to protein still circulating today and questions about the value of plant-based protein.

In this chapter, you will find the essentials related to a healthy vegetarian diet, as well as a discussion on important nutrients and lifestyle points that one must pay attention to when deciding to become vegetarian.

Let's start with a basic healthy composition of the healthy vegetarian diet. In the course of a day, you will want follow this general idea: start your diet with those foods that are going to give you protein (see Chapter 6 to calculate your ideal amount of protein), high quality fats (essential fatty acids), quality fibers, antioxidants, and phytonutrients, in this order. So each day, I make sure that I include beans (see Appendix C for protein content of key vegetarian foods, including beans), since they are a quality source of protein *and* fiber, as well as some antioxidants and phytonutrients. Beans are highly versatile, and it is ideal to have many varieties on hand in your pantry. We will speak more about this a little later in the chapter.

Once you have your beans, then you have your grains, which must be whole and unrefined. You will want to have at least nine different grains on hand for use in soups, salads and stir-fries. See the list later in this chapter for ideas. Grains offer complementing amino acids to beans plus fiber. You will want to make sure that you have these each day. By the way, the nice thing about beans and grains is that they can all be made in one day and frozen to be used later in the week.

In addition, you will want to make sure that you have some powders, like hemp, split-pea powder, rice powder, and non-GMO soy powder. You can add powders to your smoothie in the morning to get anywhere from 20-30 grams of complete protein, which is the equivalent of two cans of beans. You are getting one-third to a half of your total protein for the day in a single scoop in the morning, so, powders are essential.

Next are nuts and seeds, which contain some protein, but more importantly, healthy fats. Consume nuts in two primary forms: first, you should never have the dry roasted, salted variety; instead, consume raw nuts, or raw, sprouted organic nut butters, which are ideal because they are already ground, making them easier to digest. Almond, pistachio, walnut, cashew and macadamia are ideal and provide critical essential fatty acids. Remember seeds and raw, sprouted organic seed butters, too: sunflower, pumpkin, and sesame, as well as sunflower butter, pumpkin seed butter, and sesame butter, more commonly called tahini. Tahini butter is made by pulverizing sesame seeds, which are so small that they don't open up during digestion, and end up passing through the body in their undigested form. So, you have a much greater chance of benefitting from the oils and lignans, phytonutrients that provide a host of benefits to the body including helping to regulate hormone levels, improve prostate health, and reduce the stress hormone cortisol[9] when you consume tahini. We will talk more about the benefits of nuts in the nut section a little later in the chapter. A closing note: always store nuts and seeds in a refrigerator, ideally in a freezer, and nut and seed butters in the refrigerator so they last longer.

You also want to get some essential oils into the diet; namely, extra virgin organic olive oil but also organic coconut oil, flaxseed oil, hemp oil, avocado oil, and sesame oil. I generally use oil on salads and add a tablespoon of coconut, flax, or hemp oil into smoothies. Oils provide crucial essential fatty acids that benefit your heart and your brain and are useful for repairing arteries and improving energy.

Next are vegetables: enjoy 9-11 servings a day, including juices. One good serving a day of squash—hubbard squash, winter squash, acorn squash, spaghetti squash—would be good, in addition to root vegetables like carrots, parsnips, rutabaga, kohlrabi, and leafy greens. In terms of leafy greens, go heavy on your sprouts. Sunflower sprouts are terrific; they're my number one favorite, but garlic, onion, daikon, other spicy sprouts, and mung bean sprouts are also great. Aim for five or six different types of sprouts. Enjoy a variety of mixed greens and micro greens twice a day. Lastly, have one serving every day of sea vegetables; see our list below. Sea vegetables provide key minerals, including iodine for thyroid metabolism.

As far as fruits, I recommend 10-11 servings a day, including juices. The lower sugar, lower glycemic fruits like grapefruits, pears, apples, and berries are best. Five servings of fruits a day means you're getting quality fiber, as well as polyphenols, phytonutrients, all of your flavonoids, and antioxidants. Fruits contain all of these superstars of healing and disease prevention. To assist you in obtaining these healing properties, I prescribe fresh berries or a berry smoothie daily. The berries I recommend are blueberries, blackberries, raspberries, black raspberries, strawberries, cherries, pomegranates, blackcurrants, and red currants. You can get them frozen and thaw them out as needed. In addition to smoothies, consider adding them to your breakfast cereals, salads, salad dressings or mixed with unsweetened coconut flakes. I suggest at least two servings of berries a day. The berries are crucial; you can never get too many berries in my opinion. Also, watery fruits like watermelon, and other melons are great for juicing.

Always have lemons on hand. You will want to start your day with the juice of two lemons in 16 ounces of coconut water; it's a terrific way to flush out toxins, and alkalize the body. Also, figs and dates, as well as dried fruits like papaya, mango, and pineapple can be used sparingly. They are great as a snack. Juices make great snacks, too: try two apples with some celery and lemon—a phenomenal concoction.

You'll want organic apple cider vinegar and balsamic vinegar on hand, and for cooking—even light temperature cooking—you'll want macadamia nut oil, mustard seed oil, and coconut oil. And always use herbs in your cooking and in your salads; see our list on p.210 of the most important culinary herbs and their nutritional profiles. Lastly, as far as vegetarian milks, I keep rice milk, coconut milk, almond milk, and cashew milk in the refrigerator, where they last about six months. Always check the expiration dates when you pull things from the refrigerator, as well as off the shelves at health food stores. Sometimes an expired product is missed by staff.

A Day in the Life...

I believe that the strongest way of getting your breakfast is a smoothie. Here's an example of what I put in my smoothies: a teaspoon of coconut oil, a teaspoon of hemp oil, a teaspoon of flaxseed oil, a tablespoon of organic walnut butter, 30 grams of vegetable protein from mixed sources, a scoop of vegetable powder, a scoop of berry powder, some fresh pomegranates, and rice milk.

If I'm hungry prior to lunch, I will have a small snack. If you have bread, make it Ezekiel sprouted bread or another brand of sprouted grain bread. Nut butters on bread or organic corn or brown rice cakes are delicious. You can also make yourself a little dipping dish with herbs and some extra virgin olive oil and a little lemon juice—delicious dipping. On this note, have no more than one slice of bread a day.

Make sure you also have plenty of living food snacks: all health food stores carry a raw food section. Here, you can get sprouted seeds, kale "chips," dehydrated crackers, raw food snack bars, and even raw chocolate. On the note of chocolate, you want to avoid chocolate made from cow's milk. One 2 ounce piece of raw cacao or vegan chocolate a day is great for your brain, your heart, and your circulation. In addition, stock up on a rotating mix of fresh raw vegetables that you can cut up and store in air-tight containers as crudité, as well as hummus, Baba ghanoush, or a fresh nut or seed pate for dipping. It will make a world of difference in your success on this program if you have ready, healthful snacks on hand.

Now let's take a closer look at some of the foods and their nutritive qualities. Dolores Riccio, author of *Superfoods for Life*, says the best foods are those given to us in nature, such as the following:

Vegetables

Vegetables contain valuable nutrients for health. Especially noteworthy are the cruciferous vegetables—broccoli, Brussels sprouts, cabbage, kale, radishes, and watercress—for their anti-cancer properties. Melatonin, for immunity-boosting and better sleep, is found in bananas, corn, and tomatoes. Chromium helps regulate insulin and can be found in apples, broccoli, grapes, raisins, mushrooms, and potatoes. Magnesium defends against asthma and heart disease, and is also a memory booster. Good fruit and vegetable sources include avocados, bananas, and dark green vegetables. Vitamin E's helper, selenium, is found in onions, shallots, mushrooms, and garlic. These foods help the heart and keep the skin elastic.

Intense color and flavor indicate health-giving properties. Dark green and orange vegetables, for example, are high in carotene, which protects against cancer. And bitter greens like dandelion, kale, and arugula help the liver. Citrus fruits, such as oranges, lemons, and grapefruits, help rid the body of free radicals, keep the skin looking young, and accelerate healing. Here is a more detailed breakdown of categories of vegetables—including something on nutritional value. As I said previously, enjoy 9-11 servings of vegetables a day.

Tubers (potatoes, sweet potatoes, yams, Jerusalem artichokes, etc.)

Potatoes are well known for their high starch content, with a medium potato providing approximately 26 grams of carbohydrate, but did you know that one medium sized white potato or yam (with the skin on) can provide 45% of the daily recommended value of vitamin C? They are also a good source of vitamin B6, potassium, and phosphorus, and contain a number of health-promoting phytonutrients, including carotenoids and polyphenols. Chlorogenic acid with antioxidant properties makes up some 90% of the potato's phenols andhas been linked to blood pressure lowering effects[10], and the link between potatoes and their possible effects on lowering blood pressure was demonstrated in a study by the Institute for Food Research that found potatoes to contain the bioactive chemicals kukoamines with blood pressure lowering properties.[11]

Like the common potato, sweet potatoes are also an excellent source of carbohydrates and rich in vitamins C and B6. In addition, their orange-flesh is a good source of vitamin A, the antioxidant beta-carotene (one medium-sized sweet potato contains a staggering 438% of the daily vitamin A requirement), and dietary fiber. Purple-fleshed varieties are also available. The purple color comes from anthocyanins, which have important antioxidant properties and anti-inflammatory properties.[12] Sweet potatoes can be baked, mashed, or eaten in wedges raw or cooked; they are also a great addition to grain or green salads in their grated form. Their smooth creamy texture is ideal for making creams, soups, dips, and due to their natural sweetness they can be added to many cake recipes.

Yams are rarely found in supermarkets in the US. They are starchy tubers about the size of a small potato and somewhat dryer than sweet potatoes. Of all the roots and tubers, the protein content of yams, together with potato, is the highest. They are rich in the amino acids phenylalanine and threonine, but limiting in cystine, methionine, and tryptophan, and a good source of potassium and vitamin K. Yams can be prepared in much the same way as potatoes, or alternatively, try crunchy, no-sugar-added yam chips for a delicious and nutritious snack.

Jerusalem artichokes are lumpy, brown-skinned tubers. They are not actually an artichoke at all, but rather a species of sunflower (the flowers are pretty similar). The white flesh of this vegetable is nutty and sweet and a good source of iron, potassium, niacin, and thiamine. These tubers contain inulins, a type of dietary fiber with prebiotic properties, and a study published in the *British Journal of Nutrition* demonstrated that inulins from Jerusalem artichoke can stimulate the activity of "friendly" bacteria.[13] Jerusalem artichokes can be cooked in much the same way as potatoes or parsnips and are excellent roasted, pickled, puréed to make a delicious soup, or thinly sliced raw in salads.

Root vegetables (carrots, radish, daikon, rutabaga, turnips, parsnip, celeriac, etc.)

Carrots have long been associated with maintaining healthy eyes due to their high content of beta-carotene; in fact, women who consumed carrots at least twice per week were found to have significantly lower rates of glaucoma than women who consumed carrots less than once per week.[14] Besides, beta-carotene, other carotenoids found in carrots, including lutein, are also being investigated for their role in vision.

Carrots are extremely versatile and can be eaten cooked or raw. Add them to stews and salads, use raw carrot sticks for dipping, try them roasted with honey, or for those with a sweet tooth, make your own carrot cake. A 100 gram serving of carrots provides more than 100% of the daily vitamin A requirement and is a good source of vitamins B6 and K and dietary fiber.

The carrot's claim to "superfood" has been supported by recent studies, which found a compound in carrots with anticancer properties. Falcarinol, a polyacetylene present in carrots, was found to inhibit the growth of human intestinal cancer cells.[15]

Radishes, with their crunchy texture and peppery flavor, are rich in folic acid and potassium and a good source of magnesium, vitamins C and B6, and calcium. The red varieties contain the antioxidant sulforaphane and are commonly added to salads; alternatively, they are good eaten dipped into creamy mild sauces, or used to make pickles. Black radishes contain four times more glucosinolates than other varieties, and have been shown to have detoxifying properties.[16] Other popular varieties include daikon, a mild-flavored white radish. Daikon is low in calories; 100 grams contains just 18 calories but 27% of the recommended daily intake of vitamin C, and is high in fiber, calcium, folate, and iron. Try it grated over dishes or added to stir fries.

Rutabaga is great added to stews and soups, and when added to mashed potatoes, it gives a subtle flavor boost. Just one cup contains 53% of the daily recommended amount of vitamin C and is also an excellent source of potassium, manganese, and the antioxidant beta-carotene. Very similar to rutabaga but smaller in size, turnips are also a good source of vitamin C as well as manganese, potassium, vitamin B6, folate, and copper. Eating just two medium turnips would meet your vitamin C needs for the entire day, and consuming foods rich in vitamin C has been shown to reduce wheezing symptoms in children.[17] Baby turnips have a sweet, delicate taste whereas winter turnips have a stronger flavor, and don't forget the greens! Turnip greens can be utilized in a wide-range of recipes to provide folic acid and four times more calcium than many other greens. What's more, the greens contain a higher content of glucosinolates than many other cruciferous vegetables; these phytonutrients can be converted into isothiocyanates with scientifically proven cancer-preventing properties.[18]

Celeriac is a root vegetable with a subtle, nutty yet celery-like flavor. It is very rich in vitamin K and phosphorus, which are important for bone mineralization and the prevention of osteoporosis. In fact, studies with vitamin K have shown that patients given vitamin K supplements had a reduced risk of osteoporotic fractures.[19] Celeriac is also a good source of dietary fiber, vitamin C, manganese, iron, copper, and potassium and is very low in cholesterol. Try it roasted, mashed, in soups and stews, or grated raw.

Parsnips contain more sugar than carrots, radish, or turnips and, therefore, have more calories (100 g provide 75 calories). Parsnips are packed with potassium and folate, important for red blood cells, and are an excellent source of soluble and insoluble dietary fibers. As for carrots and other members of the apiaceae family, parsnips contain polyacetylene antioxidants such as falcarinol, shown to protect against colon cancer.[20] Try them roasted with honey, added to stews and soups, or mashed–they combine particularly well with carrot and rutabaga.

Bulb vegetables (onions, shallots, garlic, leeks, scallions, chives, etc.)

The aromatic vegetables of the *Allium* family are low in sugar and fat, and contribute flavor to any savory dish without adding calories. They are also well-known for their medicinal uses.

Onions contain several important phytonutrients, such as polyphenols, with shallots having the highest amounts. Other phytonutrients include flavonols, the predominant pigments in the onion family and also found in chocolate. These compounds have antioxidant properties and have been associated with lowering blood pressure, and a diet rich in these compounds was associated with a reduced risk of death from cardiovascular disease in postmenopausal women.[21] Red onions have a considerable content of anthocyanins, which as previously mentioned have been shown to possess important antioxidant and anti-inflammatory properties. Furthermore, a study in *The American Journal of Clinical Nutrition* found that garlic and onion consumption was associated with a lower risk of some common cancers—colorectal, breast, prostate, ovarian, and others.[22] Garlic also contains over 20% of the recommended daily amounts of vitamins B6 and C, and manganese and is considered to be one of nature's "super foods."

Chives, usually sprinkled in small amounts over soups, salads, or in sandwiches, also contain the beneficial allyl sulfides common to the onion family and, according to the National Cancer Institute, are believed to be responsible for the lower incidence of cancer in people who consume large amounts of bulb vegetables,[23] in addition to being rich in vitamins A, C, and K, folic acid, iron, and calcium. Don't forget the chive flower! Not only is it pretty, it is edible, providing a mild flavor, and can add a decorative touch to dishes.

Stalk vegetables (celery, swiss chard, asparagus, kohlrabi, fennel, bamboo, etc.)

Celery is often used in weight-loss diets, as it is low in calories but high in dietary fiber. However, celery contains a surprisingly large number of antioxidants, including coumarins that also have appetite-suppressing properties, and lutein, which was found in a study published in the *American Journal of Clinical Nutrition* to prevent colon cancer.[24] Celery is commonly used as a base for soups and stocks, and raw for dipping. Try celery sticks filled with peanut or almond butter for a protein-rich snack.

Swiss chard is a rich source of omega-3 fatty acids and the vitamin B complex. It contains many phytonutrients, such as betalains, also found in beets, which have antioxidant and anti-inflammatory properties,[25] and kaempferol, demonstrated to possess a wide range of potential anti-cancer properties.[26] In addition, chard is one of the excellent vegetable sources for vitamin K, whose adequate levels in the diet help to limit neuronal damage in the brain and, thus have been associated with the treatment of patients with Alzheimer's. Young, tender leaves can be added to salads; alternatively, gently steam or sauté the leaves or add them to stews, stir fries, grain dishes, or even try making some Swiss chard pesto.

Asparagus is a delicacy that can be boiled, steamed, and is delicious lightly cooked in the oven drizzled with olive oil and added to pasta. Add it to soups or try it in a warm salad. It is very low in sodium and has high levels of vitamins A and C, potassium, iron, calcium, magnesium, and zinc, and is a good source of dietary fiber. Asparagus is a diuretic, giving urine an unmistakable aroma and also contains prebiotic inulins[27], which are soluble dietary fibers that pass through the small intestine and ferment in the large intestine. Through the fermentation process, the inulin becomes healthy intestinal micro flora (bifidobacterium).[28]

Kohlrabi has a mild, sweet flavor and a crisp, crunchy texture and is a very good source of dietary fiber, vitamins C and B6, and potassium, copper, and manganese. It is a low calorie, high carbohydrate food that can be eaten raw or cooked. Try it sautéed with garlic and lemon juice, boiled and added to mashed potato, grated in coleslaw, or roasted.

Fennel, an aromatic bulb, whose leaves, flowers, and seeds are also edible, contain dietary nitrates, which have been found to lower blood pressure[29] and protect the heart due to their vasodilatory and vasoprotective properties. Fennel has an aniseed-like flavor and is delicious added to salads, braised, or added to risottos; alternatively add it to blueberry and apple juice for an interesting twist. Fennel, and particularly its seeds, is often used to naturally freshen the breath. It also has moderate levels of carbohydrates (17 grams per bulb), and provides a good source of potassium, calcium, vitamin C, and iron.

Bamboo shoots are commonly used in Asian cuisine, either cooked or pickled. They are a very good source of vitamin B6, potassium, copper, and manganese, and the shoots contain rich essential fatty acids. Chlorogenic acid, with antioxidant properties and blood pressure lowering effects has been found in bamboo.[30] Try adding them to stir fries, curries, salads, or soups.

Leafy vegetables, including dark green leafy vegetables (kale, cabbage, spinach, bok choy, collards, lettuces, arugula, watercress, etc.)

The dark leafy green vegetables in this family are all high in fiber and antioxidants. They are also particularly enriched with glucosinolates, which have been shown to reduce the risk of developing lung, colorectal, breast, prostate, and pancreatic cancers.[31]

Kale is currently hot on the health food scene and this is no surprise when you take into account its nutritional value. One cup of kale contains more than 100% of the recommended daily amounts of vitamin C and A, is rich in calcium and iron, and a great source of the omega-3 fatty acid alpha-linoleic acid (ALA), essential for brain health. But it doesn't stop there; kale also contains an impressive range of phytonutrients, such as quercetin, a flavonoid with antioxidant and anti-inflammatory properties[32], which may help reduce atherosclerosis (plaque buildup in arteries that can lead to heart attack or stroke).[33] Kale is delicious sautéed with garlic, lightly blanched and added to a warm salad, chopped as a salad; or, alternatively, try kale crisps for nutritious, tasty snacks.

Cabbage, like kale, is packed with high concentrations of antioxidants, glucosinolates, and anti-inflammatory phytonutrients, in addition to being rich in vitamins B and K. A study led by Michigan State University and University of New Mexico researcher Dorothy *Pathak* reported an impressive reduction of breast cancer risk in women who consumed four servings of cabbage a week compared with those that ate it once a week.[34] Try it sliced raw with carrots, toasted nuts, raisins, and olive oil and lemon juice dressing for a crisp salad.

Spinach is particularly rich in iron, vital for the function of red blood cells that transport oxygen around the body, and is an excellent source of vitamins A, C, and K, and folic acid. The dark green color of spinach leaves indicates they contain high levels of carotenoids, such as beta-carotene and lutein. Lutein is concentrated in the macula, a small area of the retina where it protects the eye from oxidative stress, and increased levels of lutein can reduce the risk of certain eye diseases, such as cataracts[35] and age-related macular degeneration,[36] which can lead to blindness. Other health-promoting phytonutrients found in spinach are the glycolipids or glycoglycerolipids, which have been shown to suppress tumor growth[37] and are under investigation for their use as anti-cancer therapeutics. Spinach can be added to soups and pasta dishes, added raw to salads and pizzas, or eaten as a dish in its own right, especially pairing well with garlic and nutmeg flavors.

Bok choy (also known as pak choi or Chinese cabbage) ranked second for nutrient density out of 41 "powerhouse" fruits and vegetables.[38] Unlike some other members of the cabbage family, these ranked nutrients include omega-3s due to their significant amount of alpha-linolenic acid, as well as the antioxidant mineral zinc, in addition to high levels of vitamins K, C, A, B6, potassium, folate, calcium, and manganese. It is a very good source of iron, vitamin B2, phosphorus, fiber, and protein. Try it steamed, sautéed, or stir fried; it is delicious combined with sesame.

Collard greens are an important non-dairy source of calcium; these greens are also rich sources of vitamins A and C, manganese, and a good source of vitamin E. Steam them to preserve their vitamin C content or add them to stir fries, soups, or stews. Also, a recent study found that steamed collard greens were the best at binding bile acids,[39] leading to a lowering of cholesterol levels when compared to other leafy green vegetables.

Lettuces are available in a vast number of varieties and textures, and all types are very nutritious. They are low in calories and high in water and fiber content as well as a good source of vitamin A, vitamin K, folate, and molybdenum. Combine mixed lettuce leaves in your salads with other stronger flavored leaves such as arugula and watercress. Arugula (or rocket) has a strong peppery flavor and besides salads, it is also commonly added to pasta or pizzas. Arugula is a good source of folic acid and vitamins A, C, and K, and was thought by the Romans to be an aphrodisiac, so get inventive and add it where you get a chance. Arugula like many other leafy vegetables contains cancer-preventing glucosinolates.

Watercress, the close family member of arugula, also has a peppery flavor and is highly nutritious, containing significant amounts of iron, calcium, iodine, folic acid, and vitamins A, C, E, and K. Watercress is also a significant source of omega-3 fatty acids and because of this, perhaps surprisingly for some, watercress tops the list of "powerhouse fruits and vegetables" compiled in a peer-reviewed CDC study.[40] Try it combined in a salad with milder leaves or with potato in a soup.

Inflorescent vegetables, meaning we eat the flower of the vegetable (broccoli, cauliflower, artichokes, cardoons, etc.)

Broccoli and cauliflower are brassicas and both contain an array of antioxidants, including beta-carotene, quercetin, and kaempferol. In terms of nutrients, while broccoli has higher levels of vitamins C and K, cauliflower has higher levels of potassium and folate. Young sprouts of broccoli and cauliflower are particularly rich in glucoraphanin. When these foods are consumed, the glucoraphanins are converted into a sulforaphane, and new research led by the University of East Anglia found that sulforaphane slows down the destruction of cartilage in joints associated with arthritis.[41] As mentioned earlier, the nutrients in these valuable vegetables are best accessed when exposed to a bit of heat. They are both great in stir fries, soups, grain salads, or on their own gently steamed with a bit of homemade dressing like tahini.

Although the flower heads of broccoli raab look like sprouting broccoli, this is actually a member of the mustard green and turnip family, and the flower heads and leaves have a slightly bitter flavor. Broccoli raab is an excellent source of vitamins K, A, and C as well as folate, manganese, potassium, calcium, and iron. Like other members of this family of vegetables, it is packed with phytonutrients, including lutein, an antioxidant that protects the retinas of your eyes from damage caused by free radicals and may slow the progression of macular degeneration and cataracts.[42] Try it sautéed with garlic and chili or with walnuts and cannellini beans.

Artichokes are a good source of folate and vitamins C and K, and artichokes are also packed with antioxidants; they're number 7 on the USDA's top 20 antioxidant-rich foods list. One medium artichoke provides 41% of the recommended daily amount of fiber, which contains inulin to promote intestinal health (as mentioned before) by stimulating the growth of good bacteria in the colon, and soluble fibers, which help lower cholesterol and maintain balanced blood sugar. Try them roasted; jarred artichokes are great on a pizza or added to salad, or why not make them into a tasty dip combined with lemon.

Fruit-like vegetables, meaning foods that we call vegetables but that are botanically considered fruits (a seed-bearing structure that develops from the ovary of a flowering plant), include a wide-range of commonly eaten vegetables such as olives, tomatoes, avocados, okra, eggplants, zucchini, cucumbers, squashes, pumpkin, peppers, peas and beans, etc.).

Olives come in many different shades from green to black, with the difference in color reflecting their ripeness. As black olives have been given longer to ripen, they have a higher oil content, which gives them a milder flavor and softer texture. Olives are rich in monounsaturated fats, which help reduce cholesterol, and research suggests that the Mediterranean diet, which is rich in monounsaturated fatty acids, can help to prevent coronary artery disease and strokes.[43] Olive fruit also contains vitamin E, particularly important for the skin, flavonoids, and the polyphenols, oleuropein and oleocanthal, which are all powerful antioxidants.[44] Olive oil forms a staple part of any diet nowadays but is especially important for vegetarians as it provides both omega-6 (linoleic acid) and omega-3 (linolenic acid) essential fatty acids at the recommended 8:1 ratio, and about 75% of its fat in the form of oleic acid (a monounsaturated, omega-9 fatty acid) that can help lower blood pressure.[45] Due to their salty taste, olives can make a great addition to dips and tapenades, and are great in salads, on pizzas, and added to pasta dishes. As a side note, organic whole grain or gluten-free pizza crusts are best, as are sprouted or gluten-free pastas made of lentils, quinoa, or brown rice.

Tomatoes are known as "functional foods," meaning they can provide health benefits beyond just basic nutrition. They are rich in vitamins A and C, fiber, manganese, and potassium, yet the majority of their health benefits can be attributed to the antioxidant lycopene, which gives tomatoes their red color. Tomatoes provide 80% of the lycopene content of the typical American diet, although apricots, guava, watermelon, papaya, and pink grapefruit are also sources. According to the American Cancer Society, some studies have shown that people who have diets rich in tomatoes may have a lower risk of certain types of cancer, especially cancers of the prostate, lung, and stomach.[46,47] For example, in one study, people who consumed high amounts of raw tomatoes had an 11% reduced risk of prostate cancer[48], and interestingly, those with a high intake of cooked tomato products experienced a 19% lower risk, with evidence suggesting that the lycopene from processed tomatoes is more bioavailable than that of fresh tomatoes.[49]

A tomato-rich diet has also been shown to improve the skin's ability to protect against harmful UV rays through the effects of lycopene and lead to higher levels of procollagen,[50] which helps keep the skin firm. Tomatoes can be eaten raw in salads, added to sandwiches, pizzas, or as garnishes. To help improve the bioavailability of lycopene, also include them grilled or cooked in sauces.

Another fruit-like vegetable that can improve the skin's ability to protect against harmful UV rays and aging is the avocado due to its high levels of free radical fighting vitamin E. Avocados are also rich in vitamins B, C, and K, potassium, copper, and carotenoids such as lutein and zeaxanthin. Although an avocado is about 67% fat, the fat is mainly the monounsaturated fat asoleic acid, and the omega-6 fatty acid, linoleic acid. Avocados also contain oleic acid, an omega-9 fat, one of the building blocks of healthy skin with a role in regenerating damaged skin cells.[51]

Okra is known for its high vitamin C, vitamin K, folate, and dietary fiber content. These ridged pods contain edible seeds that produce a sticky thick liquid when chopped and cooked, which has led to it being used to thicken soups and stews, and its subtle flavor means it is often accompanied by spicier ingredients. Try it pickled, add it to curries, or Southern fried, a favorite in Creole cuisine.

Eggplants are very low in calories and fats but rich in soluble dietary fiber and copper, and a good source of manganese, B-group vitamins, potassium, and vitamin K, and their consumption has been linked to the effective control of cholesterol.[52] Their purple skin contains significant amounts of the antioxidants anthocyanins, linked to protection against cancer and inflammation. One potent anthocyanin found in eggplant skin, nasunin, was found to protect human colon cells from DNA damage.[53] Try them roasted or cubed and added to stews. Or why not try making baba ghanoush, mixing pureed roasted eggplant with garlic, tahini, lemon juice, and olive oil.

Zucchini and cucumbers are members of the squash and pumpkin family. Cucumbers are 95% water, making them great hydrators; but they are also rich in vitamins B, C, and K, and copper, potassium, and manganese. Cucumbers contain an anti-inflammatory flavonol called fisetin that appears to improve memory and may protect from Alzheimer's-associated memory loss.[54] Try cucumbers fermented or raw in salads. They are also a great base for juices due to their mild flavor and high water content.

Squash and pumpkins are a rich source of beta-carotene that our bodies use to make vitamin A, and pumpkins are also rich in the antioxidants lutein and zeaxanthin associated with vision and the prevention of cataracts. Squash also contains omega-3 fatty acids in the form of alpha-linolenic acid. While squash only contains about one-third the level of omega-3 as say walnuts, less than 15% of the calories in winter squash come from fat. Try squash or pumpkin baked, roasted, stuffed, puréed, or added to soup. Similar to melon seeds, pumpkin seeds make a nutritious snack; one serving provides high amounts of protein (equivalent to a similar serving of peanuts) and more than 20% of the recommended daily intake of iron.

You may be surprised to know that bell peppers contain more vitamin C than oranges and are also good sources of fiber, vitamin E, and antioxidant and anti-inflammatory carotenoids such as beta-carotene and zeaxanthin. Both the vitamin C and carotenoid content of bell peppers increases with ripening: A cup of red pepper contains nearly three times the vitamin C of an orange, whereas a cup of green pepper contains 200% of the recommended daily intake of vitamin C. Of all the peppers, however, chili peppers contain the highest levels of vitamin C. Also, capsaicin, the compound that makes chilies hot, can bind onto nerve cell receptors and change the pain sensation,[54] relieving joint and muscle pain. As such, a little liquid cayenne added to lemon water or a few shakes of cayenne powder used in everything from salads to soups will support increased circulation and lower inflammation in the body. Sweet red peppers make a delicious addition to juice, particularly in combination with oranges, or eat them raw for dipping, and chili peppers can add spice and nutritional content to a huge range of dishes.

There are many types of peas and beans, all of which are good sources of dietary fiber. Peas are a low-fat food yet they contain an impressive range of nutrients, including both omega-3 alpha-linolenic acid (ALA) and omega-6 fatty acid, linoleic acid, beta-carotene, and small but valuable amounts of vitamin E. Peas also contain a polyphenol called coumestrol, and the daily consumption of peas was recently shown to protect against stomach cancer.[56]

Fava beans (or broad beans) are also particularly nutrient rich. They are high in protein, low in fat, and an excellent source of folate, with 100 grams providing more than 100% of the recommended daily amount. They also contain good amounts of other B-group vitamins, phosphorus, iron, copper, manganese, calcium, magnesium, are one of the highest plant sources of potassium, and are rich in phytonutrients such as isoflavones. Fava beans make delicious additions to soups, stews, pasta dishes, and stir fries.

Sea vegetables

Sea vegetables rank high as sources for the basic essential minerals as do green vegetables such as dandelions and watercress. They all contain calcium, magnesium, phosphorus, potassium, iron, iodine, and sodium. Most Westerners dislike the idea of eating seaweed. If they were to sample what they're missing, though, they'd find a new world of taste and high-quality nutrients—especially trace minerals—in the six varieties of sea vegetables available in most natural food stores and food co-ops.

Sea vegetables contain the following macro nutrients in a highly bio-available form; in other words, the human body "understands" how to absorb and utilize them. Major minerals examples are:

- Calcium (for skeletal health, healthy heartbeat, nervous system function)[57]
- Magnesium (activates enzymatic activity, essential for healthy heartbeat)
- Potassium (naturally prevents high blood pressure, provides cellular energy)
- Sodium (essential for the correct balance of body fluids — our internal "ocean")
- Phosphorous (builds strong bones and teeth)

Trace elements are especially essential to the body's countless enzymatic functions.[58] Examples are:

- Chromium (works with insulin to regulate blood sugar)
- Iodine (thyroid health)
- Copper (protects nerve sheaths, builds supple arteries, required for iron absorption)
- Iron (transports oxygen to cells and enzymes, needed for healthy brain development and immune function)
- Manganese (assists in bone formation, builds cartilage and improves immune system response)

- Molybdenum (works with riboflavin to help use iron to make red blood cells)
- Selenium (works with vitamin E as an antioxidant, protects cells and supports immune function)
- Zinc (supports enzymatic reactions, healthy immune system and skin integrity, promotes cell reproduction, tissue growth, and repair, and helps better utilize vitamin A).

I cannot overstate the importance of sea vegetables in the plant-based diet. However, you don't need to overdo them; use them a couple of times a week or better yet make a salad with ginger dressing. Be sure to rinse the sea vegetables at least one time and perhaps two to reduce the amount of salt. You can try any number of these, but arame, hijiki, wakame, kelp, and dulse are some of the most popular. As mentioned previously, sea vegetables from the Atlantic are best until it is determined the effects of Fukushima on the Pacific coast vegetables.

Agar

Agar, or agar-agar (called kantan in Japanese, and also known as Ceylonese moss) is a translucent, almost weightless seaweed product found in stick, flake, or powdered form. You can use it like gelatin to thicken fruit juices or purees. Agar also can be used to make aspics and clear molds of fruit juices, fruits, or vegetables. It is a good source of vitamin E (Alpha Tocopherol), vitamin K, pantothenic acid, zinc and copper, and a very good source of folate, calcium, iron, magnesium, potassium and manganese.[59] With 81.2% of its content as fiber, it is one the highest among all foods for this nutrient.[60]

Dulse

Dulse is the only commercial sea vegetable that comes from the Atlantic Ocean (specifically, the Canadian Maritime Provinces). This ready-to-eat seaweed can be chewed in its tough dry state, but a short soaking to rinse it and to remove any small, clinging shells is worthwhile. Dulse can be added to miso soup. This red algae is particularly rich in omega-3 fatty acids, EPA and alpha-linolenic acid, as well as omega-6 fatty acids, AA and linoleic acid, and relatively high levels of oleic and palmitic acids.[61] What's more, an 8 gram serving of dry dulse provides more iron than 100 grams of sirloin steak, provides more than 100% of the recommended daily amount of potassium, and is packed full of protein, folate, and vitamin B12,[62] which—being mostly found in animal foods—makes dulse an excellent source of this vitamin for vegetarians and vegans.

Hijiki (Hiziki)

Another Japanese seaweed is the jet-black hijiki or hiziki. This stringy, hair-like seaweed contains 57% more calcium by weight than dry milk and has high levels of iron as well. Dried hiziki should be soaked in several cups of water for about 20 minutes, then strained in a colander and lightly pressed to squeeze out excess moisture. Once reconstituted, hiziki is best when sautéed together with other vegetables—especially onion and leeks—or cooked with beans and grains. Hijiki, as well as other seaweeds including kombu, bladderwrack, and wakame, contains fucoidan, a sulfated polysaccharide (similar to starch or cellulose) with important anti-inflammatory properties and reported effects in preventing tumor progression.[63]

Kombu (Kelp)

Kombu is the Japanese term for several species of brown algae. In English, these are usually referred to collectively as kelp. Kombu is especially rich in iodine, vitamin B2, and calcium. When using the dried form of kombu, rinse it once and soak for 10 to 15 minutes. Note that all dried seaweeds increase greatly in size when reconstituted. For example, 1/4 cup of dried hiziki will yield 1 cup when soaked. Save the water in which the seaweeds are soaked and use it as soup stock. Reconstituted kombu strips can be used whole in the cooking water for beans and grains, or can be cut into thin strips or diced for use in soups and salads. It was suggested that kelp might decrease the likelihood of estrogen-dependent diseases in humans, such as breast cancer, and vigorous studies of the Japanese diet have been undertaken. Earlier reports showed that Japanese women had longer menstrual cycles and lower serum estradiol levels than their Western counterparts. It is believed that these factors contribute to the lower rates of breast, endometrial, and ovarian cancers in Japan. It is documented that longer menstrual cycles are associated with a lowered risk of breast, ovarian, and endometrial cancers. In addition, and particularly interesting for those trying to lose weight, a recent study published in the journal *Food Chemistry* found that alginate—a fibrous material found in sea kelp—can suppress fat absorption in the gut.[64]

Nori (Laver)

Nori is the most popular Japanese seaweed, also known as dried purple laver. It is sold in the form of paper-thin purplish sheets, with 8 to 10 sheets per package. Laver has been used as food by many peoples. The Japanese and Koreans are the only people to cultivate these plants and dry and press the mature leaves into sheets. The nori sheets are toasted over a flame until crisp, during which their color changes from black or purple to green. They are then crumbled or slivered and used as a condiment for noodles, grains, beans, and soups. Remarkably rich in protein, nori is also high in vitamins A, B2, B12, D, and niacin.

Wakame

Wakame is a long seaweed with symmetrical and fluted fronds growing from both sides of an edible midrib. Although generally used fresh in Japan, it is only available dried in the West. It is reconstituted in the same manner as kombu: rinsed once, soaked, and pressed of excess moisture. If the midrib is particularly tough, it can be removed. When used in soups, wakame should be cooked for no more than a few minutes and should therefore be one of the last ingredients added to miso soup. This delicious vegetable is rich in protein and niacin. In its dried state, it contains almost 50% more calcium than dry milk. Fucoxanthin, the pigment that gives wakame its brown color, is being investigated for its fat burning and anti-cancer effects[64] among others.[65]

Fruits

Berries are small, juicy fruits with thin skins, such as raspberries, strawberries, blackberries, cranberries, blueberries, and grapes.

Strawberries are excellent sources of vitamin C, a good source of manganese, and their seeds (achenes) contain the essential omega-3 fatty acid alpha-linolenic acid. This fatty acid is also provided by raspberries and blackberries, which are some of the fruits richest in omega-3 fatty acids. Strawberries also contain a flavenoid called fisetin, which has been shown to improve memory and can help treat symptoms of Alzheimer's.[66]

Blueberries contain an impressive cocktail of antioxidants, including anthocyanins, resveratrol, and tannins. Like strawberries, the consumption of blueberries has been shown to improve memory and concentration. One study found that just one 200 gram blueberry smoothie was enough to increase powers of concentration by as much as 20% over the day,[67] and their daily consumption for 12 weeks improved the memory of older adults.[68]

Cranberries have a tart, fresh flavor and like the other berries are a rich source of vitamin C, fiber, and antioxidant phytonutrients. Cranberries are well-known for helping prevent urinary tract infections, and this property has been attributed to their proanthocyanidins, which act as a barrier against infection-causing bacteria.[69] In the same way, these compounds can protect against the stomach bacteria that can cause stomach ulcers.[70]

For a fruit, mulberries are an unusually high source of protein, containing some 4 grams of protein per serving. Both mulberries and boysenberries—large, reddish-purple berries—also contain high amounts of vitamins C and K, iron, calcium, and are an excellent source of anthocyanins, and resveratrol, shown to have neuroprotective effects against Alzheimer's, in addition to cardiovascular disease, diabetes, and cancer.[71] Raspberries, strawberries, cranberries, and boysenberries also contain the phenolic compound ellagic acid, shown to slow the growth of some tumors.[72]

Grapes are botanically classified as a berry, and like several other berries, the consumption of grapes has been shown to bring cognitive benefits. For example, elderly participants that drank a glass of grape juice daily over three months showed memory and verbal learning.[73] Grapes are a very good source of vitamin K and C, riboflavin, manganese, potassium, and copper. However, it's the content of antioxidant and anti-inflammatory phytonutrients that stands grapes apart. They contain hundreds of antioxidants, the majority of which are found in the skin, and several of which—such as resveratrol—are believed to play a role in longevity.

According to a study published in the *American Journal of Clinical Nutrition,* blackberries were ranked as being the most antioxidant-rich food based on a typical serving.[74] They are also rich in vitamins C, A, and K, manganese, and dietary fiber, and their dark blue purple color means they are packed with phytonutrients such as cancer-protecting ellagic acid[75]—and antioxidant anthocyanins, also shown to have anti-bacterial activity against pathogenic microbes such as *Salmonella* and stomach ulcer-causing *H.pylori.*[76] Add berries to breakfast smoothies, or eat them with natural yogurt, muesli, and nuts for an antioxidant packed start to the day that will also boost your cognitive levels.

Pit fruits contain a hard stone in their center surrounded by a soft fleshy fruit and are covered by a thin outer skin. They include cherries, apricots, nectarines, peaches, and plums.

Apricots, with their orange-colored flesh, are an excellent source of vitamin A in the form of beta-carotene and lutein, both shown to be important for vision and are also a good source of vitamin C, iron, copper, dietary fiber, and potassium. Apricots are an important source of catechin (associated with the health benefits of green tea), potent anti-inflammatory phytonutrients.[77]

Plums are a very good source of the B-group vitamins and vitamin C and contain a range of antioxidants such as beta-carotene. Prunes (dried plums) are a good source of concentrated energy and nutrients, including calcium, magnesium, potassium, fiber, and iron due to the loss of water. Plums and prunes are particularly well-known for their laxative effect. Both contain insoluble dietary fiber whose bulk helps to prevent constipation, but also has important prebiotic effects in the intestine. Prunes also contain soluble fiber that helps to lower cholesterol levels by binding to and removing bile acids.[78] Finally, prunes consist of 15% of the natural sugar sorbitol and isatin, both of which have constipation relieving properties.

Cherries are rich in vitamins C, E, potassium, magnesium, iron, folate, and dietary fiber, and contain more antioxidant beta-carotene than blueberries or strawberries, as well as anthocyanins scientifically linked to the prevention of cardiovascular disease, cancer, diabetes, and inflammation among others.[78] What's more, cherries are one of the few food sources of melatonin[79], important for the regulation of sleep, and whose levels reduce with age.[80]

Pit fruits are delicious fresh or dried, making excellent energizing snacks, and are also commonly available canned or in jams.

Core fruits, such as apples and pears, have a seed containing core surrounded by a thick layer of flesh.

Apples rank among the fruits with the highest content of antioxidants, important free radical scavengers that help prevent cancer, including quercetin. One study carried out by researchers from the UK Department of Public Health Sciences found improved lung function among middle-aged men who ate an apple a day, another study found that people who regularly ate apples cut their lung cancer risk in half, and one group of researchers who tracked the food consumption of over 9000 study participants for 28 years found that those who ate more apples had a lower risk of stroke, all effects associated with apples' rich source of antioxidants.[81-83]

Apples are also a good source of vitamin C. Since almost half of an apple's vitamin C content is found just under the skin, as well as the apple's fiber, it's best to eat apples with their skins on. Apples and pears make delicious additions to salads, are excellent juiced, or alternatively, try them stewed and served with yogurt for an antioxidant-packed dessert.

In comparison to apples, pears contain more pectin water-soluble fibers associated with lowering cholesterol levels.[84] Pears are also rich in vitamins A, B, C, and K, copper, phosphorus, potassium, and boron, which helps the body to retain calcium. Pears also contain an array of beneficial antioxidant phytonutrients, although importantly, the skin has been shown to contain three to four times as many as the flesh as well as about half of the pear's dietary fiber. Due to their rich flavonoid content, apples and pears were shown to help protect against development of type 2 diabetes[85] and to lower the risk of esophageal cancer.[86]

Citrus fruits are divided into segments and have a thick outer rind. They include oranges, tangerines, grapefruits, kumquats, lemons, and limes. All citrus fruits are excellent sources of vitamin C, a powerful antioxidant that scavenges harmful pro-inflammatory free radicals from the blood.

Well-known for being an excellent source of vitamin C, oranges contain an array of phytonutrients that are also important for antioxidant protection. They also offer another important yet lesser-known group of nutrients called citrus limonoids, which come from the compound–limonin glucoside—present in citrus and citrus juices in about the same amount as vitamin C. In laboratory tests with In laboratory tests with human cells, human cells, citrus limonoids have been shown to help fight cancers of the mouth, skin, lung, breast, stomach and colon.[87] Oranges are also a good source of dietary fiber, folate, vitamin A (in the form of carotenoids), B-group vitamins, potassium, copper, and calcium. In fact, the World Health Organization's recent draft report, "Diet, Nutrition and the Prevention of Chronic Disease," concluded that the folate, potassium, antioxidants, and vitamin C contained in citrus fruits such as oranges can protect against cardiovascular disease.[88]

Pink and red colored grapefruits contain the antioxidant lycopene, demonstrated to decrease the risk of prostate cancer[89] and probably protect against other cancers. Grapefruits are also rich in vitamin C—half of a grapefruit provides about 78% of the recommended daily intake—and a study published in the *Journal of Medicinal Food* found that eating half a grapefruit before meals without making any other dietary changes led to an average weight loss of 3 and a half pounds over 12 weeks.[90]

The bitter taste of grapefruit comes from an antioxidant and anti-inflammatory known as naringenin, which was shown to prevent kidney cysts from forming[91] and is also found in lemons and oranges. In addition, lemons can help prevent the formation of kidney stones due to their high citric acid content, which can dissolve kidney stones and aids digestion.

Lemons and limes contain limonoids, which have been shown to help fight cancers of the mouth, skin, lung, breast, stomach, and colon. Scientists from the US Agricultural Research Service (ARS) have shown that our bodies can readily absorb and utilize the limonoid in citrus fruits, which can remain active in the body for up to 24 hours.[92] Drink a refreshing glass of lemon water, or combine lemon juice with olive or flax oil, freshly crushed garlic, and pepper to make a light yet nutritional salad dressing.

Melons *are large, juicy fruits with thick skins and many seeds, and include cantaloupe, casaba, honeydew, and watermelon varieties.*

The orange-colored flesh of cantaloupe melons is high in vitamins A and C, and is a very good source of manganese and potassium, as well as B vitamins, magnesium, antioxidants, and fiber. Moreover, the phytonutrients, such as oxykine, contained in cantaloupe melon may improve insulin resistance.

A wedge of refreshing honeydew melon provides more than half the recommended daily allowance of vitamin C as well as important sugars, dietary fiber, and potassium, all while being low in calories. For something different, why not try making a delicious fruit salsa with chopped honeydew, tomato, onion, jalapeno pepper, cilantro, and lime juice.

Watermelon contains about 91% water, sugars, and is a good source of vitamins C, A, and B6. The red watermelon pulp is also one of the best sources of cancer-combating lycopene. Drinking watermelon juice before an intense workout was shown to reduce next day muscle soreness.[93] This effect was attributed to the citrulline found in watermelon, which can be converted by our bodies to the amino acid arginine that helps to improve blood flow.

Try watermelon seeds dried and roasted; they are commonly eaten to by the Chinese for New Year celebrations and have a nutty flavor. Like other varieties of melon seeds, they are a good source of the essential omega-3 fatty acid alpha-linoleic acid.

Tropical fruits, considered to be exotic as they are generally grown in warm climates, include coconut, bananas, figs, dates, guavas, mangoes, papayas, pineapples, pomegranates, and kiwis.

Coconuts are highly nutritious, being rich in fiber, vitamins B, C, and E, iron, selenium, copper, sodium, calcium, magnesium, zinc, and phosphorous. As mentioned in the oil section, coconuts contain significant amounts of fat, but mainly in the form of medium chain saturated fatty acids, such as lauric acid. Lauric acid can be converted in the body into monolaurin, an antiviral and antibacterial compound that may help protect against infections and viruses.

Try coconut milk as a cow's milk alternative; it is lactose-free, vegan, and makes a great base for smoothies or milkshakes. Coconut water makes a particularly refreshing drink that is packed with electrolytes, containing more potassium than four bananas and is cholesterol free. A study recently published in *Journal of the International Society of Sports Nutrition* found that coconut water replenishes body fluids as well as commercial sports drinks and without the harmful chemicals.[94]

Bananas are a good source of vitamins B and C, manganese, dietary fiber, and copper. However, they are perhaps most famous for being a provider of easily digestible sugars—although they have a low glycemic index value—and potassium. One medium-sized ripe banana contains 14-15 grams of total sugar and more than 400 mg of potassium, important for maintaining normal blood pressure and protection against atherosclerosis and stroke.[95] Bananas also contain small amounts of sterols that can help our cardiovascular health by blocking the absorption of dietary cholesterol, and also contain probiotic indigestible fructooligosaccharides that help maintain "friendly" bacteria.[96] In fact, their daily consumption was shown to lead to significant increases in beneficial *Bifidobacteria* and a reduction in digestive problems.[97]

There are many varieties of bananas, differing in sweetness and also some that are starchier, such as plantain. Plantain is usually cooked and has a higher beta-carotene concentration than other sweet bananas.

Papaya is a fruit that has more vitamin C than oranges and is also rich in dietary fiber, vitamin B, potassium, copper, magnesium, calcium, and antioxidants such as prostate-cancer protecting lycopene,[98] and the flavonoids, beta-carotene, zeaxanthin, and lutein. Despite having a sweet flavor, papayas have a low sugar content and glycemic index, and studies show that papaya extract can have a protective effect on patients with type 2 diabetes.[99] In addition to the dietary fiber they contain, papayas can also help digestion due to the protein-digesting enzyme papain that they contain, which is extracted to make digestive dietary supplements.

Pineapples, like coconuts, are also high in fiber and an important source of natural sugars. In addition, pineapples contain unique protein-digesting enzymes collectively known as bromelain, which help to digest protein-rich foods. Our stomach's hydrochloric acid is essential for protein digestion; however, the production of this acid by the body usually declines after the age of 35 and protein breakdown can be impaired. Therefore, the particular benefit of pineapples and their bromelain may help. Bromelain has also been shown to reduce the severity and duration of colds and flu as they reduce inflammation of the nasal cavity and help prevent excessive mucus in the respiratory system[99], and may be effective in relieving the pain associated with arthritis.[100]

Pomegranate seeds are a good source of many vital B-group vitamins, vitamin K, calcium, copper, potassium, and manganese, and the US Department of Agriculture ranks pomegranate juice as the fifth strongest antioxidant (behind chocolate, elderberries, and two different varieties of apples). Pomegranates also contain ellagitannin antioxidants compounds, such as punicalagin, shown to reduce heart-disease risk factors such as lowering blood pressure and increasing the removal of atherosclerosis.[101,102] Sprinkle them on salads or add them to your juices and smoothies.

Among the thousands of whole foods in the USDA nutrient database, figs make the top ten for fiber content, providing 20% of the daily value, and thus are often recommended as natural laxatives. Figs are also good sources of potassium, calcium, magnesium, iron, and copper, as well as vitamins A, E, and K.

Dates are the fruit of the date palm tree and provide several nutritional benefits when eaten fresh. People often avoid dates because of their high sugar content, however a study published in *Nutrition Journal* found that despite their high amounts of natural sugars, dates are a low-glycemic index food and did not significantly raise blood sugar levels after they were eaten.[103] Their consumption was also shown to lower blood lipid levels and protect against oxidative stress.[104] Like figs, dates are fiber rich, and according to the USDA National Nutrient Database, just one pitted date contains 6% of the recommended daily intake. Dates are also an excellent source of B-group vitamins, as well as A and K, potassium, copper, manganese, magnesium, calcium, phosphorous, iron, and zinc. Figs and dates make a nutritious addition to breakfast oatmeal, are delicious combined with cheese, almonds, or walnuts in salads, or can be poached in red wine for a tasty dessert.

Grains

These fiber-rich foods keep our digestive tracts healthy. They are high in B vitamins, which work to support the brain, and rich sources of vitamin E, making them good for the heart and skin. In addition, whole grain fibers such as brown rice contain zinc for nourishment of the male reproductive system and repair of the body.

Whole grains are cereal grains that contain bran (the hard outer layer of cereal grains) and germ (the heart of the cereal kernel), in addition to endosperm (nutritional tissue found in the seeds of most flowering plants). This differs from refined grains, which retain only endosperm. Plant a whole kernel of any grain and, given the right combination of earth, water, and air, it will naturally sprout and grow to maturity. Not so with refined grains, which are robbed of the vital minerals and vitamins found in the discarded outer layers. Nearly all of the B vitamins, vitamins E, unsaturated fatty acids, and quality proteins are found in whole grains, but refining removes most of these nutrients. Many people mistakenly believe that whole grains are nothing more than fiber. Research shows that whole grain foods play a significant part in reducing the risk of many chronic diseases. Whole grains contain a plethora of beneficial health substances such as vitamins, minerals, phytonutrients, and fiber.

In spite of this, 90% of Americans do not meet the suggested 3 daily servings of whole grains. Whole grains' unique blend of vitamins, minerals, carbohydrates, antioxidants, and fiber seems to work synergistically to lessen the risk of heart disease and some forms of cancer. One study, published in the Proceedings of the Nutrition Society in 2003, reported that 160,000 people who consumed extra whole grain foods considerably lessened their risk of type II diabetes. In addition, whole grains helped maintain healthy blood sugar levels in non-diabetics. Whole grains are a healthy way to shed undesired pounds. Studies report that individuals who eat more whole grain foods have a lower body mass index and are more likely to maintain their proper weight.[105] Whole grains are low in fat and high in fiber and complex carbohydrates, making you feel fuller for an extended period of time. This can help you avoid the munchies and make you less likely to reach for unhealthy snacks. Several guests on my radio show over the years have speculated that upward of 50% of health problems originate in the digestive tract. Whole grains can help in this area because they are an important fiber source that enables you to "be regular," thus having a healthy bowel, as we discussed in the fiber section before.

In addition to their beneficial effects on the digestive system, a diet rich in fiber can prevent the risk of coronary heart disease and help stabilize blood sugar levels.[106] A study found that people who ate a diet higher in fiber had lower levels of sugar and insulin in their blood.[107]

Here is a list of grains as well as notes on their beneficial nutrients:

Amaranth

Amaranth is a native grain. It has been cultivated in the American Southwest for hundreds of years. The plant yields a tiny seed that should be prepared similarly to rice. When cooked, it has a very soft, nutlike consistency. Numerous studies have shown the health-benefiting properties of this grain, including its potential benefits for patients with cardiovascular disease. A study by the US Department of Agriculture found that amaranth can lead to a lowering of LDL cholesterol levels due to it being a rich dietary source of cholesterol-lowering phytosterols.[108,109]

Barley

Barley has much to offer as a solo grain dish. Some of the best barley in the world—consistently high in protein and minerals—comes from the rich soil of the Red River Valley of North Dakota and Minnesota. Since unhulled barley is almost impossible to cook, practically all barley available in food stores has been "pearled" so as to remove its tenacious hull. The factor to consider here is just how much pearling has taken place; too much results in a whiter product robbed of the nutrients in its outer layer. Look for the darker barley available in most natural food stores. Barley is a very good source of molybdenum, manganese, dietary fiber, and selenium, and contains eight essential amino acids. Recently, researchers have found that barley, eaten daily, is successful in lowering cholesterol levels by 25%.[110]

Buckwheat

Buckwheat is actually not a true grain but a grass seed related to rhubarb. When raised commercially as a grain crop, buckwheat is unlikely to have been fertilized or sprayed. Fertilization encourages too much leaf growth; spraying stops the bees from pollinating. The best buy is whole, hulled, unroasted (white) buckwheat grains, known as groats. Roasted (brown) and cut groats are less nutritious, and the roasting can easily be done just before cooking without disturbing the flavor or the B vitamins. Buckwheat is a low GI food whose consumption, as buckwheat bread, induced significantly lower blood glucose and insulin responses than wheat bread.[111]

A Japanese pasta called soba is now readily available in natural food stores and in Asian markets. It contains anywhere from 30 to 100% buckwheat flour. Its subtle flavor and light effect on the stomach should encourage pasta enthusiasts to give it a try. It needs no heavy sauces; try a simple garlic or onion and oil topping.

Corn

A staple food for thousands of years, corn has changed from a small shrub with only a few kernels to today's hybrid varieties with 6-foot stalks bearing several ears that contain over 100 kernels apiece. Before we get into our discussion on corn, I wanted to comment about corn's place in the world. In its dried form, it is considered a grain, while in its fresh form, it is considered a vegetable. Both white and yellow varieties of dried corn are readily available, but in the American Southwest the blue and varicolored older types of corn are still grown. "Sweet" corn is normally boiled or steamed in water and consumed as a vegetable, as I just noted; field corn is likely to be ground into meals and flours.

Corn is a good source of the B vitamins folate, thiamin, and B5, and of all the grains, it contains the highest levels of riboflavin, B6, and the antioxidant lutein. In addition to lutein, different colored corn varieties have different antioxidant combinations, with yellow corn packed full of carotenoids, blue corn with anthocyanins, and purple corn with protocatechuic acid, a particularly effective antioxidant with anti-inflammatory properties.[112] Recent studies have shown that corn has prebiotic effects in the intestine, with one study finding that the regular consumption of whole grain corn-based breakfast cereals like Kashi Organic Simply Maize Corn Cereal or Arrowhead Mills Puffed Corn Cereal supported the growth of friendly bacteria in the intestine and helped improve digestive health.[113, 114]

Millet

The many virtues of millet are often overlooked because of its reputation as "the poor person's rice." Being the only alkalinizing grain, millet is the most easily digestible. It is also an intestinal lubricant. Its amino acid structure is well balanced, providing a low-gluten protein, and it is high in calcium, riboflavin, and lecithin, not to mention rich in antioxidants.[115] Millet is a highly versatile stuffing for anything from hollowed-out zucchini halves to mushroom caps, and millet meal and flour are quality protein additions to any baked good. Millet meal also makes a good hot cereal.

Oats

Oats must be hulled before they can be eaten; after hulling they are cracked or rolled into the familiar cereal forms. Rolled oats are shot with steam for a number of seconds and then passed through rollers; thus some nutrients are lost. Rolled oats will cook faster than whole oat groats, but whole oat groats are the most beneficial. Known variously as Irish oatmeal, Scotch oats, or steel-cut oats, whole-oat groats are soaked overnight before being cooked as porridge. Whole oats are wonderful in soups. You can add both rolled and whole groats to all sorts of breads and patties. Oat flour, available at most natural food stores, can be used in equal proportions with whole wheat flour to bake up a tasty batch of muffins. Oats contain more soluble fiber than any other grain, making them particularly "filling" and satisfying.[116]

Quinoa

Quinoa (pronounced keen-wah), a staple of the Inca Indians, is a delicate, light-textured, high-protein pseudo-grain that resembles tiny granules of tabouli or couscous. Known as "the mother grain," it is actually not a grain but a seed. It is high in complete protein, cooks in 10 to 15 minutes, and approximately triples its volume when cooked, somewhat mitigating its current high price in health food stores. It can be particularly useful for those following a gluten-free diet; in fact, its inclusion was shown to improve the levels of protein, iron, calcium, and fiber in a gluten-free diet.[117] It also provides more than 20% of the daily recommended values of the B vitamins thiamine, riboflavin, folate, and B6, and is a rich source of iron, magnesium, phosphorus, and zinc. A study at the Universidade de São Paulo in Brazil found that quinoa was rich in the antioxidant quercetin and had the potential to help in the management of the early stages of Type 2 diabetes.[118]

Rice

From a nutritional standpoint, we are speaking of brown rice—whole grain rice which, unlike white rice, has not had its bran (and, therefore, much of its nutrition) removed.

Brown rice is available in short, medium, and long grain varieties, the difference being largely aesthetic. The shorter the grain, the more glutinous it is, which by the way does not imply that it contains the kind of gluten present in wheat products that is dangerous to people with Celiac disease; it does not. It simply means that short grain rice cooks up stickier and long grain comes out fluffier. There's even a sweet rice grain, which is the most glutinous of all but, again, is gluten-free. There are so many varieties of rice that this is a wondrous category to explore. Try Jasmine, Basmati, black, red, wild, Wehani, and purple Thai rice for variety. Be careful about your source of brown rice; commercially produced rice is among the food crops most heavily treated with chemicals. Comparative nutritional studies have shown that rice has more magnesium and phosphorus than the other grains, and the pigments in red and black rice varieties offer nutritional benefits: these anthocyanins are powerful antioxidants and have been suggested to reduce the formation of atherosclerotic plaques.[119]

Rye

Rye is mostly known in its flour form, and used in bread loaves often flavored with caraway seeds. Especially in its sprouted form, rye is rich in vitamin E, phosphorus, magnesium, and silicon. Like wheat sprouts, rye sprouts sweeten as they lengthen because the natural starches turn to sugar. For salad purposes, use the rye sprout when it's the same size as the grain. Allow it to lengthen up to 1 inch for a sweeter intestinal-cleansing sprout and for cooking. Rye flakes can be added to soups and stews, or used as a cereal if soaked overnight. Rye flakes, like wheat and oat flakes, make good homemade granolas. For cream of rye, somewhat coarser in texture than rye flour, add 4 parts water to 1 part grain and simmer it over a low heat for about 15 minutes. In one European study, a high intake of whole grain rye was associated with decreased LDL cholesterol and an improved LDL to HDL ratio.[120] Another study at the University of Kuopio in Finland found that subjects eating a low glycemic meal of rye and pasta demonstrated lower rates of inflammation than those who consumed a high glycemic meal comprised of oats, wheat bread, and potato. The results suggest that certain cereal grains are important for reducing diabetes risk, especially in those who already have metabolic syndrome, which is a cluster of conditions—increased blood pressure, high blood sugar level, excess body fat around the waist, and abnormal cholesterol levels—that occur simultaneously, thereby increasing the risk of heart disease, stroke, and diabetes.

Triticale

This highly nutritious grain with relatively high protein content (approximately 17%) and a good balance of amino acids, can be cooked whole in combination with other grains, especially rice (2 parts water to 1 part triticale). Sprouted, it can be used in salads or breads; flaked, in granolas and casseroles. Triticale flour has become a favorite of vegetarians because of its unusually nutty sweetness and high protein content. As a flour, it must be mixed with other flours containing higher gluten contents, since its own protein has a low gluten content. Triticale originated from a cross between wheat and rye and compared to these whole-grain flours, contains more protein--almost double that of rye flour—and significantly more lysine, the main limiting amino acid in cereal grains.[121] It also contains more dietary fiber, magnesium, and folate, providing double the folate found in wheat and triple the amount found in rye whole-grain flours.

Whole Wheat

Today, whole wheat holds a pre-eminent position among grains because of its versatility and high nutritive qualities. Containing anywhere from 6 to 20% protein, wheat is also a source of vitamin E and large amounts of nitrates. These nutrients are distributed throughout the three main parts of the wheat kernel or berry. The outer layers of the kernel are known collectively as the bran; there is relatively little protein here, but it is of high quality and rich in the amino acid lysine. The dietary fiber of wheat bran is also the site of about half of the 11 B vitamins found in wheat, as well as the greater portion of the trace minerals zinc, copper, and iodine. Next comes the endosperm, the white starchy central mass of wheat kernel, which contains some 70% of the kernel's total protein, as well as its calorie-providing starch. Finally, there is the small germ found at the base of the kernel, which, in addition to containing the same B vitamins and trace minerals as the bran, is the home of vitamin E and the unsaturated fatty acids. Whole wheat has significantly more vitamin E, niacin, selenium, manganese, copper, and zinc than the other grains.

Wheat bran has been shown to accelerate the metabolism of estrogen, a known promoter of breast cancer. In one study, pre-menopausal women who consumed high levels of wheat bran showed decreased levels of blood estrogen compared to those who ate corn or oat brans.[122] Furthermore, whole wheat contains lignans, phytonutrients that can occupy the hormone receptors in the body and thus protect against high levels of estrogen. As such, the components of wheat have a dual function in protecting against breast cancer.[123]

Bulgur is a variety of whole grain wheat that is parboiled, dried (often in the sun), and then coarsely cracked. This Near and Middle Eastern staple has found its way to America in a distinctive salad called tabouli. Bulgur does not require cooking but is simply reconstituted by spreading the grain an inch deep in a shallow pan and pouring enough boiling water over it to leave about half an inch of standing water. Once the water is absorbed, stir the grain several times with a fork until it is cool. It can then be chilled, combined with greens such as parsley, fresh mint, and watercress, and marinated in a dressing of sesame oil, lemon juice, and tamari.

Couscous is a form of soft, refined durum wheat flour ("semolina") that has been steamed, cracked, and dried. It can be prepared for eating by adding 1 cup of couscous to 2 cups of boiling salted water with a teaspoon of olive oil if desired, reducing the heat and stirring constantly until most of the moisture is gone. Remove the couscous from the heat and let it stand covered about 15 minutes, fluffing it up several times with a fork.

Wheat also makes an excellent sprout, containing substantially larger amounts of all the vitamins and minerals found in the dormant kernel. The sprout, which sweetens as it lengthens, can be used in dessert preparations.

Whole wheat flour can be made from hard wheat (high protein, high gluten) or soft wheat (lower protein and gluten, high starch), or from spring or winter wheats. Hard wheat is excellent for making bread. The spring wheat contains a higher gluten content than the winter wheat. Soft wheat, either spring or winter, is known as pastry wheat because it yields a fine, starchy flour. Wheat flours are available at natural food stores in many pasta forms—from alphabets to ziti—often combined with other flours such as buckwheat, corn, rice, soy, and Jerusalem artichoke. Whole grain flours can become rancid. Rancidity occurs when the unsaturated fats in the flour are exposed to the oxygen in the air. The vitamin E in the whole wheat flour acts as a natural preservative, but within 3 months it is exhausted. This problem can best be handled by storing the flour in a cool dry place immediately after milling. There are a number of small natural food companies like Arrowhead Mills and Bob's Red Mill that mill and distribute their fresh-ground flour through health food stores. There are also numerous online sources.

Beans and Legumes

The members of the bean family are important, inexpensive sources of protein, fiber, minerals and vitamins. In a meat-free diet, in addition to dark green leafy vegetables, they are particularly important sources of iron: One cup of soybeans can provide 49% and one cup of lentils 37% of the daily requirement. More notably, according to NutritionFacts.org, studies show that legumes may be the most important predictor of survival in older people from around the globe. "They looked at five different cohorts in Japan, Sweden, Greece, and Australia. Of all the food factors they looked at, only one was associated with a longer lifespan across the board: legume intake… only for legume intake was the result plausible, consistent, and statistically significant from the data across all the populations combined." In terms of amounts, the research noted an 8% reduction in risk of death for every 20 gram increase in daily legume intake, which is approximately two tablespoons worth.[124]

Legumes can be cooked whole, flaked like grains, sprouted, ground into flours, even transformed into a variety of "dairy" products. As a general rule, 1 cup of dry beans will make about 2 ½ cups of cooked beans, enough for 4 servings. Many beans should be soaked, preferably overnight; these include adzuki beans, black beans, chick-peas (garbanzos), and soybeans. As an alternative to overnight soaking, you can bring the beans (1 cup) and water (3 to 4 cups) to a boil, remove the pot from the stove and cover, let the beans sit for an hour, then cook the beans by simmering after first bringing them to a boil or by putting them in a pressure cooker. When using beans for a soup dish, allow five times as much water as beans at the beginning of the cooking process. Don't salt the water until the beans are soft (or after the pressure in the cooker has come down), because the salt will draw the moisture out of the beans. If you wish to use salt, add it once the beans are cooked; consider a dash of Celtic sea salt, Himalayan pink salt, or Herbamare—an organic herb and vegetable seasoning with sea salt.

Adzuki

Adzuki are small red beans that have a special place in Japanese cuisine as well as in traditional Japanese medicine, where they are used as a remedy for kidney ailments (when combined with a small pumpkin called hokkaido). They have also been shown by Japanese researchers to help lower cholesterol and blood pressure.[125] Very high in B vitamins and trace minerals, adzukis should never be pressure-cooked because it makes them bitter. After overnight soaking, simmer adzukis with a strip of kombu (a kind of kelp) for about 1 to 1 ½ hours until tender, with 4 to 5 cups of water to each cup of beans. One favorite preparation: add 1 cup each of sautéed onions and celery to the tender beans and then puree them together in a blender. The resulting thick, creamy soup can be thinned with water or bean juice and flavored with a dash of lime juice, tamari, and mild curry.

Black Beans and Turtle Beans

Black beans and their close relative, turtle beans, have served as major food sources in the Caribbean, Mexico, and the American Southwest for many years. These beans should not be prepared in a pressure cooker since their skins fall off easily and may clog the valve. A smooth, rich black bean soup, a specialty of Cuba, is made by cooking the soaked beans until tender, adding sautéed garlic, onions, and celery, and then pressing the mixture through a colander (or, more easily, quickly blending it in an electric blender). A small amount of lime juice may be added to lighten the taste.

Black beans are high in folate and magnesium and a good source of the essential nutrients potassium, zinc, manganese, and iron, as well as alpha-linolenic omega-3 fatty acids. The black coat of the bean is a magnificent source of the antioxidant and anti-inflammatory anthocyanin flavonoids.[126] Additionally, black beans were recently shown to provide a larger indigestible fraction than lentils or chick-peas, an important source of bioactive molecules, and supportive for friendly bacteria in the intestine.[127] Studies indicate a protective effect against colon cancer in populations with higher legume consumption.[128]

Black-Eyed Peas

Black-eyed peas, a Southern favorite, provide a delicious complete protein-balanced meal. Among the quickest-cooking beans, they become tender in 45 minutes to an hour. Eating this bean on New Year's Day is said to bring good luck throughout the year. Black-eyed peas, like other legumes, are a low-fat low-calorie food, yet their high fiber and protein content keeps you feeling fuller for longer. As a high potassium, low sodium food, they can help to reduce blood pressure. They are also an excellent vegetarian source of zinc, a trace mineral that is essential for the vision and the functioning of the immune system and wound healing, and vital nutrients such as B vitamins, vitamin E, copper, phosphorus, manganese, iron, and potassium.

Chick-Peas (Garbanzos)

Chick-peas, or garbanzos, are so versatile that they have been the subject of entire cookbooks. High in protein, they are also good sources of calcium, iron, phosphorus, potassium, magnesium, B vitamins, especially folate, and the omega-6 fatty acid, linoleic acid. The FDA and the Food and Agricultural Organization of the United Nations/World Health Organization (FAO/WHO) gave chick-peas one of the highest protein digestibility scores for a non-animal based food, rating them extremely high in protein quality.[129] The consumption of chick-peas for at least 5 weeks was shown by investigators at the University of Tasmania to result in significant reductions in total and LDL cholesterol levels.[130] They can be roasted like peanuts or boiled. After a very thorough roasting, chick-peas can even be ground and used as a coffee substitute. Hummus is a thick paste that combines mashed chick-peas, hulled sesame-seed tahini, garlic, and lemon juice. Bean patés using chick-peas as a base offer many creative opportunities for plant-based proteins. Cooked grains, ground seeds and nuts, raw vegetables, herbs, and miso may all be combined with the cooked beans to produce a sophisticated and appealing paté or paste.

Great Northern Beans and Navy Beans

Great northern beans and their small counterpart, navy beans, cook in less than an hour and require no presoaking. They are often used for hearty soups. Cook the beans with 5 to 6 parts water or stock to 1 part dry beans. Firmer vegetables, such as carrots, rutabagas, or turnips should be added one-half hour before the soup is finished; other vegetables, such as onions, celery, and peppers, should be added 15 minutes later, either sautéed or raw. These beans are one of the most abundant plant-based sources of phosphatidylserine yet known.[131] Phosphatidylserine is a cell membrane component whose consumption may reduce the risk of dementia and cognitive dysfunction in the elderly and has been shown to have mood-enhancing properties.[131, 132]

Kidney Beans

Kidney beans, standard in all sorts of chilies, will cook in about an hour, after having been soaked overnight. The fragrant brown bean juice produced in cooking the beans makes the addition of tomato virtually unnecessary. Once the beans are tender, try dicing onions, garlic, and red and green peppers; sauté them lightly in sesame oil until the onions are translucent, then add them to the beans. Season them to taste. Rich Mexican chili powder seems to lend more flavor to the beans than does a scorching Indian one. Tamari, a dash of blackstrap molasses, or fresh-grated ginger root can further enhance the beans. For a perfect final texture, add dry wheat flakes to the chili about 20 minutes before serving; this allows time for the flakes to cook and disintegrate, thickening the dish while complementing the protein of the beans. In addition to being a good source of protein and dietary fiber, 100 grams of kidney beans can provide 99% of the daily recommended intake of folate and over 30% of that for iron, magnesium, potassium, and zinc, and more than 100% of the recommended intake of molybdenum, an important antioxidant that helps activate cells to produce energy and activates enzymes that are required for the removal of toxins.[134]

Lentils

Lentils come in a rainbow of colors, but generally only the green, brown, and red varieties are available in the United States. On a gram-to-gram basis, lentils contain more protein than beef, and are inexpensive and nutritious sources of phosphorus, magnesium, zinc, calcium, potassium, cellulose, vitamins K and B (particularly folate), and an important source of iron. Lentils, like other beans, are rich in both soluble and insoluble dietary fibers, with positive effects on digestive and cardiovascular health, having three times more fiber than a serving of bran flakes for example. One study that followed food intake patterns across seven countries found that those who ate a diet rich in legumes had an impressive 82% reduction in the risk of death from heart disease.[135] Scientists have demonstrated that lentil-based diets can lead to the lowering of cholesterol levels and reduced inflammation.[136, 137]

Lentils require no presoaking and disintegrate when cooked, leaving a smooth base to which you can add fresh or sautéed vegetables (including carrots, turnips, onions, and peppers). They sprout well in combination with other seeds and produce large quantities. The flavor of the uncooked sprout is similar to that of fresh ground pepper on salad; when cooked it has a more nutlike taste. The sprouts should be harvested when the shoot is as long as the seed.

Mung Beans

Mung beans are probably best known in their sprout form, eaten raw or lightly sautéed with other vegetables. They can be cooked as a dry bean, using three times as much water as beans, and then pureed in an electric blender into a smooth soup. The result is rather bland and benefits from the addition of tamari and fresh or dried basil. But as sprouts, mung beans really come into their own. Mung sprouts are rich in vitamins A and C and contain high amounts of folate, calcium, magnesium, phosphorus, and iron. The hulls are easily digestible and rich in minerals. Regular consumption of mung beans may help control blood glucose levels. In one study, a group given a 50 gram portion of mung beans exhibited a 45% lower glucose response than those who ate equivalent amounts of grains, and the beans were able to lower the glucose response in individuals with Type 2 diabetes.[138, 139]

Mung sprouts can be harvested any time from the second day, when the shoot has just appeared, to the third or fourth day when the shoot is about 4 inches long. Mung beans make a good first choice for beginning sprouters.

Peanuts

Peanuts, though commonly grouped with seeds and nuts, are actually members of the legume family. Their high protein content is well known. In the United States, eating peanut butter is virtually a national pastime. Peanut butter can—and should—contain 100% peanuts; sugars, colorings, stabilizers, added oils and preservatives are neither necessary nor desirable. A single grinding under pressure extracts enough oil from the nut meal to give the peanuts a creamy texture.

Peanuts are rich in monounsaturated fats, such as oleic acid, the healthful fat found in olive oil associated with the benefits of a Mediterranean diet. In fact, one study found that a diet rich in peanuts and peanut butter decreased cardiovascular disease risk by an estimated 21% compared to the average American diet due to the positive effects of these fats.[140] Peanuts are also good sources of vitamins B and E, manganese, and the antioxidant resveratrol, also found in red grapes and red wine. However, it's best to consume peanuts in moderation as they can contain toxic fungal aflatoxins, which may grow on them if they're not stored properly in a cold, dry environment. Aflatoxins can negatively affect the liver and can even lead to liver cancer. [141]

Peanut allergy is one of the most common food allergies, and it can cause a severe, potentially fatal, allergic reaction (anaphylaxis). For those who arc allergic, strict avoidance of peanut and peanut products is essential. Always read ingredient labels to identify peanut ingredients. Allergies to peanuts appear to be on the rise in children. According to a Food Allergy Research & Education (FARE)-funded study, the number of children in the US with peanut allergies more than tripled between 1997 and 2008.[142]

Since peanuts are a legume and grow underground, they are not the same as tree nuts (almonds, cashews, walnuts, etc.), which—as the name suggests—grow on trees. Moreover, an allergy to peanuts does not mean that you will have a heightened sensitivity to other legumes, including soy; in fact, there is no greater risk for this than a person without a peanut allergy.

Pinto Beans

Pinto beans are popular in American Southwest dishes and lend themselves especially well to baking. Naturally sweet in flavor, they adapt to many types of seasonings, and once cooked tender, they can be used in casseroles. Pinto flakes cook quickly and reconstitute themselves into tender round beans in about 40 minutes (2 parts water to 1 part dry flakes). Cumin blends nicely with these beans, if used sparingly. One cup of pinto beans can provide approximately 30% of the required daily protein intake and 60% of the daily fiber requirement, plus their regular consumption was demonstrated to lower both LDL and total cholesterol.[143]

Soybeans

Soybeans, unquestionably the most nutritious of all the beans, have been the major source of protein in Asian diets for centuries and are increasingly viewed as the most realistic source of high-quality, low-cost protein available today. In addition to high-quality protein, soybeans contain large amounts of B vitamins, minerals, and unsaturated fatty acids in the form of lecithin that help the body emulsify cholesterol. Following the analysis of 29 clinical trials, soybean protein was shown to reduce both LDL and total cholesterol levels.[144] Even the Food and Drug Administration has recognized their value, saying that 25 grams of soy protein a day, as part of a diet low in saturated fat and cholesterol, may reduce the risk of heart disease. Soybeans also contain significant amounts of the essential omega-3 fatty acid, alpha-linolenic acid, and choline, diets high in choline have been associated with reduced inflammation.[145] In addition, soybeans contain important phytonutrients, including the antioxidants isoflavones and saponins, which have been linked to protection against osteoporosis in both young and post-menopausal women.[146, 147]

The soybean is the most widely grown and utilized legume on earth, but sadly more than 94% of soybeans grown in the US are genetically modified; you must purchase organic soy if you wish to avoid GMOs.[148]

Thanks to their bland flavor after cooking and their high concentration of nutrients, soybeans can be made into an amazingly diverse array of foods. Western technology in recent years has focused on creating a wide range of synthetic soybean foods. There are protein concentrates in the form of soy powder containing from 70 to 90% moisture-free protein, isolates (defatted flakes and flours used to make simulated dairy products and frozen desserts), spun protein fibers (isolates dissolved in alkali solutions for use in simulated meat products), and textured vegetable proteins (made from soy flour and used in simulated meat products and infant foods).

The soybean can be enjoyed in many ways, as tofu (see below), or as a fresh green summer vegetable, simmered or steamed in the pod. Roasted soybeans are now available in many varieties: dry-roasted, oil-roasted, salted, unsalted, and with garlic or barbecue flavors. They contain up to 47% protein and can either be eaten as a snack or added to casseroles for texture.

Tempeh

An interesting soybean preparation called tempeh is made from cooked, hulled soybean halves, to which a *Rhizopus* mold is introduced. The inoculated bean cakes are then fermented overnight, during which time the white mycelium mold partially digests the beans and effectively deactivates the trypsin enzyme, which could inhibit digestion. The soybeans have, by this time, become fragrant cakes bound together by the mold; you can then either bake them or add them to a stew as a vegetarian meat substitute. Tempeh is rich in protein (from 18 to 48%) and like the other fermented soy products and sea vegetables, it is one of the few nonmeat sources of vitamin B12. It is also a very good source of manganese, copper, phosphorus, magnesium, and calcium. Tempeh is highly digestible and the nutrients it contains are highly absorbable due to the fermentation process. For example, one study found that calcium from tempeh was equally as well absorbed as calcium from cow's milk.[149] Tempeh can be made easily in any kitchen with a Tempeh starter kit (containing dried *Rhizopus oligosporus* spores), which is commercially available.

Tofu

Tofu (soy curd or soy cheese) is among the traditional East Asian soy products. Tofu is a remarkable food. It is very inexpensive when purchased at Asian markets or natural food shops and even more so if made at home. Two other related products, tamari soy sauce and miso (fermented soy paste), will be discussed later in this chapter. You can make your own tofu by grinding soaked soybeans, cooking them with water, pouring the resulting mixture into a pressing sack, and collecting the "milk" underneath by squeezing as much liquid as possible from the sack, leaving the bean fiber behind. The soy milk is then simmered and curdled in a solution containing sea-water brine (called nigari), lemon juice, or vinegar. Any of these three solidifiers will work well, although commercial nigari is most often used for this coagulation process.

Tofu is easy to digest and low in calories, saturated fats, and cholesterol. When solidified with calcium chloride or calcium sulfate—as in most commercial American tofu—tofu contains more calcium by weight than dairy milk; it's also a good source of other minerals such as iron, phosphorus, and potassium. Since it's made from soybeans, tofu is free of chemical toxins. One comprehensive analysis by Chinese scientists of 28 studies showed that soy in the form of tofu (and soy miso) was better at reducing the risk of stomach cancer than soybeans.[150] Since the majority of tofu is made from GMO soybeans, it is generally free of chemical toxins because GMOs are more pest-resistant. Nonetheless, if you want to avoid GMOs, stick to organic tofu; sprouted varieties are even better.

Edamame

Young soybeans eaten fresh and generally still in the pod are gaining popularity and are known by their Japanese name, edamame. Unlike other soybeans, according to the National Soybean Research Laboratory, all edamame are non-GMO.[151] These soybeans are eaten raw as a nutritious snack, particularly by the Japanese, where they are simply served in their pods and sprinkled with salt. Like other soybeans, edamame are a complete protein, meaning they contain all the essential amino acids and are high in dietary fiber and healthy polyunsaturated fats, especially omega-3 alpha-linolenic acid. They are also rich in folate, magnesium, vitamin K, iron, potassium, phosphorus, calcium, and manganese.

Nuts and Seeds

Nuts and seeds are fine sources of protein, minerals (especially magnesium), some B vitamins, and the antioxidant vitamin E. Nuts and seeds contain antioxidants and a good source of vegetarian protein. In addition, linoleic acid, an unsaturated essential fatty acid, is abundant in many nuts, fatty seeds (such as flax, hemp, poppy, and sesame seeds) and their derived vegetable oils. Nuts can help to reduce the levels of inflammation in your body, according to the Linus Pauling Institute, and research has shown that those who regularly eat nuts are at a lower risk of death from cancer and cardiovascular disease, with an 11% and 29% reduction, respectively, than those who do not eat nuts.[152, 153] The Institute also reports that nut consumption correlates with a reduced risk of type 2 diabetes. Throw some on top of your favorite vegetarian dish or salad.

Nuts can be eaten as snack foods or used with other foods to add interesting flavors, textures, and nutritional values. A general sprouting procedure for seeds and nuts is to soak the dried seeds for about 8 hours (approximately 4 parts water to 1 part seed). Don't throw away the soaking water; use it as a cooking liquid, or water your houseplants with it. Rinse the seeds with cool water and place them in a sprouter; the nuts can be used right away and either dehydrated as snacks or pulverized into nut patés or "cheezes," (spelled this way to impart that they are dairy-free) or simply add them to salads. Keys to successful sprouting include keeping the sprouts moist but never soaked, keeping them moderately warm, rinsing them several times a day, and giving them enough room so that air can freely circulate around them. They have a refrigerator life of 7 to 10 days, and can also be dried easily for use in beverages, nut butter, and spreads.

Alfalfa

Many people think of alfalfa as a barnyard grass, which it is. Because its roots penetrate deeply underground to seek out the elements it craves, alfalfa is one of the best possible fodders. But the fresh, mineral-laden leaves of this plant are especially nutritious for humans when juiced. Alfalfa seeds purchased at a natural food store may seem expensive, but a few of them go a long way—½ teaspoon of dry seeds yields an entire trayful of sprouts. The sprouts have a light sweet taste and are particularly rich in vitamin C, as well as in chlorophyll (when allowed to develop in light). They also have high mineral values, containing phosphorus, chlorine, silicon, aluminum, calcium, magnesium, sulfur, sodium, and potassium. Alfalfa seeds sprout well in combination with other seeds and have a high germination rate. They can also be used when dried.

As many readers will know, there have been outbreaks of salmonella poisoning and E. coli with sprouts, but they are not limited to alfalfa. I'm placing this note here because the alfalfa outbreaks are the ones that have made American news. In the US there have been at about 40 outbreaks since 1990 according to Bill Marler, a personal injury attorney who specializes in food-borne illness.[154] So, yes, it is an issue. Yet because these contaminants can get into cracks in the seeds, there is little that can be done outside of radiation to handle the problem entirely; radiation, by the way, doesn't just kill the germ, it kills the enzymes in the food too. If you want to take precautions, I suggest that you swish the seeds for 10 minutes in a solution of water and 10 drops of grapefruit seed extract prior to sprouting.

Almonds

Almonds are a wonderful nut, one of the lowest in fat in the nut family. They can be eaten raw, pulverized into a pâté, or soaked overnight and then used to make almond milk: use 1 cup of soaked almonds blended with four times as much water. Then strain the mixture through a nut bag or cheesecloth to get the milk; reserve the pulp for almond cheeze or a savory or sweet nut spread. Almonds, which have an exceptionally high mineral content, are delicious raw or roasted with tamari. The raw nut can be sliced, slivered, or chopped, and even can be ground into almond butter.

Almonds are a particularly good source of vitamin E, copper, and magnesium, in addition to a lot of bioactive phytonutrients. Scientific peer-reviewed studies conducted by the Loma Linda University and University of California, Davis, have shown their consumption can lower cholesterol levels and reduce the risk of colon cancer.[155,156]

Brazil Nuts

Brazil nuts, like other seeds and nuts, have a high fat content and contain the highest amount of saturated fat of any nut, although they are a very rich source of omega-6 fatty acids. Because they are also high in protein, they are actually not much higher in calories per gram of usable protein than are whole grains. They also offer unusually high amounts of the sulfur-containing amino acids and are a very good source of magnesium, copper, manganese, phosphorus, zinc, and selenium, which we need for thyroid function and immunity. In fact, you only need three to four Brazil nuts to get the daily recommended amount of this mineral. Recent studies have also shown that a diet rich in selenium can help prevent the development of pancreatic cancer, the fourth leading cancer in terms of mortality in the US with some 80% of patients dying within 12 months of diagnosis.[157] For this reason, you can serve them to good advantage as a chopped garnish for fresh vegetables such as brussel sprouts, cauliflower, green peas, and lima beans. These vegetables are all deficient in the sulfur-containing amino acids but high in the amino acid isoleucine lacking in Brazil nuts.

Cashews

Cashews are also popular nuts that can be added to many dishes. They are a good source of copper, iron, zinc, magnesium, phosphorus, manganese, potassium, selenium, calcium, and vitamin K, and have a lower fat content than most other nuts, two-thirds of which are "healthy" monounsaturated fats such as those found in olive oil. What's more, these nuts were shown by researchers from the University of Montreal to be beneficial in the control of blood sugar, important in reducing the risk of developing diabetes, due to the presence of anacardic acid in cashews, the release of which improved the ability of sugar to enter into cells and decreased the amount in the bloodstream.[158] Use them as a layer in a casserole or simply roast them lightly and toss them in a bowl of steamed snow peas. Cashew butter, from both raw and roasted nuts, is growing in popularity and is well-suited for use in sauces, where it can be diluted with water and miso paste. You can mix it yourself in a nutritious soy "milkshake." Blend 2 cups of plain or sweetened soy milk with 1/2 cup of cashew butter; add 2 tablespoons of carob powder, a pinch of salt, and a dash of vanilla extract and nutmeg. Cashews are readily used in raw food preparations such as raw "cheezes," pie crusts, and patés.

Chia Seeds

Chia seeds, now available in natural food stores, have long been a staple in Mexican and Native American diets, where they were traditionally used to increase endurance on long hunts and migrations. Although a member of the mint family, chia seeds have a mild flax-seed-like taste. They can be chewed raw or sprinkled into hot or cold cereals or fruits. Chia seeds are mucilaginous by nature, which means they become sticky mucous-like when soaked in water. As such, they are frequently used in raw food preparations such as puddings, pies, and smoothies. Their sprouting procedure is also slightly different. To sprout, sprinkle the seeds over a saucer filled with water and allow to stand overnight. By morning, the seeds will have absorbed all the water and will stick to the saucer. Gently rinse and drain, using a sieve if possible. Then, as with other seeds, rinse twice daily. Also try sprouting the seeds in a flat, covered container lined with damp paper towels. Harvest the chia seeds when the shoot is one inch long.

Chia seeds are rich in the omega-3 fatty acids, alpha-linolenic acid, high in antioxidants, and are 40% fiber by weight, making them an excellent dietary source of fiber. They are also good sources of calcium, phosphorus, magnesium, and manganese. One study found that the consumption of chia seeds by patients with type 2 diabetes improved blood pressure and other important health markers.[159]

Clover

The red variety of clover makes a delicious sprout similar in taste to alfalfa. In its sprout form, this forage plant can be an excellent source of chlorophyll. When the primary leaves are about one inch in length, spread them out in a nonmetallic tray and dampen them. They should be covered with clear plastic to hold in moisture and placed in a sunny spot for 1 to 2 hours.

Cress Seeds

Cress seeds are tiny members of the mustard family. They add a zesty taste to salads when used in their sprout form. They too are mucilaginous seeds and are sprouted in the same way as chia and flax. Harvest the sprouts at about 1 inch long and use them in sandwiches instead of lettuce. They provide an excellent source of iron and are rich in folic acid, calcium, vitamins C, E, and A, and both arachidic and linoleic fatty acids. Cress has long been given to lactating mothers because it boosts milk production.[160]

Fenugreek Seeds

Fenugreek seeds were first used by the ancient Greeks to brew tea. This strong tea is an excellent mouthwash, as well as a tasty and nutritious addition to soy or nut milk. The ground dry seed is one of the components of curry powder. When sprouted, fenugreek can be added to soups, salads, and grain dishes. The sprout should be harvested once it is 1/4 inch long, for it will become very bitter soon afterward.

Filberts (Hazelnuts)

Filberts or hazelnuts are tasty nuts that, once chopped, make a delicious garnish for both greens and creamy tofu pudding. These nuts, however, contain an excess amount of calories for the amount of protein they provide, although they are a good source of folate.

Flax (Linseed)

Flax, also known as linseed, is a versatile plant. The fiber of the mature plant is used to make linen and pressed to extract its oil. As a sprout, flax has been used for centuries. At Greek and Roman banquets, flax sprouts were reportedly served between courses for their mild laxative effect. Flax is also a mucilaginous seed and has a variety of uses: Sprinkle them over salads, or grind and use them as a thickening agent for dressings, sauces, soups, or smoothies. Ground, they are also an excellent substitute for eggs in vegan baked goods.

Flax seeds are high in magnesium, manganese, B-vitamins, omega-3 fatty acids, and fiber. They are also high in phytochemicals, particularly lignans, which may help prevent cancers, including breast and prostate, and type 2 diabetes.[160-163]

Mustard

The small seeds of the common black mustard plant will sprout quite readily and are usually available at herb and spice stores. Small amounts of these sprouts add a spicy flavor to salads and sandwiches. Harvest when shoots are about an inch long.

Pecans

Pecans are nuts that are cultivated organically in Texas and New Mexico. Like filberts, pecans are not good sources of protein as they contain too many calories for the amount of protein they offer. However, they are high in potassium and B vitamins, as well as rich in antioxidants, including polyphenolic antioxidant ellagic acid, vitamin E, beta-carotene, lutein and zea-xanthin. Research studies suggest that these compounds help the body remove toxic oxygen-free radicals and thus offer protection from diseases, cancers, and infections.[164] Pecans also contain concentrated amounts of plant sterols, effective at lowering cholesterol levels.[165] They are also high in oleic acid, the healthy fat found in olives and avocado. Pecans are delicious as tamari-roasted nuts: Dry-roast in a heavy skillet and when they begin to emit a pleasing fragrance, remove to a plate and sprinkle lightly with tamari.

Pignolias (Pine Nuts)

Pignolias, or pine nuts, have an unusual flavor but are a poor source of protein. However, for each ounce of pignolias, they provide the entire recommended intake of manganese, over 20% of the daily magnesium intake, approximately 20% of the intake for zinc, and vitamins E and K, and 9% of the recommended daily iron intake. They are also a rich source of the fatty acid pinoleic acid, proven to be an appetite suppressant.[166]

Found in the cones of the small pinon pine, which grows in the American Southwest, these nuts have been used by many Indian tribes as a food staple. Most of the pignolias consumed in the United States, however, come from Portugal. Pan-roasted pine nuts are delicious with green vegetables like peas and beans, and are also tasty in bread stuffings. They are also a main component in pesto.

Pistachio Nuts

Pistachio nuts are familiar to many as an Italian ice cream flavor. For snacking purposes, use the naturally grown pistachio rather than the dyed varieties. Like other nuts, pistachios should be consumed only in small quantities, since they are high in calories, although they contain fewer calories than other nuts. However, they're the only nut to contain moderate levels of the important antioxidants lutein and zeaxanthin, due to their unique green and purple colored flesh, as well as being a good source of potassium, magnesium, vitamin K, and fiber. Pistachios also contain L-arginine, which can make the lining of the arteries more flexible[167] and have been linked with various positive effects to protect against heart disease, including lower levels of cholesterol.[168]

Pumpkin Seeds, Pepitas, and Squash Seeds

Pumpkin seeds, pepitas, and squash seeds are delicious seeds rich in minerals that can be eaten as snacks or ground into a meal for use in baking and cooking. One serving provides a high protein content (equivalent to a similar serving of peanuts), more than 20% of the recommended daily intake of iron, and is a good source of the essential omega-3 fatty acid alpha-linoleic acid, zinc, manganese, phosphorus, magnesium, and copper. Eastern Europeans, who eat many more pumpkin seeds than do Americans, use them to help prevent prostate disorders and several studies have shown the protective effects on the prostate[169] of pumpkin seed oil's phytosterols. Also, the lignans in pumpkin seeds have been shown to have antimicrobial and anti-viral properties.[170] Save the seeds from a pumpkin or squash and sprout them. Harvest when the shoot is just beginning to show (after 3 or 4 days). If allowed to lengthen any further, the sprouts will taste bitter.

Radish Seeds

Radish seeds, both black and red, make wonderfully tangy sprouts. They sprout easily and work well when combined with alfalfa and clover seeds. They're relatively expensive compared to most sprouting seeds, but you don't need many of these peppery-tasting sprouts to perk up a salad. Harvest these shoots when they're about an inch long.

Sesame Seeds (Benne)

Sesame seeds, or benne, are popular around the world because of their taste and high nutritive content, with one ounce providing 23% of the recommended daily intake of iron. Most sesame seeds available in the United States are grown in southern Mexico, where few sprays are used. They are available hulled or unhulled. The unhulled variety is nutritionally superior since most of the mineral value is found in the hull. Sesame seeds are an excellent source of protein, unsaturated fatty acids, copper, manganese, calcium, magnesium, iron, B vitamins, zinc, selenium, and vitamins A and E. In addition, sesame seeds contain two unique cholesterol-lowering lignans—sesamin and sesamolin—and sesamin was shown to be particularly effective in protecting against hypertension, as well as having antioxidative properties.[171,172]

The protein in sesame seeds effectively complements the protein of legumes, because both contain high amounts of each other's deficient amino acids. Therefore, an especially good addition to a soy milk shake is tahini, or sesame butter. Used extensively as the whole seed in breads and other baked foods, in grain dishes, and on vegetables, the unhulled seeds can also be toasted and ground into sesame butter, which has a stronger taste and higher mineral content than sesame tahini. Tahini, made from toasted and hulled seeds, is a mild, sweet butter. Tahini is used in the

Middle East, where the oil that separates from the butter is used as cooking oil. Tahini is an excellent base for salad dressing and acts as a perfect thickener for all sorts of sauces.

Sunflower Seeds

Sunflower seeds are sun-energized, nutritional powerhouses rich in protein (about 30%), unsaturated fatty acids, phosphorus, calcium, iron, fluorine, iodine, potassium, magnesium, zinc, several B vitamins, vitamin E, and vitamin D (one of the few vegetable sources of this vitamin). Sunflower seeds are a good source of several mood affecting minerals, including magnesium—and just a handful delivers half the recommended daily amount for magnesium. Magnesium deficiency has been linked to anxiety and mood disorders, and supplementation of magnesium has been shown to be beneficial in treating depression and irritability.[173] The seeds also contain good levels of the amino acid tryptophan, critical for the body to produce serotonin, which helps maintain a calm and relaxed mood.[174]

Their high mineral content is the result of the sunflower's extensive root system, which penetrates deep into the subsoil seeking nutrients. Their vitamin D content is partially due to the flower's tendency to follow and face the sun as it moves across the sky. Sunflowers were cultivated extensively by American Indians as a food crop. In their raw state, sunflower seeds can be enjoyed as snacks or included in everything from breads to salads. The seeds are also available as toasted, salted nut butter. Sprouted sunflower seeds should be eaten when barely budded or they will taste very bitter. However, it usually takes 4 to 5 days for the shoot to appear. Unhulled seeds, or special hulled sprouting seeds, are used when sprouting, but the husk should be removed before eating.

Walnuts

Walnuts are a good source of protein and iron. Black walnuts contain about 40% more protein than English walnuts (also known as California walnuts in the United States). Walnuts will keep fresh much longer when purchased in the shell. This is true of all nuts. It also brings down the price considerably. Walnuts are packed full of omega-3 fatty acids, with half an ounce of walnuts providing the recommended amount of omega-3 oils, in addition to antioxidants, tryptophan, and folate. Walnuts also provide vitamin E, particularly in the form of gamma-tocopherol, and studies have shown that increased levels of gamma-tocopherol (and not alpha-tocopherol, the other form of vitamin E) are associated with a reduced incidence of cardiovascular disease.[175,176]

Miscellaneous Vegetarian Additions

Miso & Tamari Miso

Miso and Tamari Miso, a fermented soybean paste, has long been a staple seasoning in the Asian kitchen. It is produced by combining cooked soybeans, salt, and various grains. Barley miso is made with barley and soybeans. Rice miso is made with both hulled and unhulled rice plus soybeans. Soybeans alone are used to make hatcho miso. These cooked and salted combinations are dusted with a fungus mold, koji, which produces the enzymes that start to digest the bean-and-grain mixture.

Tamari is naturally fermented soy sauce. Originally considered excess liquid, it was drained off miso that had finished fermenting. Today it is a product in its own right and is made from a natural fermentation process of whole soybeans, natural sea salt, well water, roasted cracked wheat, and koji spores, all aged for 12 to 18 months.

Miso and tamari are useful in all cuisines, but because of their high salt content—11% for the saltiest of hatcho miso and 18% for tamari—they should be used sparingly. However, one study of over 40,000 Japanese participants over more than 10 years, found that miso-containing diets lowered the risk of cardiovascular disease, a result that is unusual for a high-sodium food.[177] Miso and tamari are probiotic foods that contain beneficial bacteria that live in the large intestine. Also, tamari contains unique polysaccharides from the fermentation process that can lessen the activity of an enzyme called hyaluronidase, whose activity is associated with inflammation and allergic reactions. By lowering its activity, consumption of tamari may be able to relieve allergy symptoms such as hay fever (although those with allergy to soy should still be careful).[178]

Salt

Controversy continues about the virtues and dangers of salt. Some people consume large quantities of salt. Many others attempt to get their salt from the juices of celery, spinach, beets, or carrots. Very little sodium, however, is derived from these supposedly sodium-rich foods. Still other people decide upon or are prescribed low-sodium or even "salt-free" diets. People on low-sodium diets have often been suffering from hypertension (high blood pressure) or kidney problems. Overconsumption of salt will lead to hypertension: the salt draws water out of blood cells and vessels, which in turn causes dehydration of the tissues and forces the heart to pump much too strenuously.

Overconsumption of salt also clogs the kidneys and creates an excess of water that cannot be properly eliminated from the body. On the other hand, moderate and intelligent consumption of salt helps the body retain heat by slightly contracting the blood vessels, which is why we tend to consume more salt in cold months. Sodium also helps maintain intestinal muscle tone. You should evaluate your own salt needs according to your physical activity, climate, water intake, and—above all—diet. People in meat-eating cultures seldom need extra salt per se, because they get all they need from the blood and flesh of the animals they eat. Vegetarian or agricultural peoples, however, tend to have a high regard for salt and use it to cook, pickle, and preserve foods.

If you want to eat salt, you should use the natural sun- or kiln-dried variety, which still contains important trace minerals. Refined "table" salt is made fine by high heats and flash-cooling, and then combined with such additives as sodium silico aluminate to keep it "free-flowing." Kosher salt is an exception. It has larger crystals due to its milder processing, and nothing is added to the better brands like Selina Naturally® and Real Salt®. Natural salt—rock salt or sea salt—is not free-flowing, but some brands add calcium carbonate, a natural compound, to prevent caking. All salt is or once was sea salt; as such all of them are composed of the minerals sodium and chloride. Different salts can have different textures and different perceived levels of perceived saltiness,[179] meaning that less could be added to food to obtain the same taste. Generally, the differences between salt obtained from inland rock deposits or from the sea are fairly unimportant. However, one study demonstrated that sea salts harvested from different parts of the world do have minor differences in their mineral contents. For example, Himalayan Pink salt, which is pink due to traces of iron, was also found to contain higher levels of calcium, potassium, and magnesium compared to table salt, and slightly lower amounts of sodium.[180]

No natural salt contains iodine, which is far too volatile a substance to remain stable for long without numerous additives. But there is an excellent source of iodine from the ocean: sea vegetables, the most common being kelp. These contain a natural, sugar-stabilized iodine—as well as about 4 to 8% salt. They are harvested, roasted, ground up, and marketed as salt alternatives. Another healthful way of adding salt to your diet is to use sesame salt, sold as gomasio. This versatile condiment can be used in place of ordinary salt on cooked greens, grains, and raw salads. Gomasio can be purchased in most natural food stores. Salted umeboshi plums also may be used. These small Japanese plums are known for the high quality and quantity of citric acid they contain. The citric acid in plums allegedly helps neutralize and eliminate some of the excess lactic acid in the body, helping to restore a natural balance.

Umeboshi plums also have many culinary uses. Use them to salt the water in which grains will be cooked or use several in tofu salad dressings instead of tamari or sea salt.

Sweeteners

Carbohydrate sugar is unquestionably essential to life; but best to get it in as unadulterated a form as possible. Common table sugar has been processed to 99.9% sucrose, devoid of the vitamins and minerals found in sugar cane or sugar beets. This refined sucrose taxes the body's digestive system and depletes its core of minerals and enzymes during sugar metabolization. For this reason and others, white sugar has understandably earned a bad reputation and the label "empty food." Carbohydrates include many sugars. The best known is sucrose, or white table sugar, which breaks down in the body into simpler sugars, glucose and fructose. There are also starches in whole cereals (together with their own component enzymes, vitamins, minerals, and proteins) that break down uniformly in the body into simple glucose molecules once they have been cooked, chewed, and digested.

Compared with these refined starches, refined sugars tend to overstrain the body's digestive system. So it would seem wiser to get the sugars you need from abundant natural stores in cereals, vegetables, and fruits. Eaten in moderate amounts, starches are not fattening, contrary to public opinion. When cooking with natural foods, you should simply replace refined sugars with the richer flavors of naturally occurring sugars.

Maple syrup, for example, or honey (in spite of the challenges associated with its consumption) or fruit juice can substitute for sugar in almost any home recipe. Maple sugar is expensive and very sweet, so use it in moderation. Use ½ cup of maple syrup instead of 1 cup of sugar and either reduce the other liquids in the recipe or increase the dry ingredients accordingly. Maple syrup is a good source of some minerals, including manganese (100 grams of syrup provides 165% of the recommended daily intake), zinc (100 grams of syrup provides 28% of the recommended daily intake), iron and calcium, and has been shown to contain some 24 different antioxidants, including resveratrol, also found in red grapes and red wine.[181] But be sure that the maple syrup you buy has not been extracted with formaldehyde.

All honeys, while not vegan, are basically the fruit sugar fructose, which consists of varying amounts of dextrose, levulose, maltose, and other simple sugars, and comprise up to 95% of the product.[182] The flavor of honey depends on the source of the bees' nectar. All honey you use should be unheated and unfiltered because pure, raw honey is antibacterial and provides small amounts of B-group vitamins and minerals such as calcium, copper, iron, magnesium, manganese, phosphorus, potassium, and zinc, providing more nutrients than sugar, and antioxidants such as flavonoids. Honey has a wide range of health benefits due to these properties not found in refined or treated honey, including an array of friendly bacteria. Manuka honey, in particular, is linked to many health benefits. It is particularly helpful in healing infections, and many hospitals around the world now keep active manuka honey on hand when nothing else works for treatment of antibiotic resistant MRSA super bugs. Methicillin-resistant Staphylococcus aureus (MRSA) is a form of bacterial infection that is resistant to numerous antibiotics including methicillin, amoxicillin, penicillin, and oxacillin, thus causing difficulty in treatment of the infection.[183]

A study published in the *European Journal of Medical Research* in 2003 claimed manuka honey used under dressings on post-operative wounds had an 85% success rate in clearing up infections, compared with 50% for normal antibiotic creams.[184] According to the Honey Center in Warkworth, New Zealand, manuka honey has also been shown to be helpful to aide in healing bed sores and other external ulcerative conditions, *Helicobactor pylori* (stomach ulcer causing bacteria), *E. coli*, *Staphylococcus aureus* (the most common cause of wound infection), and *Streptococcus pyogenes* (stubborn, often antibiotic resistant bacteria that inflame and cause sore throats). It is also very healing, they note, when used externally on the skin for conditions such as burns, wounds, dermatitis, eczema, abscesses etc., and "medical-grade" manuka honey has been approved by the FDA for use in wound management.[185] Additionally, it can decrease the duration of bacterial diarrhea, and studies show that it assists in rehydration of the body during diarrhea sickness.[186]

However, there are other challenges with honey that make it a less than desirable sweetener option. The practice of commercially farming bees for honey is hazardous to bee populations, and the diversity of these populations, and is responsible—along with toxic pesticides like Neonicotinoids—for bee colony collapse. Like all factory farming, beekeeping has morphed into an industry that puts profits ahead of animal concerns. Commercial farmers take all or nearly all of the honey, and feed the bees sugar water instead, leading to health problems for the bees. A team of entomologists from the University of Illinois has found that when bees eat the replacement food instead of honey, they are not being exposed to other chemicals that help the bees fight off toxins, such as those found in pesticides. In other words, the bees' immunity is compromised.[187]

Moreover, queen bees will often have their wings removed and are subject to artificial insemination. They are also frequently destroyed far earlier than their usual lifespan. And it doesn't stop with the queen bee: Malcom Sanford, an Extension Apiculturist in the Department of Entomology and Nematology at the University of Florida, and Roger Hoopingarner, a Professor in the Department of Entomology at Michigan State, explain why some beekeepers choose to kill off their colonies in the fall rather than care for them over the winter:

> "The other option is to kill colonies in the fall, extract and sell most of the honey that would have been consumed during the winter months and start with package bees the following spring. This appears practical since the 60 or so pounds of honey that would have been consumed by an over-wintering

colony more than offset the cost of the package of bees. The labor savings seen also support the conclusion that using package bees has advantages. When analyzed more completely, however, the cost savings from selling honey that would have been used in winter may be offset by the reduced success rate of colonies started from packages. Package bee colonies may also have reduced value in pollination and honey production as compared to an overwintered colony." Sanford and Hoopingarner.[188]

Remember, bees are highly sophisticated creatures, they feel pain, and we are dependent upon them for our food. In spite of its many benefits, the choice to eat honey is an ethical one but it is also one unquestionably linked to our own survival. If you do decide to consume honey, choose local ethical purveyors. One study conducted by *Food Safety News* found that more than three-fourths of the honey sold in US grocery stores isn't exactly what the bees produce; through high-level filtering system, much of the "good stuff"—the pollen—is filtered out.[189]

Granulated date sugar, available in many natural food stores, is indispensable when your recipe specifically calls for a granulated dry sugar. This sugar has the distinctive flavor of whole dry dates. Another dry sweetener is carob, or St. John's bread. This powder comes from the dried pods of the carob tree and can be purchased roasted or unroasted. Use the unroasted variety and toast it yourself for a fresher taste. In addition to its natural sugars, carob is especially rich in potassium, iron, and calcium, and low in fats. Also, being a member of the legume family, it is a source of protein and dietary fiber due to its content of pectin and cellulose, shown to help lower cholesterol, and also contains significant amounts of antioxidant polyphenols.[190,191] Only a small amount of this strong sweetener is necessary; either mix with the dry ingredients or dissolve in a little water or soy milk before adding to the other liquids.

Coconut sugar, made from the dried sap of the coconut palm, has been traditionally employed as a sweetener in South East Asia for generations. It has impressive amounts of nutrients like zinc, potassium, magnesium, and iron as well as antioxidants and B vitamins. Coconut sugar also contains good amounts of inulin, a type of dietary fiber that acts as a prebiotic, feeding your intestinal bifidobacteria.[192] At 78% sugar, its glycemic index was determined at about 35, officially ranking it as a low-glycemic sweetener, and one study, published in the *Diabetes & Metabolism Journal*, found that inulin could improve glycemic control and antioxidant status in women with Type 2 diabetes.[193] What's more, coconut sugar is considered to be a sustinable sweetener since its production uses less water than other sugar crops, such as sugar cane, and coconut palms can keep producing for approximately 20 years.[194]

From the starches, two grain sweeteners are available: barley malt (also made from other grains and containing the sugar maltose) and a rice syrup called *ame* in Japanese. These grain syrups are produced by combining the cooked grains, rice in this instance, with fresh sprouts from whole oats, barley, or wheat.

So-called raw sugar, or turbinado, is available in many stores, but is only slightly more nutritious than white sugar. It is 96% sucrose, compared with the 99.9% sucrose in white sugar. The only refining step to which it has not been subjected is a final acid bath that whitens the sugar and removes the final calcium and magnesium salts. This "pure" sugar was, as a juice from either sugar beets or sugar cane, only 15% sucrose. In its final form, all natural goodness has been lost.

Several sweeteners produced in the intermediate stages of sugar refining can be used somewhat more nutritionally than white table sugar. Once the cane or beet juice has been extracted, clarified to a syrup form, and crystallized, it is then spun in a centrifuge where more crystals are separated from the liquid. This remaining liquid is molasses, which is then repeatedly treated and centrifuged to extract more and more crystal until the final "blackstrap" form contains about 35% sucrose. Blackstrap molasses also contains B vitamins and trace minerals, for example one serving (two tablespoons) contains approximately 18% of the recommended daily intake of manganese, 14% of copper, 13% of iron, 12% of calcium, 10% of potassium, 7% of magnesium, and 3% of selenium, an important antioxidant. In addition to selenium, a study published in the *Journal of Agricultural and Food Chemistry* found molasses to have the greatest antioxidant capacity compared to other sweeteners, including honey and maple syrup.[195]

Another variety of molasses is known as Barbados. This milder, dark-brown syrup is extracted from the processes described earlier, resulting in a lighter-tasting product with a higher sucrose content. Sorghum molasses is produced by a similar process, but uses a raw material, the cane from the sorghum plant. It has a distinctive, rather cloying taste and is best used in baking, especially cookies.

Fats and Oils

Contrary to common trends, we all need some fat in our diets. A teaspoon a day of monounsaturated fats is essential for keeping the brain and heart functioning properly, for protecting our appearance, for raising HDL (good) cholesterol and lowering LDL (bad) cholesterol, and for keeping our hair and skin from becoming dry. A good source of monounsaturated fats is olive oil.

Olive oil forms a staple part of any diet nowadays, but is especially important for vegetarians because it provides both omega-6 (linoleic acid) and omega-3 (linolenic acid) essential fatty acids at the recommended 8:1 ratio, and about 75% of its fat in the form of oleic acid (a monounsaturated, omega-9 fatty acid) that can help lower blood pressure.[196] Numerous scientific studies have found that people who regularly consume olive oil are much less likely to develop cardiovascular disease, and one study found regular consumers to have a 41% lower risk of stroke compared to people who didn't consume olive oil.[197,198] Evidence suggests that it's the polyphenol antioxidant components of olive oil, such as *hydroxytyrosol*, that impart these anti-inflammatory properties and cardiovascular benefits.[199] For example, in one study, healthy men took 1½ tablespoons of high- or low-polyphenol olive oil daily for three weeks, and those consuming the high- polyphenol olive oil showed reduced levels of "bad" LDL cholesterol, high levels of which are a strong predictor of heart attack.[200] What's more, the study found that the greater the polyphenol content of the olive oil, the greater its ability to increase "good" HDL cholesterol levels. Most polyphenols are lost in the refining process, so choose virgin or extra virgin oil rather than a refined one. The polyphenols in olive oil, such as oleuropein and hydroxytyrosol, have also been shown to inhibit the growth of bacteria in the gut that are responsible for digestive tract infections.These include the *Helicobacter* bacteria that can cause stomach ulcers.[201] In addition to its positive effects on cardiovascular health, 25 studies on olive oil intake and cancer risk were analyzed and diets high in olive oil intake were associated with a reduced risk of breast, colorectal, and other types of cancers.[202] Some studies have also shown the potential of oleocanthal to help protect against Alzheimer's, and rates of Alzheimer's are much lower in Mediterranean countries where consumption of olive oil is higher than anywhere else in the world.[203]

In terms of foods that contain fat in their natural state, avocados, nuts, seeds, and cured olives are excellent sources, again not to be overdone.

Avoid saturated fats—those found in potato chips, meats, cheeses, and palm oil—with the exception of unprocessed coconut oil. An important and beneficial saturated fat, coconut oil, has scientifically demonstrated health benefits, including support for the heart and brain. Despite the belief that consumption of coconut oil can lead to weight gain, quite the opposite has been shown to be the case. Studies have shown that the consumption of medium chain fatty acids, such as those found in coconut oil, can actually help to burn calories and promote weight loss.[204] What's more, multiple studies on Pacific Island populations, who obtain 30-60% of their total caloric intact from fully saturated coconut oil, have all shown nearly non-existent rates of cardiovascular disease.[205]

Coconut oil is a good source of medium chain fatty acids, such as lauric acid, an antiviral and antibacterial compound, and capric acid, which shares some of the same antimicrobial benefits.[206] They are particularly easy to metabolize and absorb, providing the body with a quick source of energy.[207] In fact, medium chain fatty acids are often included in intravenous drips and infant formula, and they are naturally present in breast milk.[208,209] Supplementation of a low-fat diet with medium chain fatty acids has been shown promising results in patients with epilepsy in terms of seizure control with no side effects.[210]

Polyunsaturated fats, like those found in flaxseed oil, are precursors for omega-3s, such as DHA and EPA, which prevent clotting of blood and stickiness of platelets. Research shows that these fats can get into the blood vessels and stabilize plaque.

Fermented Foods

Sandor Katz, the author of *Wild Fermentation: The Flavor, Nutrition, and Craft of Live-Culture Foods* (Chelsea Green, 2003), is a self-described fermentation specialist. Sandor is a graduate of Brown University and a former urban planner and policy analyst. He has been living with AIDS for more than a decade and considers fermented foods an important part of his healing. He explains:

> My fermentation fetish grew out of my overlapping interests in cooking, nutrition, and gardening. I am also an herbalist and an activist. I have always

> loved fermented foods. As a child, sour, brined pickles were my favorite food. I loved sauerkraut. Then in the late 1980s, I spent a couple of years following a macrobiotic diet. That was the first time that I became aware that there were certain health benefits to fermented, live-culture foods.

"Living" fermented foods contain bacteria or yeast that feed on the natural sugars and produce compounds such as lactic acid or alcohol, helping to preserve the foods and their nutrients content. Fermented foods can help digestion, absorption of nutrients and immune function. This is well established in medical and scientific literature.

For example, fermentation can help improve the food's nutritional content by reducing some substances, such as phytic acid, that prevent your digestive tract from absorbing important nutrients. A 2003 study found that the phytic acid found in soy could be reduced by 31% following the soybeans' fermentation.[211] The bioavailability of some nutrients, such as the amino acids lysine, methionine and cysteine, can be improved following the fermentation of legumes and cereals.[212] In fact, the fermentation of some foods can even increase their vitamin content, as in the case of tempeh (fermented soy), which has over 100 times the levels of vitamin B12 as unfermented soy.[213]

The fermentation process can help to "release" beneficial compounds from our foods. According to the author of one study, "fermented cabbage could be healthier than raw or cooked cabbage, especially for fighting cancer," due to the increase in glucosinolates,[214] enzymes found to prevent cancer, resulting from the fermentation of cabbage. Similarly, fermented rice and beans were shown to contain increased levels of antioxidants, important cancer preventing molecules.[215]

Since fermentation relies on bacteria or yeast, fermented foods are filled with "friendly" bacteria such as those commonly found in probiotic products. Friendly bacteria help form a defense barrier in the gut from pathogenic bacteria and have been shown to prevent diarrhea and benefit children and adults with irritable bowel syndrome, and Crohn's disease.[216–219]

Live-culture foods are available on a small-scale commercially at your local health food store. Most of what you find in the mainstream supermarkets is not live-culture foods. The most reliable way to get live culture foods is to make them yourself. And when you make them yourself, they have the added benefit of containing the bacteria that you are sharing your specific ecological niche with. So it's a way of inviting your environment into your body and becoming one with that environment. And this is the best way to get health benefits from this type of food. There are plenty of other books on the market today that teach how to make fermented foods; they are not only fun to make, but a delicious addition to your diet.

Culinary Herbs

ANISEED or ANISE are the aromatic seeds from star anise, an aromatic spice that imparts a distinct flavor of licorice. Besides imparting flavor, anise is rich in B-group vitamins, as well as vitamins A and C, calcium, potassium, iron, magnesium, phosphorus, zinc, manganese, and selenium. In fact, just 20 grams of dry seeds would provide over 100% of the recommended daily amount of iron. Interestingly, this spice contains anethole, a compound that gives anise anti-fungal,[220] anti-bacterial, and anti-viral properties, and anise has been shown to be effective against growth of the yeast *Candida albicans,* responsible for candidiasis (thrush), the herpes virus, and several drug-resistant bacteria.[221,222] Anise can be added to an array of different cookies and cakes, and pairs particularly well with citrus fruits. Try a sprinkling of anise on a fruit salad or add some seeds to fruit pies or relishes.

ALLSPICE is the hard berry of an evergreen tree native to the West Indies and Central America that is also commonly known as Jamaican pepper or pimento. It is normally sold in ground form, although the whole berry—similar in appearance to a brown peppercorn—is available in spice shops and is used in pickling and to flavor soups and marinades. Allspice works well with sweet chutneys, apple desserts, and banana breads and also complements squash, pumpkin, or sweet potatoes particularly well. Allspice contains a very good amount of vitamins A, B, and C, potassium, manganese, iron, copper, selenium, and magnesium. What's more, allspice contains several bioactive phytonutrients, including eugenol, which is responsible for its aroma—composing 60-90% of the essential oil from allspice berries—and has been shown to help alleviate pain and to stimulate digestive enzymes.[223]

BASIL is a delicious herb best used fresh, although dried forms are commonly available. Its name derives from the Greek for "royal," and it has held an important place in many cultures through the ages. Fresh basil is the main component of pesto sauces and works particularly well with tomato. Dried basil is also good in soups, marinades, and vinaigrettes. Basil is a good source of vitamins C and K, copper, manganese, calcium, iron, folate, and magnesium, as well as omega-3 fatty acids and phytonutrients such as flavonoids and bioavailable beta-carotene, lutein, and zeaxanthin antioxidants.[224]

BAY LEAVES are the whole, dried leaves of the bay laurel tree and are best used in slow cooking recipes to give the leaves time to release their warm flavor—and complement tomatoes, potatoes, and beans. Although the leaves themselves are generally not consumed, one study published in the *Journal of Clinical Biochemistry and Nutrition* found that bay leaves may be beneficial for people with type 2 diabetes.[225] Participants who consumed a few grams of ground bay leaves every day for a month experienced a drop in both blood glucose and cholesterol levels.

CARAWAY SEEDS are crescent shaped and have a nutty, anise-like flavor. They are best known for adding zest to rye and pumpernickel breads. These seeds are an excellent source of dietary fiber, as well as the vitamins A, B, C, and E. They pair particularly well with potatoes, parsnips, turnips, and cabbages.

CARDAMOM, an essential ingredient in Indian cuisine, is available in whole or ground form. These seed pods can provide an intense aromatic flavor for grain dishes and curries and work well with squash, pumpkin, or sweet potatoes. A single tablespoon of cardamom contains 80% of the recommended daily intake of manganese, as well as smaller amounts of iron, calcium, magnesium, potassium, zinc, and the vitamins A, B, and C. One study published in the *British Journal of Nutrition* found that cardamom can be protective against skin cancer,[226] as it reduced the activity of genes linked to the growth of skin cancer cells.

CAYENNE PEPPER is perhaps the hottest is perhaps the hottest of the spices, ground and ground and dried from a very hot variety of a pepper of the Capsicum genus. A small amount goes a long way and is used to give fiery flavor to Mexican, Indian, and some Southeast Asian cuisines and is also useful in spicing Creole and Cajun specialties. Cayenne pepper lends itself to vegetable or bean stews, curries, chilies, spicy cold noodle dishes, and hot-and-sour dishes.

CHILI POWDER is a blend of dried, ground red chili peppers, and can vary from milder to hotter varieties. Chili flakes are now available in most supermarkets and combine the seeds with the dried flesh of the pepper. Chili powder is an obvious addition to tomato-based enchilada sauces, but can also be used to flavor bean stews and soups and to add a warm note to tomato-based pasta sauces and Oriental-style sauces. All chili peppers contain capsaicin, which gives them their characteristic punch; the hotter the chili pepper, the more capsaicin it contains. The topical application of capsaicin is now a recognized treatment for osteoarthritis pain.[227]

CHIVES, like garlic, are a bulb vegetable and a member of the lily family, whose relatives include onions, scallions, and garlic. Rich in vitamins A, C, and K, folic acid, iron, and calcium, fresh chives are readily available in markets today and easily grown in the kitchen garden—in fact, they proliferate quickly. Their flavor is much like that of scallions, yet more delicate, which makes them delightful to use raw when available fresh. Fresh chives add flavor to potatoes, potato salads, and almost any fresh vegetable salad. Dried chives are also commonly available; use them in dips, dressings, soups, and sauces, where they will have a chance to reconstitute. See p. 157 for more on the nutritional qualities of chives.

CILANTRO, sometimes referred to as Spanish or Chinese parsley, is the fresh herb whose seeds are the spice coriander. Cilantro has a unique flavor and aroma and is used widely in Mexican, Indian, and Asian cuisines. Since both flavor and aroma are lost when the herb is dried, the leaves are best added raw as a garnish or near the end of cooking in order to maintain their delicate flavor and texture. Cilantro has high concentrations of vitamin K, as well as vitamins A, folate, potassium, manganese, and choline. Cilantro leaves contain high amounts of antioxidants such as beta-carotene, lutein, and zeaxanthin. Furthermore, cilantro leaves are effective chelators of heavy metals and may help remove toxic heavy metals, such as lead and mercury, from the body. Add it to green leafy salads, fruit salads, or to juice to benefit from its detoxification properties. Cilantro can also add a zest to bean stews, Mexican dishes, tomato sauces, and creamy vegetable dips.

CINNAMON is one of the earliest spices recorded and is obtained from the bark of cassia evergreen trees that forms the rolls or “quills” as it dries. Cinnamon has a sweet, aromatic flavor and is commonly used in cakes, puddings, and fruit pies. It particularly complements cooked apples and pears, other stewed fruits, squash, pumpkin, and sweet potato and is also a common component of curry blends. Try it sprinkled on your oatmeal or yoghurt to add a sense of sweetness without adding sugar. It is also delicious added to rice or grains, particularly in combination with dried fruit. One recent study found that cinnamaldehyde, an antioxidant in cinnamon, was more potent than other antioxidants found in spinach, chard, and red cabbage.[228] In another study, cinnamon was shown to improve serum glucose, triglyceride, LDL cholesterol, and total cholesterol levels in people with type 2 diabetes, which suggests that the inclusion of cinnamon in the diet of people with type 2 diabetes will reduce risk factors associated with diabetes and cardiovascular diseases.[229]

CLOVES are the dried flower buds of the evergreen clove tree and have a strong yet sweet flavor and aroma. Historically, they have been used as a natural numbing agent especially for toothache, but did you know that cloves are rich in polyphenols with antioxidant activity[230] and that just half a teaspoon of ground clove contains more antioxidants than half a cup of blueberries? Ground cloves (you might not want to bite into a whole clove, they are somewhat bitter) are also a good source of copper, manganese, iron, magnesium, and calcium. Whole cloves can be added to slowly simmering stewed fruits or mulled wine, and ground cloves can be added to baked goods, oatmeal, or recipes with apples, pears, bananas, squash, sweet potato, and pumpkin.

CORIANDER is the aromatic seed of the herbal plant whose leaves are known as cilantro and adds both a different flavor and nutritional value to dishes than cilantro. Coriander contains a good amount of vitamin C and B-complex, is rich in dietary fiber, is an excellent source of iron, and contains significant amounts of copper, magnesium, manganese, calcium, potassium, and zinc, as well as important fatty acids and an array of phytonutrients including antioxidants.[231] Coriander is usually one of the main components of curry mixes and is commonly used in Indonesian cuisine as a seasoning for tempeh recipes. Try adding ground coriander to bean dishes or soups, and cabbage or sautéed spinach, or add it to vanilla soymilk with honey for a delicious drink.

CUMIN seed is used extensively in curry blends and is an important spice in Indian and Mexican cuisines. In European cuisine, a pinch was traditionally added to bread. Its spicy hot flavor is a great complement to the hearty flavor of legumes, spinach, and tempeh dishes. Try adding it to flavor sautéed vegetables or vegetable stews, in combination with black pepper. Cumin seed is a very good source of the essential minerals iron and magnesium, which aid the absorption of calcium, manganese, phosphorus, and vitamin B1.

CURRY POWDER is a blend of spices used in Indian cuisine. The exact mix can vary according to the store (and in India would vary according to the dish and region), but will most probably contain cumin, coriander, and turmeric, and may include fenugreek, cinnamon, ginger, chili powder, and cardamom. It will typically be available in mild or hotter versions. Why not try mixing and grinding your own preferred spices? Curry powder can be added to a wide range of dishes to give spice and color, including dishes of potato, beans, or grains.

DILL WEED is a feathery green herb with a strong distinctive taste similar to fennel and celery. The seeds can also be used and are often chosen as a milder substitute for caraway seeds. They are popular for adding to pickled cucumbers, and are delicious in breads or as a topping for potato, cabbage, or casseroles. Fresh or dried dill weed pairs especially well with tomato and cucumber. Try adding some to a cucumber salad topped with cool yoghurt or soured cream, or combined with broad beans and rice, like in Iranian cuisine. Dill weed is a good source of calcium, manganese, and iron, and also contains antioxidant and anti-inflammatory flavonoids. Dill weed has been used as a digestive aid in many cultures, and may help to inhibit acid secretion.

FENNEL SEEDS, the small dried seeds that come from the fennel herb, have a subtle anise-like flavor. Nutrients in fennel seeds include essential fatty acids, vitamins C, B, and E, calcium, choline, iron, magnesium, manganese, phosphorus, potassium, and selenium, and certain amino acids. They are used in some traditional Italian bread recipes and in the Chinese five spice mix, and they add a pleasant flavor to vegetable dishes, stews, curries, and chutneys. To maximize their flavor, grind the seeds yourself or dry fry them for a couple of minutes. Fennel seeds have also been found to be a promising diuretic, helping the kidneys excrete urine and sodium.[232]

FENUGREEK is a less common aromatic spice with a somewhat bitter flavor and strong aroma. It is actually a member of the legume family and rich in dietary fiber, vitamins A, B, and C, copper, potassium, calcium, iron, selenium, zinc, manganese, and magnesium. Fenugreek is also a source of choline and the amino-acid 4-hydroxy isoleucine, which has glucose uptake stimulatory activity and is thus recommended in the diet of diabetics.[233,234] Fenugreek is a principal element of Indian cuisine, and the seeds can be found in most Indian specialty stores. Grind or dry fry the seeds to obtain the optimal flavor when adding to curries, stews, and dips, or try sprouting them to add to vegetable and lentil dishes.

GARLIC is well known and almost universally loved by good cooks across a multitude of cultures. As noted above, garlic is a bulb vegetable, a member of the lily family, and related to onions, shallots, and the like. It contains over 20% of the recommended daily amounts of vitamins B6 and C, and manganese. Fresh garlic is almost always preferable, and is excellent in dips, dressings and meals of all kinds. Fresh or powdered garlic can be used in just about any dish; note that the fresh garlic is stronger than powdered. See more about garlic on p. 225.

GINGER root is the underground rhizome-like root of a tropical plant. Like turmeric, it is frequently used dried and ground in both baking and cooking, and is commonly used as a spice for pumpkin and squash pies, as well as an enhancement for apple desserts, and sweet potato dishes. However, the uses for raw ginger are numerous. Add a one-inch piece in your juices, or mince it and put it in soups, salads, and entrees. There's much to say about fresh ginger, so it is under a separate entry in the *Rhizomes* in our "Superstars of the Vegetarian Diet" section on p. 223 for more about ginger's highly nutritional profile.

MARJORAM is a culinary herb from the same family as oregano. They have a similar taste, but marjoram is slightly sweeter and subtler than oregano. Fresh marjoram is one of the richest herbal sources of vitamin K, and an excellent source of iron. The leaves also contain high levels of vitamins A, and C, manganese, potassium, copper, zinc, magnesium, and calcium, besides, numerous antioxidants, such as beta-carotene, lutein, zeaxanthin, and anti-inflammatory eugenol and terpinenes.[235] Marjoram pairs well with peas, beans, spinach, carrots, potatoes, and cauliflower and with tomato-based sauces and stews.

MINT is a well-known and highly aromatic herb. There are many different varieties, but the most common are peppermint and spearmint, which is most widely used in Western cooking. Fresh mint is an essential ingredient in Moroccan teas, Middle Eastern taboulis, and Indian palate-cooling dips. Mint leaves contain a considerable amount of vitamin A, and smaller amounts of vitamins C and B. Spearmint is also a good source of iron and manganese, and peppermint a good source of copper and manganese. All mints contain the essential oil menthol, which has been shown to be effective in relieving the general symptoms of irritable bowel syndrome.[236] Try adding fresh mint to fruit salads, steamed green peas, or smoothies.

MUSTARD SEEDS are available in a range of different colors and pungencies; the black seeds tend to be the most pungent whereas the white seeds tend to be milder. The ground seeds are mixed with water and vinegar to make the popular condiment. The Greeks and Romans used mustard seeds for medicinal purposes, and scientific studies have shown that, as a cruciferous vegetable, they contain cancer-combating glucosinolates,[237] and are an excellent source of selenium, a nutrient that has been proposed to help reduce the severity of asthma, as well as a good source of omega-3 fatty acids, vitamin C and many of the B-group vitamins, and contains smaller amounts of potassium, phosphorus, magnesium, and calcium. Once ground, mustard seeds release their warmth and pungency, and mixing with water initiates an enzymatic process that further enhances their pungency and heat. Add mustard seeds to soups, salad dressings, grain dishes, bean dishes, potato dishes, and curries.

NUTMEG is the brown nutlike seed of the evergreen nutmeg tree. The nutmeg tree produces two spices, nutmeg and mace—mace is the red membrane that grows around the seed, which is dried and ground. For the best flavor, grate the whole nutmeg seed, although the ground form is also commonly available. Nutmeg is commonly added to puddings and cakes, but also pairs particularly well with broccoli, cauliflower, spinach, potatoes, and squash. The spice is rich in vitamins A, B, and C, and is a good source of manganese, copper, magnesium, potassium, calcium, iron, and zinc, and as well as antioxidants like beta-carotene. Nutmeg also contains several volatile oils, including eugenol and myristicin, which give the spice stimulating effects (that can be hallucinogenic in high doses).[238]

OREGANO is a well-known culinary herb, thanks to its prevalence in Italian dishes such as pizza and tomato-based sauces and Greek cuisine. Its green leaves are rich in phytochemicals and vitamin E and have a surprisingly powerful antioxidant capacity. Oregano has 12 times more antioxidant activity than oranges and 4 times more than blueberries, according to the US Department of Agriculture (USDA) study.[239] Importantly, research by the UCLA School of Medicine reported that the dried form of oregano, and many other herbs retained their antioxidant capacity following drying.[240] Oregano is also an excellent source of vitamin K and a good source of manganese, magnesium, potassium, iron, calcium, and dietary fiber. Add it fresh to salads and sandwiches, or use to enhance the flavor of bean or grain dishes, pasta sauces, stews, and soups.

PAPRIKA is made by grinding a dried, sweet Capsicum pepper. It adds a rich red color and a sweetish, warm flavor to dishes. Paprika is a good source of vitamins A and E, as well as iron, and the health-promoting carotenoids lutein and zeaxanthin, which are responsible for its color. Lightly coat potatoes in olive oil and paprika before roasting, add to chick-peas or try it paired with cooked carrots, squash, sweet potato, or pumpkin.

PARSLEY is probably the world's most popular herb due to its mild flavor and is highly nutritious too. Parsley is an excellent source of vitamins K and C, and a good source of vitamin A, folate, iron (providing twice as much as spinach), copper, potassium, manganese, and calcium. Parsley is also rich in dietary fiber and chlorophyll, and contains an array of antioxidant phytonutrients, including beta-carotene, zeaxanthin, and apigenin, which was shown to slow the progression of certain types of breast cancer.[241] Freshly cut parsley works well as a garnish for most plates and can be added to salads, soups, vegetable dishes, grains and bean dishes. Or why not try making a parsley pesto with walnuts for a change from the basil version? It's quite delicious.

PEPPERCORNS are the whole, dried berries of an evergreen vine. Black pepper is an excellent source of manganese and vitamin K, as well as copper, iron, manganese, chromium, calcium, and dietary fiber. Pepper has been shown to increase the metabolic rate, and piperine, an active compound naturally found in peppercorns, was shown to suppress the development of new fat cells, leading to suggestions that black pepper could help weight loss.[242,243] Interestingly, piperine was also shown to prevent the proliferation of rectal cancer cells.[244] Buy whole peppercorns and grind them when required to add flavor to an infinite number of dishes.

POPPY SEEDS are the tiny, round seeds of the beautiful opium poppy that are commonly added to bagels, muffins, or other bread products. Poppy seeds have a mild nutty flavor but are also packed full of dietary fiber and a good source of calcium, iron, copper, phosphorus, zinc, and folate. Why not add them to salad dressings, or sprinkle over cabbage dishes or those with root vegetables, noodles, and casseroles?

ROSEMARY is the name given to the slender leaves of a small evergreen shrub of the same name. It imparts a robust, piney flavor when added to dishes. Generally used just to flavor dishes and then removed, crushed rosemary is a good source of vitamins A and C, iron, calcium, and manganese. Furthermore, several studies show that rosemary can inhibit the growth of foodborne pathogens, including *E.coli*, and researchers from the University of British Columbia found that rosemary extract could inhibit the proliferation of ovarian cancer cell lines.[245,246] Use it to flavor vegetable stews, soups, and casseroles or sauces. Used sparingly, it also works well in fruit salads and sorbets.

SAFFRON, meaning yellow in Arabic, is derived from the crocus flower and is the most expensive spice in the world as it has to be painstakingly plucked, piled and dried. It is rich in vitamin C, iron, magnesium, potassium, phosphorus, B-group vitamins, calcium, and zinc, not to mention a whole host of carotenoids—including beta-carotene, zeaxanthin, and lycopene—that give it its distinctive color and delicate flavor. Interestingly, saffron has been found to help alleviate depression.[247] Saffron is predominantly added to rice dishes, particularly Spanish paella, but try adding it to give both color and intensity to other grain and potato dishes too.

SAGE is from the leaves of a small evergreen plant that has an aromatic earthy taste and is normally consumed in a dried form. Sage is rich in B-group vitamins and vitamin K and contains good amounts of vitamins A and C, potassium, zinc, calcium, iron, manganese, copper, magnesium, and antioxidants such as beta-carotene. Scientific studies have provided evidence that sage could help improve the cognitive function of patients with Alzheimer's disease, and the consumption of sage oil was associated with improved memory recall.[248] Tofu and tempeh are tasty seasoned with sage, which can also be added to grain dishes and vegetable soups and pairs particularly well with pumpkin and squash.

SAVORY has a subtle flavor, somewhere between parsley and thyme, with summer savory giving a milder flavor than the winter savory variety. This herb is a good source of vitamins A, B, and C, as well as potassium, iron, calcium, magnesium, manganese, zinc and selenium. Fresh summer savory can be added to salads, or in its dried form it can be added to soups, stews, and bean dishes.

TARRAGON has a sweet anise-like flavor and is popular in Mediterranean cuisines. Tarragon is rich in vitamins A, B, and C, and a good source of calcium, manganese, iron, magnesium, copper, potassium, and zinc, as well as having one of the highest antioxidant values among the common herbs. Tarragon adds a distinctive touch to salads, salad dressings, and tomato dishes, or why not try sprinkling some on cooked peas, beans, asparagus, or Swiss chard?

THYME is a woody shrub with an aromatic and earthy flavor, popular in Mediterranean and Creole cuisines. Thyme is a good source of vitamins A and C, dietary fiber, iron, manganese, and copper, not to mention its variety of antioxidant flavonoids, including breast-cancer inhibiting apigenin.[249] What's more, thyme's volatile oils have been shown to have antimicrobial activity against a number of bacteria and fungi, including pathogenic strains such as *E.coli* and *Shigella.*[250,251] It's quite strong flavor pairs well with tomatoes, celeriac, mushrooms and carrots. Add thyme to soups and grain and bean dishes.

TURMERIC, like ginger, is typically used dried and ground as the product of a fleshy root; however, it is also excellent raw, added to juices and soups and grated on salads. It is prized for its brilliant yellow color, and is highly effective in reducing inflammation in the body. Turmeric is heavily utilized in Indian cooking, and is one of the main components of curry mixes. Use it to brighten rice pilafs, curries, and other vegetable dishes or to add color to a dish as it does when making black mustard seed look as if it were yellow as in most mustards sold in retail today. See *Rhizomes* in our "Superstars of the Vegetarian Diet" section on p. 224 for more about turmeric's highly nutritional profile, and other health benefiting properties. For example, according to Cancer Research UK, although "there is no research evidence to show that turmeric or curcumin can prevent or treat cancer… early trials have shown some promising results."[252]

Superstars of the Healthy Vegetarian Diet

Before we close this presentation on specific foods of the plant-based diet, I wanted to revisit a few of the standouts of the vegetarian world, sharing a bit more science supporting their tremendous benefits to those on a plant-based diet. Some of these items have already been discussed earlier in the chapter but are worthy of a second mention for the special place they hold in the diet and their importance to healing.

Cruciferous Vegetables

The reason why cruciferous vegetables have not yet been mentioned is because we chose to present the foods of the plant-based world based on their botanical rather than their health/culinary classifications. You will see in the list below that cruciferous vegetables include root vegetables, as well as leafy and influorescent vegetables. Here is the list; it's a long and tantalizing one:

> kale, collard greens, Chinese broccoli, cabbage, Brussels sprouts, kohlrabi, broccoli, broccoflower, broccoli romanesco, cauliflower, wild broccoli, bok choy, mizuna, Rapini, flowering cabbage, Chinese cabbage, turnip root and greens, rutabaga, Siberian kale, wrapped heart mustard cabbage, mustard seeds, tatsoi, Ethiopian mustard, radish, daikon, horseradish, wasabi, rocket (aka, arugula), watercress, garden cress, komatsuna.[253]

Raw cruciferous vegetables are delicious on their own and offer a wide variety of nutritional properties. They should not be underestimated as sources of fiber, vitamin C, vitamin K, folate, and omega-3 fatty acids, and there is no other vegetable group as rich in vitamin A carotenoids (such as beta-carotene, lutein, and zeaxanthin). As to the phytonutrients contained in these varied greens, let me mention the chemicals I3C and DIM. These help in the conversion of the sex hormone estradiol (found in both men and women) to 2-hydroxyestrone, and are derived from glucosinolates, which are found in cruciferous vegetables.[254] They have been shown to aid in the protection against certain cancers and also to decrease the number and size of tumors once they form.[255,256] Indeed, health writer Byron Richards reports on a study that shows that eating a mere half-cup of broccoli or cauliflower once a week can stave off cancer. Scientific studies have demonstrated that just three servings of this vegetable group per week decreased the risk of developing prostate cancer by 41%, one daily serving was shown to reduce the risk of breast cancer by over 50%, and the more cruciferous vegetables breast cancer survivors ate, the lower their risk of cancer recurrence.[257-259]

Here's something to note when you eat them: The health-promoting compound of cruciferous vegetables, glucosinolate, is not released until the plant cell wall is broken. Chewing will shatter this cell wall, though hardly as efficiently as juicing or lightly steaming. Dr. Joel Fuhrman recommends juicing a wide variety of organic vegetables two or more times a day, including especially the green cruciferous vegetables like kale.[260] He also recommends eating sprouts as a way to enhance phytonutrient intake. Cruciferous vegetables contain important phytonutrients such as lipoic acid, which plays a role in energy production and is being investigated as a possible regulator of blood sugar.[261,262]

Some feel that supplements are necessary to achieve the full benefit of the helpful compounds in cruciferous vegetables, as cooking may destroy them to some extent, and chewing can't release them all. When cooking cruciferous vegetables, to maximize the glucosinolates, steaming for three to four minutes is recommended.[263]

Dark Green Leafy Vegetables

Dark green leafy vegetables are the nutritional powerhouses and should be a mainstay of any healthy vegetarian diet. They are rich in vitamin K; just one cup of cooked greens far exceeding the minimum recommended intake, as well as vitamins A, C, E, and B and minerals including potassium and magnesium. They are particularly important for vegans because they are an excellent source of calcium and iron.

They are also packed with phytonutrients—particularly abundant in chlorophyll, which alkalinizes the blood and may reduce the diseased state or morbidity—have dietary fiber, which keeps the colon healthy and can help prevent colon cancer, and carotenoid antioxidants, whose regular consumption is associated with a decreased risk of age-related macular degeneration and cataracts, and according to AICR's second expert report, *Food, Nutrition, Physical Activity, and the Prevention of Cancer: A Global Perspective*, foods containing carotenoids probably protect against cancers of the mouth, pharynx, and larynx.[264-267] In addition, researchers from the Rush University Medical Center have recently found that eating green leafy vegetables regularly can help keep the brain functioning optimally. Martha Clare Morris, leader of the research team, said "Since declining cognitive ability is central to Alzheimer's disease and dementias, increasing consumption of green leafy vegetables could offer a very simple, affordable and non-invasive way of potentially protecting your brain from Alzheimer's disease and dementia."[268]

While the USDA recommends eating one-half cup of green leafy vegetables each day to prevent nutrient deficiencies and serious illnesses, I, as well as many other healthy leaders in the health profession, recommend consuming much more green leafy vegetables daily. As a side note, it is my contention that the USDA's recommendations on all plant-based food groups are grossly wrong and border on the edge of criminal negligence. We should be having at least eleven servings of fresh organic fruits and vegetables per day. As far as edible green leaves, there are many varieties, and they are most nutritious when eaten raw, in salads, smoothies or juices, or lightly steamed.

Here are examples of what to look for:

Lettuces: romaine, green leaf, arugula, and butterhead

Cruciferous leafy greens: kale, mustard greens, collard greens, cabbage

Amaranthaceae family: Swiss chard and spinach

Other edible dark green leafy vegetables: dandelion, red clover, plantain, watercress, and chickweed

Sea Vegetables

As I noted in the previous section on sea vegetables, Americans are generally lacking in important minerals; this means that sea vegetables offer crucial support to those participating in the vegetarian diet. One dangerous example of this is magnesium—a deficiency that according to a report in *Life Extension* is linked to cardiovascular disease.[269] One government study reported by *Life Extension* showed that a whopping 68% of Americans do not consume the recommended daily intake of magnesium; another study places the deficiency as high as 80% in Americans.[270] Even more disconcerting was that 19% of Americans do not consume even *half* of the government's recommended daily intake of magnesium.[271]

Another prevalent deficiency noted by *Life Extension* is iodine, which they say has increased fourfold in the developed world over the past 40 years.[272] The article goes on to state that nearly 74% of normal, "healthy" adults may no longer consume enough iodine. Dr. Ryan Drum, noted herbalist and author of *Therapeutic Use of Seaweeds* (Proceedings of the 2001 Pacific Northwest Herbal Symposium) states: "Seaweeds, eaten regularly, are the best natural food sources of biomolecular dietary iodine... no land plants are reliable sources of dietary iodine."[273] *Maine Coast Sea Vegetables* notes that a person would have to eat about 40 lbs. of fresh vegetables and/or fruits to get as much iodine as they would from 1 gram of whole leaf kelp.[274]

Consuming sea vegetables a couple of times a week addresses the issue of under-mineralization in a healthful, plant-based way. Plus, they are often hand-harvested, which is easy on the environment.

Rhizomes

Ginger Root

The benefits of ginger on patients suffering from arthritis and other conditions of inflammation have been well documented for decades. A group of powerful antioxidants unique to ginger, called gingerols, a relative of capsaicin, are responsible for ginger's anti-inflammatory properties.[275] One study of patients with painful arthritis in the knee found that those given ginger experienced significantly less pain and swelling.[276] Ginger root has also been shown to be effective in preventing nausea and vomiting during pregnancy.[277]

Ginger gives a special zest to dishes and is delicious added to herbal teas. Try it grated with lemon juice and water for a refreshing drink, or add it to soy sauce, olive oil, and garlic for a tasty superfood salad dressing.

Turmeric

Turmeric is a common spice, also known as Indian saffron, which gives dishes a distinctive yellow color and is an excellent source of manganese and iron. As a relative of ginger, turmeric has long been used as an anti-inflammatory in Chinese and Indian traditional medicine, due to the anti-inflammatory properties of the pigment curcumin.[278] Curcumin has been suggested as an effective treatment for inflammatory bowel diseases such as Crohn's and for rheumatoid arthritis among others.[279,280] In addition, results of several studies indicate curcumin exhibits powerful anti-cancer activity. For example, a phase I clinical trial monitored the progression of pre cancerous changes in different organs in 25 patients who were fed turmeric during three months and found that curcumin could stop the precancerous changes becoming cancer.[281]

Ginseng

Ginseng is a potent adaptogenic herb that has been used the world over throughout history. There are several different types of ginseng, all adaptogens, including Korean, Chinese, Siberian, and American. Adaptogenic herbs primarily act as stress fighters by restoring homeostasis. A growing body of peer-reviewed literature supports that ginseng possesses a large variety of therapeutic effects on the body, including benefits to the central nervous system, cardiovascular system, and endocrine secretion, immune function, enhanced physical performance, stress, aging, etc.[282-286]

Green Tea

Widely hailed for its medicinal qualities, green tea possesses numerous compounds that promote joint health and mitigate the impact of various types of inflammation, possibly due to its high flavonoid content.[287] Decaffeinated is best. Also, the consumption of green tea was shown to significantly reduce blood pressure and cholesterol levels.[288]

Super Foods

Chlorella

Chlorella is a type of algae packed with more chlorophyll than most plants along with a diverse set of detoxifying agents, vitamins, and minerals, including calcium, iron, and amino acids. It has been observed in studies to reduce various forms of inflammation and hypertension.[289,290] One study even found that its antioxidant effects could prevent the decline of age-related cognitive ability.[291]

Garlic

According to John Milner, director of the Human Nutrition Center at the Agricultural Research Service at the USDA "Garlic has some significant health benefits."[292] Individuals looking to prevent and treat chronic diseases are advised to incorporate this superfood into their diet; consuming garlic raw is best. Garlic is abundant in anti-inflammatory sulfur compounds such as diallyl sulfide (DAS) and thiacremonone.[293] What's more, a number of studies have demonstrated a link between garlic consumption and a decreased risk of cancer, especially cancer of the colon and stomach.[294] There is also some research to suggest that garlic may protect against breast cancer too.[295]

Spirulina

Also known as blue-green algae, spirulina contains a number of anti-inflammatory phytonutrients, including zeaxanthin and beta-cryptoxanthin, which hold great promise as a natural means of curbing arthritis and other inflammatory conditions while promoting healing throughout the body.[296-297] Added to juices and smoothies, spirulina can increase antioxidant and protein content, with protein making up about 60-70% of spirulina's dry weight, as well as provide B-complex vitamins and vitamin E, manganese, calcium, zinc, copper, iron, potassium, selenium, and essential fatty acids.

Acai berries

Acai berries (or Açaí, and pronounced ah-sigh-ee) are small, round berries, similar in appearance to a blueberry, from Brazil. Their taste is often described as a mix of wild berry and chocolate. Acai berries are low in sugar and are excellent sources of iron, calcium, dietary fiber, and vitamin A. They are one of the fruits with the highest antioxidant content, higher in fact than strawberries and blueberries. They are particularly rich in anthocyanin phytochemicals, including resveratrol, known to protect against cardiovascular, diabetes, Alzheimer's, and cancer, with levels at least ten times higher than those found in red grapes.[298] In addition, they contain beneficial fatty acids such as oleic acid, one of the oils found in olive oil.

One study with overweight adults found that taking 100 grams of acai twice daily for a month led to reductions in insulin levels and total cholesterol, and acai berries reduced the levels of selected metabolic disease markers in the overweight subjects.[299]

Generally, acai berries are sold freeze-dried and in powdered form. This is because they are so low in sugar and acid—which protects most fruits—that if left unprocessed, the fruit would oxidize and lose its beneficial micronutrients. Add them to juice or smoothies or use them to make a delicious tea.

Goji berries

Also known as wolfberries, goji berries are from the same family as the tomato and eggplant. On the vine, they somewhat resemble a miniature tomato; however, they are generally sold in their sun-dried form. Goji berries are rich in vitamins A, B, and C; are an excellent source of dietary fiber and linoleic acid, an omega-6 fatty acid (found in the seeds); and contain all the essential amino acids, a property unique among fruits. What's more, 100 grams of dried fruit provides 100% of the recommended daily intake of iron and copper, 91% of the daily recommended allowance of selenium, and 24%, 18% and 9% that of potassium, zinc, and calcium, in that order. Furthermore, as a member of the tomato family, goji berries have a high carotenoid content, including beta-carotene, lutein, zeaxanthin, and lycopene.

Goji berries have a high antioxidant capacity, higher than citrus fruits, grapes, and many types of apples, but not as high as acai or blueberries in their raw form, according to the USDA database (although the dried berries are supposed to have even higher levels).[300] The high antioxidant (especially zeaxanthin) content of goji berries has been attributed to their beneficial effects on vision. In fact, a 90-day study with elderly subjects consuming the berries daily showed increased antioxidant levels, as well as protection from hypopigmentation and protection of the macula.[301] A small study also found that the daily consumption of goji berry juice led to improved feelings of wellbeing.[302] However, the study only involved 34 people, so the results are not entirely conclusive.

Dried phytochemical-rich goji berries are often added to soups or rice dishes in Chinese cuisine, where they have been used for centuries as a medicinal plant, or boiled as herbal tea. Alternatively they are delicious eaten in their dried form as a snack or added to muesli or oatmeal. They can also be soaked for a couple of hours in just enough water to cover them and then added to juices and smoothies.

Pomegranate seeds

Pomegranate seeds are a good source of many vital B-group vitamins, vitamin K, calcium, copper, potassium, and manganese. They contain ellagitannin antioxidants, shown to reduce heart disease risk factors, such as lowering blood pressure and increasing the removal of atherosclerosis.[303,304] Sprinkle them on salads or add them to your juices and smoothies. In fact, the US Department of Agriculture ranks pomegranate juice as the fifth strongest antioxidant (behind chocolate, elderberries, and two different varieties of apples).

Juices

Consuming fresh squeezed fruit and vegetable juices is one of the best ways to prevent and reverse inflammatory diseases—and all disease has an inflammatory component. Health-boosting antioxidants, vitamins, minerals, enzymes, phytonutrients, and chlorophyll found in fruits and vegetables promote and maintain healthy cells and reduce chronic inflammation that results in degenerative diseases. It is one of the quietest but more formidable revolutions occurring today, and for good reason. According to *Barron's*, juicing, as a meal replacement or refreshment, has become a $5 billion business in the US, and is projected to grow by 4% to 8% a year.[305] While juice fasts, or juice cleanses, have long been used to shed unwanted pounds, the latest craze seems to be reflective of a national movement toward healthier eating and greater consumption of raw and organic produce—in this case, conveniently packaged and on the run.

Nutrients are much more easily absorbed by the body in the form of juices rather than if we were to consume these foods whole, especially because many of us do not chew our foods well enough to receive their full nutritional offerings. This is particularly true with plant-based foods since they are comprised of cellulose, which needs to be broken down through the process of mastication in order to extract all of the food's nutrients.

If you think about what you might put into on 16 oz. juice—2 cucumbers, 4 stalks of celery, 3 or 4 stalks of kale and one whole apple, and perhaps a bit of fresh raw ginger—and then think about eating all of these foods in one sitting, you will start to get a sense for what I'm saying. Juices provide a convenient way of ingesting large quantities of nutrients, and in a "pre-digested" form—meaning that we need not masticate the actual plant foods to receive the nutrients. (Although, it is absolutely important that we "chew" our juices, too; this promotes optimal absorption. By this, I mean allowing the juice to mix with the digestive enzymes rather than gulping them down.) This allows the beneficial constituents to work synergistically with our body's systems.

Juicing as a healing therapy is also a very useful tool. Since we utilize up to 30% of our energy in a day consuming, chewing and digesting our food, juicing when we are ill rather than eating makes perfect sense. We are, in essence, freeing up the energy that would typically be spent on digestion and assimilation, which can be redirected toward healing. I've known many people to use this therapy at the first sign of a cold, for example, and completely avoid its onset. The trick is to take your rest day (or two) the moment that you notice the scratchy throat, running nose or the lethargy associate with colds. By taking a day or two of complete rest, sleeping as much as needed and consuming only juices, you are allowing your immune system to refortify itself while preventing more serious symptoms from setting in. In the American culture, however, we typically wait until the symptoms are so bad, perhaps out of fear that we will be judged for taking off of work, as one example, when we are "not really that sick." However, what is better: one or two days away from work, or an entire week or more, which can occur if we push ourselves and not allow our bodies the rest that they need?

Juicing is also helpful when we are feeling lethargic or fatigued, or low on sleep, for example. In these cases, we might be inclined to reach for sugar and caffeine when a mixed vegetable juice with a little fruit may be all we need, and is far healthier. Plus, if we choose the juice, we won't have to deal with the rebound tiredness associated with sugar consumption (low blood sugar), or adrenal fatigue. Plus, there is the chance that the high quantities of nutrition will actually energize us.

The juices you drink should always come from fresh organic produce; you can make them at home with your own juicer, or order at your favorite juice bar. For convenience sake, you can make all of your juice on one day of the week and place in airtight containers in the refrigerator for a couple of days, or freeze them in plastic bags, simply thawing them the night before the day you are planning on consuming them.

By having three 16 oz. glasses of juice a day, you are flooding your body with essential nutrients that promote your health in powerful ways. For example, the chlorophyll in these juices acts as a natural chelator, removing toxic heavy metals from the body, while the sulfur compounds found in cabbage juice help guard against cancer. If you don't mind the taste of garlic, push a few cloves through your juicer to create a potent antiviral, antibacterial blend.

To help stimulate healing in the gastrointestinal system and stomach, add a teaspoon of probiotic powder along with 1000 mg of buffered vitamin C and 2 oz. of aloe vera juice. You can also mix in different supplements like green tea extract, curcumin, or astragalus to further enhance its functional food healing value. One day a week, it's a good idea to add a scoop of non-GMO brown rice, pea or hemp protein powder into your juices and use that as your fasting day. By restricting calories in this way, you are detoxifying the body and contributing to the health of your cells.

For many years, I've incorporated juicing in my health protocols. One study with arthritis patients, lasting for 28 days, included up to 6 fresh juices a day; the results were very impressive.[306]

Other Important Factors for a Healthy Vegetarian Diet

Here, also, are some general rules to follow that will increase your success, health, and happiness when it comes to the basics of a food program:

- Vary the amount of food you eat according to the time of day: Eat like a king at breakfast, a prince at lunch, and a pauper at dinner.

- Drastically reduce overall fat and sugar intake. All oils, including olive oil needs to be used as a condiment. Experts say that total fat intake should be no more than 30% of your weekly total calories.
- Eliminate refined carbohydrates from your diet and substitute complex carbohydrates that have lots of fiber, such as oats, barley, bran, beans, soy products, apples, cranberries, currants, and gooseberries.
- Reduce your use of salt. While certain variety of salt like Celtic sea salt, Himalayan pink salt, and certain Hawaiian salts provide essential nutrients, salt dehydrates tissues. Consumption of sodium-rich vegetables like celery, beets, spinach, Swiss chard and carrots.
- Keep alcohol consumption to a minimum. Alcohol, even in small amounts, will destroy folic acid, B6, and B12. That, in turn, makes you more susceptible to homocysteine, which is a greater predictor of heart disease than cholesterol levels. We know that homocysteine leads to the pathogenesis of the aging of the heart.
- Eat a variety of fruits, vegetables, and whole grains in their least processed forms. These foods are the building blocks of good health. Include such foods as fruits, vegetables, sprouted, whole-grain breads, cereals, wholegrain pastas, starchy vegetables, and beans.
- Have lean or nonfat *protein* at every meal. Though important, we now know that more protein is not better. (Protein, including vegetarian sources, will be discussed in entirety in Chapter 6). Rather, we should distribute small amounts of protein throughout the day. This will keep our energy levels high and eliminate that "sinking feeling" that sometimes occurs in the late afternoon.
- Consume as much *organically grown food and locally grown food* in your diet as possible. Yes, organic foods cost more at the grocery store, but the trade-off is obvious: health is good, chemicals are bad. A meta study published in the prestigious *British Journal of Nutrition* in July of 2014 showed that organic crops are between 19% and 69% higher in a number of key antioxidants than conventionally-grown crops, which is the equivalent of two portions of fruits and vegetables a day without additional caloric intake.[307] Pesticide residues in organic foods are 10-100

times lower than in non-organics. Eating foods with chemicals burdens the body. Even small amounts of toxins accumulate and eventually wear it down. See our section on page 271 re: chemicals in food products. Be kind to your body by keeping your diet as pure as possible. Organic produce is now more commercially viable, and many local farms are using organic methods, even if they are not organically certified. Visit your local farmer's markets and speak with the farmers directly about your preferences for safe food.

There are plenty of books, including many that I have authored, that can give you a complete run-down of the best foods to eat as well as delicious-tasting recipes.

Basic Supplementation on the Vegetarian Path

Supplements can be taken with protein shakes throughout the day or with food for people with sensitivities. Here is a list of basic daily supplements that I recommend to start off in becoming a healthy vegetarian:

✓ Vitamin B12, 800 micrograms

This vitamin helps in metabolism of all proteins and amino acids and cell reactions called methylation. See my complete discussion on vitamin B12 on p. 246.

✓ B-vitamin complex with folic acid, 25 mg of B-vitamin complex and generally 500 micrograms of folic acid

The B-vitamin complex consists of an array of different components that have been individually identified through research. **Vitamin B1** (Thiamine) is essential to normal metabolism and normal nerve function. It converts carbohydrates into glucose, which is the sole source of energy for the brain and nervous system. B1 helps the heart by keeping it firm and resilient. **Vitamin B2** (Riboflavin) helps promote proper growth and repair of tissues, and enhances a cell's ability to exchange gases such as oxygen and carbon dioxide in the blood. It helps release energy from the foods we eat, and is essential for good digestion, steady nerves, assimilation of iron, and normal vision. It is vital to the health of the entire glandular system, most particularly the adrenal glands, which are involved in stress control. **Vitamin B3** (Niacin) is essential to every cell in the body. It is the fundamental material of two enzyme systems and helps transform sugar and fat into energy. **Vitamin B5** (Pantothenic Acid) also works in all our cells. It converts carbohydrates, fats, and protein to energy, acts as an anti-stress agent, and manufactures antibodies that fight germs in the blood. **Vitamin B6** (Pyridoxine) nourishes the central nervous system, controls sodium/potassium levels in the blood, and assists in the production of red blood cells and hemoglobin. It helps protect against infection and assists in manufacturing DNA and RNA, the acids that contain the genetic code for cell growth, repair, and multiplication. **Folic acid** works mostly in the brain and nervous system. It is a vital component of spinal and extracellular fluid. It is necessary for the manufacture of DNA and RNA and helps convert amino acids.

✓ Vitamin C, 3000 mg

Vitamin C has many benefits. It strengthens the immune system, keeps cholesterol levels down, combats stress, promotes fertility, protects against cardiovascular disease and various forms of cancer, maintains mental health, and ultimately may prolong life. Its presence is necessary to build collagen, the "cement" that holds together the connective tissue throughout the body.

✓ Vitamin D3, 3000 units

Vitamin D helps the body utilize calcium and phosphorus, and form strong bones and teeth, and healthy skin. Its action also is vital to the nervous system and kidneys. An article in *US News & World R*eport noted that if you're fair skinned, experts say going outside for 10 minutes in the midday sun—in shorts and a tank top with no sunscreen—will give you enough radiation to produce about 10,000 international units of the vitamin.[308]

- ✓ Vitamin E, 400 units

  Vitamin E is basically an antioxidant; that is, it protects our fatty acids from destruction and maintains cellular health and integrity. It is especially important for promoting the health of our muscles, cells, blood, and skin. It is a primary defense against respiratory infection and disease. Vitamin E also is an excellent first aid tonic for burns. It is believed that vitamin E's antioxidant effects make available larger amounts of fats for metabolism, providing the body with extra energy for muscle contractions as is important for exercise.

- ✓ Coenzyme Q10, 100 mg

  Though we naturally produce coenzyme Q10, our output decreases as we grow older. Coenzyme Q10 is important in supplying energy directly into the muscles, which helps fight combat fatigue. In addition, it is vital for the health of the heart.

- ✓ Zinc, 15 mg

  Zinc plays an important role in the body's production of growth and sex hormones, and in its utilization of insulin. As a coenzyme, zinc helps start many important activities and sparks energy sources. It is an important element in the body's ability to remain in a state of balance, keeping blood at a proper acidity, producing necessary histamines, removing excess toxic metals, and helping kidneys maintain a healthy equilibrium of minerals. Zinc works in the protein production system, blood cells, circulatory system, and nerves.

Essential Nutrients in the Vegetarian Diet

B-Vitamins

Related to the question of the B vitamins is the level of the amino acid homocysteine in the body. The B vitamins regulate and (when necessary) lower the levels of homocystine. Too much homocysteine in the body has been tied to a number of disease conditions and imbalances, including:

- increased levels of low density lipoprotein (LDL), which is the blood-vessel-clogging form of cholesterol;
- epileptic seizure;
- the death of neural cells due to blood vessel shutdown, as well as other diseases of neuronal regression;
- problems during aging: homocysteine can cause a reduction in nitric oxide (NO) activity, which can then affect the arteries and veins, reducing their carrying capacity. This can wreak havoc on circulation as one ages, and can bring about other ill effects and
- reproductive problems have been associated with high homocysteine rates, including abnormal pap tests and arterial occlusion, which results in the need to use drugs such as Viagra.

To get back to the topic at hand, which is that meat readily provides the B vitamins that regulate the amino acid homocysteine while vegetables and fruits do not, it should be acknowledged that one study has shown that meat-eaters had lower homocysteine levels than vegetarians. Further, vegans, who eat no animal products whatsoever, had the highest levels of all. So here meat eaters do have the advantage over vegetarians. However, as we've seen, this advantage is offset by the many other harmful effects associated with meat-eating.

Still, this lack is one that can easily be remedied. For vegetarians, who take folate supplements together with other B vitamins which have been shown to decrease homocysteine levels, and we offer a suggested daily *Anti-Homocysteine Formula* just below.

I suggest taking folate (the naturally occurring form of folic acid) with vitamin B because this chemical also plays a part in homocysteine regulation and is a substance lacking in the diets of vegetarians. One reason an individual may have too much homocysteine in the blood is that this amino acid is not being converted to methionine. Folic acid is involved in this conversion, a biochemical process called methylation, an essential process connected to the formation of proteins and important brain chemicals such as serotonin. If the methylation process is interrupted in the liver, it can lead to free radical distress. Free radicals are roving electrons, molecules, or atoms that can damage bodily organs and processes, as well as decrease levels of the important organic chemicals superoxide dismutase and glutathione peroxidase.

Given the importance of folic acid, along with the already discussed B vitamins, in lowering homocysteine levels, the concerned vegetarian should supplement with folate as well as the vitamins. The folate can be combined with B6, and B12. Folate, however, works best with B12, and low B12 levels may be the reason some vegan dieters have higher levels of homocysteine than the general population.

Here is the homocysteine reduction formula I promised, one useful for all vegetarians.

Anti-homocysteine Formula (once a day)

B6	50 mg
B12	800 mcg
B1	25 mg
B2	25 mg
Folic Acid	1,000 mcg
TMG	500 mg

I might also add here that folic acid is not hard to come by in a plant-based diet. According to the *Vitamins and Health Supplements Guide*, folate can be found in the following:

> Arugula, asparagus, avocados, beans, dried beans, beet greens, beets, bok choy, brewer's yeast, broccoli, Brussels sprouts, cabbage, cauliflower, chard, chick-peas, citrus fruits, dandelion greens, escarole, garbanzo beans, kale, leafy green vegetables, lentils, mache, mustard greens, orange juice, oranges, peas, pinto beans, radicchio, rapini, savoy, soybeans, Swiss chard, turnip greens, and wheat germ.

Even with all these sources of folate, I still feel it's a nutrient that a vegetarian needs to be make certain they obtain fully; thus, my recommendation is to supplement with 500 mcg of methyl folic acid daily.

Fiber…YES! It's a Nutrient

I've already touched on the value of fiber content related to a food's digestibility, but let me now speak about its numerous other benefits.

As we are learning, one of the great advantages of vegetables over animal protein is that it contains fiber, which provides the following health benefits:

- aids in digestion;
- absorbs fluids such as saliva and gastric secretions, and expands and scours the intestinal walls, removing some potentially toxic agents, which would otherwise accumulate;
- aids in weight-control by giving a feeling of fullness without the calories;
- works as a natural laxative;
- is a non-nutritive substance that is not itself used by the body, so it slows the digestion of the parts of the food that are being broken down. The end result is that it makes for a slow, steady release of energy in contrast to the sudden spurt and subsequent slump you get from high-sugar, refined foods; *and*
- is now recognized across the medical establishment as playing a large role in preventing colon and prostate cancer.

Let's contrast all the benefits that come from eating high fiber diets to the results of eating a lot of meat, which contains no fiber at all, and refined foods, whose fiber content is minimal. On this healthy vegetarian diet, instead of having what is eaten quickly flushed through the intestines, spurred by fiber, there is likely to be internal stagnation, allowing the meat to sit in the digestive tract for up to three days, and perhaps indefinitely when there is not enough fiber, overall, in the diet. In these cases, stagnation can cause constipation (of which 40% of Americans suffer from[309]) and the release of toxins can lead to diverticulitis and may even be a major factor in some forms of cancer.

By the way, the measure of healthy bowel function is dependent on how many bowel movements you have in a day, and when you have them. Vegetarians with healthy diets (limited number of process foods, including breads) will typically have a bowel movement after each major meal. A minimum of two movements a day is necessary (three is ideal); it's how our bodies are designed to operate and essential for health. Remember, however, it takes time for the health of your GI tract to rebound during a transitioning from an animal-based to plant-based diet. So stay intentional and be patient.

According to the Dietary Guidelines for Americans 2010, men should aim for 38 grams of fiber daily, while women need 25 grams of fiber each day.[310] As you can suspect, most Americans are consuming nowhere near the level of fiber necessary for a healthy diet given their standard American fare. Vegetarians, on the other hand, have a much easier time meeting fiber requirements. Raw and sprouted preparations contain slightly more fiber than cooked foods, and more water, which is a necessary component for the body in using fiber.

In an article appearing in the *Huffington Post*, Selene Vakharia, a holistic nutritionist and lifestyle consultant, shows us the realities of what it takes to meet our fiber requirements by sharing the top 14 foods high in fiber:[311]

> *Apples:* As with other fruits and veggies with edible peels, eat your apple au naturale. The peels are an important source of fiber and nutrients like phytochemicals. One medium apple (with peel!) has 4.4 grams of fiber.
>
> *Pears*: One medium pear has 5.5 grams of fiber, which definitely goes a long way towards keeping our intestines healthy.
>
> *Parsnip*: Parsnips are like white carrots but have a distinct (and unique!) taste. You can use them all the same ways you'd use a carrot, or even use it as a substitute for potato, and they taste great mashed! A nine-inch-long cooked parsnip has 5.8 grams of fiber.
>
> *Broccoli*: There is a reason why parents harp on their children to eat broccoli! A cup of chopped raw broccoli has 2.4 grams of fiber, along with a huge dose of vitamin C and vitamin K. It is best to lightly steam or sauté broccoli in a tiny bit of water, until it becomes bright green. When steaming, wait for the water to boil and then add the broccoli, otherwise you won't get that bright green effect.

Brussels Sprouts: Another member of the power-packed cruciferous family that I will be speaking about a little later. Sadly, Brussels sprouts are often overcooked, which lends to a mushy and unappealing texture. Give this veggie is a whole different experience by oven-roasting, or even shredding and added it raw to salads. Each cooked sprout has 0.5 grams of fiber, so that adds up quickly.

Carrots: Along with being a great source of beta-carotene, carrots are a very good source of fiber—a ½-cup serving of raw baby carrots has 2.9 grams of fiber, and a half cup of cooked carrots has 2.3 grams.

Spinach: Raw is the best way to assimilate this beneficial dark-leafy green, and a bunch of it has 7.5 grams of fiber! Throw a handful in your smoothies or combine it with salad lettuces for extra fiber. This is another great benefit for vegetarians—extra iron.

Whole Grains: As mentioned before, in order to be a good source of fiber, grains must be in their whole, *unprocessed* form. Processing removes the bran and leaves a product that doesn't have the fiber content. As one example, cooked long-grain brown rice has 1.8 grams of fiber per half a cup, while the same amount of cooked long-grain white rice has just 0.4 grams. Big difference. On this note, avoid bread as a general rule, and instead cook up some kamut, wheat berries, or barley, and add them to your salad.

Quinoa: Quinoa is technically a seed, not a grain, but it's a great source of fiber with 5.2 grams in a one-cup serving (cooked). It's also a source of protein, with 8.1 grams per cooked cup. If you haven't tried this superfood yet, now's the time!

Amaranth: Like quinoa, tiny amaranth is a seed but acts like a grain and can be used like one in cooking. It's another fiber superstar, with 5.2 grams per one-cup serving. Try adding it to soups, where it'll cook quickly, absorb the flavors, and add some protein. It's also great for breakfast cereals; add some fruit, nuts, and a tiny bit of natural sweetener and you have a well-balanced start to your day.

Legumes: These are a vegetarian's dream: great source of fiber and protein. For example, quick-cooking red lentils have 4 grams of fiber per half-cup serving. Next time you get Indian food, try the dal instead of a meat dish—you'll get the same flavors but with more fiber and less fat.

Beans: Beans, beans, they're good for your heart... and your colon. These nutritional superstars are full of fiber—for example, cooked black beans have 15 grams per one-cup serving and white beans have a whopping 18.6 grams in the same amount. Up your bean intake slowly if you're not used to eating them to give your digestive system time to adjust.

Flax Seeds: One tablespoon serving of ground flax seeds has 1.9 grams of fiber. Consider adding a teaspoon of ground flax to your oatmeal or cereal in the mornings. If you pre-grind your flax, or buy it ground, keep it in the fridge or freezer. Grinding releases oils in the seed that can oxidize at room temperature.

Chia Seeds: These tiny seeds have a whopping 10.6 grams of fiber per ounce, and the gel coating that forms around them when they come in contact with liquids helps waste move through your digestive tract. Try adding chia seeds to your non-dairy yogurt or smoothies.

So, as you can see, a plant-based diet is the only way that you would satisfy the recommended daily need for fiber.

Omega-3 and Omega-6

Benefits of Omega-3; Dangers of Omega-6

We've been talking about the dangers of high protein intake when those proteins are from meats and other animal products as well as about other risks that come with this dietary emphasis. I also pointed out that a vegetarian eater is seldom at risk of getting too much protein. For one, this seldom happens since one would have to eat quite a few legumes, sprouts or wheat grass to boost one's protein intake too high. But, as I said, even if it did, this would not pose much danger since vegetarian protein is of a different quality from meat protein.

But are there any health dangers from vegetarian eating? One that needs to be looked at carefully does not involve ingesting toxins, but rather the possibility of not getting enough of a vital fatty acid. Vegetarians' diets can get skewed towards overconsumption of omega-6 fatty acids. The vegetarian diet is typically high in linoleic acid, an omega-6, which is readily available in polyunsaturated vegetable oils. It's not that the omega-6s are bad for you, but that if you are depending too much on them, you may not be getting sufficient omega-3 fatty acids (in scientific terms, alpha-linolenic acid or ALA), which as I pointed out previously are available in flaxseed, walnut and canola oils. Omega-3s can also be obtained by non-vegetarians via fish oils, which actually convert more readily to necessary internal body chemicals than do plant-obtained oils. However, one word of caution about taking fish oil supplements. A report published in the July 2013 issue of the *Journal of the National Cancer Institute* found a higher risk of prostate cancer among men who regularly ate oily fish or took fish oil supplements, although some have suggested this study had some significant flaws.[312,313] Still, plant omegas do work well. The Vegetarian Society recommends you get roughly 4g of ALA a day.

Both these oils (3s and 6s) are needed to maintain optimum health, as has been shown particularly in studies of children and older people. One study of the former looked at 117 children (aged 5-12) with developmental coordination disorder (DCD). The clumsiness associated with this disease is seen in children who have trouble with simple tasks that involve use of large and small muscles, tasks such as buttoning buttons or forming letters. The group in the study registered significant improvements when treated with dietary supplementation of omega-3 and omega-6 fatty acids. As the study stated, the children improved "in reading, spelling and behavior over 3 months of treatment."[314]

The same type of findings, a marked improvement after supplementation, was found in a study of 75 children and adolescents (aged 8–18) with attention deficit hyperactivity disorder (ADHD). As the findings showed, "Children and adolescents with ADHD… treated with omega 3/6 fatty acids for 6 months responded with meaningful reduction of ADHD symptoms."[315]

On the other end of the age spectrum, in a study dealing with older people, as reported in the *British Journal of Nutrition,* it was found that there were "significantly lower" levels of omega-3 fatty acids EPA and DHA in Alzheimer's patients than in control subjects without the illness. It was further learned that "DHA levels were progressively reduced with severity of clinical dementia."[316] In other words, the less of the omega fatty acid in the subject, the more likely he or she was to have this disease. Additionally, high levels of omega-3 fatty acids were found to be required in order to benefit from the protective effect of B vitamins on brain tissue. Incognitively impaired elder subjects were treated with a daily dose of folic acid, vitamin B12, and vitamin B6 for two years. Their omega-3 levels were determined by blood tests at the beginning and end of the study and their brains were scanned. The study found that subjects with low omega-3 levels at the beginning of the study did not appear to benefit from B vitamin; however, supplementation with B vitamins of the subjects with higher omega-3 levels reduced the rate of brain tissue loss by 40% compared to the control group.[317]

There are a host of other studies affirming the benefits of omega-3 in addressing certain lifestyle diseases. One study found that men who had higher levels of omega-3 fatty acids had a reduced risk of developing prostate cancer.[318] They elucidated the molecular mechanism receptors whereby EPA binds to and activates a fatty acid receptor (called fatty acid receptor 4) (FFA4), which led to an inhibition of cancer cell proliferation in human prostate cancer cell lines. "This kind of knowledge could lead us to better treat or prevent cancer because now we know how it works," said Kathryn Meier, professor of pharmacy at Washington State University Spokane and lead researcher of the study.[319]

Lastly, a study involving 374 patients recovering from heart attacks found that those supplemented with omega-3 fatty acids for six months experienced less deterioration in heart function in comparison to the control group.[320] It was discovered that "Omega-3 fatty acids may have anti-inflammatory effects and also promote better cardiac healing," commented Dr. Kwong, study co-author.[321] "Giving a high dose of omega-3 fatty acids soon after a heart attack appears to improve cardiac structure and heart functioning above and beyond the standard of care," Dr. Kwong concluded.

I have cautioned that non-fish-oil-consuming vegetarians should be very aware of the need for omega-3 fatty acid intake (ALA) as compared to omega-6s, which you will probably be getting in abundance. To assure yourself that you are getting the full measure of 3s, avoid using oils like safflower, sunflower, peanut, palm and canola oils with a lot of 6s, that is, with high quantities of linoleic acid (LA), thereby reducing the ratio of LA to ALA (i.e., omega-6 to omega-3). The Vegetarian Society makes this easy for you by setting out the following dosages of plant omega-3, in the form of ALA, found in certain foods, and the concurrent amounts of linoleic acid or omega-6, found in the same foods[322]:

Flaxseed oil	1 tablespoon (14g)	provides 8g of ALA and relatively insignificant levels of LA
Flaxseed, ground	1 tablespoon (24g)	provides 3.8g of ALA and equal amounts of LA
Walnuts	1 oz (28g)	provides 2.6g of ALA but also four times as much LA
Tofu	4.5 oz (126g)	provides 0.7g of ALA but also seven times as much LA

Other plant foods provide omega-3 fatty acids. If you wish to increase your intake of these important fatty acids, make sure to consume copious amounts of: fruit, most green leafy vegetables, non-green leafy vegetables, grains, legumes, chia seeds, flax seeds, hemp seeds, and walnuts.

Omega 3s and Arachidonic Acid

I don't know if as a child you played the game Pick-up sticks; a series of sticks were thrown on the ground, all interlacing and lying on top of each other. The object of the game was to remove a stick without disturbing any others. Well, the body is like an unplayable game of Pick-up sticks. There's not a single element you can remove without affecting the others. As an example, I mentioned how certain chemicals found in cruciferous vegetables were advantageous, not because they necessarily have a big role in and of themselves, but because they are essential in aiding conversion of the sex hormone estradiol to another significant body chemical.

Along these same lines, I now want to return to a subject already given in some detail—the omega fatty acids. Some of the intricacies of their involvement in human physiological processes weren't mentioned before, but are worth looking into. In that earlier discussion, I talked about the fatty acids and the danger of imbalances in vegetarians. Rather than paraphrase what I said, let me simply repeat it, since it relates to this as-yet-unconsidered aspect. Vegetarians' diets can get skewed toward overconsumption of omega-6 fatty acids because of unhealthy oils. As long as you stay away from the processed oils like canola oil, peanut oil, cotton seed oil, safflower and sunflower seed oil, and stick with the organic extra virgin olive oil, coconut oil, macadamia oil, avocado oil, and almond oil in small quantities you'll be fine. The vegetarian diet is typically high in linoleic acid (LA), an omega-6, which is readily available in polyunsaturated vegetable oils, and in foods such as potato and corn chips, grain-based desserts, salad dressings, breads, pastas, and French fries.[323] It's not that the omega-6s are necessarily bad for you, but if you are depending too much on them you may not be getting sufficient omega-3 fatty acids, and it's the ratio between omega-6/omega-3 that actually determines health. These omega-3s are called in scientific terms, alpha-linolenic acid or ALA.

It might seem that I have already exhausted this subject. At this point, nonetheless, I'd like to revisit this discussion from a more positive side. I don't want to dwell again on the danger of vegetarians having a fatty acid imbalance, but on a special danger, one aggravated by current eating patterns. This is a risk that I have not mentioned previously but is appropriate now that we have been looking in greater depth at various nutrients and their effects on the body.

The problem here is arachidonic acid. For those of us in the Western world who are not careful—even vegetarians—it's easy to get too much refined sugar in our diets. Dietary sugar is either released as blood glucose or converted into fat, which contains arachidonic acid. Too much arachidonic acid can lead to inflammation problems.

I haven't mentioned the fatty acids yet, but a little more dialogue here is necessary for a complete understanding. This arachidonic acid-containing fat, which was converted from excess blood sugar, is part of a chemical chain of reactions involving *series two prostaglandins*.[324] Prostaglandins are similar to hormones in that they facilitate communication in the body. While hormones communicate between cells, prostaglandins facilitate communication *within* individual cells or close by the cells.[325] There are three series of prostaglandins: series-1 is from omega-6, series-2 from arachadonic acid and omega-6, and series-3 from omega-3. Series-2 is thought to induce swelling and inflammation in tissue—especially damaged tissue, while series-3 ameliorates the effects of series-2 prostaglandins, helping to protect the body against heart attacks, arthritis, lupus, and asthma. Prostaglandins also increase and decrease certain bodily functions relating to clotting and relaxation of blood vessels, etc.[326]

Series three prostaglandins, in particular, are important in our context because they inhibit the production of arachidonic acid.[327] These prostaglandins are made from omega-3 fatty acids. The starting point for the synthesis of these valued prostaglandins is the omega-3 eicosapentaenoic acid (EPA). Researchers differ over how much ALA is converted into its usable forms EPA and DHA, but for our purposes, the salient point is that this conversion is occurring from the omega-3s.[328, 329]

See the connection now? If you don't have enough omega-3 fatty acids, you don't have enough series three prostaglandins. When you don't have enough of these, arachidonic acid is unregulated, and the body will likely give way to some type of inflammatory disorder. Remember the Pick-up sticks analogy? It applies here in spades.

I wouldn't bring this up except that omega-3 fatty acid deficiency is widespread in American society among meat- and plant-centered diet eaters alike. Insufficient intake of omega-3, which is a precursor to chronic states of inflammation, can lead to multiple problems, as the following explains:

> Omega three deficiencies have… been tied to dyslexia, violence, depression, memory problems, weight gain, cancer, heart disease, eczema, allergies, inflammatory diseases, arthritis, diabetes, and many other conditions.[330]

The list indicates that trouble is brewing if your deficits in omega-3 fatty acids reach quite a distance beyond the simple inability to control arachidonic acid.

I must believe this is because of the broad role these fatty acids play in the body's composition and function. A report by Dale Kiefer of *Life Extension* magazine points out that three-fifths of the brain is comprised of fats. An omega-3 called DHA is an important part of nerve endings in brain cell receptors. Further, as Dr. Ronald

Hoffman explains, DHA is important for healthy brain development in babies and is a critical component of eye health.

The *Life Extension* article notes a point that I brought up in the earlier discussion of the topic, which is that many people get their omega-3s from fish.

They are plentiful in fatty cold-water fish such as salmon, tuna, bluefish, sardines, herring, and king mackerel. A three ounce serving of salmon, for instance, yields roughly three grams (3,000 mg) of combined EFA's [essential fatty acids].[331]

But the same article points out that those who don't eat fish can get their EPA and DHA directly from the same source the fish do, namely seaweed and edible marine algae.[332]

According to the University of Maryland Medical Center, "dietary sources of ALA include flaxseeds, flaxseed oil, soybeans and soybean oil, pumpkin seeds and pumpkin seed oil, purslane, perilla seed oil, walnuts and walnut oil." In fact, most flaxseeds won't even open for the average person; they go right through the body without getting the benefit. So it's best to purchase flaxseed meal, or use the flaxseed oil, or a combination of both, because it's the oil that we're getting the benefit from. Both the meal and the oil should be refrigerated, and it's okay to freeze the flaxseed meal to prevent spoilage. Not that we needed more evidence of the benefit of omega-3s, but a more recent meta-analysis examined how a plant-based diet offers protection against cardiovascular disease; the results were published in the peer-reviewed journal *American Journal of Clinical Nutrition*. They found after a review of twenty-seven studies and over 251,000 subjects that higher ALA levels correlates to a lower risk of cardiovascular disease.[333]

Let's close this chapter on the health effects of varied nutrients with two important points. First, let's simply note the unfathomable complexity of the human body, and how varied components of the vegetarian diet minister so well to its needs when correctly applied and moderated.

Second, I want to reinforce what might be a hidden point of my Pick-up sticks analogy that's worthy of mention. Currently, the thinking by most trained in the modern Western medicine paradigm is to treat a symptom and/or isolate and annihilate a "bad guy"—whether a pathogen or tumor or some other deleterious "intruder." The typical approach for this is to use drugs and/or surgeries to remove the protagonist, without paying attention to the bunch of Pick-up sticks surrounding that one (issue).

Remember what I said a few pages back: *There's not a single element you can remove without affecting the others.* However, today in this country, we practice "medicine" by removing something—a tumor, a knee, or an organ, and expect that we've "handled" the "problem," all the while living with a mistaken perception about the actual origin of the problem.

What most in our society and in our medical community almost certainly miss is this extremely fundamental point: The farther and more consistently we live *away* from our true nature—as loving, compassionate human beings whose bodies thrive on pure water, a plant-based diet, a little sunshine, exercise, positive thinking, etc.,—the more *dis*-ease we will experience, and the more *disease* we will manifest. It is this simple. Like the Pick-up sticks, everything is intertwined; all affects the one.

More importantly, can you imagine a world where we utilized the science related to the superiority of plant-based nutrition and re-created our "green" planet? Can you imagine a world where everyone received, as a benefit of human experience, the basics of a *sustainable existence*: clean water and air, food, shelter, clothing, satisfaction of purpose by serving one's community and fellow human beings, and love? What really do we need beyond these things? Let's take an honest look at this now…

Vitamin B12

Those that harp on the health dangers of a plant-based diet do one important service. They keep those of us who follow this green path aware of the fact that there are a few things that can very well be lacking in a vegetarian diet. This is especially true for diets that are not well planned, heavy in processed vegetarian foods rather than whole-foods, or where the practitioner does not know how and when to use supplements.

I talked quite a bit early on about vegetarians' need to watch that they get enough vitamin B12, a nutrient abundant in meat and absent in vegetables, but I didn't go into the second nutrient that can be found missing in green diets, iron; and like B12, it is an essential component in being a healthy vegetarian. I'll go into that in a minute. First, let me say something, as yet unmentioned, that makes B12 deficiency such a threat.

The crucial difficulty here is that deficiencies often don't show up for five to ten years, since B12 is a storable vitamin and a supply is kept in-house in the body to take up slack when not enough is coming in through food. The most disturbing thing about B12 deficiency is that it may go undetected until there has been irreversible damage to the nervous system or spinal cord. The body requires B12 to make red blood cells and a deficiency puts a person at a greater risk of pernicious anemia. Also, B12 is necessary for cell repair as it is an essential component in DNA synthesis, and is required for normal motor function, regulation of heartbeat, and mental functions like memory. If it is not present in adequate amounts, all these areas may suffer weaknesses. This might present itself with such symptoms as facial swelling, weakness, fatigue, weight loss, depression or thinning hair. Importantly, without enough B12, the capacity for your body to rejuvenate cells and heal wounds are seriously compromised.

Although a person wouldn't want to rely on emergency procedures, it is true that if people are not ingesting sufficient doses of this vitamin, their bodies will resort to recirculation of this water-soluble vitamin and, possibly, intestinal manufacturing of B12 by bacteria. In fact, a comprehensive study of vegans in England showed no signs of vitamin B12 deficiencies, and many of the subjects hadn't eaten meat in 30 years. This was probably because they relied on supplements as well as taxed their bodies to make and recycle the vitamin. Nevertheless, this last comment shouldn't be read as if I were downplaying the hazard of doing without B12—far from it.

To offer more insight and a wider perspective on the somewhat contentious and confusing vitamin B12 issue, let me refer to an interview featured on *Natural News* with Gabriel Cousens, M.D., founder of the Tree of Life Rejuvenation Center in Patagonia, Arizona and health blogger Kevin Gianni. In the interview, Dr. Cousens asserts that the vitamin B12 derived from vegetable protein and microalgae are inactive B12 analogues that actually block the uptake of vegan B12. He found in a review of 18 studies of vegans and live food aficionados, that about 80% were vitamin B12 deficient.

At one time, we believed that a serum analysis of B12 would provide relevant diagnostic information. However, according to Dr. Cousens, a simple urine test has proven to be the gold standard for measuring human active B12. Previously, it was believed that 200 micrograms was adequate to lower homocysteine levels.

(Homocysteine is an amino acid and breakdown product of protein metabolism that, when present in high concentrations, has been linked to an increased risk of heart attacks and strokes. Elevated homocysteine levels are thought to contribute to plaque formation by damaging arterial walls.)

With the updated protocol for measuring B12, we see that the level required for lowering homocysteine is 400 micrograms. For those of you who have studied the subject, the test measures the metabolite methylmalonic acid (MMA), which is used by the body along the human active homocysteine levels pathway. When MMA is elevated it means that your body is not properly utilizing homocysteine levels and this indicates a deficiency.[334]

How can vegetarians be sure to get enough vitamin B12? I talked about this with some general ideas on what to eat when the topic came up earlier. However, I did not make a specific recommendation at the time and will here. I will precede this by again making some positive comments about tempeh and miso as they both contain B12, albeit small amounts. Additionally, there is some indication that the sea vegetable dulse contains B12, but further testing would be necessary to conclude this as an adequate source.[335] Miso contains about .17 micrograms of B12 per 100 grams (.03 mcgs. per tablespoon) while tempeh has 3.9 mcgs. per 100 grams.[336] Depending on the type of miso, protein quantity can range from 12 to 20%, and this offers more usable protein than found in beef. Compare miso's net protein utilization rate of about 72% versus that of a hamburger, which weighs in at 67%. In Japan, miso isn't the dominant protein consumed; it does, however, play an important role, accounting for 10% of the protein intake in modern Japan, and is relied upon as a primary food staple.

As discussed above, the sea vegetable dulse has been shown to contain B12. An investigation by two researchers in Great Britain in the 1950s confirmed the presence of cyanocobalamin (vitamin B12) in dulse, but could not find the mechanism by which the plant might be metabolizing it. According to the reporting site, "The two scientists speculated that it was made 'perhaps by bacteria living in the surrounding seawater or on the surface of the plant.' (It is well known that various species of bacteria, or epiphytes, use the plants' surface as their substrate)."[337] VeganHealth.org notes that dulse contains .3 to .39 μg of B12 analogue per 3 g serving, but notes with caution that until it is shown to lower MMA levels, it should not be considered a source of active B12.[338]

As to my recommendation, I believe vegetarians should supplement with methyl B12 sublingually, 800 mcg daily.

Iron

As noted a moment ago, in terms of nutrients, obtaining sufficient iron is probably the second most pressing dietary concern for non-meat-eaters. It is also true that iron from plant sources is slightly different from the iron in meat, and plant-derived iron is not so readily absorbed as iron from meat. Yet, with some judicious juggling of nutrients, vegetarians can keep themselves adequately supplied with iron.

Iron from plant foods is called non-heme iron, and its absorbability is influenced by other foods in the diet. The absorption of heme iron (from meat) is unaffected by outside factors. It stands to reason, then, that a vegetarian must find the component of the diet that makes the non-heme iron absorbable and eat that. It turns out this is not so challenging. For vegetarians, vitamin C is the magic ingredient that boosts iron's absorbability. Green eaters need to incorporate lots of vitamin C-rich foods into their diets, such as leafy green vegetables, dried fruits (such as apricots, figs, and raisins), blackstrap molasses, and yeast in order to guarantee proper iron absorption.

Since I've already said to limit your intake of dried fruits, your best option is leafy greens, such as spinach, kale, collard greens, etc. Plant-Based Physician, Michael Klaper, M.D., suggests squeezing a little lemon juice on steamed kale or over your salad daily to help with iron uptake. Dr. Klaper summarized a study published in the *International Journal of Vitamin and Nutrition Research*: "Vitamin C increases the absorption of iron in two ways: (1) by preventing the formation of insoluble and unabsorbable iron compounds, and (2) by contributing electrons to the iron atoms (the chemists would say "reducing" them from a +3 to a +2 state), which seems to be a requirement for the uptake of iron atoms into the mucosal cells."[339]

Zinc

Zinc a macro mineral is absolutely necessary, and plays an important role in the body's production of growth and sex hormones, and in its utilization of insulin. As a coenzyme, zinc helps start many important activities and sparks energy sources. It is an important element in the body's ability to remain in a state of balance, keeping blood at a proper acidity, producing necessary histamines, removing excess toxic metals, and helping kidneys maintain a healthy equilibrium of minerals. Zinc works in the protein production system, blood cells, circulatory system, and nerves.

Excellent vegetable sources include peas, soybeans, mushrooms, whole grains, most nuts, and seeds, especially pumpkin. Lack of taste or smell is a sign of zinc deficiency. Skin problems also may indicate zinc deficiencies. Stretch marks are an indication that elastin, the fibers that make skin springy and smooth, are not incorporating enough zinc to keep skin healthy. Acne and psoriasis can result from zinc deficiency, as can an abnormal wearing away of tooth enamel. Other signs of zinc deficiency include opaque fingernails, brittle hair, and bleeding gums. The daily zinc requirement for adults is 15 milligrams for men and 12 milligrams for women. Most zinc can be obtained from the diet; wheat germ, spinach, pumpkin and squash seeds, cashews, dark chocolate and cocoa, beans, legumes, peas, mushrooms, and avocados are all good sources of zinc. As far as for ensuring that children raised vegan get enough zinc, it's really simple; all you have to have is a good quality diet for children with a simple supplement.

More on Vegetarian Health Enhancements

Advocates of the American way of eating, such as the misinformed dietician in my previous example, can depend on so-called "common knowledge"—such as the widespread and erroneous belief that meat and dairy are our only protein sources—to back them up in their assertions and practices. After all, one has to look no further than the Food Pyramid for their answers, which by the way as I've noted in a number of my other books was originally developed by the dairy industry. A vegetarian, on the other hand, even in our increasingly green-eating-tolerant society, frequently must be well informed (or good at sidestepping debates) and defend his or her beliefs to the core, while risking being judged and even ostracized.

Remember my conversation earlier in the book on epistemology, which considers *how we know what we know*? Well, because common knowledge regarding diet and health has been linked for centuries to consuming animal products, most people (including the vast majority of dieticians) actually believe this is true, *and without having looked into the facts of the matter whatsoever*! When challenged on the superiority of animal-based proteins, you may hear responses like well "that is just known," or "that is what I learned in my college programs." Further, the inertia surrounding the issue makes it is astoundingly difficult for plant-based initiatives to gain traction, regardless of the mounds of data supporting their superiority. That is, until now.

If one were to talk to an *open-minded* meat advocate—they still exist—one thing to mention is how vegetarianism stacks up against the typical meat-based diet. When the British Medical Association and the World Health Organization compared non-vegetarian and vegetarian diets, they found that the latter met the recommended daily allowances for all nutrients, and *in a healthier way*.[340] Vegetarians took in fewer calories, less fat, and more complex carbohydrates and fiber. Even though calcium and riboflavin intake tends to be lower, the vegetarian diet is closer to the dietary guidelines of the USDA than the average American diet.

Along these same lines, and adding support to vegetarians' claims that green eating has significant advantages over meat eating, was the 1954 study that found no significant difference between the physical, blood, and biochemical tests of vegetarians and omnivores but noted that the vegetarians had significantly lower levels of serum cholesterol than the other groups.[341] A high level of this cholesterol has been associated with heart problems. Later studies showed that levels of folic acid, often deficient in omnivore control groups, were usually higher in vegetarians, as the best sources of this nutrient is fruits and vegetables.[342] Folic acid is necessary to many bodily processes. It should be reiterated that many vegetarian mainstays are not only economical sources of protein but are replete with other nutrients as well. A meal of whole grains, beans, potatoes, carrots, cabbage, spinach, and watercress, for example, provides a wide variety of nutrients.[343]

Let's say, however, that an individual (the open-minded meat eater) is not swayed by the points about comparing meat- and green-centered diets, and throws in the old canard, one we've discussed a bit earlier, that non-milk-drinking green eaters suffer from lack of calcium. The informed veggie will counter that with proper planning; even vegetarians who take in no dairy products can get more than enough calcium in their diet. While a cup of whole milk contains 288 mg of calcium and 0.1 mg of iron, a quarter cup of sesame seeds has 580 mg of calcium and 5.25 mg of iron—far more than the dairy source.[344] Sesame seed butter—known in the Middle East as tahini—can be used to make a delicious, rich-tasting, high-protein sauce to serve with salads, vegetables, or pasta. Collard greens and kale and are also excellent sources of calcium, offering a whopping 357mg and 137mg, respectively, per 1 cup serving in a highly absorbable form,[345] and all of these come without the harmful side effects of consuming dairy.

Health in Plants

At this moment, let me drop the framework I have temporarily adopted of considering how to address a person who wants to learn more about the health benefits of vegetarianism vs. a meat- and dairy-based diet, and take up a topic that has been touched on lightly but not given full expression yet: the health yields of green eating. This will serve as a prelude to a discussion of some of the workshops and study groups I have conducted on vegetarianism. In these sessions, I have seen the connection between going green and improving one's health with my own eyes.

As we've seen, vegetarian diets depend heavily on four groups of plant foods: grains and cereals, legumes (including beans and peas), fruits and vegetables, and nuts and seeds. Including something from each of these groups at every meal guarantees maximum nutrition. Additionally, when you cook plant foods from scratch, you avoid the additives so often found in processed and packaged items.

So, let's look at the healthful nature of plant foods. They contain a variety of helpful chemicals, including ones that regulate hormones, and phytonutrients that act as free radical scavengers, protecting against the oxidation effects of normal bodily processes and cell degradation by environmental pollutants. Plant food fiber, in its various forms, as noted earlier on, helps the digestive system run smoothly, partly by blocking the development of fermenting, toxic pockets of undigested food in the bowel.

With all these good things in their makeup, it is natural that in scientific studies, eating plant-based foods and avoiding animal products correlates with lower serum lipid levels (noted a moment ago), less hypertension, lower body weight, fewer cardiovascular complications, fewer problems with processing of blood sugar, fewer malignancies, and less early death. One study indicated that African-Americans, many of whom unfortunately, follow the Standard American Diet with its emphasis on meat and dairy, have high levels of lifestyle-associated diseases. The study also indicated that they are able to lower early death rates *more than a third* by including fresh greens, nuts, and fruit in their daily diets.

Along with the phytonutrients, plants also contain phytoestrogens (plant compounds that can influence the human sex hormones and, in studies so far, seem to have positive effects on diabetes and heart disease). A key group of phytoestrogens is the lignans, which are under intense study by a growing number of researchers that are looking at the benefits they may offer to the body's hormone systems. One online source notes about the broader phytoestrogen group, "Evidence is accruing that [they]… may have protective action against diverse health disorders such as prostate, breast, bowel, and other cancers, cardiovascular disease, brain function disorders, menopausal symptoms and osteoporosis."[346]

Other phytoestrogens, ones found more in the Asian diet, are soy isoflavones. These are lignans' counterparts and have received good press for what some have found to be their beneficial health effects. According to findings by Dr. M.J. McCann and others, published in *Nutrition and Cancer*, one reason rates of prostate cancer may be much lower in East Asia than in the West is the inclusion in the Oriental societies of much soy, with its phytoestrogen, in the diet.[347]

For those who don't eat much in the way of soy-based foods, let me add—as noted by Dr. M.S. Morton and others in an article in another cancer journal—cereals, grains, and other plant matter may have effects similar to that of the rich phytoestrogen-containing soy compounds found in Asian diets.[348]

Plant lignans take a number of forms, and many of them are metabolized (broken down) by human intestinal bacteria into two compounds, enterolactone, which supports prostate health, and enterodiol, which may reduce risk of cardiovascular disease. The lignin precursors for these compounds are found in many vegetarian foods, including seeds (flax, pumpkin, sunflower, poppy), whole grains (rye, oats, barley), bran (wheat, oat, rye), fruits (particularly berries), and numerous vegetables.

Following up a remark I just made, which is that these lignans are now under intense scrutiny for their health effects, let me highlight a number of other studies targeting the lignans present in specific plants.

One study showed that flaxseed lignan extract reduced cholesterol and blood sugar levels in human patients.[349] Sesame lignans, on the other hand, in some trials are shown to enhance the antioxidant effectiveness of vitamin E.[350] (As I mentioned earlier, antioxidants curb free radicals, which are atoms, electrons, and molecules that are running loose and colliding with one another, damaging healthy tissue.) Sesamin and sesaminol are the two most abundant of the sesame lignans. Once the antioxidant effects of sesamin are activated in the liver, research shows that, "it works to improve liver function and accelerate the decomposition of alcohol… lower high blood pressure, reduce the blood cholesterol level and prevent breast cancer."[351]

Another lignin byproduct, enterolactone, was found to reduce risk of death from coronary heart disease and cardiovascular disease when it was found in elevated levels, according to a study of Finnish men.[352]

Introducing the Vegetarian Lifestyle

Vegetarianism in its best incarnation is not just a dietary plan but a lifestyle, and most dedicated vegetarians see well beyond the dinner plate when it comes to living a healthy life. Exercise and stress-reduction methods like meditation are part of the full-scale vegetarian routine. Studies show further that "vegetarians usually abstain or are moderate in their use of alcohol, caffeine and tobacco."[353] This cuts down their chances of developing alcoholism, emphysema, lung cancer, and heart disease. Because vegetarians often opt for natural healing methods over invasive ones, they are also generally able to avoid the dangers of getting hooked on pharmaceutical medications. Further, they tend to ask and research the deeper questions in life; they do not accept common knowledge as true until they have looked into it themselves. They also tend to support initiatives founded in unification rather than separation, and are typically active in efforts to preserve the value of life for all living beings.

And to take up the remark I made earlier about some vegetarians feeling defensiveness in relation to children and green eating, let me say this: while it's important to make sure that children eat a wide variety of foods and get all the vitamins, minerals, and protein they need, a *carefully monitored* non-flesh diet can lower children's risk of disease. Dr. Scharffenberg, of San Joaquin Hospital in California reports, notes: "Seventeen percent of sixth to eighth graders have serum cholesterol levels greater than 180 mg/dI, an obvious result of the usual so called 'good' American meat diet." This is a recipe for ill health a little bit further down the road for these youth, and, as he sees it, a low-fat, high-fiber vegetarian diet might be a child's best health insurance.[354]

Specific Vegetarian/Vegetarian-Based Diets

The Macrobiotic Way to Health

In a previous chapter, I discussed the work of George Ohsawa, the Japanese health practitioner who drew on the philosophy of yin and yang to create a dietary regimen called macrobiotics, which is primarily a plant-based diet, but allows for some fish, weekly, and some dairy and other meat on very rare occasion or not at all. I didn't, however, mention that this style of eating is controversial in many circles.

Many people have embraced the principles of the macrobiotic diet, some hoping to overcome illness, others simply trying to reach and maintain optimum health. They see it as a firmly rooted practice that has helped them deal with diseases as serious as cancer. On the other hand, doctors and others warn against forsaking traditional medical care in favor of dietary-based protocols. They say that by the time you can assess whether a particular diet is helping to alleviate a condition, it may be too late to turn to effective medical intervention.

Given these opposing views, it makes sense to take a closer look at macrobiotics.

In my previous discussion, I've explained how macrobiotics draws on principles found in Zen Buddhism, applying them particularly to foods, which are classified as either yin or yang. The diet advised avoiding any food that carried extremes of either of the energies. Another important dietary rule of macrobiotics is to strive to eat mostly locally grown, in-season foods.

This last element of the program would link an eater directly to their own particular region, suggesting that in a particular geographic zone, both the human and vegetables and other green foods grown there share a common template, of weather, seasons and other broad components. The theory is that by eating foods locally produced at their time of harvest, the individual vegetarian is placing them self fully in sync with the land.

In talking about the value of eating one's regional cuisine and eating in tune with nature, Michio Kushi, who was instrumental in bringing the macrobiotic way to the US, explained that different climates are responsible for such varying food qualities as mineral, protein, and fat content. In fact, different weather and rainfall patterns produce diverse soils, which certainly impact the chemical composition of the foods grown in them. Macrobiotics holds that the most beneficial food qualities for any given consumer are then found in the seasonal foods grown in that consumer's native region since both have been molded by that environment and contain its yin/yang profile.

I share the general opinion that it's better to eat from what your region has to offer, though for different reasons than those given by the macrobiotic practitioners. It is a colossal waste of energy to have locally picked wool sent halfway around the world to be processed. I would say the same about the bananas that I consume, for instance, even though I love them as much as the next vegetarian. However, cross-country shipping is an expensive endeavor. Locally farm-raised foods are the best option, saving the most resources overall.

Macrobiotic practitioners do not share my viewpoint on this second concern—eating from one's region *to conserve the world's energy*. They argue that if essential or desired foods cannot be found locally, they may be imported from a different region, provided that it is in the same general climate zone. The "temperate zone," for instance, includes most of the US, Europe, the Soviet Union, China, and Japan. According to macrobiotic practitioners, foods from anywhere in these countries are okay for those living in the temperate zone, but one shouldn't eat food if at all possible from a totally different climatic zone—such as a tropical zone like most of Central America.

For some people, shifting to this diet has worked wonders with their health. Although certainly a healthy choice, I do not have enough evidence to judge macrobiotic eating and its ability to forestall or turn back diseases, so I will simply report the anecdotal evidence here. Many people who adopt macrobiotics say that they sleep better and for fewer hours than before, feel more vital when awake, have better health, higher energy, and participate more fully in life than they ever thought possible.

A number of writers tell stories of how the adoption of a macrobiotic eating plan helped them beat back disease assaults. In *Macrobiotic Miracle*, Virginia Brown, a mother and nurse from Vermont, tells of her recovery from fourth-stage melanoma cancer, an illness few survive. She was told that without surgery, she would die in six months, but she refused that option and took up macrobiotics instead. Brown is not only still alive, but directing a support group in the Kushi Foundation, a macrobiotic educational center located in Becket, Massachusetts.

Another cancer sufferer who swears by macrobiotics is Elaine Nussbaum. She underwent three painful years of chemotherapy for advanced uterine cancer before hearing about macrobiotics from one of her children. She decided to give it a try and eventually the cancer went into remission. She went on to study nutrition, earning a master's degree in the subject. Even Jesse Jones, the spokeswoman for the Kushi Foundation, used macrobiotics to overcome throat cancer.

You will have to decide for yourself whether the macrobiotic diet has these disease-disabling qualities, but I can say with conviction that the plan is simple, easy to follow, and reasonable.

Here are the basic guidelines: 50% of the food in any meal should be grains. About a third should be fresh vegetables; 10%, soups; another 10%, beans and bean products; and the last 5%, sea vegetables. Although fish, fruit, seeds, and nuts are not recommended, the eater may partake of them sparingly. Remember the principle guiding macrobiotic food choice is not vegetarianism per se, but the avoidance of foods overly powerful in yin or yang, which include most meats. With regard to drinking, the diet's prescriptions say that any beverage should be mellow, non-aromatic, and non-stimulant. Most of the food should be gently cooked, though a portion of the vegetables may be eaten raw. All food should be organically grown, natural, unprocessed, and unaltered.

As you may know, macrobiotic eating has caught on, at least in a small way in the US. Health food stores and Asian food marts should have most of the foods you'll need to get going. It's also possible to find macrobiotic restaurants in many cities throughout the country.

Try a macrobiotic restaurant, and you will enjoy a delightful eating experience. From there (even if you don't become a full-fledged adherent of this form of near vegetarianism), you will be ready to try some of your own macrobiotic meals.

Now, you may have caught on that I have some reservations about the macrobiotic way of eating. For one, as I made clear, the healing benefits of following a macrobiotic regimen are mainly anecdotal as opposed to empirical, of the sort I've already discussed. But, it is a plant-based diet and, therefore, holds merit.

One of the few scientific experiments so far is one where researchers from Harvard University collaborated with Michio Kushi on an attempt to study the effects of macrobiotics on blood, cardiovascular strength, and overall condition. Approximately 200 Boston residents following the macrobiotic diet were the subjects of the study. They were asked to relax their strict eating habits for several weeks, and to eat more standard American fare, with meats and heavy sauces, sweets, processed foods, and the like. The results showed that the subjects' cardiovascular systems and blood conditions suffered with the switch to the all-American diet.

While whatever was causing the higher cholesterol in the American diet was not pinpointed, we do know that in the Harvard studies, the macrobiotic diet led to lower cholesterol levels and lower blood pressure, hence better circulatory and heart condition. Once you're following the program, it's a good idea to keep in mind Kushi's observation that the macrobiotic diet is not a narrow one, even though it is a strict discipline. Make your own food selection, preparation, and dining the type you would expect in a good macrobiotic restaurant. Avoid the unimaginative, austere, and boring. Vegetables have many brilliant and stimulating colors—use them to dress up your meals and make them visually appealing. Use a variety of foods. Don't just get your 50–60% grains from the same pasta every day or from brown rice. Rotate: use rice one day; millet another; oats, sprouted wheat, bulgur, corn, and so on. Practice variety, and rotate that variety.

The first shortcoming of the macrobiotic diet is its lack of focus on nutritional supplements. Largely due to decreasing soil fertility, you can't really get all of your necessary nutrients from your food, as proponents of this diet argue. Secondly, there is a lot of sodium in this diet which brings its own health concerns. At the same time, the diet discourages drinking water or other beverages or eating fruit which is high in water content that could help with the aforementioned issue of sodium. Thirdly, the diet tends to ignore dark, leafy greens, which are prime sources of critical nutrients. Fourthly, the lack of fruit in the diet is a concern in itself, as fruit contains important enzymes that aid digestion. Finally, the macrobiotic diet encourages eating the foods grown in your climate, which is problematic from a health perspective because not all regions offer enough of a variety of foods to reach and maintain optimal health, and problematic from a social responsibility perspective because the diet encourages eating foods that are shipped from other places with climates similar to your own.

The macrobiotic way has given us great insight into the relationship between nutrition and health. It is not intended to displace medical therapies, but to complement them. Its emphasis on live, whole foods and its rejection of meat, dairy products, and processed foods are fundamental postulates of healthy living that we should all embrace. Further, its inclusion of sea vegetables on a daily basis is highly beneficial for providing necessary minerals to the majority who are suffering from a lack of proper mineralization today.

Macrobiotics asks us to attain health and happiness through avoiding extremes, the outriders of yin and yang food, and to discover the harmony and balance within ourselves and our environment, to learn the way of gentleness and calm, vitality and clarity. These are all the laudable broad goals and practices, which lay out the royal road to good health, longevity and joy. Of course, a fundamental benefit to this diet is the aspect of eliminating many toxic foods that you may be consuming; so despite my reservations about this diet, macrobiotics does capture the essence of the healthy vegetarian lifestyle.

The Raw Vegan Diet

I said earlier in the book that 75% of the diet should be raw (uncooked) plant-based foods. Eating foods as close to how Mother Nature delivers them to us, and uncooked, is the healthiest possible way; consuming living foods over dead and denatured foods is *vitalism*—the act of creating vitality in the body. Why raw foods? In short, because all foods contain valuable enzymes that help us digest foods making it easier for our bodies to assimilate its nutrients, and these are essentially destroyed when foods are heated at temperatures above 125 degrees Fahrenheit.

Enzymes, which are molecules that accelerate, or catalyze, vital biological processes in the body and are vitally important—we couldn't exist without them. Here are the three primary categories of enzymes—digestive, metabolic, and food. We've already spoken about food enzymes, so let's take a quick look at the others:

Digestive enzymes also break down foods, allowing nutrients from these foods to be absorbed into the bloodstream and used in body functions, ensuring that we get the maximum nutritional value from foods; Metabolic enzymes spark reactions within the cells, and are involved in facilitating all other body processes—from our heart beat to thinking to the blinking of our eyes.

For the reason that raw foods are so vital and nourishing, the movement has gained tremendous momentum in our country. The ability of raw food preparations and fresh raw juices to thwart disease and literally turn back the hands of time is tremendous. Consuming foods either raw or only slightly cooked (steamed) has many benefits including strengthening the immune system, purifying the blood, detoxifying our cells, improving digestion (since raw or slightly cooked plant foods are some of the easiest to digest), clearing up skin issues, reversing the effects of oxidative stress, elevating mood, enhancing cognitive performance and memory recall, regulating hormone balance and weight, and, of course, reducing pain and inflammation.

Some of the people advocating the raw diet have become fanatical about it, saying things like: "You must drink your juice within 20 minutes or the enzymes leave and it's worthless." This is simply not true. As a scientist, I take these things to the laboratory and I test them; time and again I've come to the decision that as long as our diet is 70% raw—with fruits, juices and salads—then we're doing great. Remember, there are some items that are much more likely to be beneficial if we heat them *lightly*—if it's through steaming, or cooking a sauce or soup; through this process, nutrient are liberated and become more bio-available to the body. Broccoli, cauliflower, Brussels sprouts, and asparagus do not digest as well in their raw forms, and the valuable nutrient of lycopene in tomatoes is better available when a little heat is applied. So it's not just the fact that something is raw, it's a question of: Is it bioavailable? If the answer is that processing produces greater bioavailability, then we should alter the form in slight ways to maximize nutritional intake.

Grains, for example, cannot be eaten raw. When you heat them in water—the process of hydrolysis—the outer shell, which is full of fiber and not digestible, opens up, allowing the inner nutrients to be available for nutrition purposes. So you actually increase bioavailability of certain beans and grains by cooking them. Nut butters are another good example. Nuts in their raw, whole form are good for you; walnuts, in particular, are phenomenal. If you eat that nut whole, you need to chew it to a cream in order to release all the available nutrients. But if you grind that nut into *nut butter*—the nutrients are instantly more available. The same goes for peanuts, which as we've said is not an actual nut but a legume instead.

Let's close in on an important note: I have counseled far too many individuals, as a nutritionist and a dietician, who were simply nutrient deprived and sick because they were on a strictly raw food diet. Again, raw foods are a piece of the puzzle—one part of the scientific laws governing the optimal functioning of the body. We need raw foods, especially when transitioning from a wholly processed American diet of deep-fried, overcooked, barbequed, and grilled foods. It's a very substantial transition for most people, and it takes time for the body to acclimate.

The Gluten-Free Vegan Diet

Gluten is the major protein found in some grains. These include all forms of wheat (bulgur, durum, semolina, spelt, farro) as well as barley and rye and a wheat-rye cross called triticale. It's also a common additive in many prepared foods, cosmetics, toothpaste, yogurt, tomato sauce, and even medicines. For the 1% of the population with celiac disease, gluten can be deadly; however, the majority of people challenged by wheat are considered *gluten sensitive*.

Gluten can cause substantial inflammation in the intestine, and that in turn and in time can lead to a chronic state of disease leading to malabsorption, constipation, polyps, allergies, yeast overgrowth, and more. So a lot of people have been advocating for a gluten-free diet. *South Beach Diet* originator, cardiologist and author of *The South Beach Diet Gluten Solution* Arthur Agatston, M.D., notes: "Gluten readily forms cross-links with itself and with other proteins. This crosslinking property makes bread chewy (viscous and elastic), but it also makes gluten difficult to digest. In people with celiac disease, gluten greatly damages intestinal villi, leading to diarrhea, abdominal pain, weight loss, fatigue, and anemia."[355]

Why all of a sudden are people sensitive to wheat? The answer lies in the breeding; however, the results of this breeding and their correlation to gluten sensitivity are still being disputed. *Life Extension* magazine presents: "Although wheat is not a GMO (Genetically Modified Organism), centuries of selective breeding and hybridization have increased the gluten content of wheat for the purpose of strengthening dough, which has led to an increase in celiac disease and gluten sensitivity."[356]

Dr. William Davis, author of *Wheat Belly,* disagrees that the rising prevalence of gluten sensitivity is due to an increase in the amount of gluten in the wheat itself. Instead, he notes a 2013 USDA study on the subject where the lead scientist writes, "In summary, I have not found clear evidence of an increase in the gluten content of wheat in the United States during the 20th century, and if there has indeed been an increase in celiac disease during the latter half of the century, wheat breeding for higher gluten content does not seem to be the basis."[357]

Mark Hyman, M.D. *New York Times'* best-selling author and director of the Cleveland Clinic Center for Functional Medicine believes that gluten sensitivities are related to three factors: a super starch called amylopectin A that is super fattening, a form of super gluten that he says is super inflammatory, and a form of super drug that is super-addictive and makes you crave and eat more. Hyman speaks of *dwarf wheat*, a genetically manipulated and hybridized version of wheat with "much higher amounts of starch and gluten and many more chromosomes coding for all sorts of new odd proteins." Regarding his point about the addictive quality of wheat, he says: "When processed by your digestion, the proteins in wheat are converted into shorter proteins, "polypeptides", called "exorphins." They are like the endorphins you get from a runner's high and bind to the opioid receptors in the brain, making you high and addicted just like a heroin addict. Bottom line: wheat is an addictive appetite stimulant."[358]

Hyman goes on to say that these super drugs can cause multiple problems, including schizophrenia and autism, but they also cause addictive eating behaviors including cravings and bingeing. What's even more alarming, notes Hyman, is that these food cravings can be blocked using the same drug that is used in the emergency room to block heroin or morphine overdose, called naloxone. Binge eaters, he says, ate nearly 30% less food when given this drug.[359]

Regardless of the causes, there is one fact that cannot be disputed: the American diet has become rife with highly processed products made with highly refined wheat flour, and the gluten-free diet is the diet of the future. As one CNN report said, "We are just beginning to appreciate gluten's impact on our health."[360]

In fact, many are in a state of "gluten overload," and experiencing such unpleasant symptoms as stomach pains, bloating, heartburn, joint pains, headache, skin rashes, fatigue, insomnia and brain fog, to name some of the most common.

And don't be fooled by those pedaling whole wheat bread as a health food; it is not. Dr. Hyman states, "There is no difference between whole wheat and white flour here. The biggest scam perpetrated on the unsuspecting public is the inclusion of 'whole grains' in many processed foods full of sugar and wheat giving the food a virtuous glow." In fact, he adds: "Two slices of whole wheat bread now raise your blood sugar more than two tablespoons of table sugar."

I think that we've got a clear enough picture of the increasing challenges of consuming wheat. While there is no need to panic, it would be wise to evaluate your experience first-hand. Dr. Agatston says: "Gluten is not something to fear. I like to tell my patients that they need to be gluten-aware, not gluten-phobic. This happens when they learn where they fit on the gluten sensitivity spectrum and discover their own level of gluten tolerance.[361] Those who don't have to eliminate whole-wheat, barley, and rye products from their lives, should enjoy them, because these whole grains are good sources of vitamins, minerals, and fiber."

What do you do if you suspect you have gluten sensitivity? The first step is to remove all gluten for a minimum of a week. Then, eat a product with gluten and see what happens: do you have any symptoms? Be on the lookout for any of the common ones noted above. If not, wait a day or two and see if you are still clear; if so, try another. Finally, if you do notice symptoms, consider trying to eat sprouted grain products. Sprouted grains like Ezekiel breads and pastas offer a wonderful alternative to traditional wheat products; there are also many delicious gluten-free pastas offered today. Make no mistake about it: reducing your wheat intake, especially refined flours, is beneficial for anyone.

Making the Vegetarian Diet a Reality

The Value of Immersion Programs

At the beginning of this chapter, I spoke about the value of making a radical change in one's diet and lifestyle when converting to vegetarianism. In my career, I have indeed seen the power and benefits of a 4-week cleansing program for stopping and reversing symptoms for anyone dealing with a health challenge. I have also seen how valuable such a cleansing program can be for jump-starting someone into healthier habits.

It's important to note that planned, administered and supported programs are incredibly helpful toward making a radical lifestyle change. Immersion programs offer the benefits of: professional education and guidance, peer support, and the opportunity to quickly feel the physical benefits of the vegetarian program. This goes a long way for inspiring people to continue on the path. I especially recommend group immersions programs for people who *are* facing a health challenge, especially a serious one.

This brings me to another point, which is: serious diseases don't "just happen." They occur, in large part, because of a lifetime of poor eating and lifestyle habits and patterns; this is why we call many of our modern diseases "lifestyle diseases." In reality, your health is very much in your hands, by the choices you make about what you eat and how you live. You can make these changes gradually or radically; that choice is up to you.

Basic Transition Guidelines

If you think that a detoxification program is best for you, try the basic one in my, *Reverse Arthritis and Pain Naturally: A Proven Approach for Reducing Pain, Arthritis and Inflammation.* In it, you will find a 3-week program for cleansing and detoxifying. I also recommend the *Anti-Arthritis, Anti-Inflammation Cookbook*: *Healing Through Natural Foods*. Both of these books will help you to get creative in your kitchen by making delicious healthy vegetarian appetizers, salads, soups, entrees, juices and smoothies. We have plans this fall for a companion cookbook to this book, which will specifically feature protein-rich dishes to support those who are transitioning to the plant-based lifestyle.

Juicing is one of the best ways to prevent and reverse inflammatory diseases, which are essentially all of the lifestyle disease. When we juice, the health-boosting antioxidants, vitamins, minerals, enzymes, phytonutrients and chlorophyll found in fruits and vegetables are much more easily absorbed by the body than if we were to eat these foods whole. These beneficial constituents work synergistically to promote and maintain healthy cells and reduce chronic inflammation that results in degenerative diseases.

The juices you drink should always come from fresh organic produce whenever possible; you can make them at home with your own juicer, or order at your favorite juice bar. For example, the chlorophyll in these juices acts as a natural chelator, removing toxic heavy metals from the body, while the sulfur compounds found in cabbage juice help guard against cancer. If you don't mind the taste of garlic, push a few cloves through your juicer to create a potent antiviral, antibacterial blend. To help stimulate healing in the gastrointestinal system and stomach, add a teaspoon of probiotic powder along with 1000 mg of powdered and buffered vitamin C and 2 oz. of aloe vera juice. You can also mix in different supplements like green tea extract, curcumin, or astragalus to further enhance its functional food healing value. One day a week, it's a good idea to add a scoop of non-GMO brown rice, pea or hemp protein powder into your juices and use that as your fasting day. By restricting calories in this way, you are detoxifying the body and contributing to the health of your cells.

More about Transition on the Vegetarian Path

The biggest transition problem I hear from people is that sometimes they feel hungry. Without meat or a chicken sandwich, they lack the satiety that can keep someone feeling full for four or five hours. The ways to accomplish more satiety on the plant-based diet are numerous and varied. As one example, you can add almond butter to a protein shake, a little bit of coconut oil, and rice milk, and a scoop of, let's say, protein powder along with your chosen fruit, and you have a meal that will stabilize your blood sugar for several hours. Or, have a meal with beans, rice, and veggies, which will settle in just fine for a few hours. As long as your blood sugar is stabilized, you're not going to have highs and lows.

This, in part, is why the high protein diets are so popular: meat—as unhealthy as it is for you—stabilizes blood sugar. When transitioning to a plant based diet, you want to be mindful of blood sugar levels. If you start eating fruits all the time, your blood sugar is going to go up and then it's going to crash down, so you don't want to overdo the fruits. You want to have seeds, beans, nuts, legumes, and tubers, because they stabilize blood sugar. Stable blood sugar allows you to control your appetite a lot better.

I always suggest to people to have a super-sized salad. Start with a whole bunch of bean sprouts, like sunflower sprouts, broccoli sprouts, mung bean or adzuki bean sprouts, all of which are great healing sprouts, and then add some sundried tomatoes, olives, pomegranate seeds, and perhaps some hearts of palm and artichoke hearts along with lots of mixed baby lettuces, and some spicy microgreens if you can get them. Top that with a nice homemade tahini or avocado dressing, for example, and you have a meal fit for a king, as they say. Now, when you eat this, you're going to have the same fullness that you would if you ate a steak, because the avocado and the olives are going to take longer to digest, and blood sugar level will remain stable. The lettuces and bean sprouts, will give that sense of fullness. Since it is low in calories and nutrient-rich, it's fortifying and cleansing, not constipating.

One final note about salads: a common error some make in transition is to make too large of a salad, or use too much dressing. It is a natural response for a short period of time to a perceived "loss," or some idea that the salad won't be filling enough. One way to test your satiety level is to eat your meals in silence, and without the distraction of TV, reading, looking at your phone, computer or talking. I know it sounds odd, and practicing it at first may feel strange, but research suggests that watching TV and even listening to music increases food consumption not only during the meal, but at subsequent meals as well.[362] The only way to regulate your satiety is to chew well and to pay complete attention to how you feel, *as you're eating*, which is not possible with distractions.

Eating in silence at the beginning of your transition will not only help you slowly savor your food, but will help you determine better portion sizes based on what your body really needs. I mentioned earlier that Americans are used to super-sizing everything; we tend to shovel our food, eating quickly, rather than enjoying a leisurely meal over a period of an hour or more—a common practice in Europe. Eating less than you think you need is a much better practice than piling it on and dealing with sluggishness and indigestion that can easily occur in the plant-based diet with meals that have too much fat, too many grains, nuts and legumes, or processed vegan fare, like soy cheeses and the such. I recommend eating slowly and leaving the table prior to becoming full. This is a must if you are aiming to drop excess weight.

What about Gas?

Sometimes when people are new to eating more fruits and vegetables, gas presents itself. The reason for this is that fruits and vegetables, grains, nuts, and seeds could be fermenting in your lower intestine. (Foods in each of these categories require different times to digest; eating fruits, for example, which typically take anywhere from 30 minutes to an hour to break down with nuts, which take closer to 3 or 4 hours, can cause fermentation—a process that converts sugar to acids, gases, and/or alcohol.)

In some people, this can be an issue. That's why I suggested earlier considering helping your body with the digestion process by soaking, blending, or lightly cooking certain foods. When you soak beans overnight, for example, you lessen the potential for gas with them, especially if you add some lemon juice and apple cider vinegar to the soaking water. If you pressure cook them, you lessen the gas even more. If you make a puree from the beans—you're helping ease the digestive process. This is also why I suggested nut and seed butters earlier; not only do they give you access to more nutrients; they are more easily digestible, which reduces gas.

More than anything, chewing your food thoroughly and eating slowly will reduce gas. What most people don't realize is that our digestive system begins in the mouth, where enzymes are secreted, initiating the breakdown of foods for fuel. Burping, a form of gas, usually occurs through the process of gulping air while consuming food too quickly; by slowing down and masticating your food well you are essentially pre-digesting your foods, and you will have better success at eliminating this problem.

A Word about Food Combining

Food combining is consuming foods in a way that maximizes ease of digestion, and therefore absorption. I wrote a book in the 1970s on food combining made easy. I had been motivated by conversations I had with Herbert Shelton, the man who really invented food combining in the United States. It made sense when I was speaking with him, but then I went into the laboratory and started to perform studies, my results showed that in many cases it wasn't true. I was so disappointed in the outcome that I asked the publisher to withdraw my book, which he did, even though it was a best-seller, because I thought I was doing a disservice.

I found that most of us can in fact eat grains, legumes, and pulses (like beans), tubers (root vegetables, like rutabaga, parsnips, and turnips and kohlrabi), and seaweeds (kombu, wakame, kelp, arame, bladdarwrack, sea lettuce) together, along with a salad, without having a problem. Where he was correct, however, was his point that items that contain saturated fat and protein take much longer to digest and leave the stomach. In fact, when you eat anything with fat, the body senses this, sends a message to the gall bladder, and starts releasing bile through the bile duct into the intestine to break down the fat into smaller molecules. Eventually, I wrote a book on this called *Why Your Stomach Hurts,* a book on digestion. (So I went from being disappointed that we had been oversold on incorrect ideas of food combining to showing people how real digestion occurs.) I came to the conclusion at the time that as long as you eat your animal proteins separate from other items, you're okay. But since we're not talking about eating *any* animal proteins, or any of these negative saturated fats except for coconut oil, then healthy vegetarians won't have this issue.

Now, some people cannot eat fruits and vegetables without getting gas; in this case, I suggest just eating one or the other at a time with at least an hour and a half in between. More importantly regarding digestion is how many liquids we consume—how much and at what temperature. For ideal digestion, we should have our beverage *before* our meal, so that the hydrochloric acid is not diluted; and at least an hour after the meal. It should be a warm or room temperature beverage, filtered or spring water or perhaps a tea that is not destructive of the body's natural hydrochloric acid pH, and core temperature.

Note that when we eat too much food and then drink a beverage, the stomach becomes so full that the pyloric sphincter muscle opens and allows partially digested food into the intestines. With too much food and too much liquid, the hydrochloric acid in our stomach becomes diluted, so it can't do its job properly. As the partially digested food passes through the intestine, it causes inflammation in the gut, which leads to leaky gut. The partially digested food literally leaks into the blood stream; the body then sends white blood cells to attack what it thinks is a foreign body (because it's not meant to be there in the blood stream), and you end up overstressing the immune system. So by eating slowly, eating less, and not drinking with the meal, you get better, easier, more complete digestion and less indigestion. That's a winning combination for health and an essential protocol for a healthy vegetarian.

Surprise Food Items Containing Animal Products

As a society, we've become tremendously disconnected from our food system and many people have no idea what they're eating. As vegetarians, we tend to ask more often, "What does this contain?" But there are all kinds of nasty surprises lurking in food, particularly in refined and processed foods, many of which are animal-based. Many seemingly meat-free products may unexpectedly contain animal components, such as vegetable soup, which often contains beef stock, and hydrogenated lard can commonly be found in refried beans, cookies, and crackers. Many vegetarian-focused websites offer a list of non-vegetarian ingredients commonly found in processed foods. In this section, we'll provide you with some ideas about the types of ingredients you may want to avoid so you'll have the basic information with which to make your food choices. Choose pre-packaged products wisely by carefully scrutinizing ingredients lists, or better still—make your own!

Firstly, for those vegetarians who don't eat fish, many products unsuspectingly contain fish, for example, Worcestershire sauce contains anchovies, as do many Caesar salad dressings. Also, be careful with omega 3- and omega 6-enriched products—which nowadays include margarine, milk, orange juice, and bread among others—as they often contain fatty acids from fish such as sardines or anchovies. Speaking of bread, you may also wish to avoid bagels and bread products that have L-cysteine listed in the ingredients. This amino acid is used as a softening agent and to extend the shelf life of the bread product but is often derived from human hair or poultry feathers.

One commonly used ingredient that the majority of vegetarians may already know to avoid is gelatin. Gelatin is often used in processed foods as a thickening or stabilizing agent and originates from the collagen of cow or pig connective tissue, hooves, and skin. Gelatin can be found in gum sweets, marshmallows, Jell-O, the coating of some peanuts, and is readily used as a coating for pills and vitamin capsules. When it comes to nutritional supplements, it's best, whenever possible, to purchase supplements made from whole food organic sources, using veggie-caps, which are not made with gelatin. Garden of Life™ is one company focused on organic, whole-food supplements, and there are others at your local health food store.

The confectionary industry commonly uses two other ingredients, shellac and carmine, which are of animal origin—both from insects. Shellac is a sticky substance that is derived from the secretions of the insect *Kerria lacca*, and is what makes jelly beans and other hard-coated candy look shiny; it can also be found in hair lacquer. Check for "confectioner's glaze" on the packaging. Carmine, also known as cochineal or natural red 4 (and listed as E120 in the list of EU-approved food additives), is a red colorant that originates from crushed beetles. It is commonly added to give a red-color to candies, bottled juices, frozen pops, yogurts, colored pasta, and "natural" cosmetics. The PETA Kids website has a helpful list of animal-free candy (http://www.petakids.com/food/vegan-candy-dandy/).

Another food additive that may be found in vanilla or raspberry flavored products—including candy, drinks, Jell-O, yogurts, or ice cream—is castoreum, a food flavoring extracted from the scent glands of beavers. Beavers use this excretion to mark their territory with a musky, vanilla scent and it is utilized both as a food additive, where it is usually just listed as "natural flavoring" in the ingredient list, and in perfumes.[363] For a comprehensive list of food additives of animal origin consult VeggieGlobal's website (http://www.veggieglobal.com/nutrition/non-vegetarian-food-additives.htm).

Surprisingly, beer and wine may contain an array of products that are unsuitable for vegetarians. Isinglass is a gelatin-like substance that comes from fish bladder and is used in the clarification process of many beers and wines. Alternatively, gelatin or bone char, from crushed cattle bones, can be used for the same process (and vegans should be aware that albumin and casein are also commonly used for clarifying). These components are often not mentioned on the label so you may want to check directly with the manufacturer. A list of vegan beer and wine alternatives can be also be found on www.barnivore.com.

Apart from avoiding animal-based products that are directly added to foods as ingredients, many animal-derived products are used in the food manufacturing process. Bone char, as we've already mentioned, may be used in the clarification of beer and wine, but is also commonly used to refine sugar. White sugar is not naturally white—the molasses (which make it brown) are removed using the crushed bones as a kind of filter to refine it. But don't let that mislead you into thinking that brown sugar is any better; it's also refined, just the molasses are added back to it! Choose organic sugar since USDA organic sugar cannot be filtered through bone char.[364]

For those vegetarians who consume cheese you may want to be aware that two animal-derived products are often used during the cheese making process: rennet (or rennin), and the enzyme lipase that rennet also contains. Both originate from calf stomach—a by-product of the horrific veal production process—and are commonly used to coagulate hard cheese. Joyous Living offers a list of cheeses that do not contain animal rennet (see http://cheese.joyousliving.com/CheeseListBrand.aspx). However, not all cheese is made with animal-derived rennet, and both vegetable and microbial rennet (often produced by fungi) exist; however, the FDA unfortunately does not require the ingredient list to specify the type of rennet used. As responsible consumers, you may also want to be aware that some rennet, known as FPC, is produced by genetically modified microorganisms—in fact, in 1999, some 60% of cheeses were made with FPC—[365] or vegetable rennet may come from GMO soy. Obviously, the cheese dilemma is not an issue for those following a vegan diet.

Other components used during the food manufacture process include porcine kidney acylase—an enzyme an enzyme from pig kidneys employed for the production of aspartame—a ubiquitous ingredient in low calorie, commercial protein powders, diet products, including soft drinks, chewing gum, and jams.

Finally, to end this section, something you may wish to consider as part of your vegetarian lifestyle is the ethical source of the ingredients used in the food you buy. For example, vegetarians that consume veggie burgers should know that they commonly contain milk and eggs, which are often sourced from low ethical farms, such as from battery farmed chickens. We should consider food in its full context and tie it to our values and lifestyle choices, and as such, buying foods containing unethically sourced ingredients is another way of indirectly supporting the meat industry. As consumers, our money is power. For example, in 2007, the manufacturer of Mars Bars was forced to replace the rennet in its chocolate bar to a non-animal sourced alternative following mass protests from vegetarians.

Hazardous Chemicals Contained in Food

Part of being a healthy vegetarian means considering all aspects of a healthy life. Most of us are well aware that pesticides are "dangerous" and best avoided, but you may be surprised to know that 96 commonly used pesticides have been identified by the EPA as potential human carcinogens and at least 10 have been linked to birth defects in babies.[366] Most alarmingly is the National Research Council's finding that many children are exposed through their diet to levels of pesticide residues above those considered safe by the government.[367] Their use in agriculture is prevalent: a study carried out by the USDA's Agricultural Marketing Service tested nearly 7000 fruit and vegetable samples and a whopping 65% of them were found to contain pesticide residues, so obviously, the best way to avoid pesticides is by buying organic produce. Alternatively, aim to grow as much of your own fruit and vegetables as possible—it would be very difficult for pesticides to sneak in there! Besides pesticides, there are many other dangerous chemicals lurking in our food products and other common household items to which we'd like to draw your attention.[368]

One toxic chemical compound that has received a lot of recent media attention is Bisphenol-A (BPA), an estrogen-mimicking chemical used in the production of hard, clear plastic and commonly found in many commercial products including food and drink containers. In April 2008, following an assessment by the Center for the Evaluation of Risks to Human Reproduction (CERHR) that found, "Some concern for effects on the brain, behavior and prostate gland in fetuses, infants and children at current human exposures to BPA" due to BPA leaching out of the plastic, BPA was classified as toxic by the Canadian government.[369] Retailers rapidly responded by withdrawing plastic baby bottles made with BPA, and in 2009, the US banned BPA in plastic baby bottles and other children's food and drink containers.[370]

Nevertheless, the ban was not expanded beyond children's food and drink containers and the use of BPA is still ubiquitous in the plastic lining of tin cans for example, where it is used to prevent the food from coming into contact with the tin. According to the FDA, 17% of the American diet comes out of cans and "BPA is safe at the current levels occurring in foods."[371]

However, the Environmental Working Group found BPA in more than half of the canned food they tested at levels "200 times the government's traditional safe level of exposure", so the leaching of BPA from canned foods is of great concern.[372] In the fall of 2014, FDA experts from across the agency, specializing in a number of fields, completed a four-year review of more than 300 scientific studies, and found no information that would prompt a revision in their safety assessment of BPA in food packaging.[373] Ironically, certain industries are now self-regulating due to consumer demand; one example of this is in the manufacture of infant formula packaging. The FDA updated a ruling abandoning the use of BPA-based epoxy resins in packing effective July 12, 2013, thanks to a food additive petition submitted by Representative Edward Markey of Massachusetts.[374] If you do buy canned food, purchase BPA-free tin cans; a resin code of 7 will indicate if the container is made of a BPA-containing plastic.

Organic Grace offers a list of common brands that use BPA-free cans (https://organicgrace.com/bpa-cans). Better still, buy fresh produce and cook from scratch.

Butylated hydroxytoluene (BHT) or Butylated hydroxyanisole (BHA) are commonly used by the US food industry as preservatives, mainly to prevent oils in foods from oxidizing and becoming rancid. However, BHT/A is also used in jet fuels, is harmful to aquatic organisms (according to its Material Safety Data Sheet), the National Toxicity Program 2005 found it "reasonably anticipated to be a human carcinogen," and its use in food is banned in the UK. So, I highly recommend that you add it to your list of ingredients to avoid as well. It can be found in vegetable oil, sausages, cereals, cookies, and potato chips.

Alarmingly for vegetarians, toxic solvents such as hexane may be used in the manufacture of soy-based foods, including veggie burgers and protein shakes, and at least two hexane-extracted ingredients are found in organic infant formula.[375] Hexane, a petroleum by-product, hazardous air pollutant (EPA), and neurotoxin, is used to process soy into its protein, fiber, and oil components. The effects on consumers of hexane residues in soy foods have not yet been thoroughly studied and are not regulated by the FDA. However, test results obtained by the Cornucopia Institute indicate that residues—ten times higher than what is considered normal by the FDA—appear in common soy ingredients.[376] Choose soy-containing products that are labeled as organic, in which case the use of hexane is prohibited, or better still, make your own patties.

Sulfites are a group of chemicals that are widely used in the food industry for their antioxidant and preservative properties. Foods which can contain sulfites include beer, wine, cider, and soft drinks; sausages; bottled sauces, canned and pickled foods; many bakery goods; fresh and frozen prawns; and particularly high levels are found in dried fruits. Some people, particularly asthmatics and those with allergic rhinitis, are sensitive to sulfites and may react with allergy-like symptoms. In some sensitive individuals, sulfites can even trigger an anaphylactic reaction. In 1999, the World Health Organization (WHO) warned that up to 20-30% of childhood asthmatics may be sensitive to sulfite preservatives, yet an Australian study found that more than 65% of asthmatic children were affected by sulfites.[377] Due to its allergenic properties, any food containing more than 10 parts per million of sulfites must list sulfites as an ingredient by law, making it easier to avoid. In the case of dried fruits, chose organic alternatives or dry your own. Dehydrators are easy to come across and can set you back around 400 dollars. Or you can do it the old-fashioned way: you thinly slice your product and put it on a screen outside with a muslin cloth over it, and in four days you've got dried fruit with no chemicals in it! I also highly recommend that you have a go at drying your own kale, which is one of the must-have items in America today in the health food movement. Use of a dehydrator will allow you to dry the food at a temperature of 125 degrees Fahrenheit to preserve the food enzymes and maximize nutritional content.

Besides organic dried fruit, almonds often form a staple component of a vegetarian or vegan's diet for their high levels of vitamin E, minerals such as manganese, magnesium and calcium, and energy richness. However, since 2008, USDA legislation demands that all almonds grown in California (and virtually all the almonds sold in the US *are* grown in California) be "pasteurized"—even the organic ones. The almonds are pasteurized by fumigation with a toxic gas, propylene oxide, which is added to jet engine fuel and antifreeze, and used to make polyurethane foams. It is not generally recognized as safe for human ingestion by the FDA, its use in food has been banned by the EU, and it has been classified as a probable human carcinogen. Hmm, organic almond anyone? To avoid fumigated almonds in the US, the only other choice is to purchase unpasteurized almonds from the farmer/grower directly via a roadside stand or online.

Monosodium glutamate (MSG) is another food additive that most people have heard of and choose to avoid for reasons we spoke about on page 73.

Besides MSG, there are many other additives used in foods, particularly colorants, whose safety have been questioned. The yellow colorant No. 5, tartrazine, is an azo dye derived from coal tar, which has been banned in Norway and Austria. Tartrazine is a potential danger in aspirin-intolerant individuals: Approximately 2% to 20% of patients with asthma are sensitive to aspirin; of these, approximately 10% are also sensitive to tartrazine.[378] Due to these possible allergic responses, the FDA mandates that all products containing tartrazine be labeled so that these substances can be avoided. In addition, tartrazine and other food additives have also been suggested as a cause or aggravating factor of hyperactivity in children. Research funded by the UK Food Standards Agency found that, "Consumption of mixes of certain artificial food colors and the preservative sodium benzoate could be linked to increased hyperactivity in some children."[379]

I hope that by highlighting a few examples of how commercial, processed foods can often contain ingredients that can unsuspectingly put our health at risk particularly that of younger children. This should make it clear why buying organic, whole foods is always best. But what about cooking our food? I'm sure many, if not most of you, have non-stick pans at home. Teflon is the brand name for the chemical polytetrafluoroethylene (PTFE), a type of perfluorinated compound or PFC that is used to coat the surface of pans and cookware. But did you know that the International Agency for Research on Cancer classifies TFE as a probable cause of cancer? The National Toxicology Program classifies TFE as "reasonably anticipated to be a human carcinogen," and tests conducted in 2003 showed that in just two to five minutes on a conventional stove top, cookware coated with Teflon could exceed temperatures at which the coating breaks apart and emits toxic particles and gases.[380] These gases can cause "Teflon flu," a real condition with symptoms of headaches, chills, backache, and fever.[381] If you must use non-stick pans, make sure they do not have a damaged coating. However, it is best to opt for stainless steel or cast iron pans. Similarly, microwave popcorn bags contain a type of PFC, known as PFOA. Although this chemical has been recognized as "likely" to be carcinogenic, the EPA "has not made any definitive conclusions at this time" with regard to the restrictions of the use of PFOA. In the meantime, I for one will be making my own popcorn—it's better to be safe than sorry.

Getting Help from Professionals

Having now just spent numerous pages within this book explaining the usefulness and reasonability of a vegetarian diet, and how it becomes a norm in various cultures without the support of specific scientific information, it's interesting to note the paradox that exists in the US. Not only is there a great deal of available science supporting this fact, those that *do* have a nutritional science background tend to hold very prejudiced and, in fact, unscientific views of the value of green eating.

Certainly, there are some in the profession, like Eleanor Williams, who recognize the value of green eating. She penned an article in the *American Journal of Nursing*, where she said, "Meat isn't the only protein source," and underlined that the discerning use of whole grains, vegetables, sprouts, and fruit will cover the Recommended Daily Allowance (RDA) of the nutrients found in meat, without the heavy cholesterol count.[382]

But, in sharp contrast to her, there are many professionals who won't admit that a vegetarian diet can be as nutritionally complete as a meat diet. Because so many registered dieticians have little or no knowledge of vegetarianism, they don't feel comfortable counseling about it. Williams' notes in this same article that many dieticians allow their personal attitudes about diet influence counseling more than knowledge of nutrition.[383] Perhaps, some dieticians don't want to appear ignorant when their clients bring up the vegetarian option, so they dismiss it out of hand. This is not only unfortunate, but has grave repercussions, and it needs to be remedied if we are to have a balanced conversation in this country. An article in the *Journal of the American Dietetic Association* gives this advice: "Dieticians and nutritionists must learn about the nutrient needs of the vegetarian," adding that the best approach to nutritional counseling "is to respect the patient's dietary individualism and freedom and try not to disrupt existing eating habits and life-styles unless they are potentially harmful."[384]

If you *do* consult a nutritionist, make sure to find one who understands the benefits of vegetarianism and is impartial about these benefits, rather than a practitioner, such as one a friend told me about, who retailed only the common myths about green eating. As an example, this ill-informed counselor said that starchy foods like potatoes or pasta are *always* fattening. They're not. If you're putting on pounds after eating those foods, it's due to excess calories, which, in the case of the aforementioned items, typically come from garnishes like butter, sour cream, cheddar cheese, and bacon—not from the potato itself. A plain, medium-sized potato has only 110 calories,[385] plus essential amino acids, vitamin C, and more potassium than a banana. Plus, it is fat-, sodium- and cholesterol-free to boot! Likewise, pasta is generally only fattening when laden with cream, meat, or cheese sauces.

Children and Vegetarianism

There isn't any reason why children cannot thrive on a plant-based diet. As long as it is a well-planned diet with a balance of the foods I noted earlier in this section, a child should thrive.

A healthy vegetarian diet is considered adequate for all stages of life, including childhood. Recent research shows some underprivileged vegetarian children (and adults) deficient in zinc and iron, which is easily remedied with consumption of fortified cereals and milk, leavened whole grains, soaking dried legumes and discarding the soaking water, and drinks, fruit, or vegetables rich in vitamin C. Using fermented soy foods and sprouting some of the consumed legumes are recommended to offset these potential deficiencies. Supplementation is also easy enough.Vegetarian children with iron deficiency are also at greater risk of lowered immunoglobulin levels (immune system), but vegetarian children without iron deficiency are at no greater risk of a compromised immune system than omnivorous childre.[386,387] In fact, research also suggests that the vegetarian diet may provide some protection against allergies. Further, a vegetarian diet in childhood can actually guard against chronic disease later in life, especially those associated with obesity as research suggests that those who consume animal flesh and animal products at the age of 5-6 have a higher BMI later in life and are more likely to be overweight than their vegetarian counterparts.[388,389]

The challenge regarding children and vegetarianism that is important to know is related to how a child's palette is "trained up." Once a child is indoctrinated to the world of animal products through processed foods—and to heavy amounts of salt, sugar, and oil like those served at the typical fast food restaurant—the less likely they will take to enjoying vegetables, in particular. This is predominantly true with dairy products and the world of tasty delights associated with it—pizza, cheese crackers, yogurt, ice cream, cake, cheese sticks, etc., but also with any number of other manufactured "foods."

My reason for citing of this example is to point out the influence of poor role models on children. Those who raise children must exert positive influence when it comes to vegetables in order for their children to like them. Portraying vegetarian cuisine as tasteless, green eating as unthinkable, or conducting a "do as I say, not as I do" household with vegetables, gives children a distorted view of the whole world of food possibilities.

On the other hand, when children have a veggie-positive role model and a minimum of processed foods, they are likely to find vegetarian eating very much to their taste. One such ten-year old boy told an interviewer from *Vegetarian Times*, "You are what you eat. If you eat a chicken, it's dead and you're putting deadness inside you. If you eat fruit, it's alive. You're putting life inside you." He continued, "You know that McDonald's commercial? They show the meat being cut up, cooked, and made into a hamburger. If they showed the first step, a beautiful cow and then a butcher chopping its head off, they'd go out of business."[390] Indeed, I often wonder if the vast majority of our population, including children, would convert to vegetarianism if they saw how the food on their plate was raised and witnessed its harvesting first-hand—let alone being solely responsible for getting a live animal to a dinner plate.

It is my sincere wish that more vegetarian role models existed in our society. Without them, why would children and young people question the health value and taste of, say, fast-food hamburgers when they have been surrounded by McDonald's commercials and billboards their entire lives and their parents and friends all seem to enjoy them? If they are not directly exposed to vegetarianism, they might not even know what the word means. And, as we've covered earlier, they're certainly not going to find out about it on TV.

Personal Taste

After talking about everything I have in the past few chapters, it may at first seem frivolous to end this phase of the discussion with a few words about taste. Yet, as I suggested in the introduction, it is our daily life habits that generally reveal more about us than the beliefs we hold intellectually.

In my book *Seven Steps to Perfect Health: A Practical Guide to Mental, Physical and Spiritual Wellness*, I contrast the food consumption manners of meat eaters versus vegetarians in the following words:

> I travel frequently on planes in the US and one thing that never ceases to amaze me in observing my American fellow passengers, the meat consumers at least, is how they eat—without passion. Most use a fork or spoon like a steam shovel to put away food, which is taken more as fuel than as a delightful experience. (You can hardly blame them: if you have ever tried to chew a piece of meat until it is well pulverized, it is a taxing experience to say the least.) In vegetarian restaurants, on the other hand, I often observe how the meals are

savored. Vegetarian diners typically eat more slowly, so they can relish each mouthful, drawing out the multiple flavors and aromas and therefore, have a more enjoyable dining experience.

To my mind, part of the reason that the vegetarians, not the meat eaters, are really enjoying their meals is because, given the endless variety of protein-providing plant foods available and the tasty ways they're being combined, seasoned, and cooked, the vegetarians simply have more to choose from and enjoy in the realm of taste. It is commonly suggested to chew your food at least 30 times before swallowing to allow for the amylase, which is the enzyme in saliva that helps to break down carbohydrates. Try chewing a piece of steak 30 times; you will likely find that it becomes tiresome and isn't as tasty or appealing.

But I am willing to concede that what one finds good to eat is not solely based on acquired tastes; on whether, that is, one has been exposed to meat- or plant-based diets and grown to like them. Part of taste is genetic. Recent research suggests the genetic makeup of our tongue may determine which foods taste good to us. Those with less sensitive tongues may crave sweets; those with more sensitive tongues may crave fatty foods. For healthy alternatives, Dr. Michael Roizen, who has looked into this topic, suggests that fat-eaters try spices and sweet-eaters try nutritional stand-ins such as cinnamon.[391]

One thing is for certain: no matter what way you've been trained to eat—whether through experience or by genetic predisposition—it is not fixed in stone. Those who feel compelled or desire to move to vegetarianism from meat eating soon begin to love the many tastes available in a vegetarian diet.

At this moment in the argument, I have given you a shopping cart full of reasons to go green, yet they all seem separate rationales (some health related, some ethical, some economic) that may on the surface seem to have no particular connection to each other. However, as the book proceeds and we move to create a view of *full-spectrum vegetarianism*, you will see all these braid together into a coherent philosophy, just as, ideally, all the items in your shopping cart become delicious, delightful, and healthy vegetarian meals.

Opening to a World of Possibilities

Let's face it: from a health perspective, most people are ignorant about food, let alone nutrition. That's why so many in the US consume meat and dairy products, as well as copious amounts of other processed foods laden with chemicals, preservatives, salt, sugar, and unhealthy fats. They don't sit down at the table and say, "Gee, I'm eating this cut of beef even though the cow that it was sliced off of had a terrible life. Oh, and by eating it, I'm contributing to world hunger and adding to human suffering." Nor does this consumer consider that the lamb chops on their plate came from a baby lamb literally ripped away from his mother's teet in order to provide food for humans, when for millions of years cows have enjoyed a healthy life in the open air and sunshine having natural impulses to run and graze in a pasture with a family and community of other cows. The person consuming these poor abused creatures is only concerned with the soft, delicate texture of the meat, and not that its origin was a young animal that never saw the light of day. Nor is it likely that this person ever thinks about the cheese they are eating and that it came from the milk of a mother cow that never got to feed its young calf and literally cried out for days after it was separated from her at birth.

No, the average meat and dairy eater would never think about such things. He or she has one thing uppermost in mind as he takes a bite, "This beef tastes damn good." Or, "I can't live without cheese; I love how it melts in my mouth."

The funny thing is that, compared to meat eaters, healthy vegetarians consume a more vast array of nutritious foods than people who consume diets predominantly of animal products. There are literally hundreds of vegetables and fruits available for consumption that meat eaters may have never tried. So, any smugness from a meat eater about flavor is due in large part because they have drastically limited their food choices for most of their life, and now suffer the consequences of severely compromised and numbed taste buds temporarily incapable of reveling in the many of the delicious flavors available when eating healthy wholesome foods (more about this shortly).

We don't think about food as a form of self-expression but it is. We can demonstrate our creativity by preparing meals that include a wide variety of natural flavors and textures, or we can express ourselves unimaginatively and narrowly by limiting our choices to only those flavors, spices, and textures we're accustomed to.

There is a rich world of food choices that only those with adventuresome minds and palettes enjoy. Many people who consume a Standard American Diet don't realize that if we always stay with the same foods, we're missing out on the fun, the adventure (and yes, the risks too) of new experiences, and we're depriving ourselves of the opportunity to explore, yet surprisingly tasty, and more healthful ways of eating.

The Healthy Gourmet

But let's get back to taste. I believe that, if the unadventurous soul—who I imagined a moment ago, exclaiming about how tasty the steak was—ever dared eat a gourmet vegetarian meal, would make another exclamation, he might say, "This *mock* beef [made from seitan] tastes pretty good."

It's an almost open secret now that vegetarian food makes for good eating. This was well illustrated in October 1979 when Franciscan Brother Ron Pikarski prepared and hosted what he called a "Pure Vegetarian Escoffier Dinner" at a Chicago Club. (The Escoffier style of preparing food is that of updated French cooking.) With the assistance of an entire retinue of chefs and food preparers, Pikarski, one of the world's finest chefs, served an eight-course masterpiece of vegetarian-style French cuisine to over 100 guests. It won rave reviews.

Two weeks in the making, the nearly two dozen dishes of wholesome and primarily uncooked vegetables and soy-based items were prepared following strict vegetarian guidelines, with no flesh, dairy, processed or salted foods on the menu.

This event was a persuasive and symbolic moment for the joys of vegetarian eating.

Brother Pikarski himself has been and is a powerful advocate of vegetarianism. From 1980 to 1996, he led his American Natural Foods team to win seven medals at the International Culinary Olympics (IKA) using only vegan plant-based foods. He was the first chef in the history of that prestigious event to do so.

He came to this dietary choice as a way to solve his own weight problem, which he did. He then started preparing green meals for his brethren in the Franciscan community where he lived and was principal chef. It was there that he learned that vegetarian cuisine is not only helpful for weight reduction and to give pleasure to the taste buds, but has health-enhancing effects. He sees his nutritious meal planning as having helped stop the high incidence of heart disease that had hit his community intensely just before the onset of his cooking. Sixteen relatively young brothers and priests, most in their forties and fifties, had died of heart disease, but there have been no such incidents since Brother Ron became executive chef.[392] Pikarski believes that "if everyone understood the basics of nutrition, they would become vegetarians."[393]

It could be said by a critic that assembling a vegetarian meal takes more work because the chef has to be concerned about balancing nutrition, protein in particular. I've already said that this is hardly the difficult task that some portray, but there's another issue to consider here. The trained chef preparing a meat-centered meal is typically unaware of the nutritional components (hardly a virtue) of what they are cooking; they are primarily concerned with balancing the four basic tastes—*sweet, sour, salty,* and *bitter.* Further, the vegan chefs with whom I've worked embody a much greater awareness of the food's nutritional values that they are preparing. Still, many of us, whether chefs or just people preparing a dish for the family, often overlook the nutritional aspects of foods in favor of the gastronomical. But a consideration of nutrition should enter into *every* chef's meal plan if we expect to create a thriving species. As the popular vegetarian cookbook *Ten Talents* puts it, "The health of this generation lies with its cooks to a great degree. But alas, how little intelligent thought and study is put into this phase of human responsibility."[394]

For the person who *is* ready to venture forth from the less than healthy meat-based menus into the beautiful, health-expanding neighborhood of broccoli and cauliflower, there are many fine vegetarian cookbooks and periodicals to help lead the way.

Here are a few pointers to keep in mind: Vegetarian foods should be whole and natural, and prepared so that their unique and subtle flavors are allowed to gently present themselves. Unlike meat, poultry, or processed foods, vegetarian dishes should not be heavy or overbearing, but subtle and balanced. They should be eaten to both enhance and perpetuate life.

Unlike the imaginary young meat eater I used as an example, the vegetarian eater is sensitive to the world within and without. Vegetarians are attuned, outwardly, to the needless suffering of their co-inhabitants, man and beast, and inwardly to the health effects of what they are consuming. As we've seen in this section, this attunement, which quite naturally is seen in a greater sensitivity to injustice, is also, perhaps, evident in an expanded capacity to enjoy life. What I said in the previous paragraph about the subtlety and intertwined flavors of vegetarian cuisine should have alerted you to the fact that the vegetarian eater has a greater appreciation for varied tastes and flavors and, it follows, in contrast to meat-centered eaters, a more discerning and educated palate.

Taste as a Healing Mechanism

I am sure the above title has attracted your attention. It's a profound concept when you think about it. I mean who would have ever thought about taste as an aspect of healing. There are some staunch vegans whose commitment to green eating is inspired by ethical reasons. This person might say, "I don't care whether I'm eating tofu that tastes like paper as long as what I'm consuming is a food that doesn't hurt animals in its creation."

Such a view, while noble in its intention, is totally unnecessary, given the wide variety of delicious taste options with green eating. It also overlooks one crucial, as-yet-unexplored component of good taste. *In a special sense*, if it tastes good, it's very often good for you as well.

Wait—I'm not giving you license to go out and buy French fries and a chocolate milk shake because you like how they taste. It's a bit more complex than that, and involves a detour into Eastern Indian medicine to understand it. I can start by saying that in general people eat the foods they were raised on—foods that their caretakers and culture told them are "good." Most people have not refined their self-awareness and appreciation enough to know if, deep down, they really enjoy the tastes of those foods.

This last statement may seem a bit off kilter, but let's explore it a bit further. What I'm saying is that our sense of taste provides an innate mechanism to help us with healthy eating, *if only we pay attention to it*. In the most banal sense, if someone were to bite into a rotten fruit, he or she would immediately spit it out because it tasted and smelled "wrong." In fact, our bodies are equipped through our senses of sight, smell, and taste to know what foods are helpful to boosting bodily processes and which ones are not. If you doubt this, by the way, just offer a glass of wine or cup of coffee to a child and watch their face *just after smelling it*. Chances are they will cringe and push the vessel back toward you in haste, without even trying it. So in essence, we come with the mechanisms and the programming to make the best choices when it comes to what we put in our bodies. This, at least, is the belief of the ancient healing system known as Ayurvedic medicine. According to this doctrine, which originated nearly 4,000 years ago, our senses lead us to the specific foods and nutrients, textures and qualities that are appropriate for our balance and health at any given time. Thus our sense of what tastes good or ill is not static but ever changing, constantly adapting to the body's ever-changing needs.[395]

If an individual accepts the validity of this basic idea, they would no longer be able to make food choices by rote, but would make better choices by deepening their sensitivity so that their taste and smell awareness would guide them to the foods that are right for them at a given moment. According to this philosophy, this person's body may really need a high-protein, high-fiber food at one point, but not at another. By being aware of the subtle changes in her internal requirements, they will find that what tastes good at the moment is what is healthiest for their body at that juncture. In fact, my conversations with people who converted to a vegetarian diet support this. Shortly after the taste buds reactivate through the introduction of unadulterated plant foods, sensitivities increase. Salt, sugar, fat and the chemical additives in foods deaden the taste buds; this is what makes shifting to a vegetarian diet difficult for some people in the early stages. Someone with advanced awareness, however, can stand before the vegetable case at the market and know exactly what their body is craving. They are not operating through thoughts at this point; they are allowing themselves to be informed by their body. Moreover, after some time on the vegetarian diet, these people tend to crave certain plant-foods, such as legumes or other vegetables, rather than junk foods.

Ayurvedic medicine was originated when a medical specialist named Charak and a famed surgeon named Susruta co-wrote two texts describing the system. This one component of the system—the linking of two seemingly separate components of food, its taste and health-giving properties, is very representative of the whole Ayurvedic medical tradition, whose hallmark is its holism.

Taking its name from the combined Sanskrit terms *ayu* and *veda*, which lends the meaning "life's knowledge," the discipline, unlike modern Western medicine, doesn't concentrate only on the body's disease states and its related symptoms. It focuses on uncovering and remedying the root causes of illness through a total approach of mental, physical, and spiritual conditions.[396] If someone has a cold, this approach might include investigating, yes, their nose and throat, but then moving beyond to look at the attitude towards work, a detailed review of their diet, and even probing their feelings about his or her purpose in life and close relationships, including the degree of harmony one has with nature.

Let's get back now to our entry point into this topic, however, the importance of taste. The Ayurvedic system holds that there are six basic tastes—the four known in the West: sweet, sour, salty, and bitter; and two others, pungent and astringent. These last two play a critical role in health. Like the warning lights on our cars, they clue us in to what we need or should avoid at any given time, but only if we pay attention to them.[397]

Additionally, there is another factor that contributes to cravings, and this is the matter that food processors work hard at… creating foods that are addictive. David A. Kessler, a Harvard-trained doctor, lawyer, medical school dean, former commissioner of the Food and Drug Administration, and author of *The End of Overeating: Taking Control of the Insatiable American Appetite* notes that foods high in fat, salt, and sugar alter the brain's chemistry in ways that compel people to overeat.[398] This is why I often suggest an initial period of cleansing and detoxification when transitioning from a meat based diet to a healthy vegetarian diet. This can go a long way in breaking some of the addictive patterns that are unfortunately all too common and well anchored thanks to a diet high in processed foods.

If you are somewhat of a healthy vegetarian, which means that the majority of your diet is comprised of leafy greens and vegetables, along with some nuts and seeds, and only a bit of processed vegetarian food, then you are likely not that far away. But, if you want a rapid, first-hand experience of the effects of a clear system, you simply need to undertake body cleansing (which I address later in the book) on fresh vegetable juices and unadulterated vegetables (no salt, sugar or oils) and greens for a week. You will literally be getting a taste of what I'm talking about here.

Certainly, there are gross cases where your body alerts you to a wrong food choice. Think of when you are dining at a Mexican restaurant and unwittingly bite into a jalapeno pepper. You may feel like smoke is pouring out of your ears, as it would of a cartoon character. Or think of when your mouth puckers up when sampling a super-sour dill pickle.

Still, beyond such obvious and infrequent events, it might seem the body's relation to food via taste has little connection to health. After all, while these cues may be hard to miss, most tastes are far subtler and do not bluntly tell us about our body's requirements.

Consider this. If you bite into a delicious dish, for instance, you are stimulating many senses simultaneously. Sight, smell, and taste all cooperate to cue your body to start digesting. When we chew our food, enzymes are released to break down the food particles, releasing a variety of flavors. The more we chew, the more flavors we receive. So in order to best "understand" what our food is telling us through the stimulation of our taste buds, we should chew thoroughly and thoughtfully. The more we chew the better we digest our food, so we get extra benefits from eating slowly, digesting properly, and sensing the effects that the food is having on our bodies.

I'm saying that your sensitivity to body signals will be enhanced by thorough mastication. I would add that many of us have gotten out of the habit of eating carefully because we have eaten processed and overly refined foods that don't allow for a complex eating experience. While wholesome vegetarian foods offer many interesting smells, flavors, and textures when chewed, over-processed and junk foods only confuse our bodies. They require very little chewing, because they have already been ultra-refined, and rather than savor them, we tend to wolf them down. With this compulsive eating style, we consume far more in far less time. To confuse our bodies even further, we try to make these denatured, mono-taste foods more interesting by heaping salt, sugar, ketchup, mayonnaise, butter, and other worthless or harmful additives on them. It is not difficult to see how the inclusion in our diets of items such as fast foods, fried foods, sugars and artificially colored, sugary soft drinks, salts, and chemically fabricated "milk" shakes—among other things—lead us to the record levels of obesity and disease that we are currently facing.

The healthy vegetarian diet will not only aide in healing the physical body, but the taste buds, too. And, once you've reached a place where enough healing has occurred, you will find yourself enjoying the comfort of these exceptional foods, without a thought about returning to your previous place and time.

Reprogramming Your Taste... *in Everything*

In summary, we begin life with senses attuned to our food's inner values, yet these senses will lose their edge and become dulled and unresponsive rather quickly if one moves away from eating natural foods. If you are a junk-food offender, for instance, you might find it difficult at first to enjoy good, wholesome grains and vegetables; I mentioned this is the last section. You are also probably not used to chewing your food well because the refined foods you have grown accustomed to have so little substance that they require virtually no effort to swallow.

Eating good, fibrous foods may annoy you as you search for familiar tastes. They may even overwhelm you in that your dimmed senses will feel assaulted by the wealth of textures and flavors in such natural unadulterated fare. If you want to be in touch with your body, however, you will persist in including these foods in your diet. As I've found in the experiences of many who have been in my study groups and who took up this direction in eating, you will ultimately find it a surprisingly pleasant sensory experience, and your body will be glad to be getting the nutrients it truly craves and requires to function optimally.

When a person has an alert palate and is able to fully experience food, the individual, according to Ayurvedic medicine, is able to monitor his or her cravings in order to get a rough guide to present health conditions. Ayurvedic medicine instructs us to listen to our urges to eat certain foods in that they could be warning us of imbalances that need correction. If we crave water-soluble foods, for instance, it may be because our body tissues, which are mostly water-based, need them in order to continue functioning properly and efficiently.[399] If we crave something alkaline, on the other hand, it may be to offset a high acidity. In reaction, it would be advisable to eat something light and easily assimilated or something particularly alkaline like tofu or a green juice or salad.

While I have shared quite a bit on the issue of taste, I feel it is imperative to understand what drives us in the relatively rich and abundant nation in which we live when it comes to food—and pleasing tastes and taste sensations, or "mouth feel" as they call it in the industry. As such, it is one of the most crucial factors as our nation is presented with the challenge of tiring *and* expiring resources and for those of us who are actively asking ourselves and others to move to a plant-based diet.

Chapter 6

Protein

"Excessive animal protein is at the core of many chronic diseases."

—*T. Colin Campbell, Ph.D., Author of the bestselling book* The China Study

What Is Protein?

Let's talk for a moment about what protein is.

At the most basic level, the human body needs a number of different items that are derived from food and drink, including fats, protein, and carbs, which each play a different part in the internal system.

The role of protein is to help build, maintain, and repair the body. It is the essential ingredient in hair, finger and toe nails, skin, muscles, cartilage, and tendons. Additionally, protein is essential for the manufacture of neurotransmitters.

At a more fundamental level, it also makes up many of our hormones, antibodies, and enzymes. Unlike carbs, for example, which are converted to sugar when the body needs more energy, protein is seldom broken down for this purpose. This conversion would only happen if a person was starving or adopted a drastically unhealthy high protein, low-carb diet.

Chemically, proteins are long chain molecules made up of individual links called amino acids. There are approximately 22 amino acids that make up all the proteins in nature, whether plant, animal, or viral. Eight of these amino acids (nine in children) have to be gotten through food since they are *not* manufactured in the human body. They are valine, leucine, isoleucine, lysine, threonine, tryptophan, methionine, phenylalanine, and histadine. This last amino acid is important for the growth and development of children.

Luckily, we don't have to eat eight different foods to get the eight essential amino acids. Conveniently enough, there are foods that contain all of these amino acids in about the right proportions for human utilization. These include both animal products, such as meat, eggs, and dairy, and a multitude of non-animal foods, from peanut butter and whole wheat to rice and other grains and beans, corn, chick-peas, wheat grass, and sesame seeds.

History of Protein

Now, let's get back to the protein story.

It seems to me the American craving for meat, given all the health risks involved in eating it, is almost irrational. The argument is sometimes made that, even if the meat sold for eating has many harmful qualities, companies provide it because, as they say, "It's what the public wants." This is a possible argument to convince the highly uninformed, I guess. And it seems to work for those held in the trance of the status quo. However, anyone who knows anything about "Manufacturing Consent" the way manipulated information / propaganda is often fed to the public, how scientists sometimes (knowingly or not) collude with big business by providing one-sided data. The politics of scientific research journals publishing only the research that makes them look good (i.e., doesn't rub too much against the status quo), and the honest voices, those voices that often times at great financial risk point out shortcomings of a commercial, industrialized practice. Unfortunately the odds are unfairly stacked in the favor of wealthy corporate interests and these courageous men and women are all too often marginalized. Critical thinkers will look with some wariness at claims that the producers are just fulfilling consumers' desires—ones that have (supposedly) not been influenced by the outpouring of ads and pseudo-scientific data that meat purveyors use to support their urgings (and we haven't even gotten to dairy yet).

Let me also say a few words here about how Americans "naturally" developed their love affair with meat since it hinges on protein. It all started back in the early 1940s when the notion of "complete" and "incomplete" proteins was popularized. This idea was not only spread through women's magazines and popular science journals but was promulgated in classrooms across America. Even years later, when I was a primary school student, I remember being shown charts of meat, dairy products, and eggs, which (teacher said) were "complete" (the hero) proteins. Then she brought out another chart on which were all the other foods: vegetables, grains, legumes, and fruits, which were called "incomplete" sources of proteins (the villains). According to what my teacher said, and she was echoing what was being taught in classrooms all around the US, complete proteins had all the essential amino acids in the right proportions, while incomplete proteins lacked certain amino acids and did not have them in the right proportions. From what has been established in this book already, you know this is nonsense.

Scientists did not develop this idea as a way to curry favor with the meat and dairy producers, but they might as well have. As you can guess, these nutritionists with their talk of complete (meat) and incomplete (potatoes) protein were playing a tune that was music to the ears of the meat and dairy producers. Another thing I'm sure you can guess without me telling you is that these producers were not slow on pushing their advertising (about how what they sell contained the right kind of protein) into dietetic and general interest journals, school books, and eventually onto television. An advertisement for the Armour Beef Company in a 1949 issue of the *Journal of the American Dietetic Association*, for instance, stated that beef is, "a rich source of *complete* protein, various minerals essential to a normal blood picture, and fuel-supplying calories. And its satiety value and thorough digestibility make it an important addition to virtually every balanced diet."[1] That last sentence is as readable (for the average person) as a page from a trigonometry text, but be that as it may, that journal soon became chockfull of various ads supporting the meat industry. The American Meat Institute of Chicago, for example, ran full-page ads resembling scientific reports of the kind usually found in medical journals.

While parallel advertising ran in consumer journals, I am highlighting these because they ran in a magazine for the dieticians who would be telling students and other audiences about proper eating and so were prime targets for the meat and dairy makers. The thrust of these ads was to give scientific credence to the idea that meat was a great food for health reasons by convincing the scientists of this and then using them as mouthpieces to spread a credible message.

But don't get the idea that the meat producers had it all their own way in the scientific world. While nutritionists with their talk of incomplete and complete proteins were giving a decidedly pro-meat view, there were other scientists, working on medical issues, who doubted the rosy view being presented on the virtues of eating meat. That's why the animal products industry not only tried to spread the word about complete protein, but had to step up and defend itself against scientific charges concerning, for instance, the possibility of a connection between ill health and meat eating. An American Meat Institute ad called "Meat and the Dietary Fallacies in the Public Mind" said scientific findings on the connections between high dietary uric acid intake and degenerative diseases were "erroneous." Uric acid is connected to high protein diets, by the way. No, it told the public, meat did not aggravate such disorders as gout, rheumatism, and hypertension, and high protein diets are not harmful.[2] Meanwhile, there are countless studies today supporting the fact that meat, indeed, plays a key role in the development of diseases, including the ones noted thus far.

Such ads hit a minor note, while the major chords that were struck in the ads were those that promoted meat as a health enhancer. One example of this last point is a 1948 ad that, in a sexist way prevalent at the time, labeled meat, "Man's preferred complete protein food." The copy goes on to say, "Meat provides protein of biological *completeness*. Requiring no protein supplementation from other sources, it instead enhances the nutrient value of the daily diet by supplementing incomplete protein foods [read veggies] to full biological adequacy."[3] Poultry was pushed in other ads as being "rich in protein, relatively low in calories."[4] So, the public was told, chicken is not only a provider of complete protein, but eating it could help you lose weight, too.

It certainly was an easy selling point for animal product purveyors that they could represent their offerings, according to nutrition "experts," as foods that contained the only complete proteins. Not only did chicken, beef, and other meat makers used this claim in their ads, but so did, for instance, the Dairy Council, which hailed milk as a high-protein food, especially necessary for children and teens. A 1964 ad, paid for by this group, pictured carefree teenagers romping on the beach under the words, "Teenage nutrition: Protein? They couldn't care less!"[5] But if these young people were oblivious to such an important dietary issue, then, the advertiser explained, it was up to the parents to make sure their kids were well supplied with that prime source of readily available, high-quality protein: cow milk. Since then, the dairy industry has put the full-court press on the American public with their "Got Milk?" ads, featuring highly paid entertainers and athletes sporting milk mustaches. This, of course, to convince people that dairy milk has bone-building and other health benefits; nothing could be further from the truth. Not to be left behind, even ice cream makers claimed their commodity was a healthy purchase.

The American Dietetic Association endorsed the sugary concoction as a good source of protein, something particularly for finicky eaters, such as the convalescent and the elderly.[6] I'm not sure where they got the boldness to make this claim in that ice cream only contains 3.85 grams of protein per 100 grams, while it does have 12.06 grams of health-endangering saturated fat. As an aside, over the course of writing this book, 10 people over four states have been confirmed with listeria poisoning, and three have died because of tainted Blue Bell ice cream.[7]

But let's get back to advertising. We've been turning back the clock to look at the first wave of pro-meat propaganda. This is not meant to suggest that widespread promotion of meat has ended. Indeed, it has not. Recently, for example, the pork industry has been promoting pork as the lean meat, ideal for dieters and packed with proteins. The ads neglect to mention that it's also a toxic time bomb packed with saturated fat, cholesterol, chemicals, and calories.

But it can be said that meat-touting ads have changed in that they no longer rely on the spurious distinction between complete and incomplete protein carriers, which claimed animal products were the only authentic examples of the former. Sooner or later, the promoters were going to have to give up this theory, which had the liability *that it is wholly unfounded*. Animal products, including eggs, are not our only sources of complete protein.

Instead of using the now-forgotten idea of complete and incomplete proteins, scientifically grounded nutritionists now evaluate a food's NPU, *Net Protein*

Utilization. NPU is the ratio of amino acids converted to proteins to the ratio of amino acids supplied by the food. As it is, it is a measure of the food's overall value as a protein source. As remarked above, this does not count how much protein is in a food, but how much of that protein can be utilized by humans.[8] This depends on both the amino acid content and digestibility of a food, as we discussed earlier. Ideally, the proteins in the food hold a complete set of essential amino acids, ones which enable them to be used with maximum efficiency by the body. Moreover, a food with a high NPU would be one that is readily digestible since, if you can't thoroughly digest a protein, it might as well not be there for all the good it is doing you.

I might throw in here that one thing that adds to a substance's digestibility is high fiber content. The indigestible fiber portion of the food sweeps quickly through the intestinal tract, inhibiting bacterial action while insulating the protein molecules within the food from the destructive chemical action of digestive enzymes. So foods that include fiber in their makeup tend to have high NPUs, which means they are great sources for proteins. I probably don't have to remind you that the richest sources of fiber in the human diet come from the plant kingdom, including whole grains, seeds, fruits, and vegetables.

While some groups, such as those at the American Dietetic Association, still support the old, superseded theory that protein is to be evaluated for its completeness, more authoritative institutions such as the United States Department of Agriculture and the Food and Drug Administration support the view of protein that judges it on the basis of its NPU.

Such a viewpoint is necessarily good for the status of vegetables, fruits, grains, and legumes in that—as John McDougall, M.D., has emphasized—with very few exceptions, they contain all the essential amino acids. Moreover, a large percentage of foodstuffs from these groups have goodly amounts of these amino acids along with high NPUs, so they have the amino acids in proportions required by the body to properly utilize them.

As most of us already know, protein is essential for animal life. It is a building block used in the construction of our bones and hair, muscles and organs. It also makes up the bulk of collagen, the glue-like material connecting all our tissue. Without it, we would literally have no structure. Proteins also play a vital role in the transportation of nutrients to and from cells and organs. Our immune system also relies heavily on proteins called antibodies to address bacteria and viruses.[9] It's very comforting to know now that professionals recognize that a well-balanced vegetarian diet can meet the human body's needs for protein.

What Are the Best Sources of Protein for Humans?

In this section, I'm going to talk about how much protein various foods have to offer the human body.

Although I've said little as yet about the amino acid content of specific foods, you should already have gotten the impression that these building blocks of protein are not that hard to come by. They are found in meat, fish, milk products, eggs, legumes, nuts, cereals, and even vegetables, and their ability to be utilized by the body (referred to as bioavailability) increases in certain foods when eaten in combination with others.

Additionally, while one particular source of protein may contain a greater number or percentage of amino acids than another, if the food with more protein is also more difficult for the human body to digest and assimilate, it would be considered a lesser quality protein. Let's start off this discussion by focusing in on those foods that are commonly known to be high in protein. This will give me the opportunity to illustrate the central topic that I hinted at in the previous section, and am bringing up now, which is the *quality* of a protein source.

If you want to start at the top, the egg ranks highest in terms of bioavailability. Not only does the egg have eight essential amino acids, it also has them in the proportions best suited to human protein metabolism. The interesting thing is that eggs do not have the highest protein content of any food; the protein that they do have can be efficiently used by the eater. In other words, a slab of meat may have more protein pound for pound than an egg, but the human body cannot use a large percentage of that meat protein because we do not have all of the necessary digestive enzymes (chemical compounds responsible for breaking food down and converting it to fuel) or the proper amount of stomach acid to digest it completely. So, the additional protein may as well not have been there since it cannot be fully utilized.

While between 91% and 97% of the protein in eggs is utilized by our bodies, this high degree of utilization is not found in other animal products, whose "net protein utilization" (NPU) rates[10] are:

Milk	82 percent
Fish	80 percent
Cheese	70 percent
Meat and Poultry	67 percent

The NPU of meat and poultry doesn't put the useable proteins in them much above that of tofu (soybean curd), which has 65% usable protein. So, you should already be able to see that the claims of meat eaters who note, vehemently, that meat is "crammed with protein," have some holes in them. It doesn't matter so much that meat products are fairly high in protein (about 20%) if, as we've learned, only two-thirds of that protein is useable to humans.

This concept of "quality of protein" should have alerted the reader to the fact that the commonly given equation, meat as a good and high source of protein, is not as credible as it at first appears. Let's develop this topic a little further.

Raw Versus Cooked Protein

By now the message is clear: A certain amount of protein is essential, but as you will soon find out, we need less than we are likely presently getting and animal sources are not the best choice.

So let me shift gears here and move away from an exposure of the disadvantages of gathering too much protein from animal products to a closer look at vegetarian proteins. First, let me stress that preparation is key to reaping the full benefits available in green protein. In order to make plant protein easier to digest and allow for its complete utilization, low temperature cooking or juicing, which break down the cell wall structure of vegetables, is best. (In some cases, cooking even lessens the chance of toxicity; beans, for example, should not be eaten raw except for their sprouts.) It's not only important to avoid high temperatures, which can eradicate some of the protein, but to stick with water and steam, as opposed to, say, charcoal-broiling and pan-frying, since the water-based methods protect protein value and preserve other vitamins and minerals.

Soy Protein

You may have noted early on that I advised, "Animal products are not our only source of complete protein." The first things I mentioned as alternatives were tofu and tempeh, both soybean products.

While the soybean has been a primary protein source in Asian cultures, dating back for at least 3,000 years, even now in the US, its main employment has been for livestock feed and pressed oil. Here ignorance is not bliss; many American eaters are using soybean oil as their only contact with this wonder bean and are missing out on many delicious and nutritious culinary uses for organic, non-genetically modified soy products.

Let me briefly review the main soy products to give you an idea of their variety and health worthiness.

Tofu, or bean curd, is an easily digestible protein source made from coagulated soy milk. It has a soft, crumbly consistency, and its mild taste and spongy texture allow it to soak up and absorb the flavor of other foods or spices added to it, making it the perfect food for many dishes. On the down side, tofu is low in the important amino acid methionine, but when complemented by any whole grain, like brown rice or wheat, it becomes a total quality protein.

The exact amount of protein in a serving of tofu depends on how firmly it is pressed. The following standards have been set for protein concentration by the Tofu Standards Committee of the Soy Food Association of America:

Soft Tofu	5-6.9 percent
Regular Tofu	7-9.9 percent
Firm Tofu	10-13.9 percent
Extra Firm Tofu	14 percent or more

A second soy product, tempeh, has an even higher protein content. This form is prepared by fermenting the soy beans and packing them together in a mold. It usually comes packaged in 3/4-inch-thick rectangular sheets or patties and has such a meat-like texture that with the proper flavorings can be passed off as the animal product. Unlike the smoothed out tofu, tempeh maintains some of the texture of the original beans as well as their full nutrient content—protein, fiber, and all. Also in distinction from tofu, it doesn't lack any of the essential amino acids. It's a good protein source. Three ounces of tempeh contain 19.5 grams of protein.

Another good soy product, one especially treasured in Japan, is miso, a fermented paste typically made from a mixture of soybeans, salt, and water. Variations of miso contain barley, rice, chick-peas or barley malt, and given this variety, misos also range in color from a tan hue to a deep brown or red. Partially, the colors depend on how long the food is steeped. The longer it's fermented, the darker its color and the stronger its flavor. Like tofu, it is highly adaptable, and can be used to flavor many dishes—soups, sandwich spreads, gravies, dressings, and dips. Because it contains live lactobacillus culture and other digestive enzymes, it is easily digested and well utilized by the body. Indeed, in Japan, eaters often begin a meal with a cup of miso soup, prepping the stomach for the digestion of what's coming in the rest of the meal. Yuko Otomo, a New York City artist who was born in Japan, notes that in her native country, "Miso soup is basically a breakfast meal to prepare the toning of the body for the day. Eating tofu and miso (soup) for breakfast has been a steady diet in Japan for centuries. Even in the 21st century, people (young and old) still enjoy this tradition."

Do We Need Meat to Be Healthy?

From the perspective of substantiating the vegetarian diet as a viable option, it might be said I could end the book here, in that I have already provided a full (if not exhaustive) rationale on why it is preferable, considering ethical, health, environmental, and practical reasons. However, this book is not only concerned with the "why's" but also the "how's" related to becoming the healthiest possible vegetarian, some of which has already been covered in detail regarding the issue of protein and in the next chapter will be covered regarding the more esoteric topic of what it means to lead a spiritual life, for example.

Though I have made my case for this green way, I am aware that a number of the topics covered so far have *not* been given the amount of detail that they deserve. So, I want to go from strictly arguing for the vegetarian alternative to a more in-depth consideration of some of the important notions previously advanced. For the reader who doesn't like to look beneath the surface, this might seem boring, but for those of you who desire a thorough knowledge of what they are studying (which I believe would be most of you who have read this far), consider following me a little further on this journey.

The first topic that deserves more pondering is whether a properly thought-out vegetarian diet is wholly adequate. We saw how the early food pyramid and the theory of complete and incomplete proteins gave short shrift to the idea that you could eat healthily without filling your meal plan with meat and dairy. I noted the weakness of this perspective, while defending green eating, but a few more comments in this vein might be useful. I will begin with a parade of experts, who recommend the vegetarian option.

Dr. Mervyn G. Hardinge, physician and researcher with degrees from Harvard and Stanford, has done extensive research on vegetarianism, of which he is a strong proponent. He writes:

> That human beings do not have to eat meat… is impressively evident to anyone familiar with even the rudiments of world nutrition. It is in countries and among peoples where diets are almost wholly of plant origin and meat eating is virtually absent that fertility is high and [the] population explosion the most threatening… On what basis can one claim a need for meat in America with its large variety of available vegetarian foods?[11]

Meat, as we've seen, has attained this preeminence in the eyes of most people—including health professionals—because it and its close dietary companions, milk, cheese, and eggs, are persistently touted by industry insiders as the only complete protein providers among foods. Let's hear from Hardinge again.

Even though the protein turnover may go through several animal bodies before it appears on the table of the consumer, the food chain, regardless of its length, always begins in the leaf or green portion of a plant. It is evident, then, that somewhere down the line the essential amino acids that go to make any protein 'complete' must be obtained from plant sources.[12]

If that's true—and in light of the many environmental and humanitarian issues (including world hunger) discussed in this book already—why not simply eat lower in the food chain and take some of the burdens off our world? Given the ease with which plant proteins can be combined to insure completeness and assimilation, and given our relatively small protein needs, Hardinge concludes, "There remains no valid reason for frightening people into eating meat for fear of protein deficiency on a non-flesh diet."[13] With the significant caveat that such a diet must involve careful planning to meet the requirements for calcium, iron, and B12, a vegetarian diet is superior, safe and replete with health benefits.

Dr. Hardinge substantiates his position with the research findings of numerous nutrition and health experts. He cites a 1959 editorial from the prestigious medical journal *The Lancet,* which even then noted the poor classification of vegetable proteins as second-class.[14] Protein expert Dr. Nevin Scrimshaw of MIT (as quoted in Hardinge) bolsters this position by noting that legumes and oilseed meals are perfectly acceptable protein sources for all human needs, including that of the infant and young child.[15] Scrimshaw does not bring up the question of feeding children a vegetarian diet because he thinks this is something not to be taken lightly. He knows that with developing humans, every precaution must be taken in food balancing, supplementation and careful monitoring to make sure the child is being fully nourished. It's rather to disarm the one constant theme of anti-vegetarians that no child should ever be subjected to a vegetarian diet, not matter how carefully planned.

Conventional pro-meat and dairy arguments emphasize that vegetarianism offers inadequate protein and is always harmful to children, and pro-green writers have struggled to combat these erroneous views. As to the first, Nobel Prize winner Dr. Arturi Virtanen states: "Lacto-vegetarians can receive easily all the necessary nutrients from fruit, vegetables, potatoes, cereals and milk low in fat."[16] And, to come back to Dr. Hardinge, he adds, "Properly prepared plant foods provide adequate protein for every age group, including infants."[17]

The Physician's Committee for Responsible Medicine further ads: "Naturally, children need protein to grow, but they do not need high-protein, animal-based foods. Many people are unaware that a varied menu of grains, beans, vegetables, and fruits supplies plenty of protein. The '"protein deficiencies"' that our parents worried about in impoverished countries were the result of starvation or diets restricted to very few food items. Protein deficiency is extremely unlikely on a diet drawn from a variety of plant foods."[18]

You can see that vegetarianism is not lacking in expert defenders.

A Closer Look at Meat Protein

Let me try a metaphor here. It's often the case that the most macho of men, when really confronted with a seriously risky situation, turn out to be all bluff. In a similar way, it turns out that meat (as it has been presented in ads and meatpackers' propaganda) as the most robust and enlivening possible food, responsible for giving he-men (and the equivalent type in women) bulging biceps, ruddy complexions and generalized health, is also mostly bluff.

It is by flying under the falsity of being the ideal provider of protein and vigorous wellbeing that meat has become the star focus of the average American's diet, whereby every meal revolves around it. The average Joe and Jane believe that meat is synonymous with robust health, strength, and, for Joe, virility and sexual potency. Their weekly meals are probably eggs and bacon, sausage or ham for breakfast; a hamburger or roast beef sandwich for lunch, and a meat with a starchy food like rice or potatoes for dinner.

Certainly, over the past decade, a few progressive individuals and organizations have raised their voices in warnings about the deleterious health effects of such habits. Even mainstream medical organizations like the American Heart Association and the American Cancer Society have echoed these warnings. But how likely is one to hear these solo singers when, at the same time, whole choruses of advertisers, celebrities, and media spokespeople are singing the praises of the meat industry.

I, for one, am not interested in joining one of those well-paid, but health-threatening choruses, but would rather join the heroic few who think aware readers are ready for the difficult but empowering truths about food, rather than the myths perpetrated by meat purveyors and other special interest groups. So, let's get down to the real story.

Let's revisit what was said in the previous section: Meat has plenty of protein though generally far less than people think in terms of dietary requirements. Beef, for example, is 20% protein; the rest is fat and water. It's also number one in calories. A 16-ounce steak has about 1,250 calories. If for a dinner, you coupled this with a baked potato with butter and sour cream, and added a dessert, you will have eaten around 2,300 calories before bed. (Remember, earlier I was talking of good daily calorie intake for a man being about 2,700 calories a day!)

I don't need to mention again that 500 of those protein calories in steak are not usable in the body. And you probably already know the threat of the saturated fat in the beef to your cholesterol count, so let's move on.

Excess Protein

Let's get back to our focus on protein. As you saw, I differ from McDougall in that I hold that protein deprivation still exists in our society, even while protein-rich foods are all around us. I agree with him, nonetheless, that due to its associated hazards, excess protein consumption far outdistances under-consumption of protein as a current health threat.

I've already broached the topic of the dangers of excess protein when I talked of the problems associated with excess urea, which can build up in the blood, and put the kidneys under strain as they attempt to flush this urea out of the system. If this strain keeps up, say from a protein-loaded diet, it can lead to kidney damage. This especially concerns the elderly, whose kidneys function less efficiently, and people with pre-existing kidney damage. Weight lifters are also prone to this outcome because in addition to the exorbitant amounts of meat they consume, they also consume toxic processed supplements and protein powders, which exacerbate the problem of overconsumption of proteins. Given that this is such an unheeded problem, a few more words on the topic would be appropriate.

McDougall argues that the real problem with protein is an *over*abundance. This primarily occurs from consistent meat consumption, but can also occur from eating too many legumes—though excess vegetable protein is far easier to process than excess animal protein. Excess protein is excreted through the liver, which then has to work harder to process the excess that it changes into urea. The kidneys then have to filter the urea and additional unprocessed protein. This results in enlarged kidneys.[19]

One result of this stress is that pressure accumulates, causing damage to the tubules, the filtering apparatus in the kidneys.

If things are as bad as this, you might wonder why you don't see more kidney damage in those who gorge on meat. But you have to balance what I've said so far with the thought that the kidneys are strong. Most people's kidneys can endure the strain, though it might impair optimal functioning.

Still, the danger of too much protein is well known to the medical profession. It is with this in mind that one of the first steps a physician will take for a kidney patient is to put him or her on low-protein diets, often as restricted as 2.5 to 5% of total caloric intake.

If a person is suffering from excess urea, arising from too much protein in the system, one way to get it out of the system is by keeping oneself well hydrated. The kidneys require a lot of water to filter excess urea out of the bloodstream, so drinking loads of it will lighten the kidney's workload. Unfortunately many people, especially the elderly, don't take in enough water to support the process. Infants, too, may not be getting enough water, especially when fed high-protein diets.[20] This can arise for babies who are fed cow's milk, which has twice the protein of human milk, and if it proceeds unchecked, it may well lead to hypernatremic dehydration. (The term "hypernatremic" refers particularly to the overabundance of sodium in the blood.) This occurs in infants when their small bodies have used up inordinate quantities of water during the urea-filtration process. Hara Marano, executive editor of *American Health* magazine, says that, "Hypernatremic dehydration is four times more deadly than the water loss that accompanies diarrhea in infants, and can lead to brain damage, shutdown of the kidneys and death within hours."[21]

Presumably on the opposite end of the spectrum from infants, who can be weak because they are in the early stages of growing and developing, are those in peak condition: athletes. Yes, surprisingly enough, this is the second group who is threatened with dehydration from excess protein intake (protein loading). Not only might athletes lose large amounts of fluid from perspiration, they also require extra water to filter urea from the blood. For a marathon runner, if there is a lack of water, this can lead to a serious heatstroke.

Besides urea, there is a second byproduct of protein metabolism, ammonia, which has been indicted by scientists as a substance that, if it builds up in our gut, can cause cancer. Dr. Willard Visek of the University of Illinois Medical School (quoted in Marano) explains, "In the digestion of proteins, we are constantly exposed to large amounts of ammonia in our intestinal tracts. Ammonia… like chemicals that cause cancer or promote its growth… kills cells, increases virus infections, affects the rate at which cells divide and increases the mass of the lining of the intestines. What is intriguing is that within the colon the incidence of cancer parallels the concentration of ammonia."[22]

Those are two significant dangers from excess protein consumption, both involving the internal increase of substances that are a threat to health. But there are additional side effects of a diet of excess protein, as I will profile in the next section.

Protein: Unraveling Other Protein Myths

1. Animal products are our only source of protein, and complete protein at that. FALSE
2. If you go on a vegetarian diet, you will become protein deficient, and then weak, sick, and anemic. FALSE
3. We cannot get too much protein, as any excess will be stored in the muscles. FALSE
4. Animal protein is low in calories and will keep you slim; carbohydrates are fattening. FALSE
5. Humans were made to eat meat. FALSE
6. Meat, fish and poultry are safe to eat. FALSE
7. Animal products are our only source of vitamin B12. FALSE

How many of these oft-repeated statements are true? None. Let's examine these commonly held misconceptions with a critical eye and a host of myth-busting facts.

1. ***Animal products are not our only source of proteins or complete protein.*** The fast food chain Arby's found this out the hard way when they tweeted "protein is better in meat form" in 2014, raising the hackles of the medical industry and prompting a complaint to the Federal Trade Commission calling for prohibiting Arby's from engaging in such deceptive practices.[23] In fact, protein is all around us. In their 2015 report, the USDA recognized soy, nuts, and seeds as non-animal protein sources.[24] Soy products, such as tofu and tempeh, are very high in protein as are the single-celled algae spirulina and chlorella. Gluten, the wheat protein in meat substitutes such as seitan, veggie chicken, and veggie hot dogs is another wonderful protein source.[25] Almost every grain and legume provides complete protein with high NPU rates. That's taking the foods alone.

Francis Moore Lappé, in her excellent treatise *Diet For a Small Planet,* has acknowledged the fact that proteins do not necessarily have to be combined to meet one's protein requirements. That notwithstanding, by combining whole grains like brown rice, quinoa, amaranth, and buckwheat with chick-peas, pinto or kidney beans you provide the full complement of amino acids that your body needs. Combining high quality vegetarian foods provides as much protein as animal products but in a form more easily absorbed and used by the body, and without the health risks accompanying animal-protein consumption. Tofu isn't linked to diabetes; lentils and split peas are very high in protein (16 g per cup) and are cholesterol free; broccoli, with 4 grams of protein in a single stalk, certainly won't hurt you.

2. *What about the idea that if you go on a vegetarian diet, you will become protein deficient and weaker?* Not true. You can get all of the protein you need from a purely plant-based diet. Protein is all around us. Cruciferous vegetables are rich with it. Some of the strongest and most creative people in the world are vegetarians, as we demonstrated in the previous list of prominent vegetarians.[26]

3. *You can never get too much protein.* Even on the surface, this seems implausible since we know that eating too much of anything is apt to cause physical trouble. Recent scientific studies show this is certainly true for protein. If more is coming into the body, it is replaced faster. This overtaxing speedy replacement can lead to cell damage and thus hasten the aging process.[27]

Today's Americans following the traditional Western diet get about twice the protein they need, which is actually harmful. Excessive protein consumption is linked to osteoporosis, cancer, impaired kidney function, and heart disease.[28] Furthermore, protein metabolism produces a byproduct called urea (as I discussed in the previous section), which is filtered through the kidneys. While urea has a part to play in excretion—carrying unneeded nitrogen out of the system—when there is too much urea, in the case of excess protein, kidney stress results.

Returning to the insightful Dr. McDougall, he notes that the earlier onset of puberty (which tends to correlate with earlier aging) experienced in some of the wealthier countries may be partly the result of too much protein in the diet, which pushes the eater through the natural human cycle at an accelerated rate.

As we've covered earlier, animal products are rich in protein but they are not good sources of protein for the human body, in part because our bodies cannot digest and assimilate these foods as well as plant-based foods, and in another part because of the excessive amount of fat and toxins associated with animal products.

4. *The next myth that is ripe for demolition is the one that claims animal protein is low in calories and so helpful in weight-loss plans.* It is claimed that carbs, on the other hand, add the pounds because of their high calories. While animal protein, if it was isolated in foods, might be low-cal, it doesn't come that way. Even in "lean" meats, the protein is normally accompanied by a large amount of fat. An average 16-ounce steak, for example, has about 1,250 calories, and about 80 grams of fat. One of the things, in addition to simple or refined carbohydrates, contributing to the US's astonishing levels of obesity is excess meat consumption.

Carbohydrates, except for those found in refined carbohydrates and sugars, are much lower in calories than animal products. (We are speaking of healthful complex carbohydrates, such as vegetables, fruits and grains.)

5. *Then we have the perennial comment that humans were designed, whether by the creator or by evolution, to eat meat.* This ignores the fact that our immediate ancestors, apes, (from which we differ in DNA by only 1.6%) are primarily vegetarians, and it disregards evidence on the type of teeth we possess, among other things, which seemed designed for vegetarian eating. I also covered other differences earlier in Chapter 5.

6. *Then, we have the idea that meat is healthy and safe for humans to eat.* As you know from what I've covered so far in the book, this is about as incorrect an assertion as you can make. You could write a medical textbook on all the physiological problems that have been associated with meat, and I'm not even talking about problems from the hormones and other chemicals that are in the meat. Much evidence suggests that meat eaters are prone to illnesses of the digestive and excretory systems as well as ones that involve generalized swelling and histamine responses throughout the body. Add to those ills prostate and colon cancer, gout, liver and kidney failure, heart disease, and which are all promoted by putting meat in the diet. And let's not overlook the massive increase in the potential for developing type 2 diabetes with a meat-based diet.[29-31] Further, fertility can be compromised in both men and women with meat consumption.[32-34]

But let's get back to the point I made about the length of time meat may stay in the intestines. For one, if ingested meat putrefies, which it is likely to do, the results are toxins permeating the intestinal walls, entering the bloodstream, and coursing through the body. Also, being slow to digest, it may cause constipation. The tiredness one feels after a meal of meat may not only be due to the body's energy being directed to digestion, but also to the not uncommon tendency of meat to bring on allergic reactions.

If you actually believe meat is healthy, then you must read chapter three in this book.

7. ***The last myth that needs to be tackled is the one that says only meat is a good source of vitamin B12.*** The half-truth concealed in this myth is that this vitamin is not normally found in fruits and vegetables. It ignores two, countervailing facts. First, a vegetarian can get the vitamin easily enough in fermented foods such as miso, soy sauce, tempeh, and, for those who eat dairy products, yogurt and eggs. Second, even if you don't do dairy, and don't like soy sauce or the other items mentioned, it's easy enough to take a supplement.

In the earlier days of the vegetarian movement, say in the 19th-century US, there was little science to back up the claims of adherents to a healthy vegetarian diet. As Karen and Michael Iacobbo write in *Vegetarian America*, "Vegetarians [in the early 1900s] needed to rely on role models like Mann and MacFadden [vegetarian athletes], especially when the scientific evidence proving the power of plants in the diet to prevent disease had not yet been established. Not that there wasn't plentiful anecdotal evidence, but until [later in] the twentieth century scientific evidence for the health benefits of vegetarianism was rare."[35]

One could say meat-eaters in those days at least had some excuse if they said that following a vegetarian diet had no basis in science. In contrast, so much scientific data has since been uncovered that indicates the health benefits of vegetarianism, that meat-eaters today must be willfully ignoring evidence. And once an individual refuses to look at the available science, it is very possible that person will turn to myths to reinforce his or her preferences and prejudices. As we've covered, an individual's tendency to believe in myths is compounded when cultural arbiters, such as authority figures and advertisers, do their best to give the myths a respectable front.

Now in the world of meat-eating, the most *respectable lie* is that meat is the best, perhaps only, source of complete protein. This central myth has been buttressed by a host of subsidiary myths, and false notions of what protein does, where it comes from, and what happens if you don't get enough of it. If you've thought about becoming a vegetarian, but held back from committing yourself, chances are you've been discouraged by those who believe these myths, who've warned you that you won't get enough protein if you go green.

Indeed, as Americans have taken one step forward in the health realm by exercising more, they have sometimes lost the value of this change by taking up a new myth, which is that to keep their body in shape they should become protein fanatics. Athletes have been led to believe that they need to consume massive amounts of protein for strength and endurance. They have been told that protein was stored in their muscles and that without lots of meat, milk, and protein powders to beef up those muscles they would be as weak as Samson was when he had Delilah as his barber.

But this can't be true, as was already suggested by the list of top athletes who won medals while being vegetarians. As I'll explain in a minute, many of today's athletes are loading up on carbohydrates rather than protein, and finding they can often out-compete their meat-eating rivals.

But why do people hold these mistaken views on protein? Well, for one, these industries invest in customers for life and they still get to us when we're young. I've already mentioned the food pyramid, as well as social programs aimed toward incentivizing children to use their products.

As another example, an ad run by the beef producers, for example, has actress Cybil Shepherd face to face with a hamburger, telling the audience that she's heard of people who don't eat burgers, but she doesn't know if she can trust them. The slogan is that beef is "real food for real people." Have you taken a look at some of the ingredients in the beef at your local fast food restaurant? As a reminder from chapter 2, the list includes: MSG—glutamate can cause neuronal excitation and kill brain cells; nitrates—add an artificial red color and, when cooked, creates nitrosamines, a known carcinogen. Suffice to say that based on Ms. Shepherd's criterion, real men will apparently have fewer brain cells and more tumors. Also, it's highly ironic and implausible that Shepherd, who has been an outspoken champion of gay rights and other causes that aid minorities, has little sympathy for animals. Typically, I have found these statements are made out of ignorance, for once people become aware of the cruelty conferred upon animals in the manufacturing process and the health hazards associated with this food source they oftentimes change their tune.

On the one hand, the benefits of eating meat and drinking milk are extolled, and on the other, the downsides of these products are left in the dark. To take one example, for years, milk ads have exploited the health and vibrancy of American youth in order to tout the benefits of their product. What these ads neglect to mention, though, is that beef and dairy products are filled with all sorts of chemicals and drugs, are high in cholesterol, and not easily digested.

Protein Needs

A History of Protein Testing

I've said that 19th and early 20th century vegetarians didn't yet have a scientific basis for their beliefs nor, for that matter, did meat-eaters have such a basis for their proclivities since scientists had not looked into the topic of the proper diet for humans.

Moreover, the first scientific work done in the field, work which became very influential in framing the debate was, as it turns out, according to later research, far from rigorous.

Some of the first scientific investigations in the US of protein were done in 1914, by scientists T.B. Osborne and L.B. Mandel. Their subjects were rats and, while I don't condone animal testing, their findings showed that the rats grew better on animal than on vegetable protein, from which it was extrapolated that humans needed animal protein to grow and develop properly. [36]

John A. McDougall, M.D., who we mentioned previously, a leading nutritional physician and author of *The McDougall Plan for Super Health* and *Life-Long Weight Loss*, has done extensive research on the history of the study of protein. He looked carefully at the Osborne and Mandel experiments and concluded:

> What came about was a classification which stuck with us. That classification was that animal protein was called class "A" protein or superior and vegetables were called class "B" or inferior protein. Nobody bothered to recall that these studies were based on rats, not humans.

Amino acids—the basic building blocks of proteins—were not discovered until the 1930s, and scientists tried to fit [the old assumptions and data, and explain the] poor growth of rats [with] the new finding of amino acids. When they started analyzing the various needs for amino acids of different animals they found that the rat could make 10 out of 20 amino acids, but that there were 10 amino acids that the rat could not make and had to get from its diet. So they called those the *essential* amino acids—that is, it was *essential* to get these from external sources in order to fulfill the body's needs. What they erroneously theorized, again looking back on Osborne and Mandel's work showing inferior and superior proteins, was the reason some of these proteins were inferior was because their essential amino acids were not in great enough quantity to meet the need of the rat. That is how those two theories were tied together.[37]

What is important in these early works is that the conclusions, which were later taught in US junior high and high schools as fact, were nothing more than conjectures and educated guesses. In other words, the experiments were taken as proven for humans, though no human trials had been carried out. It was simply assumed that what was learned about rodents would apply equally to humans. But, as it turns out, that's just wrong.

It took until the late 1940s before a scientist, Dr. William Rose, looked into humans' protein needs. He recorded his results in 1952, and to date, they remain the definitive authority on protein requirements for human beings.[38]

Rose fed healthy young men diets of corn starch (maize), sucrose, butterfat, vitamins, and purified amino acids to determine their protein requirements. He was quite surprised to learn that they required a mere 20 grams of protein a day, which is the equivalent of a cup of beans.

His next step was to find out which were the essential amino acids. Would they be the same 10 that rats needed? First off, he learned that adult humans could synthesize both histadine and arginine, something that could not be done by rats. Rose's actual procedure was to systematically withdraw the amino acid he was testing for from the diets of the young men. He found that if the amino acid was essential, within two days the men would become debilitated, losing their appetite and becoming nervous, irritable, and depressed.[39]

The next step Rose took was to look at what quantities of the amino acids were required for optimal human functioning. His findings on this topic are still considered valuable and, to a degree, still valid today and will be presented in the next chapter. Later scientists, as we will see, have modified some of his thoughts. But the main point here is we require far less protein than we think we do.

How Much Protein Do We Really Need?

As we saw, Rose used the rough and ready method of determining the need for amino acids simply by depriving subjects of some of them and noting his subjects' reactions. He went about determining the protein minimum in the same way. At the time, this work was groundbreaking, if rudimentary.

A more sophisticated approach is to measure the amount of nitrogen an individual uses and loses daily. Given that protein is thc only nutrient that supplies us with nitrogen, then how much nitrogen we use per day would allow a researcher to see how much protein an individual needed to replenish his or her nitrogen supply. Scientific studies conducted over the last 30 years have measured the body's "nitrogen balance." One study reached the conclusion that 20 grams of protein—only 70% of which was high quality—would be enough to maintain the body's nitrogen balance. However, finding the nitrogen balance is a complex and time-consuming process so there have been no large-scale studies to assess, for instance, the requirements of particular age groups or weight classes. And, in the same way, if one wanted to find out his or her own protein requirements, this would not be a feasible method. For this, the individual could look at a table of "guesstimations" of daily protein requirements available from health organizations, based on caloric intake and/or body weight.

Let's look at some of these "guesstimates." (By the way, the word guesstimates should *not* be taken to imply wild conjectures, but rather tinkering within a range of broadly accepted figures.) Since we have already looked at the investigations of McDougall and Rose, let's continue with their ideas before noting the requirements suggested by various world health organizations.

McDougall gives numbers on the low end of the protein requirement scale. He believes an average person's protein requirements are somewhere around 2.5% of his or her total calorie intake. If you want to find out your own requirements: start with your total calorie intake for a day. (Various online sources can give you the amount of calories of different portions of different foods.) If, for example, you burn 3,000 calories a day, your protein intake, 2.5% of the total, would be 75 calories. Since each gram of protein contains 4 calories, simply divide by four to get the number of grams of protein you would need, in this case, 18.75.[40] These figures are about the same as the *minimum* requirements determined by Dr. Rose in the 1940s, which represent about half of what he labeled as "recommended requirements."

To my own way of thinking, McDougall's minimal figures do not take into account such things as the possibility that our demands on our bodies vary, and we sometimes require more protein to meet heavy demands on the body's functioning. So, I don't think it is wise to lowball the protein requirements. Personally, I would triple Dr. McDougall's calculations, calling for 7.5% of the body's total caloric intake as an ultra-safe requirement. That way you're ready for whatever the day may bring.

Further scientific work caused the World Health Organization (WHO) to put Rose's suggested amounts of needed protein in the middle range of recommended figures. The WHO took account of the fact that people under stress or suffering from infection or injury would have higher requirements so the top edge of its recommendations are about double McDougall's numbers. The WHO sees feasible protein intake for health as generally 5% of calorie intake. Pregnant women should have 6% and 7% for nursing women. So to do a sample calculation using these figures, a non-pregnant, non-nursing adult burning 3,000 calories a day would require around 37 grams of protein. If you consume 2,300 calories a day, you'd need around 29 grams of protein. Athletes, on the other hand, need more protein and this demand is easily met since exercise increases appetite.[41]

Since we are on this topic, it might be helpful to note that other health organizations have different daily protein recommendations, usually a bit higher. A group affiliated with the National Academy of Science suggests a protein intake of .8 grams of protein per kilogram of body weight.[42] (They would be definitely referring to average weights based on a healthy individual, not overweight Americans.) This is not the same way of looking at the recommendations we have seen so far, in that it is basing the figure not on how much you eat but on how much you weigh. To get the recommendation for you, begin by converting your weight in pounds to kilograms. (If you are overweight, please refer to the chart in the back of this book in Appendix D to determine your best weight based on your height and frame size; use that for the following protein calculations.) A kilogram is equal to 2.2 pounds. This calculation gives a higher requirement for protein intake than the earlier models.

Lastly, a very complete list of protein recommendations has been worked out by the National Academy of Science. This group almost seems to be made up of protein fanatics compared to, say, McDougall. Where McDougall called for around 2.5 of one's total calories from protein, the Academy ups this by a figure four to six times, advising individuals to obtain from 10 to 15% of total calories from protein. This would give the eater approximately 0.9 grams of protein per each kilogram of body weight. The scientific institution has provided a concise table to give a general idea of suggested protein intake. Note, though in the first category of newborns, whose requirements keep changing as they grow, and who (it is assumed, but hardly accurate) are getting their protein from breast milk, the amount needed should be arrived at by multiplying kilograms of body weight by 2.2. For older ages, their recommendations are as follows:

Six months to 1 year:	kilograms of body weight times 2.2
Children, 1 to 3 years:	require 23 grams
4 to 6 years:	30 grams
7 to 10 years:	34 grams
Males, 11 to 14 years:	45 grams
15 to 51 years and over:	56 grams
Females, 11 to 18 years:	46 grams
19 to 51 years and over:	44 grams

Pregnant women need 30 extra grams per day.

Lactating women need 20 extra grams per day.

It's fairly easy to grasp why the National Academy of Science would carefully distinguish the protein needs of children and pregnant or lactating women from that of regular adults. Children require more than adults because they are building bones, muscles, and teeth until they've reached their peak growth, around the age of 18-24. Adults normally require protein primarily for maintenance and repair. Pregnant and lactating women, however, also have higher protein requirements since they are carrying or nourishing another life. Not given in their breakdown, however, are the special needs of those engaged in a regular, strenuous exercise program, especially if it includes bodybuilding. Such adults require 10% more protein than they would otherwise need. So, for example, if you would normally need 40 grams, you'd need an additional 4 grams when you embark on a serious exercise regimen.

The most striking fact is that even with the inflated figures of the National Academy of Science, we really require only moderate protein intake, especially as compared to the enormous amounts some "experts" have thought necessary. I am also trying to present a broader framework in which to determine your own unique needs. All the calculations and weight conversions may seem a bit daunting, but you will find a clearer presentation of this in the next section.

I also somewhat offhandedly mentioned that the protein amounts in different servings of food can be garnered from the Internet. If you Google "protein content of chick-peas" (as an example), you arrive at a page that provides the amount in a light grey box; there is a Wikipedia entry to the right side of the page containing more data, for which the USDA is a source. Additionally, let me say that many foods list their nutrient breakdown on the packaging, making it easy to calculate the gram amount of protein they contain. Also very handy is the United States Department of Agriculture (USDA) Handbook #8, which gives the breakdown of various nutrients in different foods and additives. It can be obtained by visiting the USDA online;[43] written copies are no longer available. Please see our reference section starting on p. 569 in this book for more information.

Calculating Your Protein Requirements

I hope the math in the last section didn't throw you. In actuality, there are only two numbers that you have to worry about, namely the percentage of protein calories your body requires and how much of your diets total calories are from proteins. In other words, how much protein do you need and how much are you getting from what you are eating?

Let's start with a rather low amount of protein, though higher than McDougall's recommendation, and look at how it works out. Say an average adult male gets 56 grams of protein from a daily intake of 2,700 calories. Let's see how many calories that protein is. Since each gram of protein has 4 calories—no matter what the source of the protein—then:[44]

56 grams (protein) x 4 (calories per gram) = 224 protein calories

Now, what percent of the man's daily consumption is protein? That can be seen by using simple division:

$$\frac{\text{224 protein calories}}{\text{2,700 calories (total intake)}} = 8.3\%$$

In this diet, which most would accept as affording a very adequate amount of protein, this man would be getting a little more than 8% of his calories in the form of protein.

Let's say our example is going to have a nice meal of lentils. He sees from the package that 100 grams of uncooked lentils will provide 24.6 grams of protein. As noted, there are 4 calories in a gram of protein, so he has 98.4 calories in the protein portion of the lentils. (There are 340 total calories in the lentils.) Now, he would like to find out what percent of the lentils are protein. He grabs his calculator and does this computation:

$$\frac{98.4 \text{ calories (protein)}}{340 \text{ calories (total)}} = 29\%$$

That's not a bad percentage of protein content, and it's also good to know that with the 98 protein calories he got from his lentils, he is well on the way to fulfilling his need for 224 protein calories a day.

Even that little bit of information should help you overcome the fear that eating a lot of lentils and no meat might quickly lead you to be low in protein and—reverting to our earlier discussion—throw you out of "nitrogen balance."[45] It's not, by the way, that protein deficiency isn't a dire problem should it occur. With "negative nitrogen balance," our bodies must break down fat or muscle tissue to release extra nitrogen. Obviously, this is not ideal, and long term effects include muscle weakness, loss of endurance, fatigue, retardation of growth, weight reduction, irritability, lowered immune response, poor healing, and anemia. Pregnant women must be especially careful to avoid this nitrogen imbalance, as it will affect not only their health but that of their unborn children as well. Protein deficiency can also cause miscarriage, premature delivery or toxemia, and its effects on the baby's development may set the stage for chronic diseases later in life.

Chilling as this thought may be, it's not something that should particularly worry vegetarians. In fact, in multiple studies in which the subjects were given only plant sources of protein, subjects were able to easily maintain proper nitrogen equilibrium.[46] Green eaters should keep in mind that eating a variety of vegetables, grains, legumes, seeds, and nuts will easily provide adequate amounts of high quality protein, even when considered from the point of view of nitrogen equilibrium. So no need for green lovers to lose sleep over protein concerns.

Still, there's something ironic about the US's recent fixation on fears of protein deficiency; in fact, problems associated with protein deficiency are rare. The irony is that many more common health problems are occurring in relation to *too much* protein in the system.

McDougall, who I am referring to regularly because he is so knowledgeable and written so eloquently on these subjects, says that the typical American diet—the one loaded with meats and sweets—could be eaten sparingly, on holidays for example, but should never be standard, everyday fare if you are concerned with good health.

It's this meat and sweets diet, promulgated by advertising and adhered to by far too many in our increasingly obese society, that makes the average American's fear of not consuming enough protein a study in absurdity.

It seems to me that one would have to be practically living on bread and water to become protein deficient. Okay, of course that is an exaggeration, but no doubt with the abundance of protein in the American diet, it is not easy to have a protein deficiency. (However, you'll see below that I differ somewhat from his views on the prevalence of protein deficiency in our society.) In fact, McDougall highlights that if someone consumed only a single vegetarian food, ate only potatoes or rice for example (two foods that are not ordinarily associated with protein), that person would still be getting 80 grams of protein in 3,000 calories of potatoes and 60 grams of protein in 3,000 calories of rice, all of which is highly usable. So if a person ate enough of these items, they would still keep their nitrogen balance.

In his book, *The McDougall Plan*, Dr. McDougall elaborates on this point, that is, on the considerable amount of protein found in foods that grace most vegetarians' diets. He provides a chart that lists how many amino acids are in each food and notes that *all* the starches and vegetables provide *all* the amino acids an individual would need.[47]

Dr. McDougall explains quite lucidly that plants have the whole package of amino acids needed to make proteins because they themselves utilize these proteins. And since McDougall sees each plant as a power-packed protein package, he does not believe that vegetarians need to worry about combining their foods in order to obtain adequate protein.

Here's one place where I take issue, in a collegial way, with McDougall. While I agree with him that knowledgeable vegetarians shouldn't be racking up sleepless nights worried about exact food combining, I do think it's important to grasp the essential key concepts of food combining. When looking at individuals, my research shows that people differ in such matters as how they metabolize foods, absorption rates, and in amino acid requirements, which may not be fulfilled by just any vegetarian food. Perhaps McDougall worries that potential vegetarians will be put off by food combining, which might seem too complex, as if it were a branch of higher mathematics. In my experience, food combining is not really difficult and, as I've seen over and over with people I have worked with, once they start eating a vegetarian diet, food combining becomes second nature. On a particularly happy note, I've also seen that the combinations that are best for individuals are usually those that taste the best to them.

One other point on which I disagree with Dr. McDougall, something I already foreshadowed in remarks given above, is his assumption that doctors no longer come across cases of protein deficiency. Several years ago, Harry Rudolph Alsiebens, M.D., and William H. Philpott, M.D., reported that in testing patients for amino acids, every single sick person they examined had severe amino acid imbalances. This was not because they were vegetarians, which they were not, but it does indicate that protein deficiencies—caused by imbalanced eating rather than too little food and too little variety of food—have not disappeared from our society.

The final point to stress is this. There would be no protein problems, whether caused by a lack or an excess of amino acids, if people had a full grasp of what foods provide the best sources of protein and ate accordingly. So let's take a closer look at that now.

The Protein Combination Project

On a couple of occasions so far, I've alluded to the fact that even if a particular vegetarian food does not have a high amount of protein on its own, when it is in a meal with other compatible foods, the combined package often has an amount of protein that is more if eating each food alone.

I began reflecting on this idea about 30 years ago. At the time, I saw the organic egg as an ideal protein provider, and used it as a blueprint against which to compare the protein resources given by high-quality proteins of non-animal origin. I chose the egg to provide a benchmark because, as I noted before, going by NPU (Net Protein Utilization), the egg knocks it out of the park with an NPU value of 94 (on a scale of 100).

Using the egg as my template, I went on to formulate the "Protein Combination Project." I looked at the distribution of amino acids in the egg and, with the help of a computer and a very savvy programmer, began to match various combinations of two or three vegetarian foods, which when eaten together would correspond to the egg's profile.

Rationale for the Protein Combination Project

What got me on the track and had me devoting years of research to this project was the simple fact, mentioned previously, that it *is* easier in one sense to get protein from meat even when its NPU is lower—one filet mignon and you're done. This discrepancy has been exaggerated by defenders of the meat diet into an earth-shaking chasm between the two diets. Vegetarians were told that by forgoing meat they risked dangerous protein deficiency. Those who weren't intimidated by this propaganda would often overcompensate by eating large amounts of particular foods, such as soy or dairy products, to get more protein into their diet.

By the 1970s, though, many vegetarians had gotten wise to this embellishment emanating from the pro-meat camp and introduced the idea of complementing vegetable proteins, combining, say, a cup of rice with a cup of beans, a grain with a legume. This was a step—but only one step—in the right direction of helping vegetarians get the full spectrum of necessary protein in their diet.

The idea of protein complementarity was developed before it was easy for the layperson, that is, someone like me who is not a mathematician, to make complex calculations, something now easy to do with the aid of the computer.

Without the help of computers, food balancing typically was addressed via the notion of the "limiting amino acid" of a protein. The "limiting amino acid" is that essential amino acid that is present in a protein in the lowest amount relative to its requirement. Though all of the other essential amino acids may be present in full measure, the effectiveness of the protein is limited to the percentage of the limiting amino acid present (relative to its requirement), since all eight amino acids have to be balanced for the protein to be effectively used by the body. So you would complement a food low in one of the eight essential amino acids, say lysine, with a food high in lysine. All the other amino acids were just presumed to fall into place.

The problem though, was that all the other amino acids might not fall into place, and then you might end up over-consuming one or more amino acids. Or if your only goal was overcoming the imbalance caused by the limiting amino acid without regard to other factors, you might end up taking in unneeded fat or calories or excess protein.

Now, however, we can use the computer to analyze how well *all* the amino acids of a given set of foods complement each other, and we can use it to rank all tested combinations in the order of those providing the highest quality protein together with the least waste of protein and calories. And that is just what we did with the Protein Combination Project. Working with mathematician Hillard Fitzky, Ph.D., we began by developing formulas for setting the computer to the task of comparing the protein patterns of over one hundred commonly eaten foods to that of the egg.

The Protein Combination Project is thus a giant leap forward from previous methods of evaluating protein quality. Instead of vague advice to mix two foods, one of which contains high amounts of the other's limiting amino acid, the project offered hundreds of food combinations in which the proportions of all essential amino acids are close to that of the egg.

Recipes Are Abundantly Available

In 1987, I devoted a book solely to this topic entitled *The Egg Project: Gary Null's Complete Guide to Good Eating*, which is now out of print, but available online. In it, I include combinations of foods that, together, provide significant amounts of complete, high-quality protein. It contains recipes which were constructed to honor the findings of the protein combination project and so replicate, in tasty, green-eating form, the measure of NPU you get from the egg.

As I mentioned previously, one of the keys to succeeding at the vegetarian lifestyle is to enjoy it, make it fun, *and* tasty, which we will explore in the upcoming chapter. The plant-based food world offers incredible potential in terms of tasty delights. One only has to visit a fine vegetarian restaurant once to know that what I'm saying is true. In fact, many of the people I have coached over the years have told me that they were surprised at the breadth and depth of this dietary program. If you aren't already one of these people that has first-hand experience with this, it is my sincere hope that you are becoming one now.

Chapter 7

The Lifestyle of a Healthy Vegetarian

"Nothing will benefit human health and increase chances for survival of life on Earth as much as the evolution to a vegetarian diet."

— *Albert Einstein, Theoretical Physicist*

In the past three chapters, we discussed the value of the vegetarian diet from a physical perspective. In this chapter and the next, we turn to investigate the mental, emotional and spiritual qualities and benefits related to the vegetarian *lifestyle*, of which the diet is one part.

I spoke at the outset of the book that health is much more than just a physical matter, even though how we feel physically day to day can make a huge difference in the quality of our life. However, the way we think about situations in life and life itself, the manner in which we process emotions common to the human experience, and our approach to resolving what happens in life and our reason for being here—so to speak—are all connected to health. So are the practices that we initiate and maintain in the healthy vegetarian lifestyle, which I will discuss in this chapter. Healthy practices lead to good health; so, the vegetarian lifestyle is an active lifestyle rather than a passive one. I know that this seems obvious, but it bears repeating since so many of us make promises to ourselves that we don't keep, or do something to sabotage any success we may be having. In Chapter 8, perhaps the most important chapter of this book, I will talk about what is needed to make and sustain change and, therefore, success in life. Entering into any new venture, including the vegetarian diet, or expanding the horizons of one's current one would not be complete without this discussion. So, I urge you to take your time with the next two chapters.

All of this, by the way, is for supporting you on your journey of healing, which comes through understanding and compassionate action. When we don't face those aspects in us that are or may be interfering with our success, we will hold ourselves back and end up being unhappy. On the other hand, when we can embrace our weaknesses, in addition to our gifts, shining a light of unconditional love and acceptance upon them, we will be naturally want to be healthier, and it becomes easier to follow through on what we set out to do.

As you will soon see, adopting the vegetarian diet is only one small aspect of living the vegetarian life. The very exciting news, however, is that by doing both *simultaneously* you improve your chances of staying on track.

We begin our discussion of the history of plant-based living by visiting both Eastern and Western traditions. As I mentioned above, understanding is the first step in addressing any situation; so, if we want to become healthy vegetarians, it would be helpful to understand the religious, social and psychological aspects that influence our choices.

How Vegetarianism Becomes a Lifestyle

Religion, Religious Beliefs, and Vegetarianism

Many people are vegetarians because they adhere to a particular religion, which practices vegetarianism. This is a very powerful environment for developing and sustaining a vegetarian lifestyle because these members are deeply entrenched in a belief system that prohibits causing intentional animal suffering. Religious values run deeply with a person, and form a cornerstone of a person's essential ideological makeup. Indeed, religious people get their primary values from their religions. Thus, if vegetarianism is one of the values of your religion, so be it. You're a vegetarian.

In my etymology of the word Ayurveda, you may have recognized the word veda, which not only means life but refers to Indian sacred texts. The links between religion, medicine and food are not accidental for, as I remarked earlier, diet has always had a place in the teachings of the world's great religions. Particular doctrines and guidelines vary, of course, but within each discipline there are specific notions taught about food. Religion has always recognized that one's spiritual awareness is affected by one's physical state; it is difficult to be pure of spirit while inhabiting a polluted body. Many religious doctrines such as Buddhism and Hinduism, and even Christianity, conveyed that a person stained his or her body by eating meat. We'll start with Western traditions since they give us the best look at why America is where it is related to the vegetarian diet.

Western Traditions

Western religions, with a few exceptions, have not and do not promote vegetarianism. Those historical figures that did tended to be the great thinkers—the doctors like Hippocrates and the philosophers like Pythagoras, Heraclitus and Plato, as well as Epicurus, the Aristotelian biologist Theophrastus, Ovid, Seneca, the poet Virgil, and Plutarch. Then, there was Plotinus, the most influential of the Neoplatonists, whose metaphysics influenced greatly the theological doctor of the Church, St. Augustine of Hippo, who believed that humans were required by divine decree to treat animals with compassion because they also suffered and felt pain and pleasure. These prophets, rather than clergy, were the ones who redirected the violence of the day toward a peaceful city state or kingdom kindness, where respect was due to all members of society, which extended to the kind treatment of animals and a preference towards a vegetarian diet over the slaughter of animals for their meat. As a side note, perhaps the most thorough early treatise in defense of vegetarianism is *On Abstinence from Killing Animals,* by another Neoplatonist philosopher, Porphyry of Tyre, in the third century of the Christian era.

Following Emperor Constantine's conversion experience to the religion of Jesus at the Battle of Milvian Bridge in AD 312, Christianity became the religion of the empire and expanded precipitously across Europe. The Pythagorean, Orphic, late Platonic, and Epicurean mysteries, which had constantly reminded humanity about its deep connection with Nature, were severed and replaced with the objective to *renounce the pull of the earth* and strive solely for a heavenly future in the afterlife. Many advocates of vegetarianism today blame the Judeo-Christian traditions for permitting violence against animals and encouraging meat as a major source of sustenance.

Interestingly, western societies at that time, including both Greek and Roman, were largely plant-based, but out of *necessity*—pure economics; most could not afford meat. Those nobility topping the hierarchy—former warriors with a learned routine of pillaging and violence—were the meat-eaters. Over time, the people of the church and mercantile classes rose in status. But that wasn't always the case. Early Christian monasteries in Europe insisted that monks refrain from animal flesh. To a great extent this expression of vegetarianism was found in the stories and legends about ascetic saints known as the Desert Fathers in the Egyptian desert, St. Anthony the Great and St. Pachomius, the founder of cenobite or community-based monasticism, being two of the most famous of early Christian mystics and vegetarians. The tales of courageous warrior monks' escapades, struggling against phantoms and demons in the desert, and seemingly transcending the limitations of the human body, became widely popular across Christianized Europe. Once heard, countless young men were inspired to leave home and join the monastic ranks seeking an everlasting life through solitude, austerities and simple meatless diets. The earlier Greek and Roman philosophers of a vegetarian lifestyle were not role models; rather, vegetarianism found its exemplar in the Biblical image of John the Baptist, who survived solely on the fruits of the land.

The monasteries would not remain simple rural refuges for prayer and contemplation. As the Middle Ages progressed, they became enormously wealthy and possessors of huge tracts of land that could encompass villages and employ hundreds of serfs and peasants. Abbots and monks also became increasingly powerful in village politics, and the practice of abstaining from meat for ethical and spiritual reasons died out. Instead this class of "monk lords" transformed into new privileged elite, a form of nobility whose lives were more in common with a banker, corporate CEO or politician today. In 1339, even the Pope had to surrender further papal attempts to enforce vegetarianism in the monasteries. There were several attempts to revive spiritually-based vegetarianism but these were marginal. St. Francis of Assisi, Catherine of Sienna, and Angela Merici are several examples of vegetarians and spiritual reformers who attempted to return the faithful to living by the virtues of simplicity and service to others.

Vegetarianism as an ethical and spiritual principle would only appear again during the Italian Renaissance. This time it was not regarded as an austere means to reach paradise, but from the rediscovery and resurrection of the Greek and Roman classical authors after the Church had consigned them to the darker regions of a forgotten oblivion. Pythagoras, Plato, Plotinus and Paracelsus again provided light to European civilization, along with the lost writings advocating the virtues of vegetarianism. Among some of the better known vegetarians during this period were Leonardo da Vinci, the astronomer and humanist Marsilio Ficino, and Giovanni Pico della Mirandola who began the Hermetic Renaissance of natural philosophy. These and many other Renaissance philosophers, humanists and scientists who revived the virtues of vegetarianism would set the course for the later paradigm shift in thought that became known as the Enlightenment and ushered in our modern industrial age. Since then, there have been a smattering of advocates, but nothing like what is rising today in secular factions of the US.

The purpose of this illustration, in part, is to set forward the contrast of Western to Eastern religions and cultures and their connection to the environment and health, which is the central theme of the next several sections. I spoke briefly at the beginning of the book about the intimate connection between man and nature fostered by Eastern religions that promote vegetarianism. This is a sharp contrast to the western reality I have just described. Bron Taylor, Editor-in-Chief of the *Encyclopedia of Religion and Nature,* a widely acclaimed tome that critically explores the relationships among human beings, their environments, and the religious dimensions of life, noted[1] in support:

> In environmental studies it has commonly been assumed that there exists a fundamental connection between a society's management of natural resources and its perception of nature. With the publication of "The Historical Roots of Our Ecologic Crisis" (1967) [Professor] Lynn White was among the first to focus more narrowly on the relationship between the state of the environment and religion, postulating a direct linkage between the two. He blamed mainstream Christianity—in particular Judeo-Christian cosmology of man's mastery of nature—for the environmental ills facing the world today.

Indeed, with the exception of peasants, who had direct and daily contact with nature which they linked intimately to their survival, most Westerners have lost their cyclic view of life and of living in harmony with nature. But there are two Western religions worth mentioning here that stand to break the curse.

Christianity: Seventh-Day Adventists

While many later Christian and Jewish denominations forgot the importance of green eating, others stayed the course and have made vegetarianism central to their belief systems. In the US, one of the more significant of these is the Seventh-day Adventist Church, a Christian denomination that, since its formal establishment in 1863, has preached the benefits of whole vegetarian foods. This faith, sharing the belief mentioned above, holds that a strong, pure body is essential to the spiritual aspirant. What one eats is as important as how one prays because both are ways of communicating with the divine.

The church grew out of the Millerites, a sect that began in the 1840s in the US, nurtured by the belief that Christ would return to earth in October 1844. When this didn't happen, many dropped out, but a younger group, including Ellen C. White, renamed the church, and introduced a number of novel practices, such as celebrating the Sabbath on Saturday and adopting a vegetarian diet. White felt, "Vegetables, fruits and grains should compose our diet… The eating of flesh is unnatural. Many die of disease caused wholly by meat-eating; yet, the world does not seem to be the wiser. The moral evils of a flesh diet are not less marked than are the physical ills. Flesh food is injurious to health and whatever affects the body has a corresponding effect on the mind and soul."[2]

It should be noted that green eating is not mandatory for church members but about half of the current church membership is orthodox insofar as they are strict vegetarians, meaning no animal products, and only vegetarian meals are served in Church-run hospitals and colleges. In fact, because green eating is not widespread in the US, the Seventh-day Adventists have been very useful to scientists studying the value of this eating style since they can investigate the church's large membership of approximately 1.1 million to determine what health effects arise from adopting life-long green eating.[3] The results are encouraging to say the least. Researchers have conducted a number of mortality studies and found strong evidence that church members are significantly healthier than America's non-vegetarian norm. Adventists have substantially lower incidence of common degenerative ailments like heart and respiratory disease and substantially lower cancer rates as well.[4]

Judaism: Hebraic Tradition

While orthodox Jews follow kosher food regulations, which were laid out in the Bible, these do not preclude the eating of meat. They do emphasize that the preparation, consumption, and even storage of food are of utmost spiritual concern. Meat and dairy products must be neither eaten nor cooked together. Likewise, meat and dairy dishes and cooking utensils are kept separate. Animals and poultry must be carefully inspected before and after slaughter, and if found imperfect, they are rejected. Slaughter follows strict guidelines, and afterwards, the blood is thoroughly drained. Food selection and handling are treated seriously, and there are moral and ethical overtones to the strict dietary awareness of all who follow the Judaic tradition.[5]

Included in these regulations are ones that direct butchers to treat animals with compassion, even though they are to be killed for food. Among the rules is one that instructs that an animal should never be allowed to be thirsty for the sake of reducing its food intake, and another that tells an owner never to shout at an animal. Linked to this compassion for animals is the religion's belief that the body is the host of the spirit, and that food is not merely a fuel but a contributor to the body's spiritual essence.[6]

Many Jews, nonetheless, go one better on the level of compassion required of the conventional Jew by becoming vegetarians. Psychology professor Dr. Louis A. Berman notes that in the Talmudic writings, Jews are taught that, "danger to life nullifies all religious obligations." He feels that this principle is one of the cornerstones of a longstanding Jewish preference for vegetarianism. Join the already noted compassion for animal life to a belief some hold that eating meat can endanger health, and you have a thoughtful basis for Jewish vegetarianism.

Eastern Traditions

Indeed, for more than 7000 years the East has had an intimate connection with nature. They were not impacted by the Dark Ages—marked by great cultural and religious strife—as Western and Eastern Europe were, nor by Christian beliefs of dominance over nature. Their cultures were largely undisturbed, that is, until the 17th-18th century when they underwent colonization at the hands of the Europeans, and were subjugated to growing crops demanded by the West, such as tea, spices, and other commodities. As such, those in the East would have continued to eat in correspondence with their religious beliefs, and what was historically popular, including a rich heritage of growing, cultivating, and fermenting foods long before there was any concept of fermentation in the West. By this time, Easterners had already been using fermented foods for more than a thousand years, and were living long lives; in fact, they were among the longest life spans on earth.

You may recall in the previous section on Western Traditions, I quoted Bron Taylor, Editor-in-Chief of the *Encyclopedia of Religion and Nature* regarding the link between Judeo-Christianity and the loss of connection to nature. Taylor continues his overview but cautions about oversimplifying an extremely complex matter:

> Asian and indigenous concepts of nature are not less complex than their Western counterparts, and it is therefore dangerous to generalize. Nonetheless, whether looking at indigenous traditions or Asian religious creeds, scholars of such worldviews have almost invariably stressed that they are what Christianity allegedly is far removed from, namely, being *eco*centric and monistic, promoting a sense of harmony between human beings and nature. Christianity in contrast is portrayed as anthropocentric and dualistic, promoting a relation of dominating nature rather than one that is harmonious. By focusing on how these traditions are different from Western ones, the non-Western religions meet the demand for new ecological paradigms that unite man and the environment as parts of one another.[7]

Swami B.V. Tripurari, an American author, poet, and guru, echoes these sentiments in his book, *Ancient Wisdom for Modern Ignorance*, by stating, "Our present environmental crisis is in essence a spiritual crisis."[8] According to HinduWisdom.info,

Hinduism "has always been an environmentally sensitive philosophy. No religion, perhaps, lays as much emphasis on environmental ethics as Hinduism. Well-known works of eastern literature such as *The Mahabharata, Ramayana, Vedas, Upanishads, Bhagavad Gita, Puranas* and *Smriti* contain the earliest messages for preservation of environment and ecological balance. Nature, or Earth, has never been considered a hostile element to be conquered or dominated. In fact, man is forbidden from exploiting nature. He is taught to live in harmony with nature and recognize that divinity prevails in all elements, including plants and animals."[9]

We've seen already that the belief in reincarnation—that one may be born again in the form of a human child, but also a wolf cub, puppy, or other animal—is widespread in Eastern religions and provides a strong, mystical backing for their vegetarianism. Westerners tend to classify this idea as quaint or outlandish, never stopping to consider that some of their own religious beliefs might seem on the quaint side to those not raised in them. For instance, Christians believe their founder rose from the dead, flew through the sky and turned water into wine, never thinking anyone would see this as outlandish.

The point here is to look at the *ramifications* of the belief, not its credibility, and we have seen that a faith in reincarnation has had the most compassionate repercussions. Those that cherish this belief find the division between human and non-human animal life arbitrary; they also recognize the value of treating fellow humans with dignity and compassion for similar reasons. Of course, they acknowledge that one has to make distinctions among various categories of living beings, such as man, animal, fish, and insects, and what we've found over history is that humans have different relationships with animals they have domesticated. Yet, as they see it, at a deeper level, every being possesses a soul. There is a basic continuum, with each being (soul) taking on various attributes at different times, in different embodiments. One of the basic axioms of Hinduism and Jainism is that the soul does not die but simply leaves the body, moving from host to host.[10] With this belief, the two religions hold that the intentional killing of animals is a grave transgression against the spiritual law that binds the universe since it is destroying the embodiment of a soul. Such killing shows a culpable disregard for the oneness of all beings, misled by their apparent and transitory separateness.

To reiterate, let's disregard what might seem quaint in this idea and hone to its deeper message, which is not very different from the concerns of universal love and kindness to fellow creatures preached in Judaism and Christianity. The inner depth of this sensibility is well presented in *Vegetarianism and Occultism* by C.W. Leadbeater. In this poignant work, Leadbeater, a former clergyman turned spiritualist discusses the reverence for life that explains the preference for vegetarianism among Eastern religions: "The man who ranges himself on the side of evolution realizes the wickedness of destroying life; for he knows that, just as he is here in this physical body in order that he may learn the lessons of this plane, so is the animal occupying his body for the same reason, and through it he may gain experience at his lower stage. He knows that the life behind the animal is Divine Life, that all life in the world is Divine; the animals therefore are truly our brothers."[11]

Today, as our world becomes increasingly global and Westernized, religious traditions are fading, as are their influences over food choice. The choice to become vegetarian in the East today is largely related to economic necessity or activism, whether for human or animal rights, or environmental concern.

In India, about 78% of the nation is Hindu,[12] just over 30% are vegetarian;[13] diets in India are largely predicated on geography and socio-economic status, and are still largely plant-based due to widespread poverty. Although vegetarianism has never been a requirement for Hindus, as Indians become more mobile, and the world becomes increasingly westernized, younger generations of Hindus who were raised in strictly vegetarian homes are now forsaking their traditions and consuming meat.

While modern Hindus eat more meat than ever before, most know that vegetarianism promotes spiritual life; in fact, it is expected that religious leaders such as Brahmins, swamis and others are strict vegetarians. However, despite Hindu beliefs that cows are sacred—and the fact that their slaughter is banned in most of the country—India is the world's fifth-largest consumer and second-largest exporter of beef.[14] It is also host, sadly, to some of the most barbaric and cruel treatment of animals known to humankind today—because of the fact that in most parts of the country it is illegal to kill cattle.

I will not go into the gruesome details of this now; however, I bring this up in support of the discussion I am forwarding in these two chapters related to the importance of adopting the vegetarian *lifestyle* as opposed to just the vegetarian diet—which in and of itself is a tremendous accomplishment in this day and age. Adopting the vegetarian diet, alone, would be a terrific start. However, without giving equal attention to growing into sustainable practices that support basic quality and equality of life for all beings while preserving the Earth's natural resources, we will not be successful in what we are aiming to accomplish, which is, essentially, the elevation of human consciousness to a level where we could improve our chances of perpetuating as a species, barring, of course, any unforeseen interstellar catastrophe.

Buddhism

Some may take aim at my previous remarks about the substantiality of Eastern Religions—that, no matter how influential they have been in the past, they probably no longer have much weight, at least in countries in the Far East that have been modernizing. However, any more than a casual look shows that vegetarianism still has its place in China and in Westernized Japan; however, it is a much smaller presence than its 1500-year Buddhist heritage might suggest. While China is host to nearly 50 million vegetarians and growing, in 2012 the nation consumed a full quarter of the global meat supply, and the practice of raising dogs for food is still prevalent in China. Every year in June, the southern Chinese city of Yulin celebrates the summer solstice with a dog-eating festival, where it is estimated that around 10,000 dogs are killed.[15]

Yet, vegetarianism in China is a popular movement, mostly because of ecologically conscious young people who are choosing veganism out of concern for health, humaneness and the environment, plus to stay thin and attractive. Putting this into perspective, however, that is less than 4% of China's population. Until recently, vegetarianism is owed partly to general food shortages is some areas, or food prices, since vegetables are less expensive than meat in these countries.

Additionally, more of a plant-based diet has persisted as a result of extremely dense populations and limited arable acreage, due to pollution as well as ongoing drought conditions in certain parts of the nation. These observers would go on to point out that fish and pork are popular, and that a growing number of people can afford them. And, China's government is helping with this: in February 2014, China's main regulatory body, the State Council, announced a new policy away from grain production toward meat, vegetable and fruit production. For the first time, the country produced less grain than consumer demand.[16] This suggests that the majority of today's Chinese are vegetarians of necessity or out of environmental concern rather than religious doctrine.

Japan is not that much different, outside of Buddhist temples and communities. The traditional Japanese diet is non-dairy vegetarian, sometimes poultry and eggs, and fish of all types, including eel and squid. But meat and dairy emerged later on the scene as the country succumbed to Western influences. While you might think there would be a lot of vegetarians in Japan, or people who care about animal welfare, this is not the case. According to the premier vegetarian magazine *Veggie* in Japan, the number is around 5% of the population and, according to an article in the *Japan Times*, most go to vegetarian restaurants because of health reasons rather than ethical or religious reasons.[17] In fact, a small contingency of vegetarians are now rallying restaurants in Japan to offer meatless fare.[18] One of the group's founders stated: "We don't want to increase the number of vegetarian restaurants; we want vegetarian food to be served in normal restaurants. This hardly exists at present. People think vegetarians are strange and only eat salad."

In spite of the culture's reluctance to embrace a meat-free diet, over the past decade there has been a rise in popularity in vegetarian and vegan foods alongside a boom in macrobiotic food, which has led to the opening of about 500 vegetarian and macrobiotic (which also serve meat) cafés and restaurants.[19] Still, while some underpinnings of Buddhism remain, and peasants in the Chinese countryside exist more so on an austere vegetarian diet, both of these cultures have largely "Westernized" their diets, and consume meat as their economic status allows, even though religious edicts promote a reluctance to sustain life by killing fellow creatures, for the same reasons noted in the previous section.

Buddhism and Macrobiotics

Japan is a very interesting case study with respect to vegetarianism because it is there that the macrobiotic diet was popularized by George Ohsawa. Ohsawa was severely ill as a teenager when he first came across the work of the late 19th-early 20th century Japanese army doctor, Sagen Ishizuka, who prescribed for his patients a traditional Japanese diet of whole, unrefined, natural foods eaten in season. Ishizuka also strongly emphasized the proper balancing of dualistic dietary yin-yang elements, especially sodium and potassium, in eating. Ohsawa's application of the diet cured him, and he went on to name it "Macrobiotics," and to develop and promote it, writing some 300 books on the subject.

The yin and yang principles were not originated by Ohsawa, but flow through many older philosophical systems such as those of the pre-Socratic Greek or Chinese Chan (Zen) Buddhism.

This last doctrine has given most attention to how these opposed yin and yang principles function in everyday life, particularly in health. Zen Buddhism holds there should be a fine balance between the sides of the opposition, which, if maintained, creates physical and spiritual harmony. These yin and yang forces do not only function in the energetics of the body, but are thought to apply in the whole universe, which is governed by these principles. Yin is the passive element, responsible for such qualities as silence, stillness, cold, and darkness. Foods with yin qualities promote relaxation and restful expansion. Yang is the active element, responsible for sound, motion, heat, and light. Foods with yang qualities promote activity.[20]

Extreme (energetic) yang foods are eggs, meat, poultry, and salt. Extreme (restful) yin foods include sugar, chocolate, honey, saccharine, alcohol, refined flour, tropical fruits, and chemicals such as most food additives and drugs.[21] Both of these extreme classes of foods, being so powerful, when consumed will tend to unbalance the body system; so, according to Ohsawa, we should try to stay away from them. We should instead look for foods in the middle of the spectrum. Ohsawa feels that grains, especially rice, are the most balanced and health-promoting of foods.

Like the doctrine of transmigration, the yin-yang system teaches that both energies are found in human, animal, plant, and inorganic substances equally, thus affirming a cosmic unity, and obligating us (humans) to foster it not disturb it.

Hinduism

As Christianity originally developed out of Judaism, so Buddhism grew out of Hinduism. And that is not the only progeny of this world religion that has been a tremendous positive force. Yoga, another offshoot, combines meditative movement and postures (both seated and standing), and breathing techniques with a vegetarian regimen. As vegetarianism was first embraced by Americans for its health effects and only later acknowledged for its ethical and environmental components, similarly yoga first became known to the West for the value of its movement component. But today many people in our part of the world embrace it also for its spiritual teachings and insights, which are rooted in the Hindu/Buddhist theory of reincarnation as well as the practice of *ahimsa*, which is Sanskrit for "not to injure." The essence of ahimsa, therefore, is nonviolence toward all living beings and things, including planet Earth. As such, it implies the same relationship to vegetarianism as discussed in the previous sections on Hinduism and Buddhism. The yogi, like other believers in the transmigration of souls, presumes that all living beings go through a series of rebirths, taking on many forms. It is not surprising, then, that meat eating and all other violent behavior, is said to bring on negative karma, and is therefore strictly forbidden for true practitioners.[22] A traditional vegetarian yogic diet may emphasize fruits or vegetables or fermented dairy products, but any of its configurations shun meat, which is felt to be toxic, both physically and spiritually. Informed modern day practitioners recognize the appalling and heartbreaking plight of dairy cows—organically raised or otherwise—today and refrain from consuming dairy products altogether.

Another Indian religious practice with close ties to Hinduism, which has gathered a significant following in the US is the New Vrindaban International Society for Krishna Consciousness. While the group has ties to the teachings of Lord Chaitanya dating back five centuries, it was founded in 1966 by his Divine Grace A.C. Bhaktivedanta Swami Prabhupada.

A key practice for Krishna devotees is to seek religious revelation and ecstasy by chanting the Maka mantra. One cannot just begin chanting, though. They must first prepare oneself by living a "clean" life, adhering to four rules of conduct: no gambling, no intoxication, no extramarital sex, and no meat eating. The last rule is similar to that of Zen Buddhism in the adoption of vegetarianism but also in its classification of food types. While the Buddhist splits between yin and yang dishes, the Krishna disciples contrast the deleterious meat foods to *prasadam* or "mercy" foods—the fruits, grains, and vegetables that possess special purifying and spiritually stimulating qualities, especially when ceremoniously blessed.[23]

A third Hinduism-related group, the Rajneesh Foundation, based in Maharashtra, India, also embraces vegetarianism. Its founder, Bhagwan Shree Rajneesh, teaches, same as the Krishna doctrine, that physical purification must precede spiritual evolution. The first step in this process is to refrain from eating anything dead, as it deadens character. Also, Rajneesh explains, eating something that has come to us through violence only instills in us a violent and aggressive nature. The vegetarian is believed to be more graceful, and more at ease with his environment and fellow creatures because his diet consists of foods that are whole and alive.

Rajneesh describes the difference between eating and abstaining from meat poetically: "Vegetarianism is a form of purification. When you eat animals, you become heavy and gravitate towards earth. A light vegetarian diet, in contrast, gives more grace and power. Rather than gravitate, you levitate towards the sky. Like a person who is going to climb a mountain, the lighter the load, the easier the ascent. Why carry more than you have to?"[24]

Islam: Sufiism

Taking a look at the Middle East, we might consider the Islamic Sufi sect. This group practices vegetarianism for a reason that might seem the utmost antithetical to ideas held in the industrialized West—that of voluntary simplicity and eschewal of materialism. The name of the group itself, originating from the undyed wool garments called "sufi" that adherents traditionally wore, symbolizes their orientation. These clothes were uncomfortable and hence demonstrated a disregard for the comforts of the flesh, a disdain that was believed to be pleasing to Allah. Modern Western Sufis are not the ascetics like their forbearers, nor do they follow all the traditional rituals. However, some still do practice the famous whirling dancing of the "dervishes"—Sufis who seek to elevate their level of consciousness beyond the physical realm through ecstatic dancing. Further, most still adhere to vegetarianism, another cherished element of simple, close-to-the-earth living. Their meatless diet, similar to that of the yogi, helps them approach unity with God and the natural world.[25]

Secular: The Vegan Society

Finally, let me bring up The Vegan Society, founded in England in 1944. While it calls itself a purely secular organization, its emphasis on nonviolence and reverence for life gives it a strongly spiritual cast. Members of the Vegan society do not eat any animal products and try to limit their diet to the most wholesome, alive, energy-filled foods. They emphasize unaltered, unprocessed, whole foods, such as raw vegetables and fruits, nuts, seeds, and grains, while eschewing alcohol, tea, coffee, soda, processed foods, and the use of tobacco.[26] This regimen stems, not from a desire to get right with God, but from a desire to promote harmony with nature and other humans.

All the aforementioned religions believe that to live in a world without connection is suicidal. But this is the world of the meat eater who believes they have NO connection to the animal's suffering, the slaughterhouses, the waste of the world's land, water and energy resources, and the starvation in poorer parts of the world when they bite into a beef steak or a chicken leg. This perception of disconnection, and separation, is incorrect, and is the real meaning of the word "sin" in the Bible. Sadly, we humans have come to think only of the word sin in moral context when its true meaning points to something far more profound and vastly consequential. It is the separation from life itself, and why I say it is suicidal. The individuals who are not aware of this connection, that they, indeed, are a part of the grand matrix, are unwittingly lying to themselves all the while committing acts of destruction, which pollute and destroy their world, and the world at large.

When we believe that our actions are not connected to all of life, it becomes possible for us to perform all sorts of life-depleting behaviors, including the unnecessary killing of animals for food.

The world religions we have been examining recognized this error long ago, and see that the mindless slaughter of innocent animals to fill an imaginary dietary need loosens the spiritual bonding of the earth's living beings. The violence, the bloodshed, and the suffering create a negative psychic wave that begins in the animal factories and slaughterhouses and ripples throughout the world through those who choose to partake of their flesh.

Amid this spiritual malaise, religions and humanitarian groups have tried to promote the vegetarian way of life as the healthful antidote required by individuals and society alike. For if the human body is a temple housing our spiritual core, how can the core remain pure if the housing is polluted? True, whole grains give us substance, sprouts and juices offer us energy, and vegetables provide the variety and vitality essential to good health. But even more, a wholesome vegetarian diet is the underpinning of the harmonious relationship of body, mind, and spirit. Where the meat eater rips away at these connections and lives in denial, the vegetarian finds and sustains such connections, intent on reweaving the bonds between all living beings and nature itself in the light of truth.

Even before scientific evidence was available, many vegetarians would base their arguments in favor of going green on anthropology, that is, by looking at the health of people in other, primarily vegetarian societies. As we've examined, religion is one determiner of vegetarianism, while cultural norms and economic status are another.

Recent scientific literature has looked into the older history of such civilizations as the Hindu and Japanese, where for thousands of years, neither meat nor dairy products were consumed. According to meat-eaters, these cultures should have disappeared as people died from lack of protein, but instead they flourished. Some historians even claim that the healthiest civilizations are those in which the people lead essentially vegetarian lifestyles, eating little or no meat.

In fact, rather than making an eater more robust than a vegetarian, there is much evidence that eating meat makes a person weaker. Dr. John McDougall, whose vegetarian diet we will further discuss below, cites evidence from non-industrialized countries with lower protein consumption indicating that their populations suffer fewer broken bones caused by brittleness.

Vegetarians Around the World

I just finished presenting world religions such as Hinduism and Buddhism that put a great emphasis on the value of vegetarianism, which, if not strictly mandated for their followers, is nonetheless considered the higher path. I brought up the topic of the general health of populations that put little or no stress on meat or dairy. My emphasis then was on the interface between religious belief, eating patterns, and overall health.

In that discussion, I hardly exhausted what I have to say about vegetarian-tending peoples and health. Although before I proceed, let me add another caveat, which is that in assessing people's health, we have to acknowledge that many factors are involved—such as genetic influence, activity and exercise levels, access to basic health and dental care, food and other resources, general stress levels, sanitation and hygiene, the physical environment, as well as community infrastructure and support that, along with diet, influence health. That said; let's look at some cases where vegetarianism is associated with positive health outcomes.

The Hunza people of northern Pakistan are often cited for their excellent health. A 1963 *Lancet* article described the life-promoting regimen of these mostly vegetarian people who live at altitudes of 2,000-8,000 feet, deep in the valley of Kaghan, Gilgit, Hunza and other mountainous areas of northwest Pakistan. Consuming the simplest possible diets of wheat, corn, potatoes, onions, nuts and fruits, and some yogurt and milk, they trudge up and down the rough mountain paths for anything up to fifty miles a day. They have existed thus for perhaps many thousands of years to ages of 130, and even 145, free of obesity and cavities, and sure to enjoy long, healthy lives.[27]

Another population that includes a good many people who eat a plant-based diet is found in Mainland China. I earlier noted that this was a kind of *involuntary vegetarianism*, since "some observers feel that this is partly owing to general food shortages… the result of extremely dense populations and limited arable acreage." According to William H. Adolph, professor of biochemistry at Yenching University in Beijing, vegetarianism was hardly one the population would have volunteered for. He wrote this in a 1938 *Scientific American* article:

> For centuries China has unconsciously been working out a vast food experiment from which the Western World can learn practical lessons. [This experiment] … involved not merely a few… human subjects sheltered in the artificial comforts of the nutrition laboratory, but it boasted several millions of Chinese peasants as experimental subjects… not over a few weeks but over a score or more of centuries.[28]

While not an experiment we'd want to replicate in total, in that low food rations, even of rice, for peasants were often imposed by rapacious landlords that in poor crop years could lead to starvation, the results are eye-opening. The conclusion is that when vegetarian food supplies were adequate, health was maintained. Even now it is estimated that Chinese peasants get 95% of their protein from vegetable sources and hundreds of millions of them have maintained good health on such a diet. The mainstay of the peasant diet is rice, and meat and dairy products are seldom counted in as part of meals. Both of these Western staples are prohibitively expensive and the large scale raising of livestock too wasteful of energy and natural resources to be countenanced.[29] This diet explains why the Chinese expression for eating, in Cantonese "sik fan," means, translated literally "eat rice."

We've spoken extensively about what it takes to heal our bodies using fortifying plant-based foods, but what about healing our mind and spirit too—our whole person. This is what we will talk about now, because any discussion on healing devoid of these topics will fall short in achieving the end desire—a fully integrated human being.

The Conscious Path: Healing Minds and Hearts

Which came first…? It has been suggested that many people become vegetarian because of the way they see and think about the world, in other words, they are sensitive to the plight of all living beings, including Mother Earth, and choose vegetarianism. Then, there are those who begin on the vegetarian path by assimilating the diet, perhaps for health reasons, and then become more sensitized to their needs and the need of others and the environment *because* of the food.

So far, we have spoken only about the healing of the body that occurs because of vegetarianism, but there are also implications to our mind, emotions, and spirit when we adopt a non-violent lifestyle.

Other Aspects of a Healthy Vegetarian Lifestyle

There are many practices associated with the vegetarian lifestyle worth noting. Essentially, it is a lifestyle rooted in actions toward what is natural, not just to the true nature of humans, but also to what is natural in the world at large. Many of these practices are inherent to Eastern religions, so reading from that genre will facilitate a more-in-depth understanding. Many of the aspects you will read about below may be obvious in terms of their role in health, but they bear repeating given the mounting challenges we face in our nation related to lifestyle diseases.

Rest & Sleep

Rest and sleep are different, but let me speak about sleep first. Sleep is necessary for repair and rejuvenation, and those with chronic insomnia must find a solution in order to maintain their quality of life. Most people don't know that chronic insomnia predisposes people to an early death. Therefore, from the perspective of having a healthy and long life, restoring good sleeping patterns is essential.

Sleep is a smooth condition made up of a series of changes that take place during the sleeping phase. Each phase has its own unique brain wave patterns. Of special interest is the rapid eye movement (REM) period, the stage when dreams occur. REM periods are, in turn, subdivided into approximately 5 periods. The deepest levels of sleep occur during the third and fourth phases. As we grow older, the length of sleep during these phases diminishes.

Insomnia can be explained as difficulty either initiating or maintaining sleep—or both. It affects millions of people and is often hard to treat. Those with insomnia feel as though they have not had sufficient sleep upon awakening, which usually results in fatigue, irritability, and decreased concentration, just to name a few symptoms. Additionally, studies indicate that stimulants such as caffeine and nicotine contribute to insomnia by making it harder for the brain to achieve the state of relaxation needed for sleep. The amount of time it takes the body to break down 50% of a dose of caffeine is between three and seven hours; larger amounts and/or repeated doses of caffeine lead to slowed caffeine clearance, causing caffeine's effects to last even longer.[30] As a result, caffeine consumption can impair sleep for many hours. Keep in mind that elderly people may need less sleep than younger adults, who should be sleeping, on average, between 6 to 8 hours per day. This is a typical change connected to age and should not be considered a sleep disorder in a healthy person.

Rest on the other hand is related to allowing the body to experience relaxation while in the waking state. The body needs regular rest intervals throughout the day, about every 90 minutes according to performance specialist Terry Lyles, Ph.D., author of the soon to be released book *Cracking the Stress Code: Eliminate Harmful Stress and Achieve Life Mastery in 4 Simple Steps*. Dr. Lyles says, "We often regard physical energy as a scarce resource that we must carefully guard and conserve. In reality, physical energy is an abundant resource that our bodies manufacture constantly through food, hydration, and work/rest cycles throughout the day and sufficient sleep. The critical issue is in how we expend our energy and in the energy manufacture/expenditure balance that we maintain. That balance determines the level and consistency of our daily performance." Speaking to the science of physiology, Dr. Lyles goes on to say: "Blood sugar and glucose levels are regulated in three-hour modules and must be balanced by regular food intake and recovery breaks. Otherwise our energy levels will diminish."[31] He also notes that mental performance is the highest just after a break. All you need is a few minutes to disengage, walk around the block or the office, stand up and do some stretches, and you will markedly increase your wellbeing and performance levels. Dr. Lyles has researched sleep as it correlates to performance in professional athletes and highly recommends that no phones, televisions, computers, clocks, or other electronic devices be in your bedroom when sleeping; they disrupt natural sleeping patterns. If you have to get up to go to the bathroom or for any reason, do not look at a clock as it will immediately take you out of a sleep state into a cognitive state, thereby disrupting the sleep pattern altogether.

Pure Water

You can go many weeks without food, but only a few days without water. Of all the components necessary for life, water is second only to oxygen in importance. It is present in all tissues, including teeth, fat, bone, and muscle. It is the medium of all body fluids, such as blood, digestive juices, lymph, urine, and perspiration. It is a lubricant for the saliva, the mucous membranes, and the fluid that bathes the joints. And it regulates body temperature. Water also prevents dehydration, flushes out toxins and wastes, supplies the body with oxygen and nutrients, and aids muscle cells in producing energy.

The average body contains 40 to 50 quarts of water, with 40% of that water inside cells. Lean people have a higher percentage of body water than heavier people do, men have a higher percentage than women, and children have a higher percentage than adults. Water is our life's blood. Indeed, 83% of our blood is water. With a loss of 5% of body water, skin shrinks and muscles become weak. The loss of less than a fifth of body water is fatal. On average, the adult body consists of between 55 to 75% water. Approximately two-thirds of a person's weight is water. Each day you must replace between 2 to 3 quarts of water in your body.

How much water do you need?

Although water occurs naturally in most vegetarian foods, it must be consciously included in our daily diets. Include 8 glasses, 8 to 10 ounces each, every day. To rehydrate after exercise, drink one glass of water every 20 minutes for the first hour, then one glass for several hours afterward. Your body will determine how much it needs; it will absorb water at a particular rate and eliminate whatever is excess. Eating a high-protein diet results in the body eliminating water. If you are not a vegetarian, it's especially crucial to keep careful track of water. Caffeine drinks like Red Bull®, coffee and iced tea also act as diuretics, resulting in dehydration.

Lastly, drinking during meals, in a sense, can "drown" your enzymes, reducing their strength. When foods are dry, it is better to allow extra salivation prior to swallowing, to moisten them, rather than washing them down with liquids. Drink before meals and then wait up to 2 hours after to drink. Eating green and succulent vegetables with a meal also will help provide natural water or lubricate dry foods.

Organic Foods

The organic food industry is one of the fastest growing industries in the country. It has grown about 20% a year for the past 7 years. Dr. Elson Haas, a practicing integrative medicine physician and director of the Preventive Medical Center of Marin in San Rafael, California, tells about the many benefits of organic food. In several studies, he says, organic foods are shown to have higher levels of nutrients, vitamins, and minerals. For example, flavonoids, which are plant by-products effective in preventing cancer, heart disease, and a whole host of other diseases, are found in higher levels in organic produce. Flavonoids work by protecting cells from free radical damage.

Also there is the taste factor; organic foods are more flavorful. By eating organic, we are preventing potential health problems that may be caused by pesticides and other toxic chemicals. Doctor Haas continues:

> I think also by supporting organics we are basically supporting an industry and saying we don't want so many chemicals in our food, we don't want so many chemicals in our environment. We are helping independent farmers, we are protecting the soil, we are protecting the water quality, and we are protecting the animals. We are protecting our future.[32]

Eating organically grown food is the best way to reduce the amount of toxins entering the body. Remember, these toxins are not limited to pesticides, but also include heavy metals like mercury and lead, as well as solvents like benzene and toluene. Heavy metals cause damage to the nervous system, play a role in multiple sclerosis, and are associated with lower IQ. Solvents have been shown to harm white blood cells, thereby weakening the immune system.

Because organic foods contain a significantly lower amount of pesticides and chemicals than conventional produce, eating organic foods automatically decreases inflammation in our body and therefore our risk of disease.

One note here: while it is commonly believed that "organic" automatically means "pesticide-free" or "chemical-free," this is not true. However, organic farmers are obligated to use pesticides that are derived from natural sources rather than synthetically manufactured compounds. They also employ creative mechanical and cultural tools to help control pests without chemicals, such as insect traps, careful crop selection, and biological controls like predator insects and beneficial microorganisms.

While organic products can cost a little more, it is often useful to participate in co-op buying, as well as other group buying clubs to reduce costs. It is also helpful, whenever possible, to buy directly from organic farmers, which can result in a lower price altogether, but at a minimum, fresher food. Lastly, in weighing the pros and cons of utilizing organics, we must consider the costs of ill-health that could occur from a lifetime of exposure to the dangerous synthetic chemical toxins in conventional produce. All in all, organic foods are far healthier than conventional produce. Choose them as often as possible to increase your chances of preventing disease.

Below is a list of the most highly sprayed fruits and vegetables. In these cases, it is absolutely essential to purchase organic if you wish to limit your exposure to poisonous chemicals.

1. Apples
2. Celery
3. Strawberries
4. Peaches
5. Spinach
6. Imported nectarines
7. Imported grapes
8. Sweet bell peppers
9. Potatoes
10. Domestic blueberries
11. Lettuce
12. Kale/collard greens

Fasting Periods

If you want to live a longer and healthier life, one proven way to do it is to consume fewer calories. Counting calories is not as important as thoughtfully choosing the kinds and amounts of food you eat. As I covered in Chapter 5, the typical American diet needs to be adjusted to include more complex carbohydrates, fewer proteins, and less fat. Begin your new eating plan by eliminating the three whites from your diet: white sugar, white flour, and salt. Then eliminate processed foods including most canned, frozen, or prepared convenience foods. Read labels and do not eat anything you can't pronounce.

The best eating plan is to eat more frequently—smaller meals, every 4 to 6 hours, so that both hunger and satiety can be experienced. Do eat breakfast, just keep down fat and sugar consumption. More people who skip breakfast are overweight than underweight. Get in touch with your eating drives. Eat your biggest meal at lunch, veggie-loaded entrees or salads with all the 'fixins,' including beans, legumes and/or nuts are great for lunch. Beware of salad dressings; most are high in fat, sugar, and calories; homemade dressings made with olive oil, (or even without oil) are best. Dinner should be light; a soup or small salad is plenty. Eat enough breakfast and lunch to take away the strong hunger drive, but not enough to feel full. If you are hungry before the next meal, have a snack. Eat only in response to hunger, not for entertainment.

Consider taking one day a week to fast on juices or juices with protein powder. Fasting allows your digestive system to rest and promotes increased metabolism.

Limit or Exclude Alcohol and Drugs

Whether wine, whiskey or beer, marijuana, tranquilizers, antidepressants, or caffeine, these are all drugs and, therefore, detrimental to the body; they also take us away from our nature. In many cases they are used to keep you from feeling the pain of your life, including excessive tiredness or listlessness. By the way, the same goes for eating an entire box of chocolates, cookies, or pie in one sitting, which is essentially a form of drug (caffeine, sugar) abuse. We talked above about moderation and restraint, which is crucial here. Someone once said a true measure of one's character is their discipline.

Take note of your addictive tendencies: what do you do when you are feeling nervous, scared, or stressed? Answering honestly is the first step in developing healthful behaviors. We all know that compensatory behaviors provide only temporary relief and don't directly deal with the underlying issues in our lives that many of us are avoiding.

Beer, wine, and other alcoholic beverages can cause fatigue and dehydration through their diuretic actions. Plus, they are not good for your heart, including red wine, which has enjoyed this beneficial status for some time because of it contains a polyphenol named resveratrol—thought to help prevent damage to blood vessels, reduce low-density lipoprotein (LDL) cholesterol (the "bad" cholesterol), and prevent blood clots.[33] However, a study published in July of 2014 in the *BMJ* (formerly the *British Medical Journal*) found that people who drank less alcohol (regardless of type) tended to have better cardiovascular health in the long run than cohorts who drank even moderately. The study, which was a collaborative effort by researchers at a number of notable institutions and co-authored by Perelman School of Medicine's (University of Pennsylvania) Michael Holmes, included a review of more than 50 studies as well as DNA study of the "alcohol dehydrogenase 1B" gene. Specifically, subjects showed a 10% reduced risk of coronary heart disease, in addition to lower blood pressure *and* lower BMI (Body Mass Index). Holmes stated, "The biggest takeaway is that people who drink less alcohol have lower risk of heart disease. In other words, if you want to reduce risk of heart disease, drink less to zero alcohol."[34]

Highly caffeinated drinks like coffee not only act as stimulants which can result in anxiety, insomnia, tremulousness, and palpitations, as well as bone loss and possibly increased risk of fractures but also act as diuretics, resulting in dehydration. So, if you are consuming caffeine at all, you need to increase water consumption.

Exercise

Lean body mass increases when intramuscular fat is replaced with muscle. Muscles have special enzymes that burn calories during exercise. The more muscle we have, the more enzymes we have that burn calories. As the amount of muscle increases, the amount of fat decreases, and the capacity for burning more calories is further enhanced. So when muscles move, they burn calories and increase lean body mass. It's a new cycle, but this time it's not vicious! Although there probably are genetic tendencies that predetermine set points, it is still possible for most people to "reset" their fat thermostats. The key to reprogramming lies in understanding and acting on the relationship between the kind and amount of exercise you do (your energy output) and the kind and amount of food you eat (your energy input). The trick lies in changing from a fat cycle to a fit cycle.

Running and other aerobic exercises can help us enter the fit cycle. Aerobic exercises use large muscles in a repetitive rhythmic pattern. During aerobic exercise, the body is fueled primarily by free fatty acids and secondarily by glycogen. While exercising, you do not use many calories. For example, you would have to walk 11 1/2 miles to burn up 3,500 calories or 1 pound. Weight loss is the effect of a cumulative process in which calories are being used on a more regular and frequent basis. This cumulative use of calories produces ongoing changes in the body's chemistry, lowering the set point, increasing the lean muscle mass with its fat-burning enzymes, and increasing the metabolism so the body burns calories at a higher rate. For hours following the exercise period, the body continues to burn calories at a higher rate. The effects of exercise on the body last long after the exercise period has ended. This will be true as long as you continue to do aerobic exercise at least 3 to 4 days a week.

Remember, duration is more important than distance or intensity. Your individual exercise program will start the same way whether your goal is overall fitness or weight management. If you step on the scale after a few weeks of exercising, you may notice an increase in pounds. Don't be dismayed. That is a good sign. It means you are increasing muscle in relation to intramuscular fat (muscle weighs more than fat). Interpret the increase as getting better and stronger, not heavier. Then throw away the scale. Pounds do not measure fitness.

On a similar note, weight itself should not be taken as the primary indicator of health. What is important is the percentage of lean muscle tissue and the percentage of fat to total body mass. Ideally, most men should be approximately 15% body fat, most women no more than 18 to 20%. However, studies indicate that most men are between 22 and 24% body fat and most women between 26 and 34%.

Both aerobic exercise and anaerobic exercise are important—not only for weight management, but also for overall good health. Doing the same exact exercises all the time, however, develops certain muscles to the exclusion of others. Runners, for example, typically have very healthy internal body systems and well-developed legs, but they lack proportional upper-body strength. Combining different forms of exercise such as walking, swimming, bicycling, rowing, jumping on the mini trampoline (rebounder) or playing tennis or racquetball can help achieve a good balance of muscle activity throughout the body. Anaerobic exercise like weight training and yoga builds strength, power, endurance, or the skill of specific muscles or muscle groups, and are excellent complements to aerobic exercises.

For maximum benefit, aerobic exercise should occur three or four times a week for at least 20 minutes, with 30 to 45 minutes being ideal. Start slowly, increasing the amount of time and intensity by about 10% every 2 weeks. Use good quality equipment, including proper foot gear. All sports require both pre- and post-game stretching. Anaerobic exercises, weight training in particular, actually break down muscle. For this reason, you need to allow a full 48 hours between weight-training sessions for the muscles to repair and heal.

Prior to starting any serious exercise or conditioning program, most people should have a complete physical exam. Some people need a stress test. During a cardiovascular stress test, your heart and blood pressure are monitored as you walk or run on a treadmill. The workload is increased at regular intervals. The results can indicate hidden or small conditions that could lead to trouble. Stress tests are done in various centers, hospitals, and some cardiologists' offices. If you are under 35 years of age, not overweight, and have no family history of heart disease, you probably do not need a stress test. A routine physical examination will do.

What time of day is best for exercise? Most people are more flexible and looser (also more fatigued after a day's work) at about 6:00 p.m. So exercising in late afternoon takes advantage of the flexibility, pumps up energy to revitalize a tired body, and reduces the tensions of the day. Exercising in early morning, on the other hand, takes advantage of a well-rested and fresh state of mind. Each person needs to be in tune with his or her own body, following the monthly rhythms that seem to affect intellect, mood, and physical energy levels. Do it when it feels good. The right time for exercise is any time you manage to find in your busy schedule.

It is important to start your routine and proceed very slowly. If any unusual signs manifest themselves, stop right away and check them out immediately with your doctor. If you feel exhausted, reduce the intensity and duration of any exercise by 50%. Your body is talking to you. Listen to it. That's good preventive sports medicine.

Relaxation, warm-ups and cool-down exercise should be used with all types of exercise: physical activity, aerobic, anaerobic, and all those in between. They maintain flexibility in muscles, tendons, ligaments, and joints, and help to prevent injury. Too much, too fast, and too soon are the most common reasons for sport injuries. Do not overdo. Less is better—at the beginning—at least until your body adapts.

There are many valuable books on exercise today. Simply consult your local bookstore, or check with personal trainers at a local fitness club for recommendations.

Balance

Health is a balance of our emotional, physical, and spiritual conditions. At the cellular level, life is a constant struggle for balance. Even when you ingest what is harmful, your cells will always defend you. They never stop and say, "*Why should we defend this guy? He doesn't care about us. He's abusing us.*" No. All of the hundred trillion cells in our body are operating on our behalf. Each of them has a separate consciousness that works in unity with the others. We overeat, and what do the cells do? They could put all that extra weight onto the nose, but they don't. In a miracle of balance, the body puts a little weight here and a little weight there. Why? To keep our center of gravity in balance so we won't fall over.

Balance is one of the keys to life. We need to look at every part of our lives to see which parts are out of balance. These will be our problem areas. When you spend more than you make, you're financially out of balance. In a relationship, if you take more than you give, you're emotionally out of balance. If you are worried and stressed a lot of the time, you are out of balance, and not able to focus on what you do have and be present to your life. When you devote more time toward work than play, or cannot exercise because "you're too busy," you cause an imbalance. If you sit at home and do not participate in causes that matter to you, meet people in your community and support community activities, or talk to or meet your neighbors, you are out of balance. All imbalances cause stress, which leads to distress that then leads to hormonal and blood sugar imbalances, which can then lead to local inflammatory conditions and pains. All of this can lead to neurological damage and premature aging, disease and in some cases an early demise. Better to balance the time in your day now *before* you are under the threat of a surgeon's knife. This way you can grow, progress, and achieve with your friends, family, and community while becoming a living inspirational example of what is possible. When you're working with too much effort, it's almost always because you're out of balance. When you're in balance, everything flows. Your mind flows. Your body flows. Your spirit flows, and you don't even have to think about being nice.

Here are a few areas to look at in terms of creating balance:

Clutter: We need to learn to stop over-cluttering our lives, whether with people, work, engagements (electronic and otherwise), stuff, whatever it might be. Clutter is a drain on energy and attention and prevents us from investing time and energy into more satisfying and fulfilling endeavors such as nurturing relationships. (See the next section on Voluntary Simplicity for more discussion on this issue.)

Time: Be realistic about the time you have and make sure you are choosing wisely. Balance comes from the correct appropriation of time to the things that you have determined are necessary for your health and well-being. Give up multi-tasking; it doesn't work. The important thing to remember is to only focus on one item at a time. If you are trying to do more, you are diverting your attention from mastering either, and attending to the details consciously. Furthermore, I am constantly working on many projects but I never lose my sense that I am my most important project. Every day I make sure that I have what I need to maintain my balance. I come first in my life because if I am not at my optimal state of physical, spiritual, and mental health, I am not of maximum benefit to others.

Make Your Self-Care, Healthcare Your Primary Ritual: Once you discover the foundational practices that support your health and wellbeing, specifically, design your life around those. As I noted above, when you take care of yourself, you can be of benefit to others.

Lastly, we can also fool ourselves that moderation is balance; that's what most people think of as balance. But think of being okay with a moderate amount of sarcasm, or negativity, or racism, or sexism. Do we ever say, "*You can be racist one day a week, you can lie to me occasionally, and sometimes you can betray me?"* No we do not! In these instances, having balance relies on our eliminating life-depleting behavior altogether.

We all wake up each day and make choices. Our choices will either create balance or imbalance, harmony or disharmony, disease or wellness, happiness or sadness, constructive or destructive thoughts. It's all in your power. You can make it happen. Where there's balance, there's harmony. And where there's harmony, there is bliss.

Voluntary Simplicity

"Voluntary simplicity" has been a way of life in several cultures for centuries. To be successful at this, people need to understand the benefits to be gained by unraveling the clutter from their lives.

The reasons people turn toward voluntary simplicity are several. First, many people are simplifying their lives to save money; they can no longer afford the upper middle class suburban lifestyle that is still put forth as the American ideal. Second, there's the environmental concern, with many advocates of voluntary simplicity feeling that America's high living, throw-away lifestyle puts a huge drain on the planet and is unfair to less developed countries and to future generations. These people tend to be heavily involved in repairing, recycling and repurposing material goods to lower their carbon footprint while helping other community members. Also, modern American life has become so complex and demanding that people get tense trying to fit everything they're supposed to do into a twenty four hour day. So it makes sense to simplify the demands and cut down on stress. Further, some are drawn to this movement for philosophical and spiritual reasons; for example, they permit themselves frequent quiet time to rejuvenate their inner happiness and peace. This in turn helps them to speak, act, and share in the most harmonious and constructive ways with their children and others.

It is also important to learn how to say no. When have you said "yes" when you really meant "no?" Think of all the times you burdened yourself with extra activities because you were afraid to say "no." Sometimes, you said yes because you were expected to or someone convinced you to. In order to achieve balance and harmony—side effects of a simplified life—you need to remain present to what is most needed, and then have the courage to unapologetically speak about those needs.

Most of us typically work toward making our lives comfortable. Comfort provides a sense of security. But it also prevents us from trying new things. We become afraid to quit our jobs and find new work, change relationships, or even change the way we eat, dress, or comb our hair. Simplifying allows us to actively engage in the growth process, and to take action on those things that are critical to our growth and happiness.

Slowing Down/Mindfulness/Meditation

Don't rush and distract yourself with things like television while you eat. Take your time and enjoy the taste of the food. Reorganize your day if you need to so that no one tells you that your work is more important than your nourishment.

Instead of enjoying our food, we're usually concerned about the next thing that needs to be done. We keep looking to the future instead of focusing on where we are or what we are doing. This distraction creates imbalance; imbalance affects digestion and energy doesn't really get to where it needs to go. Slow down, create a meal that honors your body, and turn off the cell phone and TV. Put away your magazines and savor the experience of eating

We need to slow down and re-cultivate healthy relationships. We must learn from the negatives in our lives and create more positives. We need to learn to stop over-cluttering our lives and seeking perfection and to become more nurturing in our relationships.

In terms of our thoughts, science abounds in support of how they affect our biology. If you are worried, stressed, and fearful much of the time, your body's functions, including your immune system, are being compromised. Not only this, but it may determine whether you manifest an illness related to a genetic predisposition. A study conducted by Massachusetts General Hospital and the Genomics Center at Beth Israel Deaconess Medical Centers found that the mind can actively turn on and turn off genes. "Now we've found how changing the activity of the mind can alter the way basic genetic instructions are implemented," stated Harvard Medical School professor Herbert Benson, M.D., co-senior author of the report. The study reported significant differences in the expressions of more than 2,200 genes between meditators and non-meditators. Some of these genes included those responsible for inflammation, the handling of free radicals, and programmed cell death, which can keep genetically impaired cells from turning into cancers.[35]

Practices for Cultivating Mindfulness

Reporting on the Herbert Benson study in the previous section, the *Washington Post* noted that researchers involved in the study said, "they've taken a significant stride forward in understanding how relaxation techniques such as meditation, prayer and yoga improve health: by changing patterns of gene activity that affect how the body responds to stress." These mind-body practices as well as others have been used worldwide for millennia to prevent and treat disease and to promote wellness; this study provides the first compelling evidence that they affect gene expression changes in practitioners.[36]

Yoga

While I spoke about yoga in spiritual contexts, I have yet to speak about its benefits to the physical body. Yoga is extremely beneficial in developing mindfulness, which means it also promotes relaxation and health. Slow stretches lubricate joints and increase flexibility while special breathing techniques expel toxins in the joints and muscles and decrease mental and emotional stress. There is no end to the studies demonstrating the health benefits of yoga. A 2013 Norwegian study showed that yoga practice results in very rapid changes in gene expression that boost immunity at a cellular level.[37] Not only did the researchers believe that the changes occurred while participants were still on the mat, the study showed that changes were significantly greater than in the control group who went on a nature hike while listening to soothing music.

The consistent practice of yoga has also been scientifically shown to reduce migraines, boost sexual performance, improve sleep, and combat food cravings, in part because yoga promotes mindful eating.[38] The Yoga Health Foundation also reports that yoga is proven to help those suffering from: chronic back pain more than therapeutic exercises; depression; diabetes, through improved blood sugar regulation and nerve pulse function; menopause, by reducing hot flashes; asthma, by improving pulmonary function in patients with bronchial asthma al symptoms; cancer and heart disease by lowering blood pressure, and decreasing blood sugar; cholesterol and triglycerides while improving coordination and reducing stress; and obesity, through increased awareness of their bodies, making them aware of bad habits such as eating because of stress, boredom, or depression.[39] Yoga has also been shown to promote relaxation and, of course, to reduce stress.

There are many different types of yoga, including therapeutic yoga, and they can vary greatly. It is best to speak to a professional prior to deciding which classes are best for your current level of physical conditioning. Some yoga styles can be an extremely rigorous and inappropriate for beginners, and movements must be done properly to avoid injury. If you are a beginner or suffering from physical challenges, let your instructor know prior to class.

Create a Healthy Relationship to Stress

Virtually all the authorities agree that if you want to get a handle on health—and heart disease in particular—you have to deal with stress. Stress or distress is a major problem for the American psyche. For a long while we have known that stress is a contributor to heart disease, but only recently have we begun to understand the physiological basis of the connection.

Richard Friedman, Ph.D., of Harvard Medical School, remarks that when we are confronted with stressful situations, constantly trying to fit square pegs into round holes, and when we find that is not going to work, we turn inward, brood, and look for ways to dissipate stress, frequently by acting inappropriately, such as overeating, drinking, or taking inappropriate drugs or medications, all of which ultimately contributes to the disease process.

Dr. Friedman says there is a link between stress and cardiovascular disease. Whether we are stressed by a fear of physical or psychological danger, the body exhibits a fight-or-flight response as it prepares to deal with an enemy. Very recent research indicates that the body readies itself not to bleed if it is cut or injured, which makes a lot of sense from a biological and evolutionary perspective. However, if the threats are psychological and you have a bad diet, you may be going through stressful incidents as many as 20 or 30 times a day, constantly triggering the fight-or-flight response. Each time this happens, the body prepares not to bleed by making the blood platelets stickier.

This internal clotting takes place every time you get angry, whether on a supermarket line or in a traffic jam. Over time this continual clotting can contribute to plaque buildup in the arteries. Stress also contributes to heart disease by increasing free radical damage to tissues and increasing spasms in the arterial walls. When you are exposed to a biochemical or psychological stress, a host of changes take place in addition to platelet stickiness. The body's ability to fight off viral and bacterial infection is lessened by the weaknesses induced by stress. Stress compromises the immune system's ability to fight off opportunistic diseases.

There is some good news, though, about our ability to fight off the debilitating conditions that lead to a heart attack. Dr. Friedman notes that just as continued stress leads to a weakening of the system, there is an opposite effect, one that has been labeled by his colleague at Harvard, Dr. Herbert Benson, as the "relaxation response." Eliciting this calming response on a daily basis makes it less likely that you will have high blood pressure or arteriosclerotic plaque buildup or a heart attack down the road.

The relaxation response should be combined with other behavior modifications to create a healthier response to stress, and all these techniques should be combined with the best medical care. That is the way to optimize your health.

Dr. Friedman tells us how the relaxation response is induced: use whatever strategy you have available to let go of any muscle tension you may be experiencing. Make sure your muscles are loose and your jaw lets go. After you feel a bit more comfortable, focus your attention on your breathing. If you find yourself having any distracting thoughts, do not let them bother you or take you away from the process. As soon as you have a distracting thought, simply say to yourself, "Oh well," and return to concentrating on your breathing and to a thought or image that allows you to stay calm, peaceful, and relaxed.

Become aware of the cool air coming in your nostrils and the warm air going out. Keep this up till you are deeply relaxed. Other ways to overcome stress are exercise, deep breathing, visualization, tai chi, yoga, meditation, qi gong, mantras, massage, Reiki, biofeedback, and aromatherapy. An essential oil blend of ylang ylang, lavender or peppermint, and marjoram added to oil and applied during massage helps calm the system and may even lower blood pressure.

Mindful Consumption & Consumerism

The people in control of the nation and economy want you to spend what you don't have on what you don't need, so they get you to believe you have to maintain an image, and this becomes part of the American Dream. But the part of the American Dream they don't tell you about is the nightmare of the payments that you can't meet and the imbalance in your own life as you devote more time to work and less to family, friends, community, and outside interests. One morning you wake up thinking, "We have everything we're supposed to have. Why are we so dysfunctional?"

Imagine how devastating it would be for the people in power if you stopped buying. They wouldn't like it, but you would have the freedom to do more. If you wanted to go on a long trip with your family, or alone, you could. If you wanted to go to other countries and enjoy different cultures, you could. For some people international travel can initiate an expansion of their horizons, enabling them to identify as a citizen of the earth instead of just a patriot of a given state, region or country. If you wanted more quiet time for meditation, you could work that into your life. You'd be able to build your life around what is essential to you.

On a global scale, selfishness is manifested as multinational corporations and governments exploiting every inch of the planet. In Africa and Asia, massive poverty exists in part due to corporate intervention. Yet do we see Fortune 500 companies giving even a small portion of their revenues back to provide proper wells for clean drinking water? Do they invest in planting trees where they have devastated the environment through deforestation? Are they building medical facilities so local residents can combat local diseases such as malaria, dysentery, and tuberculosis? In almost all cases, there is little to no effort.

One confusing factor is that the heads of the multinational corporations, who are creating so much pain and devastation worldwide, are usually considered as respected individuals in their local communities. Most are religious people who donate large sums to their churches and synagogues. Almost every one of our politicians in Washington claims some form of religious belief or affiliation, and while they may hold sincere and legitimate belief in their faiths, their actions in the public sphere rarely demonstrate that they are even remotely spiritual or authentically compassionate. True decency involves helping other human beings and attempting to improve the lives of those who have been wronged, not being the wrong doer.

Letting go of the American Dream involves a new mindset. It means that we have to content ourselves without many of the toys we are addicted to. But those toys can be replaced with any number of meaningful activities including community development.

So before you purchase anything, you want to ask yourself the following questions, "Why do I need this? What is the likely outcome of me owning this? Is this a temporary purchase or is it going to be more permanent? Is there a downside to owning this? Does the company from which I am purchasing this have a level of consciousness that I'm willing to support? Do they have a track record of upholding human rights and caring for the environment?" Remember, what we own we have to maintain, and there is time, energy, and effort required towards this.

Environmentalism

We really do not have an authentic environmental movement in the US today. We have a small number of authentic individuals who are contributing what they can to different social and environment issues like protesting against gas hydro-fracking, nuclear power proliferation, the genetic engineering of our crops, and such. However, there is no central environmental consciousness in America, so much of these efforts go for naught. Some changes can be accomplished, but these are so minute they have very little effect on the whole. A good example of this is the Keystone pipeline, which remains in limbo in large part because of support from activists. However, building for the transport of crude is still going on behind the scenes. We didn't stop the problem; we just diverted attention. An AP report posted on March 16, 2015 notes: "Overall, the network has increased by almost a quarter in the last decade. And the work dwarfs Keystone. About 3.3 million barrels per day of capacity have been added since 2012 alone—five times more oil than the Canada-to-Texas Keystone line could carry if it's ever built."[40]

What do we do about this? In short, unless we are actively engaged in the healthy vegetarian lifestyle and getting off the grid, protests do not hold all that much weight. Using the example above, the question comes down to, "Are you over-using fossil fuels that you are also protesting the expansion of?" The honest answer in most cases is yes. So how do we as individuals handle this reality or hypocrisy from a place of integrity?

In a true environmental movement we need to look at *everything* we are doing and make the necessary choices: Are we purchasing clothing from sweat shops in Bangladesh that exploit women and children? Are we eating animal products and ingesting alcohol? Are we heating our house with electricity rather than solar power? Are we buying produce that has been shipped from California rather than growing our own food, or purchasing locally? Are we collecting and utilizing rain water, or recycling our water? Are we buying the things we need instead of the things we want? Are we taking our money out of national banks and placing them in credit unions or local community banks? Are we creating debt by over-utilizing our credit cards? Are we conscious of our use of plastics, and doing everything we can to recycle, repurpose and, or, reuse what we have? Are we stopping our participation in big politics and voting people into congress and into the presidency who are willing to take real action?

Yes, it's a lot to consider. But every small step, like bringing a reusable bag to the grocery store, ads up when duplicated by millions of people. We have to step back far enough to see and address the entire problem. We have to stop fractioning and compartmentalizing these issues: we need a complete solution from the Gaia perspective—the interrelationship between all things. Many scientists have been contemplating this interconnectedness, and for some time now. The Gaia Theory was developed in the late 1960s[41] by Dr. James Lovelock, a British Scientist and inventor, and has gained support ever since. The theory asserts that living organisms and their inorganic surroundings have evolved together as a single living, self-regulating system. It suggests that this living system has automatically controls environmental conditions to maintain its own habitability. The Gaia paradigm can help us model human activities after the living systems of our planet and offers lessons for the design of economic, energy, social, and governmental systems.

Coming back to the topic at hand, it does no good to attend to a couple of issues without addressing them all. This is a key reason why I've chosen to write this book. If you just choose a vegetarian diet, for example, but continue to consume resources at the levels customary to Americans, we will not realize the level of change required to reverse the tide. We need a much greater group of individuals to not only embrace the vegetarian diet, but to also embrace all of the practices of a sustainable existence now. In this case, being the change we wish to see does, indeed, require a far broader application than most of us have taken up to this point.

Moderation & Restraint

The Jains (a separate religious group in India often mistakenly linked to Hinduism) talk about the importance of becoming discriminating in relation to character. They encourage not following anybody blindly but to check things out for one's self, and determine what is best for you. Along the same lines, the teachings stress the importance of not succumbing to peer pressure, and of building and maintaining our own identities, shunning dogmatic thinking about anything. This is an important aspect on the healthy vegetarian path, as a key reason why people revert back to eating meat after becoming vegetarian is social pressure,[42] including relationships where partners eat meat and limited offerings at restaurants.

Take your time to understand what you are doing and why. This understanding joined with a bit of research and some good communication skills will help you respond well to the questions and criticisms you may receive from others on the path. Be prepared; anticipate questions and push-back because it will likely come, since we humans are very defensive about our positions. When something is presented that is out of the norm, it is likely to bring up discomfort in others that will be directed at you.

In terms of restraint, refrain from defending your position or battling back. You certainly can present some facts to inquisitive people, but to try to convince someone who isn't open doesn't work. Some eager vegetarians on the path can be perceived as, and in fact sometimes do become, righteous and judgmental of others who have not chosen the vegetarian lifestyle; this too is damaging.

Most importantly, be yourself; don't become a stereotype. Be authentic and truthful with yourself about how you want to live your life, and be this way with others in a kind, compassionate way. Most of all, find time to play and have fun; be spontaneous. Moderation also applies to making sure we aren't overworking and missing out on playtime! I offer more support for you in chapter 8 related to discovering your authentic nature, which is an essential aspect of the vegetarian path.

Spend Time in Nature

I really love nature. The crisp atmosphere is undisturbed by city lights or pollution, and the sky often holds magnificent cloud formations and exquisite sunsets, giving the sensation of immensity and expansion. When people spend time in nature, they are free of the stress and worry of daily life, free from any conversations and distractions, have shared with me that they have a feeling of oneness with the environment around them. They are able to just connect with the consciousness of the moment.

Fortunately, it's an easy issue to address. No fancy equipment or expense is necessary to reconnect with the outdoors. If you can, spend time in the woods, at the beach, or hiking a mountain trail. If that's not possible, because, for instance, you're stuck in the metropolis, then get to a park, trail, river, lake, beach, or urban garden.

Not only does this bolster reconnection, it's soothing. Being in a situation where we're not threatened, intimidated, judged, or feeling pressured to perform, that's when our positive energy manifests. No one makes unreasonable demands, yells at us, or puts us on holds endlessly.

That's why nature brings us such peace and joy. We love being around all animals, plants and water, the oceans, mountains, lakes, and rivers. We love pastures. Not only in such landscapes are we outside of judgment, we are inside of the balanced ecology of the natural world. As we lose ourselves in nature, we find our own true nature. There is a link between moving in sympathy with the cosmos in a relaxed and uncomplicated way and emotional fulfillment.

Create Supportive Communities

Equal in importance to self-love through these practices is the love we share with others. Connecting with family, friends, and community gives us a sense of belonging that is invaluable to our well-being. Recently, a link between social bonds and heart health was reported in Natural Health. The magazine summarized 30 years of research on the town of Roseto, Pennsylvania, and concluded that the most important risk factor for heart disease is a lack of community and intimate relationships.[43] In this town, people lived in three-generation households with grandparents, parents, and children. There was a lot of interaction among families and much participation in community organizations. The incidence of heart disease was virtually nil even though residents ate high-fat diets and did not go out of their way to exercise. In fact, there was less coronary heart disease in Roseto than in any other population in the United States.

Moreover, like-minded community will be invaluable to you on your journey of health and healing, especially at times when you are in need of encouragement, or in need of accessing people with more experience to shorten your learning curve.

Use Good Natural Healthcare Practitioners

Did you know that more people are visiting natural health practitioners now in record numbers? A healthy vegetarian should have a physical once per year including a cardiovascular stress test, and a basic SMAC-24 test (Sequential Multiple Analysis

Computer), which is a panel of blood tests that serves as an initial broad medical screening tool. Have your lipid profiles assessed (HDLs and LDLs—high density and low density lipoproteins), as well as your cholesterol, C-reactive protein (CRP) level, homocysteine levels, fibrinogen levels, and your aging hormones like DHEA. This will tell you if your biochemistry is manifesting the health that you are feeding it. These levels should be checked annually.

Ultimately, you are responsible for your own well-being. Having access to proper health care practitioners is an important element in health maintenance. Their educated guidance and treatment can be invaluable in times of uncertainty and crisis, and for prevention and awareness-building. Selecting the right health care professional can be an important decision that will benefit you for the rest of your life.

Let me say a few words about selecting a healthcare professional. A good alternative medical practitioner will perform at least these three basic types of analyses before prescribing any treatment plan: (1) take a detailed medical history, including lifestyle questions, including exercise, stress, and level of happiness in jobs and relationships; (2) perform a physical examination that goes beyond conventional methodologies; and (3) study carefully the results of appropriate laboratory tests taken at the time of the history taking and the physical examination. In addition, you will find that good health practitioners include some or all of the following in their practice:

- as many noninvasive diagnostic techniques as possible;
- an awareness of the potential diagnostic value of even very minor signs and symptoms in the prevention of major dysfunction;
- a preference for noninvasive over invasive techniques (for example, substances will be administered orally rather than intravenously, except when a condition calls for the more direct route);
- a recognition of the importance of strengthening the body's resistive capacities and an interest, wherever possible, in attempting to repair any malfunctioning organ or gland;

- a tendency, whenever possible, to treat the *primary* weak link first if more than one has been discovered (for example, if the stomach is producing insufficient hydrochloric acid, resulting in the malabsorption of calcium, among other substances, the resulting calcium deficiency could lead to osteoarthritis, periodontal disease, or skin problems; by treating the hydrochloric acid insufficiency, the physician would be treating the primary weak link);
- an approach that treats the person as a whole person, not just a collection of ailing parts;
- the demonstrated ability to listen carefully and to skillfully classify any relevant symptoms to arrive at the best possible diagnosis;
- an orientation toward optimal health and sensitivity to dysfunctions that signal an imbalance in the individual;
- familiarity with a combination of approaches to help the person regain balance (for example, in addition to orthodox treatments, the physician's recommendations may include advice about stress reduction and lifestyle changes to reduce or eliminate causative factors in the environment);
- a willingness to refer the individual, when the condition warrants, to other medical practitioners whose specialized knowledge in a given area may be necessary to provide the most valuable restorative program; and
- a demonstrated awareness of the importance of the individual's own attitudes toward health and disease, and a willingness to communicate openly with the individual.

They are a living example of what they preach. In other words they are not obese, or ill-tempered, nor do they look stressed out. A good health practitioner listens thoughtfully and provides sound thoughtful advice.

The key to remember is this: In general, the majority of the modern medical community remains ignorant of the critical role of a whole-foods diet and healthy lifestyle in the creation and maintenance of optimal health. Physicians in training are required to take few courses on nutrition. Once they are in practice, they are barraged by pharmaceutical company reps most often very attractive and highly skilled in manipulative sales techniques. With convincing messages of powerful drugs claimed to alleviate symptoms, which is "good enough" right now – in the sense that you aren't actually dying. My colleague Dr. James N. Dillard, M.D., D.C., L.Ac., says it this way, "Medical doctors spend most of their education identifying and treating things that are going to kill us quickly as opposed to the things that are killing us slowly. It simply would be considered 'bad form' for a doctor to miss something so obviously life threatening."[44]

For this reason, your use of medical care professionals should be wise and well-chosen. You need to be an active, committed participant in the process. Do research and ask questions of your doctors, such as, "What, specifically, is being treated? How do you know that that's the problem? What are some realistic goals in my situation? What is the time frame? Does every individual with this condition get exactly the same tests and treatments? What are my weak links? Are these tests and this treatment relevant to my body and my condition?" Taking an active role in your healthcare is an important aspect of being a healthy vegetarian.

Nonviolence & Non-Harming

We've already discussed the inherent nonviolent nature of the vegetarian lifestyle. It bears repeating for the main purpose of remembering that violence comes in many forms; even though we may not be consuming animals, if we harbor negative or violent thoughts, speak these thoughts, or simply judge others, it is an act of violence.

Practicing vegetarians respect all life. In an essay regarding Jainism and the practice of nonviolence, Mr. F. J. Dalal states:

> All life is precious. All living beings have their place and role in the scheme of things. Thus we should protect and preserve life. "Survival of the fittest" might be nature's way but we should not interfere with nature. We should respect life." The Jains believe that a religious life is one that causes as little suffering as possible, in doing as much good as possible and in showing love, compassion, truthfulness and purity as often as possible. Mahatma Gandhi summed it up when he said: "There are many causes I would die for. There is not a single cause I would kill for."[45]

In the gross sense of the word, not physically harming people and other living creatures through dietary choice are obvious acts of peacemaker. However, another key aspect of the vegetarian practice is not harming others' spirits by judging them and making them wrong for what they do, even when their behaviors are obviously life-depleting. Growing our compassion toward others by fostering an understanding of why people do what they do, while standing firm in and acting upon our truth, we become a force of peace and love in the world. Through this, great change can only continue to occur.

A Word about Practice

What we do every day in life are our practices. If we want a healthy life, it stands that we must employ healthy practices, and consistently. For the same reasons that dieting is largely ineffective, incorporating healthier ways of living as a stopgap measure is counterproductive. Health for the healthy vegetarian is a way of living. I've reviewed a number of the practices above that are included in the life of a healthy vegetarian. Decide how to incorporate them all into your life. These things will go a long way toward creating the healthy life you are imagining. When we neglect our emotional, intellectual, and creative growth during times of relative stability, we are unconsciously increasing the magnitude of our loss when a crisis appears.

Spiritualism, Vegetarianism, and Holism

Spiritualism is essentially defined as a system of belief that promotes unity with our divine nature. The National Spiritualist Association of Churches (NSAC) defines spiritualism as a religion and philosophy of life focused on joy, harmony, and a fear-free understanding of the *continuity of life*. It is different than religion because it is based on the idea that we form a *direct relationship* with God, or Source, whatever you call the mysterious entity from which all life comes, rather than an indirect relationship, such as through a priest, minister, rabbi, guru, etc.[46] From this connection, we obtain guidance through reflection and interaction, and accept responsibility for our actions based on our interaction with that guidance, which is akin to a deep knowing inside us that defines our essential self, and our moral compass, which I will be speaking about in the next two chapters.

The important thing here is not to get stuck so much on terms but to understand the essence to which I am speaking, which is that each of us determines how we operate in the world and in relation to life itself. From our ideas of what it means to be human, we form a set of beliefs from which we operate on a regular and consistent basis—in essence we create our own operator manual by defining what is valuable about a human being. This translates, essentially, into a *choice* we make in any moment on how to treat ourselves and others.

Let's illustrate this point. If we believe that all humans are essentially "good" at their core, and made "bad" by circumstances or lack of proper nurturing and support, we treat them differently than if we believe that there are "good" and "bad" people. The belief informs not only how we treat people on an aggregate basis, but how we operate in relation to others. In the case of the latter, we will not trust people as readily and therefore will tend to have more fear in our dealings with them. In another circumstance, if we believe that all life forms deserve an equal amount of respect and consideration, we will do things like adopt a vegetarian diet and lifestyle and boycott circuses and other institutions notorious for adding to the suffering of animals, as examples.

In closing this section, I wish to make note that consideration of the whole, indeed, requires us to realize that suffering of one *is* the suffering of another. Nobel Prize winner and civil rights activist Martin Luther King Jr. aptly stated that an, "injustice anywhere is an injustice everywhere." A humane ethical life means respect for others. Albert Schweitzer, M.D. (1875-1965), the Alsatian physician theologian philosopher, was a peace activist who received the Nobel Peace Prize in 1952 for his philosophy of "reverence for life," which he expressed in many ways, but which is especially well reflected in his founding of the Lambaréné Hospital in Gabon, West Central Africa, in 1913. Schweitzer taught that society is "full of folly" that will deceive us about consideration for the lives and happiness of others. Respect for life, resulting from contemplation of one's own will to live, leads us to live to serve other people and every living being. Dr. Schweitzer found many ways, big and small, to put his theory into practice in his daily life. For example, Schweitzer was left-handed, but he would write with his right hand rather than awaken the cat who loved to sleep on his left arm.

We might think this is a small act, but do we really know? So, what we might think of as trite might be the grandest expression of reverence and love. There is no need to visit a spiritual advisor in the form of a religious leader to determine the value of our actions, each of us need to reconcile the value based on our personal experience: was my thought or action enhancing the flow of life or depleting it? This is a simple question that can be the mainstay of practice steeped in consciousness and spiritualism. Then, we become the master of our destiny while simultaneously creating it. I will speak more about this in Chapter 8.

What it Means to Live a Conscious Life

Essentially, a conscious life is one lived fully present in the moment, and with deep awareness of one's interconnectedness with everyone and everything. Living consciously also means living spiritually, or with awareness of the continuity of life; it also means paying attention to other people's needs. Consciousness, then, depends on one's understanding that actions are either life-enhancing or life-depleting, and that these actions have ripple effects.

Slowing down is an inherent part of a conscious life; we must become aware of everything that we are doing and consider the effects of these actions upon us and others. If we make choices—to lie or steal, for example, or to work excessive hours and be away from our family—we are affecting ourselves and others in life-depleting ways. Similarly, if we are working excessive hours and are away from our family often, that too is life-depleting. Even if we are *aware* of our actions and of the negative effects of them, it does not constitute consciousness in the way that I'm defining it here. Only awareness with *life-giving action* is consciousness.

We must also learn to stop constantly trying to escape the emptiness we feel nagging at our lives. The emptiness isn't real, of course, but we don't even allow ourselves the chance to slow down enough to discover its illusory nature and the truth of our vibrant connection to the world. One of the most common ways to avoid facing an empty sensation is to occupy ourselves with something or immerse ourselves in our habitual routines. Everything we do to remain busy, including all of our addictions and dysfunctional behaviors, is based upon anxiety and fear of that emptiness, which we would rather avoid or fill than confront. How we busy ourselves depends upon our earlier conditioning, our intellect, and our unique disposition. For example, some people are afraid of exposing their true motives to others so they present façades to cover up their intentions. They might try to fill their emptiness with beauty, surrounding themselves with beautiful possessions or obsessing about their appearance. But there is a fundamental flaw to such strategies; they have an expiration date. Eventually, due to life circumstances, our strategies reach the end of the line, so to speak. We may lose our financial wealth or some of our physical beauty to aging, and then what? For some, the answer is cheating others so they can continue to experience financial wealth, albeit false, or endless amounts of plastic surgery, as in the second case. Do you see the insanity? We are chasing after something that doesn't exist—a sense of comfort and safety in a world of impermanence.

In a conscious life, you surrender busy-ness but also your need to define yourself through your ego with all of its cultural conditioning and let go of your need to be right. It is a "we" state more than an "I" state. The more you do this, the more you discover yourself aligned with the correctness of the universe, which offers a far more extraordinary connection than anything you could discover when being led by the ego.

So be conscious and be present. Surrender everything that imbalances you and replace it with something that creates an authentic, sustainable life. Love, joy, hopefulness, vulnerability, and a pure belief in your self are qualitative energies of an authentic life. When you connect to those energies you support your growth as well as harmony in your world.

How a Conscious Life Heals the Mind and the Heart

You can slow yourself down. You can ask yourself, "Why am I doing this? Why am I saying that? Why am I eating that? Why am I having the same phone conversation for the hundredth time? Why am I spilling out my guts when it will change nothing?" You can confess your life and your problems one thousand times over to everybody who wants to listen, and they'll cry with you; you can put yourself on the journey of finding someone who will suffer with you and who will bear witness to your suffering; but what really changes? Little to nothing. How many people want to share pleasure compared to those who want to share suffering? Isn't it amazing? There are no limits to what you can tell a person when it comes to your suffering, but what you can say about your pleasure is so very circumscribed. We've got it all wrong. Make a point to share your positive energy and pleasure, and see what happens. Experience the healing power of this first-hand.

Our Illusions of Identity

If we work at a certain job and earn a certain amount of money, we can buy a certain type of clothes, usually expensive ones. But do your clothes define you as a better person? No, that's an illusion. We can live in a fancy apartment, we can eat in fancy restaurants, not necessarily better, but perceived as better because they're more expensive and more unique. We might even get wealthy enough to be invited to exclusive places by people considered to be elite, but the idea that they're better is an illusion too.

I counsel all types of people. I counsel some of the wealthiest and most famous people and also some of the poorest people in New York, and I want to tell you something I have noticed. People have a very specific idea of their value. More often than not, their value is based on what they possess, on their reputation, or on what they've achieved. Everywhere you look we're trying to separate people by such illusions, and eventually we get a collective mindset by which people believe in a common illusion together.

If you want to heal your mind, which by the way is a good place to start, it takes courage to step aside and say no to these illusions. After you become aware of the thoughts in your mind, you need to challenge them. One effective way of doing this is with Byron Katie's work. It happens to be called *The Work.* Katie suggests that we ask four questions when we encounter a thought that is creating a life-depleting emotion in us.[47] Here are the questions:

1. Is it true? (Yes or no. If no, move to 3.)
2. Can you absolutely know that it's true? (Yes or no.)

3. How do you react, what happens, when you believe that thought?
4. Who would you be without the thought?

There is hardly a quicker way to determine that most of the thoughts running around in your head are from conditioning and that they are largely uncreative and unhelpful in terms of health and healing.

Healing the Heart

In terms of healing the heart, this occurs when we find the proper place for our mind. We are heavily trained toward cognition in our society, and as such, the heart gets shoved down. For example, we choose a vegetarian diet for the benefit of the animals, but the moment a friend challenges us, we forego the diet because we become afraid of what are friends may think of us. Why? Because our minds say something along the lines of, "You won't be accepted by this person or this group for those silly values; don't be a fool!"

If we are constantly overriding our heart's wishes with our overbearing mind, we are setting ourselves up for a life of dissatisfaction and unhappiness, based on living an inauthentic life. Our heart is what rouses us into action because it is that part of us that helps us identify our passions as it relates to life and our expression in it. I have seen time and again that the happiest people are those who live their heart's passions and dreams. They are not always successful with these endeavors, but they are engaged in life in a formidable way compared to those who are living by the dictates of their minds, which are inherently limited because of fear.

A Word about Emotional Health

As I said earlier in the book, emotional health and well-being promotes greater happiness in life. It also occurs as we meet and exercise our authenticity in the world.

Emotions can be defined as energy in motion. Keep in mind that life is a flow of energy, and emotions are our guideposts. You can block your own energy or you can let the energy flow. Everything in life is about constricting or flowing. Let me give you an example: You look at your bank balance and see that you've overspent.

The first thing you do is constrict. You may then start feeling insecure because there's a shortage: you can't buy what you need; you may also think this means you lack abundance, which makes you more apprehensive and may cause you to overreact, or pick a fight with anyone else who may have participated in the overspending: Why did we buy that?! You are in reaction.

Emotions like sadness, fearfulness, discomfort, or anger aren't "bad"; instead, as pointers, they give us clues about what is important to us. If we pay attention to them, we can learn a lot about ourselves, and use that learning to lead more authentic lives. Taking the previous example, if you recognize the extreme discomfort you experience when overdrawing an account, you can put practices into place for avoiding that, thereby honoring your needs for comfort and security in life.

A helpful practice in cultivating the awakened, emotionally-centered life I am talking about is to *slow down*; watch your thoughts and emotions carefully. There is no need to *react out* of emotion, and in fact that often gets us into more trouble; it's far better to take a moment to understand what is going on so that you can mindfully and intentionally *respond to* the situation. Think about what would *really* cause the energy to flow again. The correct answer to this may not come right away; you may have to wait until you've calmed down and are in a centered place. Otherwise, you might make a choice that temporarily assuages the ego or the discomfort you are experiencing, but does nothing, in effect, toward creating a more positive outcome.

Emotional health comes from practicing *responding* rather than *reacting*. It requires a commitment to mindfully and patiently investigate your emotions to discover the jewels hidden beneath them. It also comes from following your bliss, which is what I will talk about next.

Embracing Our Bliss

I was first exposed to the concept of bliss in Bill Moyers' PBS series, *Joseph Campbell and the Power of Myth*. Campbell talked about bliss. That's not a concept that I grew up with, so I began to wonder: What is bliss? What does it mean? What keeps us from our bliss? What manifests bliss? I came to determine that bliss is about having the courage to release immature notions and actions that make us toxic to our self and others.

I began to understand that bliss has more to do with what we must *undo* or *not do* than with what we must do. It's about letting go of fear, for instance, instead of drawing our defense mechanisms out like samurai swords. When we live in fear we tend to bury our head in the sand indefinitely like an ostrich. While taking a brief vacation to regain perspective can be helpful, like fasting from the news every so often. Consistent withdrawal will soon leave you unprepared for the adventure of life as it unfolds. In the same way, when we neglect our emotional, intellectual, and creative growth during times of relative stability, we are unconsciously increasing the magnitude of our loss when a crisis appears. So bliss is not something that is *achieved*, per se, but it is a byproduct of engaging openly and joyfully with life and all that it brings.

Bliss is our natural state, conditioning is not. Your conditioned responses act as a firewall to separate you from bliss. No baby is ever born with a negative attitude, but over time fear, psychoses, neuroses, depression, and anxiety develop that give rise to limitations, biases, and prejudices, which are conditioned responses. Fortunately, anything that is a result of conditioning can be reversed.

In this case, you want to ask yourself: Am I willing to release my conditioned beliefs? Jesuit priest and psychotherapist Anthony de Mello said: "There is only one cause of unhappiness: the false beliefs you have in your head, beliefs so widespread, so commonly held, that it never occurs to you to question them." In truth, we believe many things throughout our lives that may not be true. Sources of false information include our families, teachers, friends, books, the church, the media, and our own misinterpretation of our experiences. However well-meaning, we must recognize that beliefs can be incredibly limiting.

So once you believe something, are you capable of changing your mind and course of action if evidence to the contrary becomes available? And, perhaps, even better, are you capable of moving forward with something that you know is right in your mind, your heart, or your spirit, *even if you haven't seen full evidence yet in your life*. If so, that is following your bliss.

Finally, bliss is not something that you have to work hard to *achieve* sometime down the road. It is available now. If you are willing to practice putting your attention in your body (away from thinking), and tune in to your senses related to the world around you, right now, you have the opportunity to connect to the transcendental nature of bliss. Just close your eyes and listen to the birds, the traffic, or the hum of an air-conditioner, or feel the warmth of the breeze, or the comfort of the chair beneath you. The experience of bliss matters not, in reality, to *what* you are witnessing but *that* you are witnessing… as a living and breathing being.

Famous Vegetarians

We end this section with a look at some more well-known vegetarians. The purpose is to provide inspiration to you on the path.

Paradoxically, while critics of vegetarianism often dismiss green eaters as undernourished weaklings who don't have the strength or staying power to live a full life, it turns out some of the greatest thinkers and doers in history, and even in the present, are strict vegetarians. This is an important thing for the vegetarian movement to acknowledge and realize they are a part of.

There is a type of existence that some humans access in their lifetimes; it is not just thinking or just doing, it is *being* or *presence*. The humans who live this way do not live by agenda, but by inspiration; they get a creative impulse and that is their directive in life. This describes the life of notable leaders, inventors, scientists, writers, and founders of great philosophical traditions, for example. Here we can place Socrates and Plato, who taught that vegetarianism was the ideal diet. These people are also the originators of world religions, such as Buddha and Mohammed, who also advised against meat consumption. And there are other geniuses, but among the greatest, I could throw in such embracers of a meatless diet as Leonardo da Vinci, Sir Isaac Newton, Ralph Waldo Emerson, Charles Darwin, Leo Tolstoy, H.G. Wells, and Upton Sinclair.

Let me just mention the names of the luminaries who have chosen this green path. Later in this section I provide a list of the more popular vegetarians, not because I love lists, but because I think you will be pleasantly surprised, as I was, by several on this list; some of whom you would not think in a million years were vegetarians, including a member of the Rolling Stones. You wouldn't think it because many vegetarians do not parade their beliefs and won't mention their green lifestyle unless asked. Going beyond mentioning their names, though, I want to highlight those who have spoken eloquently of their beliefs.

Let's listen first to Gandhi, the Indian leader and pacifist, who overcame numerous obstacles in fighting for his country's independence. He felt such a strong kinship with animal life that he couldn't bear the thought of using innocent creatures for food. "To my mind," he said, "the life of a lamb is no less precious than that of a human being. I should be unwilling to take the life of a lamb for the sake of the human body."[48]

Albert Schweitzer, theologian, musician, and philanthropist, believed that Western civilization was going downhill because it had lost its reverence for life. True reverence involved vegetarianism. He wrote in describing how he came by his green eating beliefs, "There slowly grew up in me an unshakable conviction that we have no right to inflict suffering and death on another living creature unless there is some unavoidable necessity for it, and that we ought to feel what a horrible thing it is to cause suffering and death out of mere thoughtlessness."[49]

George Bernard Shaw, a caustic wit and one of Ireland's major playwrights, was an avid propagandist for vegetarianism. As against the disparaging comments of the meat eaters, whom, as I said, thought vegetarians tended to be puny, unproductive weaklings, he riposted, "I flatly declare that a man fed on whiskey and dead bodies cannot do the finest work of which he is capable." He added, "I have managed to do my thinking without the stimulus of tea or coffee," and in doing so, he boasted he felt, "seldom less than ten times as well as an ordinary carcass eater."[50]

As to his propaganda for the green cause, I refer you to his very readable and tart-tongued book, *The Vegetarian Diet According to Shaw*. In it, he takes to task not only those who imagine that the equation eating meat = nourishment indicates the only possible route to good nutrition, by saying, "An underfed man is not a man who gets no meat, or gets nothing but meat. He is one who does not get enough to eat, no matter what he eats. The person who is ignorant enough to believe that his nourishment depends on meat is in a horrible dilemma."

He also anticipated, by decades, science's findings in the realm of phytochemicals, which are chemicals found in plants that have many health-enhancing and disease-eliminating properties, by praising plants in these words, "Think of the fierce energy concentrated in an acorn! You bury it in the ground, and it explodes into a giant oak. Bury a sheep and nothing happens but decay."[51]

However, since I am an American, I don't want you to think our country has been behind in giving to the world great people who combined a vegetarian lifestyle with strong contributions to society. As you probably know, Henry David Thoreau was a pacifist and early advocate (in the 1830s) of simple living. Famously, when he went to jail because of a refusal to pay his taxes because of his opposition to slavery, his friend Emerson came by and asked him what he was doing in jail. Thoreau then asked Emerson what he was doing *out* of jail (given the slavery issue).

Aside from his principled civil disobedience, Thoreau was a strong spokesperson for vegetarianism. He felt that, "It is a part of the destiny of the human, in its gradual improvement, to leave off eating animals, as surely as the savage tribes have left off eating each other when they came in contact with the more civilized."[52] Like Shaw, Thoreau felt that avoidance of meat improved his work.[53] In his masterwork, *Walden*, he wrote, "I believe that every man who has ever been earnest to preserve his higher or poetic facilities in the best condition has been particularly inclined to abstain from animal food." His abstinence from meat, coffee, and tea was not so much for health reasons as because, as he put it, "They were not agreeable to my imagination."[54]

Another example of Americans who combined retreating from the hustle of the metropolis to retire to the country and a dedication to vegetarianism are the well-known modern-day meat-shunners, Helen and Scott Nearing. They wrote several books in which they recount their experiences with the vegetarian lifestyle, books exuding much joy and reverence for life. And no wonder: both reaped the health benefits of the practice, living long and productive lives (Scott lived to be a hundred, while Helen lived to be 91). Their meals consisted of wonderful concoctions of fresh fruits, whole grains, vegetable soups, nut butters, and molasses.

Their story is more than a tale of amazing longevity, however. Nearing was a professor of economics at the University of Pennsylvania. His pacifist and socialist views got him fired in 1915. Pacifism didn't go over big during World War I. After years of fighting for justice and peace, in the 1930s he and his new wife left busy city life and settled in the peaceful atmosphere of Maine, where they worked hard together to become monetarily independent, self-sufficient and "rich," rich on their terms, which meant—"rich in fresh air, fresh water and sunshine." Growing most of what they ate, the Nearing's enjoyed a freedom that those dependent on commercially packaged meats and other foods could never imagine: the freedom of "being master of your own destiny."[55] And not only did they inspire others by their writings, but in the 1960s when many young people joined the "back to the land" movement, moving away from cities and homesteading on farms, there were many of them who made pilgrimages to the Nearing house, not only for encouragement but to get practical advice on growing food.

To turn to more recent examples, let me mention Oscar-winner Cloris Leachman. She is one of those people who doesn't make a secret of her vegetarianism, but stands up for it, basing her belief in green eating on both political and health reasons. She turned to vegetarianism after reading "about what's wrong with meat," and is outspoken about the US political and economic system that foists meat on unwitting consumers without clueing them in to its noxious effects. She points out that the meat industry has a very powerful lobby in Washington whose tentacles reach even into our schools, where you'll rarely hear about the value of vegetarianism. Moreover, people have been led to feel that a steak on the table is a symbol of prosperity and success. Why? "Because they have been indoctrinated to believe this by the meat industry."

Leachman isn't all politics, though. One of the reasons she eats only wholesome, low-fat, natural foods is to avoid the problem of controlling weight through calorie counting, which usually leads to nothing but frustration and failure. She puts this very poetically, saying, "I'm interested in an approach to eating that is a way of life, where the road just unfolds before you and leads you into good feelings and uplifting experiences."[56]

Many actors share Leachman's penchant for vegetarianism, though not necessarily her political sensibility. Other vegetarian actors include Dennis Weaver, a veteran vegetarian of over 20 years, James Coburn, Paul Newman, Cicely Tyson, Gloria Swanson, and Susan St. James. Musicians who have taken the green path are, among others, Bob Dylan, George Harrison, Paul McCartney, Ravi Shankar, John Denver, the now slim Chubby Checker, Gladys Knight, and the members of the B-52's.[57]

Let me just add, since the theme of this book is to intertwine all the elements of the vegetarian lifestyle into one package, that many vegetarians do just that, create a way of living in which all the components of a healthy regimen, including exercise, good eating and detoxification, combine into a synergistic unit. Susan Smith Jones, a health writer, lecturer, and physical education instructor, is a good example of someone who has consciously crafted such a well-rounded life. She incorporates vegetarianism into a holistic lifestyle that includes a ten-mile morning run and an hour of meditation every day. She believes that, "The tangibility and reality of a full life is not only what you know, but how you apply it to every day… We are not victims of circumstance or fortuity, but rather architects of our lives, ourselves, and our feelings." To those who imagine that a well-thought-out regimen of healthful living is too time consuming, Susan simply says, "If we don't take time for health, in whatever capacity that might be, we must take time for sickness."[58]

Here is a list of well-known vegetarians, both old and new, filled with names, some of which you will expect, such as Buddha, and others that will probably leave you a bit surprised. Here it is:

Adam Ant	Berkeley Breathed	Charles Darwin
Al Gore	Bill Clinton	Charlie Watts
Alanis Morissette	Bill Ford	Charlotte Bronte
Albert Einstein	Bill Maher	Chelsea Clinton
Albert Schweitzer	Billie Jean King	Cher
Alec Baldwin	Billy Idol	Chevy Chase
Alice Walker	Bo Derek	Chris Evert
Alicia Silverstone	Bob Barker	Chris Martin
Ally Sheedy	Bob Marley	Christie Brinkley
Alyssa Milano	Brad Pitt	Claudia Schiffer
Andy Kaufman	Brigitte Bardot	Corey Feldman
Anna Paquin	Brooke Shields	Dan Castellaneta
Annie Lennox	Bryan Adams	Danny De Vito
Anthony Hopkins	Buddha	Danny Garcia
Anthony Perkins	Candace Bergen	Daryl Hannah
Anthony Robbins	Captain and Tennille	David Bowie
Barbara Walters	Carl Lewis	David Carradine
Belinda Carlisle	Carrie Underwood	David Duchovny
Benjamin Franklin	Casey Affleck	Dr. Dean Ornish
Benjamin Spock	Casey Kasem, DJ	Debbie Arnold

Demi Moore
Dennis J. Kucinich
Dennis Rodman
Dizzy Gillespie
Doris Day
Doug Henning
Dr Albert Schweizer
Dr. Benjamin Spock
Dr. Dre
Dustin Hoffman
Dweezil Zappa
Ed Begley, Jr.
Ellen Burstyn
Ellen Degeneres
Elvira
Elvis Costello
Emanuel Swedenborg
Emilio Estevez
Eric Stoltz
Erykah Badu
Evelyn Glennie
Forrest Whitaker
Frances Moore Lappé
Franz Kafka
George Spitz
Grace Slick
Gwyneth Paltrow
H.G. Wells
Hans Christian Andersen
Harriet Beecher Stowe
Heather Mills
Henry Heimlich M.D.
Hillary Swank
Ian McKellen
Isaac Bashevis Singer
Jack LaLaine
James Taylor
Janeane Garofalo
Jean Jacques Rousseau
Jeff Beck
Jennie Garth
Jerry Garcia
Jerry Seinfeld
Jiddu Krishnamurti
Joan Armatrading
Joan Baez
Joaquin Phoenix
John Cleese
Jorja Fox
Josh Hartnett
Joss Stone
Jude Law
Julia Stiles
Julian Lennon
Julianna Marguiles
Kate Bush
Kate Moss
Kevin Eubanks
Kim Basinger
Kirk Cameron
Kristen Bell
Larry Hagman
LaToya Jackson
Laurie Anderson
Lenny Kravitz
Leo Tolstoy
Leonardo Da Vinci
Linda Blair
Lindsay Wagner
Lisa Bonet
Lisa Marie Presley
Little Richard
Liv Tyler
Loretta Swit
Dr. Lorraine Day
Louisa May Alcott
Lynda Carter
Mahatma Gandhi
Margaret Cho
Mariel Hemmingway
Marilu Henner
Mark Twain
Marlo Thomas
Martha Plimpton
Martin Luther
Martina Navratilova
Mary Shelley
Mary Tyler Moore
Meatloaf
Mel C of the Spice Girls
Melissa Etheridge
Meredith Baxter
Michael Bolton
Michael Eisner
Mick Jagger
Milo Ventimiglia

Milton Berle	Richard Pryor	Tiffani-Amber Thiessen
Moby	Ricki Lake	Tippi Hedren
Moon Zappa	Ricky Martin	Tobey Maguire
Naomi Watts	Ringo Starr	Todd Oldham
Nastassja Kinski	River Phoenix	Tolstoy
Natalie Portman	Robert Kennedy, Jr.	Tom Petty
Nikola Tesla	Rodin	Tracy Chapman
Noah Wyle	Ru Paul	Upton Sinclair
Norman Cousins	Rue McClanahan	Uri Geller
Olivia Newton John	Russell Simmons	Vanessa Williams
Orlando Jones	Sara Gilbert	Vanna White
Ovid	Sarah McLachlan	Vaslav Nijinsky
Ozzy Osborne	Seal	Victoria Beckham
Pamela Anderson	Seneca	Vince Vaughn
Patti Davis	Shania Twain	Vincent Van Gogh
Paula Abdul	Shaun Cassidy	Voltaire
Penélope Cruz	Sinead O'Connor	Whitney Houston
Persia White	Sir Isaac Newton	Whoopie Goldberg
Peter Bogdanovich	Smokey Robinson	William Blake
Peter Gabriel	Sophie Ward	William Shakespeare
Peter Sellers	Surya Bonali	William Shatner
Peter Singer	Stella McCartney	William Wordsworth
Phylicia Rashad	Steve Perry	Woody Harrelson
Piers Anthony	Steven Jobs	Yasmin Le Bon
Plutarch	Steven Seagal	Yehudi Menuhin
Prince	Stevie Nicks	Ziggy Marley
Pythagoras	Stevie Wonder	Zoroaster
Rain Phoenix	Sting	
Ralph Nader	Susan B. Anthony	
Ralph Waldo Emerson	Susan Richardson	
Reese Witherspoon	Suzanne Vega	
Rhea Perlman	Ted Danson	
Richard Gere	Thomas Edison	

In touching on prejudices that exist against green eating, I brought up the stereotype that vegetarians, who, it is claimed, don't consume the red meat they need for strength, are all weaklings. The best argument against that canard is the host of world-class athletes who walk or, often run, the vegetarian path.

For some, vegetarianism was not their original choice as a way of eating – they grew up believing that top performance required them to "pump" iron into their bodies with massive amounts of red meat – but it was something they arrived at after considerable thought and experience. Among this group, who eventually became firm advocates of vegetarianism are "green" body builders, such as the legendary Gilman Low, who in 1903 set nine world records for strength and endurance; Roy Hilligan, the first vegetarian "Mr. America," and more contemporary competitors, including Ron Gleason, a contender in the 1972 Olympics.[59] Vegan bodybuilder Jim Morris won London Mr. Universe Tall class and placed 2nd overall in 1977.

Other star athletes have also been vegetarians. John Marino set a transcontinental bicycling record in August 1978, riding—after three years of training—from Los Angeles to New York in just 13 days, 1 hour and 20 minutes! Marino maintains that his vegetarian diet was the primary factor in his record-breaking ride.

Describing his training, he had this to say, "The first step is detoxification of the body. Unnatural foods, chemicals, drugs, alcohol, artificial flavorings, and preservatives bring on a toxic buildup in the body, which can lead to disease, lethargy and, in extreme cases, death. Our bodies are designed to consume organic foods in the natural state."[60] Another athlete who renounced meat is Norwegian skier Arden Haugen, elected to the Skiing Hall of Fame after winning four national and three world skiing championships. He maintained that giving up meat in favor of a diet of whole grain cereals and breads, vegetables, fruits, and soy milk, cleared his skin, increased his stamina, and made breathing easier.[61]

And there are many more vegan star athletes: Triathlete Madi Serpico was names Off-Road Triathlete of the year in 2010; Dave Scott 4 time Iron Man world Champion, David Smith (para rower & cyclist) helped his team to a gold medal at the 2009 World Rowing Championships; Maureen (Mo) Bruno-Roy is a cyclocross cyclist and was the overall winner of the USA National Cyclocross Calendar in 2009; vegan bodybuilder Billy Simmonds won Mr. Natural Universe in 2009; David Meyer, vegan martial artist, has competed for years at the top of the martial art of Brazilian Jiu Jitsu; over the years he has won numerous international titles at the top level including two World Championship Gold medals, four American National Golds, an American Open Gold and two Pan American Golds; Austin Aries, an American Pro Wrestler, has competed with the nation's best and won numerous World Titles; Keith Holmes was the World WBC Middleweight boxing champion for two periods in the 1990s; and Cam Awesome, outstanding Super Heavyweight amateur boxer, has been American National Champion eleven times, and ranked 4th globally.[62]

I have spent this time drawing your attention to renowned women and men, not because I want to indulge in celebrity worship, but for two other purposes. For one, I wanted to dispel the myth that vegetarians are underachievers. People who believe that couldn't be more wrong, as I think I have shown. Second, I've tried to underline that these famous people did not take up vegetarianism blindly (in the way people adopt a meat-eating diet), but usually gave thought to their health and the planet's health in making this choice.

Chapter 8

Change... It's Essential to Health and Healing

> "I wanted to change the world. But I have found that the only thing one can be sure of changing is oneself."
>
> –*Aldous Huxley,* Point Counter Point

This is possibly the most important chapter in this book.

I didn't place it as the first chapter because it wouldn't make a lot of sense without some background and, therefore, perspective related to how far off-track we have become and how remote we are from what is natural or even sensible in terms of real health.

In reality, humans very much want the benefits of change *without actually changing.* We want to be slim and to lose the belly fat or the extra pounds without eating properly; we want to feel vital and alive and have a strong sex drive but we won't give up the cigarettes, the drugs, or the stressful job; we want to have a substantial savings but instead continuously spend money on things we don't need; or, we want to have a job that we love and enjoy but won't let go of the one that we have. Many of us, also, don't want humans or animals to suffer as they do, and we are sickened by gross displays of cruelty and violence, but we continue to eat meat, wear leather and fur, play the lotto and bet at the dog track; we might also want a better functioning, more equitable government, banking system, and a corporate climate where many are served and not just an elite few, but we are unwilling to vote, to support credit unions, or to boycott or find alternatives to products and services that aren't in alignment with our values.

In truth, we want all of this—and more. How in the world do we get the benefits of change, without changing? We don't. So we live in this duality—of wanting something that we are not willing to surrender our ideas, behaviors, or positions to get. As such, we are in perpetual conflict with our self! No wonder we have so much dissatisfaction and disease, and our world is in such a state of disrepair. As one example, a 2013 Gallup poll found that 70% of American workers are *disengaged* or have "checked out" from their jobs.[1] According to the report, this costs the US as much as $550 billion in economic activity annually. The most shocking thing noted by the researchers is that the level of employee engagement over the past decade has been largely stagnant. So why don't more of us find jobs that we enjoy enough to be actively engaged? Why are we so stuck?

In one aspect change *is* hard; it requires us to look at our self—our "dark side," our weaknesses, our shortcomings and our failures—and to ask and answer some difficult questions, among them, "*Why am I in this situation again?*" In another way, we perpetuate a trivial existence—by thinking mostly or only about our self and our own wellbeing and that of those closest to us, we suffer endlessly in jobs that we loathe for the sake of paying bills, and we work tirelessly to sustain the familiar, *no matter how sad, lonely, frustrated, angry, or suffering we are about it.* The status quo, to which we humans cling, is far more "comfortable" than dealing with the fear of stepping out into the unknown. We also tend to choose what is easy or pleasurable (even if it isn't "right") and find clever ways of justifying it.

Ultimately, though, we are forced to look at some imbalance in our lives at some point. For many of us, this typically comes on the heels of a tragedy or catastrophe—a serious diagnosis, divorce, bankruptcy, loss of a loved one, or near-death experience, to name a few possibilities. These moments of truth tend to be highly uncomfortable; we have realized the weight or impact of a negative situation or occurrence and that some major changes must occur if we are not to recreate the same pain down the road. Either way, the resulting epiphany is a sort of "wake-up" call in which we realize the truth of the matter or gain some life-changing insight into the reality or essential meaning of something in life. It is an opportunity, as I noted before, for us to come clean and admit weakness or failures, realizing that in most cases we had something to do with the current situation. But there can be tremendous fear and distress in acknowledging the path that got you to where you are and not having a clear path upon which to focus in order to regain balance.

Learning doesn't have to be so painful. Instead, if we can train ourselves in the art of living—to understand what is most important to us, attend to these priorities with conviction and love, and be open to change in the face of our fears and weaknesses—then we have the possibility of an authentic life. German philosopher Friedrich Nietzsche said, "He who has a why to live for can bear almost any how." What we need more than anything to be healthy is to find our "why." We need to ask questions like, "*Who am I? Why am I here? What is the meaning of my life? What is missing? What do I need to achieve to feel whole and complete, not lonely and sad? What do I need to do to develop patience and compassion with others, instead of just thinking about how I feel?*"

And there are plenty of deep questions to ask in terms of food and eating, "*Why do I eat what I eat? What am I avoiding by overeating? How can I justify supporting organizations linked to cruelty to animals? How do I really feel about this? How important is it that I feel physical good and energized?*"

Being in conversation around the big questions takes us out of the mindset of "me" and connects us immediately to something much larger—and *that* becomes the motivation for change. Without it, frankly, the changes we make will be precursory, unimpactful, and unsustainable. I've seen it time and again in my nearly 50 years of working with people around diet and nutrition and creating vital lives.

How I Learned What Inspires People

I did a study many years ago in New York City for the purpose of understanding why people who were obese could not make the dietary changes that were necessary to drop weight and improve their physical health. There were five separate groups; each would come one night per week for six months. The people in the first group received a host of information on various diets that could help reduce weight; the second group received information on exercise information only, a third group was taught everything for de-stressing—from mindfulness to Tai Chi to journal writing and deep breathing; we focused only on nutrient information for the fourth group—what foods contained the specific nutrients they needed to achieve a healthy weight. Then, we had a fifth group. The people in this group got none of this; instead, we talked about the meaning of life. It was very interesting, because of all the groups, the people in this group for the first two weeks were very argumentative. We also had the largest number of drop-outs from this group—nearly 80% quit within two weeks; none of the other groups experienced this level of attrition. So, we proceeded to continue to interview candidates for the group to replace those who left. Eventually, we got a group together who continued for the six-month program. At the end of the six months, those in the first four groups had a failure rate of about 90-92%, while those in group five who focused on the meaning of life had a 95% *success rate* in adopting the lifestyle changes they were provided at the beginning of the program.

In my entire career, one thing has become clear: doing something because someone else says you should or is a good idea won't work; you've got to really want the benefits of the change in order to change. In a paper titled, *Influencing Patient Adherence to Treatment Guidelines*, Susan W. Butterworth, Ph.D., M.S. writes: "In translating theory to practice, people change because their values support it, they think the change will be worth it, they think they can, they think it is important, they are ready for it, they believe that they need to take charge of their health, and they have a good plan and adequate social support."[2]

So I come back to my primary question: Do you know your *Why's*? Why you are doing the job you are doing; why you are in the physical shape you are in; why you are in the relationship you are in and have the money that you have; why you are choosing to be a healthy vegetarian; why you're happy or unhappy. Do you know these answers, intimately? If not, this is the place to start. In reality, information without understanding, without reason, without the "why," changes no one. In fact, we have too much information nowadays; what we need is action that is linked to the essence of who we are—our core foundation—and beyond *persona* or identity. "*Who am I really, and what kind of life do I want to live?* "These are just two questions that you might ask yourself to gain clarity about your choices and direction in life.

Before moving on to *how* you actually create your healthy life, I want to return for a brief summary on Nietzsche's central philosophy. This is "the idea of 'life-affirmation,' which involves an honest questioning of all doctrines that drain life's expansive energies, however socially prevalent those views might be."[3] His suggestion to question and evaluate *anything* that is draining our vitality (and inhibits being in a free, creative, open state) is a very good one. I spoke about this in the previous chapter when talking about the beliefs we inherit in life from others. When we have the courage to face our discomforts head on, we can make conscious choices about what to include in our lives and work toward or not—regardless of cultural or social norms. Undertaken consciously, this evaluative process leads to a life of self-mastery.

Living Life in Reverse

As talked about in my book *Spiritual Authenticity*, if you live life according to the goals that have been handed to you, you will never be happy, you will never know—much less live in accordance with—your authentic self.

Assessing Your Life - Your Authentic Self

The best way to figure out *how* to change your life is to discover your authentic self and to decide what kind of life you want to live, rather than the life you have been programmed to live. The best way to figure out your priorities and what is most important to you is to envision living your life in reverse. Take one day and turn off *everything*: cell phones, land lines, and computers. Don't schedule activities; don't meet with any friends, family, or colleagues; clear your schedule.

You need to go somewhere where there is nothing to distract you from the task at hand. For some people, that means a quiet corner of the local park; for others, it is an out-of-the-way table at the local coffee shop or library. Bring a notepad and pen with you and using that old-fashioned technology, write down the most important *themes* of your life—a theme is very much like a premise, subject, or an idea that you believe in deeply. The difficult experiences that created insecurity as well as the positive experiences that left you feeling strong and capable and what you learned about yourself, will guide you to determine your themes. List everything of significance.

As an example, you may have been raised by a single parent and witnessed them struggle without much help in raising you and your siblings; this could have had you create a theme related to the importance of having a solid partner and community of support for helping you raise your children.

Or, as another example, you may have seen one of your friends bullied at school and, even though you were scared, stepped in to help them fend off the bully; this could result in a theme that you would do everything you could to stop violence and help those in need.

Once you have identified your themes, develop a chart of your life, from a young age on up to your current place. Reflect on each significant event: What happened, how did it play out, what long-term effects did it have on your life? Consider the effect of these remarkable moments on your career, friendships, and relationships. Think as broadly as you can.

After you've written everything down, then analyze it. Look for any patterns from throughout your life. Do you see negative patterns? For example: Do you become sad and lonely if you're home alone on a Friday night, or when you don't have a boyfriend/girlfriend? Do you react to the situation by eating a pint of Rocky Road ice cream, having a few too many beers, watching pornography, or perhaps leaving an inappropriate or overly emotional phone, text, or email message? Then, do you remember the next morning? Did you find that you regretted your evening's activities? Did you feel overstuffed with food, hung-over from alcohol, or just generally embarrassed by your behavior? Did you feel the same sadness, loneliness, or remorse that set you off on Friday night? Did you find that your actions the night before had only compounded the problems, the sadness, and the disappointment? Or, is this something that you are actively experiencing now?

By analyzing your actions, responses, and emotions to your life situations, you can see self-destructive patterns that, when addressed, will improve the quality of your life substantially. You can also see some of the events that caused you pain, particularly in your childhood, and the beliefs that you adopted about yourself and life as a result. Maybe you had a parent who never gave you the attention you needed.

Maybe your parents offered you money only, rather than time. I have found that when people overdo something, they are often overcompensating for some deep-seeded subconscious fear or need. We are composites of both constructive and destructive inputs in our lives.

By living your life in reverse and by accounting for all the major events in your life and analyzing them for patterns, you can figure out why you are the way you are and why you are where you are. Most importantly, these insights can help you determine how to change the situations in your life where you are currently not experiencing fulfillment. With a little bit of work, you can improve most situations immeasurably.

Who Are You, Really?

Finding Your Authentic Self

What if you don't know what your authentic self is?

Let's say you find you have trouble getting up in the morning, but there is nothing physically wrong with you. You just don't look forward to going to work because at your place of employment you have no chance to use your creativity, develop skills, or work harmoniously with others. It doesn't take a psychiatrist to tell you what would be in the interest of your authentic self in this situation. You should either find a way to reconfigure your workplace to suit your talents or start sending out resumes.

Similarly, if you want to take the measure of your authentic self, then ask yourself what you feel in your heart. What do you feel when you think about what you would like to do with your life, where you would like to be, the work you'd like to do, and who you would like to share time with? What are your innermost thoughts? You will probably find that your authentic self is much bigger than you expected and, perhaps, that much of what you are doing—your job, relationships, and goals—are lacking.

If so, then your choices belong to the narrower self that is defined by all the prohibitions and lessons you learned throughout your life. To move forward, you have to challenge your existing beliefs. You must ask yourself, "Are my beliefs allowing me to be happy and in balance?" If not, then we need to challenge ourselves to go further. We need to learn to stop and think about the choices we make; are they actually choices, or are we just acting out of patterns and rituals?

The more you shift from the conditioned self, the more confidence you will have in the choices you make and the happier you will become, regardless of outcome. This is because you are following your heart.

Learn to Trust the Voice Inside

If you want to live from your authentic self, you need to open yourself to the divine, creative energy within you. It's there; all of you have to do is be sensitive enough to listen to it. It will tell you what is right and what is wrong for you, what should be included and what should be excluded, and what should be joined with and what should be separated from.

It is by *taking action* on this internal *knowing* that we build confidence within ourselves and lead more authentic lives.

See the Good in Yourself

It is useful to consider both the goodness *in you* and the things that you are *good at*. By "*goodness in you,*" I mean virtues such as loving, honest, trusting, caring, adventuresome, open, and the like. It's helpful to identify and acknowledge yourself in specifics; for example, if you exhibited patience and kindness during a difficult situation. Doing this gives us courage to practice those virtues more and more in the world.

Further, by examining a list of things that you are good at (and even like to do), you may see some patterns emerge about your authentic self; this will help you sort out what you enjoy doing in this world. The more you reflect upon your goodness and strengths, the stronger you become—which, in turn, will make it easier to resolve conflicts and navigate through difficult times but also to enjoy life.

Address Your Essential Needs

We all have needs; denying this or thinking otherwise will only get us into trouble. When you think about how to change your life, make sure that you are addressing your essential needs. You may be afraid that you will feel bad about yourself if you fail at a new endeavor, or you may worry that others will judge you by such failures. If you know this, you can incorporate actions into your plan to address these needs.

A great way to learn about your needs is from your relationships. Examine the constructive and destructive aspects of your current and past relationships and ask yourself which essential needs were met and which were not. Look at other areas of your life as well—your jobs, your hobbies, and how you spend your time, in general—and strive to understand the needs that are most important to you. Once you identify what you truly need, it will be easier to walk away from nonessentials.

Remember, our essential needs tend to change as we progress through life. What is important to us at 20 years old is not so much at 40. Remain alert to your changing needs, and you will have an easier time navigating life.

The Importance of Being True to Your Self

Our success in life depends on us understanding and being true to our self. Moreover, our emotional set-point is closely accepting and celebrating who we are rather than trying to be someone we aren't or comparing ourselves to others. We would all have more harmony if we could accept and embrace these different energy types and see the value of each one to the whole.

How do you know that you're being true to yourself? You'll feel it at the heart level. If you have the sense that what you're doing is not who you really are, and if you have the nagging feeling that there is something else in life that you should be doing, it's a pretty sure sign you have tried to live in a way incompatible with your inner patterns. I have met people who try to be leaders when they are better as followers. By the same token, a dynamic person who wants to lead but has been conditioned to be adaptive may experience depression and anxiety.

My point is that by holding back your natural inclination, your energies become blocked. A person can fake their behavior, but they can't fake-out their body and mind, so they pay a price. Typically, that price is anxiety-related illness such as depression or lifestyle illnesses (obesity, heart and lung disease, cancer, etc.) that come about as a result of life-depleting coping mechanisms such as food and other addictions.

Selecting a Goal

Once you assess your life and gain a better understanding of yourself, the next step is to rethink your goals for yourself and your life. You will likely never find bliss if you follow someone else's goals or try to be someone who you aren't, and may end up resigning yourself to a life of misery or at least apathy. When you select a goal, ask yourself, "Is this my goal, or is it someone else's?" As often as not, the goals you pursue are someone else's handmedowns that they passed on to you. They may, in turn, have received their goals from someone else. It may be that the goals were created generations before you came along; they may not fit you or your needs and desires at all.

Once you determine your goals for your own life, you need to develop a long-term strategy to achieve them. When you think about this, though, focus on one goal at a time; pace yourself with small, slow steps. If we take on too much, it's harder to achieve any one goal; it also provides a built-in excuse for failure: there was "too much to do;" or, "It wasn't reasonable or even possible." If you just work on one goal, that excuse is out the window. And your chances of success are that much greater.

Make sure that each goal you select is something you really truly want to achieve; that it will be meaningful when you've achieved it. After all, if you are going to put in the effort, it should be worth it to you *personally*, and that goes for having children, which is an unconscious choice via an unexamined paradigm for a lot of people in the world. (I will speak more about this in the next section.) At the same time, though, be very patient with yourself and what may turn out to be inevitably slow-but-steady progress. If you become distracted, review your goal list and the *reasons why* you made this goal in the first place; it will motivate you to continue to make progress. If you find yourself making excuses, do the same thing, and solicit support from friends, family, or a professional coach to keep you on track.

Following the Culturally Accepted Paradigm

Let's say you and your partner plan to have a future together, a simple life where you can both do all the things you've always wanted. It is lovely that you've found someone whose life goals are in sync with yours. But perhaps the two of you anticipate that achieving those goals is going to be rough, perhaps it will require putting in seventeen-hour work days, spending less time together, and being stuck with nights of exhaustion, all with no end in sight. Yet you decide that this is all right with you and your partner because the incredibly strong social paradigm tells us we are supposed to get married, have children, buy a home, overwork, create debt, stress ourselves, and make superficial friends.

The paradigm tells us that we will find security by doing what most everyone else is doing and closing our eyes and tolerating the illusion. So we embark on our lives, confident that the plan will give our days meaning. We work hard, fully believing that our efforts will pay off in a meaningful life.

Unfortunately, this plan isn't ideal; in fact, it is severely flawed. However, since we are indoctrinated into it, we plod along and like most couples in our society we often follow it for years—and then wake up one day and realize I'm overweight, divorced, alcoholic, incredibly unhappy, or seriously ill, and I've been sublimating my true needs and desires from the frustration of not living an authentic life. We've been wasting our time…time our most limited and precious time on this earth, without even realizing it.

The good news… we can change the paradigm, and consequently the outcome.

How Open Are You to Change?

Are you willing to release your conditioned beliefs? We believe many things throughout our lives that may not be true. Sources of false information may include our families, teachers, friends, books, the media, and our own misinterpretation of our experiences.

Once you believe something, are you capable of changing your mind if evidence to the contrary becomes available? A renowned professor was visiting a Zen master who asked, "Tea?" "Yes," said the professor. The Zen master began to pour the tea and continued pouring. As the hot tea began to run over the rim of the cup, the professor, shocked, cried, "Enough!" There was nothing that could be added to the professor's cup. When our minds are full of dogma, there is no room for fresh knowledge. Keep emptying. Is your cup already full, or are you ready for refreshing new insights?

Do you cling to the notion of permanence to resist change? Life is impermanent. That's not what we are taught to believe early in life, however. Teenagers don't worry about impermanence because they do not usually have to come face to face with that impermanence unless they lose a pet or a grandparent dies. They're told what's happening, but it doesn't really register. There is sorrow and there is grief, but buoyancy soon returns ushered in by hopefulness of the future.

The older we get, the more impermanence haunts us because we envision death encountering us somewhere on our path, though we never know how or when it will come. So we resist it or try and push it away. One of the greatest obstructions to authentic living has been our obstinate, unreasonable clinging to the notion of permanency. Remember: if you wait for certainty and security, you will never really do anything in your life. Once you allow yourself to realize and accept that life is impermanent, however, you can get on with *living* and getting to know your true self.

Change Happens in the Moment

Our lives are a compilation of moments. Each individual moment is all we have to affect change—through the choices we make *in that moment*. Are we turning away from uncomfortable feelings and eating a couple of doughnuts instead? Are we yelling at someone and blaming them for our troubles rather than asking the question, "*What did I do to cause this?*" Are we allowing negative thoughts about our self to occupy our mind, or are we thinking positively about our contributions? The *how* of change comes down to few simple practices: identifying what we really want (our goal), learning actions and practices that will support the attainment of that goal, and making choices in each moment that support what we are creating. All of this requires awareness. We can focus on what's important or we can distract ourselves with the unimportant—things that are not related to our goals, do not add to real enjoyment in life, or, worse, thoughts that are counterproductive.

How much of our time is spent on unimportant moments? Most of the time, if we really examine our lives, we're doing the nonessential altogether too often. Instead, we need to learn to live a *purpose-driven* life from moment to moment. If we give our attention to each moment and to our goals rather than to a set of thought patterns about how we *should* be behaving or what we *should* be doing in relation to the roles we have taken on (wife, husband, father, mother, employee, etc.), our authentic selves will emerge. But as long as we are holding on to one particular energy flow (from an entrenched paradigm, for example), a different energy flow cannot take its place. In other words, if we are holding onto a way of living and being that is not entirely meaningful, it becomes difficult to create a way of living and being that would be more suitable and significant, more authentic.

This is the reason that we tend to think at higher levels yet act on lower impulses. We think light yet choose actions that are heavy; we think spiritually but act materially; and we think positively but act negatively. We keep exchanging the energy for what we ideally want because we're not willing to let go of the particular energy we have become.

We must learn to be present in this moment because when we're in the moment and conscious of the movement of energy within (thoughts, feelings, emotions, etc.) we can make choices with utmost clarity. We can exchange any negative energy for positive focuses. We can speak our feelings out loud, even if it's just to our self, and know they are honest and authentic ones. We can also observe things and situations for what they *actually* are rather than what we *think* they are or *wish* they would be.

Conditioned responses no longer exist in this moment because we see and hear everything clearly and take things at face value. When, I'm doing this, I am not vetting, interpreting, or editing what I am seeing through any particular filter or belief system. I am conscious, aware, and in control of my life. Our belief systems cause us to ignore facts, take things out of context, and blow things out of proportion; they are the reason we are able to continue justifying violence, racism, sexism, and our personal dysfunctions. Whenever we exchange truth for an illusion, we are allowing ourselves to continue to think and act in negative, life-depleting ways.

But when we exist in the present moment, there is only clarity, authentic control, and the ability to surrender illusion. We act only on what is in front of us rather than our stories about it. This is where we gain enlightenment, because in these moments we make authentic choices. Enlightenment in life is fundamentally about the quality of non-judgmental awareness we have about what is happening in and around us in any given moment, the quality of the choices we make in those moments in terms of their ability to enhance and elevate our energy and the energy of those around us), and our willingness to stand for them.

Use Conscious Creating

At the end of the day, we all yearn for a simple, uncomplicated, pleasant life. But our day-to-day choices often remove us from our ideal life. Where we live and the work we perform routinely often times can remove us from our ideal life. Even our friends and associates can remove us from what we need most. By existing in opposition to our ideal, we generate anxiety, depression, and resignation. And these emotions lead to drinking, smoking, overeating, or taking medications to distract us from our sense of incompleteness.

One way to live at an enlightened level is by engaging in what I call conscious creating. You do this by starting to develop wonderful ideas while being conscious in the moment. You must avoid the habit of convincing yourself you do not have enough money to do this, or that you are not educated enough to make good decisions. All you have to do is trust that the universe will help you manifest an idea and you will suddenly find your energy starts to lighten up. Creative energy is a rapid, vibrating energy. Try to be creative with everything you do, in every area of your life. Have fun with the energy. Play with it.

If you're not creating, your energy stagnates. Stagnant energy is negative energy; it drains you and leaves you with even less energy. The less you create, the less positive energy you have at your disposal. The more you create, the lighter your energy becomes. But we must be creating in a way that allows us to rebalance ourselves and lead a simpler life every day; this way we experience sufficiency as we are and discover the enlightenment possible in each moment. If we invest time and thought into these practices, we will reap the benefits and so will those around us, in time.

Putting the Real You to Work in Our Troubled World

How did we reach this point in history when we can no longer discern what the truth is, when reason has been subverted by ignorance, where insecurity, instantaneous pleasures, and the rejection of personal responsibility for uplifting others have become the norm? This book is intended to be a mirror to help answer these questions and to go beyond. I hope by reading so far you will have perceived accurate reflections of what we have become. I am also hopeful that we can equally observe the signs pointing to our authentic, true nature. This book is not meant to make us feel bad or angry about ourselves and others; rather its purpose is to spell out the often shocking facts that will support more of us to make the changes that are so desperately needed today. The contemporary theologian Matthew Fox outlined succinctly the predicament of our personal responsibility toward ourselves and others. It is no longer sufficient for us to simply say, "Forgive us for we know not what we do." Rather, the mantra today should be, "Forgive us for we do not do what we know we should do." It is our apathy, complacency, and deep seated fear of change that prevents us from taking that initial step forward to act as we ought to act.

Dr. Alberto Villoldo, a medical anthropologist and shaman, describes two coexisting universes: the universe of predators and the universe of creators. The world of corporate and political greed that we are witnessing today, the lack of ethics among investors and journalists, and the "me first" wealth-hungry values of our youth embody this predatory world. Alternatively, there is the world of creators, individuals who are gradually becoming the harbingers of a new culture based on enlightened reason, spiritual principles, and the restoration of social ethics based upon compassion, community, and personal responsibility for one's actions. One of the salient reasons for composing this book is to provide readers with some hardlearned inspiration to become a creator of harmony—in part through choosing a healthy vegetarian lifestyle. When we are able to become creators in a predatory society and can remain in balance while doing so, we then have the capability for implementing genuine change.

No major social issue such as poverty, the drugging of our nation and children, the war in Iraq and other global conflicts, and all the political, health, and educational crises, can change for the better until we as individuals change. Our systems for social and environmental sustainability are collapsing. Our nation is utterly bankrupt, borrowing more than we even hope to pay back; and, our environment is heavily poisoned. Brutal reality television programs have become postmodern gladiatorial sports, sanctioned by our culture because they provide us with a means to escape our hectic, busy lives and to give us an excuse for not awakening from our cultural dream.

The mistake we make is thinking that what any one of us does won't be enough to turn the tide. In reality, the only tide that you really have to worry about turning is your own; the rest of the world will respond accordingly.

Taking Responsibility for Your Life

Take a look at your life today. Remember that nothing gets better on its own. We have to take control of everything in our life and create balance. From balance comes harmony. From harmony comes bliss. When you have harmony, bliss, and balance, you surrender disease, conflict, and anxiety.

As I said earlier in the chapter, don't wait for a crisis—whether in the form of an illness, divorce, or job loss—to wake up; that is a more stressful way to learn. Crisis is the universe warning us to make necessary course corrections, and you will find that it is usually preceded by earlier promptings for change that went unheeded. It's the universe's way of getting you to listen, and it can teach us something if we pay attention and are willing to learn. Better to pay attention now and make changes proactively—even if that is scary—lest we repeat these painful experiences. What areas of your life are you not honoring? Only you can answer that for yourself, and only you can arrange pieces of your life's puzzle in a way that will bring you joy and enable you to share that joy with others.

Remember, don't hesitate: start now.

Ask Transformative Questions

If we really want to change our lives, to experience the excitement of change, we have to ask ourselves perspective-shattering questions. We have to consider, "Do I really want to keep this job or even stay in this line of work?" Or, "Am I really happy in the bucolic countryside or do I want the hustle and bustle of living in a major city?" Or maybe even, "Am I really happy in my relationship or marriage? Do I need new friends, stronger—or weaker—family connections, or a different partner?"

But we can only ask those questions if we don't fear the answer. After all, if you are entertaining the idea that you are in an unrewarding profession or unsupportive relationship, you are opening yourself not only to the possibility of putting effort toward change, but also, possibly, to confronting and discarding some of the beliefs you have been living by.

Making changes in life, though, is a good thing if you think carefully about what you are doing. If your goal through change is to eliminate stress and anxiety and experience more joy in life rather than to simply seek permanence, you are on the right track.

Overcoming Fear

Most people view crisis through a prism of fear. When crisis is absent from our lives, what should we be paying attention to? Are there changes still to be made, and if so, what are they? In most cases, people do nothing when their lives are crisis free because safety is found in predictable patterns, in clinging to the same habits. When an opportunity arises to make a change and try something new, we so often stop in our tracks and refrain from taking advantage of the opportunity. Beneath our hesitation is a deep fear about what is unpredictable if we become our real self. We are fearful of where an important change will lead us, and we fear our resources for managing the consequences are limited or unavailable. Most often this translates into a belief that we simply do not have the capability to undertake a major change.

Fear constricts you in every way you can imagine. It constricts your body and it narrows your mind. When the mind constricts, it fears taking chances and when enough behavior becomes conditioned to avoid taking chances, growth ceases and fear wins. The cycle of avoidance spreads into other areas of our lives and pretty soon we stop trying anything new or different to avoid being criticized, laughed at, or simply thought of as different. Staying safe and comfortable becomes the modus operandi and risk aversion the primary purpose. The problem is that this living in fear of change leads to stagnation and grave imbalance.

You must put aside your fears and build your confidence instead. When we go to a deeper level of the self, we are identifying with our true authenticity as a human being, instead of our fearful mind. Then you will be able to assert yourself in any situation. However, be careful not to confuse arrogance with confidence. Arrogant people act out of a need to feel superior; they too are motivated by fear and insecurity.

When you are truly confident, you feel good about your actions. If we become accountable for our thoughts, our words, and our deeds, and then realize the positive or negative effects these have upon our authentic self, we can begin to live authentic and virtuous lives. We can improve our own day-to-day existence and through that improve society as a whole.

Preparing for Change

Ask yourself whether you have the determination and motivation to seek truth regardless of how deep you must dig. Do you have the courage and fortitude to stand up as a freethinking human being and challenge the artificial social environment and the people who wish to curtail your growth and imprison you in their false belief systems? It takes impeccable honesty to acknowledge that something that appears to be real is inherently false. These are the essential qualities—determination, courage, fortitude, and honesty—to create authentic self-esteem. When you learn to become an aware observer, you will discover truth and meaning in everything.

Remember, it is vital to accept yourself completely, all of your gifts and all of your foibles. There is no better way to enhance self-esteem and harness its benefits for living an authentic life than by accepting the self, because then we are not centered in our ego and trying to legitimize the ego's desires. You can begin by forgiving everything that has prevented you from accepting yourself fully and pursuing your full potential.

Now Do You Really Want to Change?

Austrian neurologist and psychiatrist and holocaust survivor, Viktor E. Frankl said in his book *Man's Search for Meaning*, "Everything can be taken from a man but one thing: the last of the human freedoms—to choose one's attitude in any given set of circumstances, to choose one's own way."[4]

With every situation, one choice is to remain unwilling to change and to stay as we are, as servants to the existing social paradigm and the powers that control it, governed by fear. According to Frankl's account of Auschwitz, this choice would have led to certain and imminent death. Thankfully, most of us reading this book are not currently in such dire situations. However, if our attitude is to get through life now and not feel any connection with or responsibility toward the society around us, then we will continue to ignore what is happening, resist conversations that could help us, and whine and complain about the injustices we witness without making the formidable changes in our own lives that are both necessary and achievable. What are those changes? Many possibilities are outlined in this book: I cannot say for you, but as I alluded to at the beginning of this chapter, they are related to your "why" for being here.

Harold S. Kushner, prominent American rabbi and author, including of the bestselling book, *When Bad Things Happen to Good People*, affirmed this in the foreword for *Man's Search for Meaning*, "Terrible as it was, his [Frankl's] experience in Auschwitz reinforced what was already one of his key ideas: Life is not primarily a quest for pleasure, as Freud believe, or a quest for power, as Alfred Adler taught, but a quest for meaning. The greatest task for any person is to find meaning in his or her life."[5]

We are only able to be beneficial and constructive members of society, as well as of the global community, if we take ownership of our role and responsibility in preserving the best they have to offer. If we only focus on our self and how we feel, we will not be able to make the leap in understanding that is essential for choosing a healthier way of living and being in this world. Therefore, it is incumbent upon us to understand how each choice we make affects someone, somewhere, something every day. The choices, then, are to commit ourselves to awakening and learning to become aware of our exchange of energies with ourselves and others; to be a cause for overcoming our weaknesses and reducing suffering in the world wherever we can, to confront our fear and refuse to let it govern our actions, and to pursue our bliss as fully actualized human beings.

It is a challenging but not impossible task.

Don't Wait to Be Saved

We cannot hand over responsibility for our happiness to someone else. We cannot wait to be rescued, to be saved. No one will save you; you have to become highly proactive. It is your life, and you're the only one who's responsible for it. You're the only one who can self-actualize.

Do you constantly seek success in the hope that recognition will overcome your insecurity, doubts, and fears? If so, then you will try to control everything that people think about you through your actions and your words. Living this way is to suffer endlessly. You are not living an honest, authentic life; you are trying to create and live up to a false image of yourself.

If we give someone else responsibility for our happiness, we are striving for external acceptance. But the only acceptance that truly matters is internal. We need to love ourselves completely and unconditionally.

It can be scary to think that we're so powerful that we can be complete within ourselves. We have been led to believe that we are nobody unless we have the right spouse, clothes, job, or friends. But if you are fully present and honest with yourself, you can look for the authentic qualities in your surroundings. You can feel complete in the moment, no matter what.

When you have faith in yourself, your spiritual and emotional roots go so deep that in any crisis you will just smile and say, "Here is another lesson to learn from. I'll be better, stronger, and wiser because of this." This is all possible once you believe in the completeness of your being.

The happy person is balanced. And balanced people appreciate what they have. This is one of the most important things I have learned about life and why I insist: Stop always thinking that there is someone or something missing from your life and that you won't be happy until you find it. When you live in the moment, when you are true to your authentic self, you will find peace and joy wherever you are, although obviously not 100% of the time as struggle, frustrations, sadness, and anger are all aspects of life. It's just that when you live an authentic life, there is far less of it.

In Closing...

I have attempted to outline clearly to you the tools, regardless of the generation into which you were born, that are needed to reclaim your dignity and become a spiritually realized member of the human race. More on these topics is available in my book titled, *Living in the Moment: A Prescription for the Soul.* As I alluded to earlier in this chapter, until you become committed to getting "right" with yourself, the changes you implement will be merely cosmetic—to appease the ego—and will not result in the real health that you desire. Real health takes work. Each of us possesses qualities of universal love and compassion, kindness and nurturance that can generate harmony throughout the world when they are brought to consciousness and acted upon. This book, therefore, is intended to provide and strengthen us with essential insights that will enable us to personally transform ourselves and thereby allow us to experience the remarkable realization of our extraordinary potential.

To this point in the book, I have detailed the healthy vegetarian diet, including supplementation, as well as many of the lifestyle practices of the healthy vegetarian and the reasons for undertaking them. We have taken an in-depth look at how harmful the practice of consuming animal products really is—to both humans and animals. We also now see how detrimental it is to our environment, and the spiritual underpinnings and implications of this choice. I also spoke about how important it is for each of us to find our W*hy*, and for *everything* in life. Bringing this level of contemplation to our existence will enable us lead an authentic, self-directed life—one where we are free from the trappings of narrow societal influences.

We also discussed the realities of creating a healthy life, including the fact that it does take work. We need to stay open and flexible while addressing our fear of change. We humans are creatures of comfort, but the comforts that we choose—among them diets high in fat, sugar, and salt—are killing us and the environment. Where is our responsibility in all of this? Well, as I said a little while ago, it is with you…and with each one of us. I quite enjoy this anonymous quote, "'I must do something' always solves more problems than 'Something must be done.'" While we may not be directly to blame for the intense pain and suffering experienced by farm animals and other humans as a result of our ways, we are responsible for it as well as our life and our health. But where does that responsibility begin and end? That is what we will explore now.

Part II:

Healing The Planet

> "Waste no more time arguing about what a good man should be. Be one."
>
> – *Marcus Aurelius,* Meditations

We are facing unprecedented challenges on this planet at this time; the threats are unparalleled, yet very few are actually interested in getting into action and doing something about it. *Planet Earth Herald* issued a top 10 environmental issues list that is more than eye-opening; I'd like to provide a short summary. When you see all of these issues on one page, it certainly seems insurmountable, daunting at best. Here are just a few of the realities. World population has increased by almost 3 times since 1950, when the population stood at 2,555,982,611 compared to today's population of 7,358,692,228 (at the time of this writing, increasing more than one person per second).[1]

Then there is the issue of climate change, about which they note, "Recently an overwhelming majority of climate scientists believe that human activities are currently affecting the climate and that the tipping point has already been passed. In other words, it is too late to undo the damage that climate change has done to the environment." As far as the specifics, 40% of US CO_2 emissions come from electricity production, and burning coal accounts for 93% of emissions from the electric utility industry. Yet, the demand for electric gadgets increases without widespread alternative energy sources. Further, our modern car culture and appetite for globally sourced goods is responsible for about 33% of emissions in the US[2] and I've already spoken about how the animal agriculture industry contributes to this.

It is wise to note that the oceans absorb as much as 25% of all human carbon dioxide emissions. The gas then combines with other elements to form compounds such as carbolic acid. Over the last 250 years, surface acidity of the ocean has increased by an estimated 30%, and expected to increase by another 150% by 2100. The report points out, "The effect of over acidification of the oceans on sea creatures such as shellfish and plankton is similar to osteoporosis in humans. The acid effectively is dissolving the skeletons of the creatures." It is thought that the negative effect to marine life is now on a scale that the planet has not seen for millions of years.

We are losing species at the rate of dozens every day.[3] Does this sound shocking to you? Let me give you the background of this so that you better comprehend the scope of this number. Although extinction is a natural phenomenon, the typical baseline rate is about one to five species per year! Scientists estimate we're now losing species at 1,000 to 10,000 times the background rate, which translates into as many as 30 to 50% of all species possibly heading toward extinction by mid-century. Research published in *Nature* confirms this deadly trend, noting that by 2050 rising temperatures could lead to the extinction of more than a million species. Many scientists agree that our planet is now in the midst of its sixth mass extinction of plants and animals and the, "Worst spate of species die-offs since the loss of the dinosaurs 65 million years ago."[4] What we don't realize is that our life, indeed, depends on the vitality of the planet and these species. We might be quick to think, "Well, we can survive without them," but with every loss to the food chain, our delicate ecosystems are interrupted and our life is affected. *Planet Earth Herald* notes that a, "catastrophic impact of loss of biodiversity is likely to affect the planet for millions of years to come."[5]

Then, there is the issue of water. Currently, one third of humans do not have access to clean, fresh water—that is approximately 2.5 billion people, 8 times the population of the United States. Unfortunately, this number is expected to increase by up to two thirds by 2050. Think about this for a moment; the experts are telling us that within 35 years, only one-third of us in the world will have access to clean water. Many of these same experts believe that water will become as valuable as gold or oil and that the new wars will be fought for access.

Other human infractions against the environment are related to the use and abuse of nitrogen, which we readily remove from the atmosphere and convert into reactive forms, such as nitrates—to the tune of around 120 million tons a year. This is undertaken for the production of nitrates for fertilizer for crops and in the use of food additives. The run-off from crops and lawn care into our oceans has a profoundly negative effect upon the phytoplankton, which is responsible for the production of most of the oxygen in our air.

The depletion of our ozone level is real. The release of chemical pollutants such as chlorine and bromide through human activities cause ozone molecules to break apart and holes to form.[6] The largest of these holes is now over the Antarctic. According to the Environmental Protection Agency, *one* atom of chlorine can break down more than 100,000 ozone molecules, which is why they have banned CFCs, but this doesn't even begin to go far enough.

Overfishing is perhaps the most sobering of all these facts. Some researchers say that in the last 60 years stocks of large fish have fallen by 90% and that we are facing the collapse of all types of fish species in less than 50 years. Currently, the ocean is the largest source of food in the world, with fish serving as the main source of daily protein for 1.2 billion people.[7] This, in my opinion, is an atrocity, and it is where the USDA did not go far enough in their recent food recommendations.

Nonetheless, let's look at this reality. In 2006, a group led by Boris Worm, Ph.D., from Dalhousie University in Halifax, Nova Scotia and his colleagues in the UK, US, Sweden, and Panama, set to determine the effects of this wide scale loss of species and its impact on human life. Their report, published in the highly reputable *Science* magazine noted among other things that species in the ocean play a vital role in our own survival. One of sea life's primary roles and benefits to human life is filtering toxins from the ocean and controlling algae blooms, which if left uncontrolled by nature, can have disastrous effects. Worm stated, "A large and increasing proportion of our population lives close to the coast. The loss of services such as flood control and waste detoxification can have disastrous consequences." Nicola Beaumont, a

PhD of the Plymouth Marine Laboratory, U.K., and one of the scientists on the study said, "If biodiversity continues to decline, the marine environment will not be able to sustain our way of life. Indeed, it may not be able to sustain our lives at all."[8]

Lastly, and not any less alarming is the rate of global deforestation. Since 1990, half of the world's rain forests have been destroyed, and the clearing of forests continues at an alarming rate. Beyond this, trees are now dying globally at a rate never before seen. A study that appeared in the December 2012 issue of the journal *Science* determined that trees between 100 and 300 years old are perishing "en masse." The cause The cause, a deadly combination of large destructive events like forest fires, and other, more incremental factors like drought, high temperatures, logging, and insect attack. This new development means that old trees are dying at 10 times their normal rate.[9]

Hear me when I say this: Our planet—and therefore all of mother earth's inhabitants, which includes us humans—are in danger, as a direct effect of our human behavior. I have taken a position throughout this book to be understanding of the forces that impact human behavior and take these into consideration with my recommendations so far. But, I must go on record to share my belief, which is that the healthy vegetarian lifestyle is not just something nice to do for our own health and the planet. In reality, it is our imperative, and we must do this now. It is no longer a luxury for the intelligent few; it is a necessity to sustain life on this planet for future generations.

Why, do you ask, should I do anything different and rally up if, indeed, the whole thing is going down in flames? Because I have seen people with stage 4 bone cancer and many other life threatening diseases who were given just weeks to live who have turned their lives around and survived. Yes, these are rare individuals; but their persistence and unwavering commitment to reversing their prognosis gives me hope that with enough proper action, our species can accomplish the same, thereby affecting the health of the entire planet positively.

Chapter 9

What is Our Obligation to Society and the Planet?

> "Wrong does not cease to be wrong because the majority share in it."
>
> — *Leo Tolstoy, Author of* War and Peace

Morality

Without offering a full treatise on the concept of *morality,* this discussion warrants a few words on the concept before proceeding. Morality is essentially our compass that tells us right from wrong, whether we are referring to behavior or thinking or both. It is a uniquely human mechanism that guides our thinking and our doing, protecting us and our surrounding world from potential harm that we might otherwise inflict. The concept has been contemplated since the earliest days of higher thinking and has seen multiple trajectories. Philosophers have connected the concept of morality to specific areas of life, such as sexuality and corporate behavior. Ultimately, though, morality ensures that our thinking and behaving is appropriate toward life, meaning it is *life-enhancing*. Abraham Lincoln said it best when he spoke these words, "I am not bound to win, but I am bound to be true. I am not bound to succeed, but I am bound to live up to what light I have."

Moral behavior reflects higher consciousness, and the greater moral responsibility in a society, the more evolved it is perceived to be. We don't tend to look kindly on nations and societies where mistreating their people through "inhumane" conditions is the status quo. This, we assert, is immoral.

Unfortunately, morality is oftentimes offset by self-serving interests: either we do whatever we want, or we do the "right" thing, or something in between. But we can feel really grateful when doing the right thing happens also to be what we want to do. More often than not, however, these two drives compete. We see this in the case of our own personal health but also with regard to the health of our planet: we choose doughnuts and coffee over smoothies and fresh vegetable juices; we continue to water our lawn and apply non-organic fertilizers and pesticides rather than use our lawn for fruits trees and a vegetable garden, using compost or a not-toxic pest solution that we made at home. In these examples, we either serve ourselves and our own immediate desires, or we set our selfish desires aside and opt for socially responsible behavior that contributes to the greater good—as one example.

And no discussion of a healthy vegetarian would be complete without some discussion of the morality of what we consume. It is purely morality that guides our abstinence (in the US) from eating the following:

- *Other humans.* We call this cannibalism, and our moral compasses points hard away from this behavior.
- *Cats and dogs.* These domesticated animals are our pets. They live outside in our yards or in our homes and sleep in our beds with us. They are our friends, and often are considered an integral part of the family. We love them, and we know that they love us. We nurture them when they are sick and are grateful for their nurturing and unconditional love when we are under the weather. They protect us from harm, and we protect them. We discipline and punish them when they misbehave, and teach them, similar to how we teach our own children. When we know them well, we can see in them the things that they understand, such as their shame when they have knowingly broken a rule. We spend time with them, and we learn their likes, dislikes, and emotional range. We can tell when they are happy or sad, and when they like something or don't like it. So, we don't eat them.

- *Birds.* Same with the types of birds that people typically have as pets.
- *Rodents.* Likewise for typical pets such as hamsters and mice, etc.
- *Monkeys, apes, and other primates.* These are our nearest physiological cousins. We look at them and despite a different exterior, we recognize their similarities with us when we look in their eyes, and see the depth of their souls. We observe their family behavior and recognize it as strikingly similar to that of humans. We watch them play with each other and with us, and if we watch them enough, we will see their emotional range. Thanks to the work of many researchers, we know that they are incredibly smart, even capable of learning language, and they have demonstrated compassion for the suffering of those they love, whether of their own species or ours. Basically, monkeys and other primates are just *too close* to us for us to justify eating. It's not exactly cannibalism, but close enough. In truth, we also don't eat them because they're not indigenous to the US and it's illegal, but even if it were legal, there aren't a lot of cultures in the world that eat monkeys.
- *Horses.* These beautiful creatures are pets for some and hobbies for others; they are like children—each with different personalities. And they display emotions as much or even more than dogs and cats.
- *Endangered species.* We know it's not right to kill species that are struggling to survive. We aren't that hungry.

So essentially, we won't eat anything that a) is too close to us physiologically; or b) lives in our homes with us as members of the family. We draw these lines because we can see the suffering on the faces of these people and/or animals we might be tempted to kill for food, and we simply can't bear it. Our moral compass points away from this behavior. If we violate it, we end up with severe internal turmoil as our conscience wreaks a bit of havoc for us. Why? Because the life that moves through them is the same life that moves through us. So, in this sense, we are one with them.

The logical next question then becomes, "Why is it okay to eat animals that don't live with us or that we're not physiologically as close to?"

Singer's Five Ethics

In Peter Singer's foray into where our food comes from in *The Way We Eat*, he outlines five ethical principles that he believes most people will share. He lists the following:

1. **Transparency.** We have a right to know how our food is produced. Some say that if slaughterhouses had glass walls, no one would eat meat. The point is that we have the right to access accurate and unbiased information about what we are buying and how it was produced.

2. **Fairness.** Food production shouldn't impose costs on others. If the method of food production imposes significant costs on others, such as emitting odors that bother neighbors, then the market is not operating efficiently and the outcome will not be fair to those taken advantage of. Any unsustainable food production contains this intrinsic injustice, since future generations will pay the price for our decisions.

3. **Humanity**. It is wrong to inflict significant suffering on animals for minor reasons. Most people agree that we should avoid harming animals through inflicting pain or other forms of distress. Kindness and compassion toward all animal life, human and otherwise, is certainly more desirable than indifference to the suffering of another feeling being.

4. **Social responsibility.** Workers should be paid a decent wage and enjoy decent working conditions. Freedom from child labor, forced labor, and sexual harassment are the most basic of decencies for employees and suppliers. Discrimination based on physical or social characteristics is wrong. Workers should receive a wage they can live on and support their families on.

5. **Needs.** The preservation of life and health is more justifiable than other desires. Meeting our most basic needs of food, survival, and adequate nourishment trumps other considerations.[1]

Currently, none of these ethics is entirely met in the United States, and we largely have corporate monstrosities to thank for this. Monsanto vehemently litigates *against* transparency every time a state's residents push for GMO and other labeling that would increase transparency about what we're putting into our bodies. You see,

Monsanto doesn't want you to know. Why else would food lobbyists be busy persuading regulators NOT to require meat manufacturers to inform you when you are buying laboratory created (cloned) meat? They know that in transparency, they will lose. Large food producers are the same; once you know what's actually in the food that you're buying, you won't buy it any longer.

If you've ever lived anywhere near a slaughterhouse, you know that the smell is downright disgusting, especially on a hot, windless day. Indeed, the reek of decomposing flesh and blood fills the air and prevents their neighbors from fully enjoying their lives. This is but one small example of how our current practices are unfair.

We definitely don't meet any sort of threshold for the humanity ethic. Eating meat violates this ethic, period. Even in the non-factory farms, where animals are free to roam and enjoy their lives, they suffer when we take their young away from them or they themselves become highly agitated when boarding the slaughter house trucks. If you eat meat, you are violating this ethic.

There is no social responsibility within the factory farm industry. Workers do not enjoy decent wages or decent working conditions. As outlined by Eric Schlosser in *Fast Food Nation*, sexual harassment among many other abuses in the industry is the rule rather than the exception.[2] It is far from an ethical industry, on any account.

As far as meeting our basic needs above other needs, sadly that is simply nonexistent as well, not only here in the US, but abroad in many countries as well. The very fact that we have to have the conversation about how food corporations twist the truth to line their pockets demonstrates clearly that not everyone cares enough about meeting humans' basic needs. Many are far more motivated by greed. Yes, we have a long way to go, but adapting a healthy vegetarian lifestyle will end some of the suffering altogether, now, while getting us to where we are going faster.

Respect for Animal Life Translates into… Respect for All Life

When we consider actually working on a factory farm or in a slaughterhouse, we can't imagine half of the human abuses that occur in those environments. Eric Schlosser's *Fast Food Nation* provides provocative insight to this industry in all of its ugliness.

The meat-slaughtering business isn't only off-putting when we think about the kill floor, the animal shit mixing in with the packaged food sold to consumers, workers wading in blood or even when we think about actually killing our fellow creatures. This is bad enough, but it's only the half of it. According to Schlosser, working in this business is not only dangerous, but inhumane. Undocumented workers dodge killing and cutting machines as a way of life, and are essentially prohibited from filing claims for on-the-job injuries when they occur because these companies know how desperate illegal workers are for work. They have no rights and risk deportation if they don't follow the rules. One bad fall or unfortunate run-in with a piece of machinery can mean an entire family's demise, not to mention possible permanent injury that prevents this injured worker from ever gainfully earning again.

This doesn't happen in some faraway land, but in everyday slaughterhouses within our nation's core across numerous states.

How is it okay to subject our fellow men and women to these sorts of working conditions, in this country and in this day and age? We rally against sweat shops in foreign lands as inhumane, yet we subject our workers to these conditions on our own soil? As for the work itself, could *you* take a knife to the throat of one chicken after another 8 to 12 hours a day, or a harmless cow or steer? Could you do it? Would you? If not, why should these workers be expected to? More critically, if not, how can you justify eating what you would not tolerate harvesting?

Animals suffer. They feel pain—physical, emotional, and psychological, as do we. When they break a leg, they cry. When they lose their offspring, most of them do cry. When they understand that they are being hunted down or shipped off to a slaughter house and that their lives are about to end, they experience fear and stress. If you've spent any time at all around cows, you know that they know more than we give them credit for; they know what's going on. They line up and observe in silent respect as any large animal gives birth. A calf will bawl in fear when it's separated from the herd, and a mother will bawl in worry when she can't find her calf. When a cow gives a still birth, she bawls in grief as she licks it and nudges it to move. They will bellow loudly and resist tremendously when the slaughter truck comes for them, in awareness of what happens once they get on that truck. A cow will bawl for days when her calf is suddenly gone, even when that calf is full grown. They know who their children are, and they suffer when their children leave as any human mother suffers when her child is suddenly ripped from her life. They feel physical pain when they get caught in the fence, emotional pain when they lose a child, and psychological pain when they board the slaughter truck because they know what fate awaits them. They feel, they love, they cherish—and they suffer.

No, cows are not human. And their range of emotions is probably not as complex as ours. Does this mean that it's okay for us to patently ignore their suffering as if it's simply not occurring, or doesn't matter? Are we capable of being sensitive to the needs of the greater good? Or are we conscienceless psychopaths hell-bent on serving our own selfish interests regardless of the suffering it wreaks? The simple fact is that we have a responsibility; and, we make choices on this matter every day and at every meal.

Nineteenth-century German philosopher Arthur Schopenhauer said, "Compassion is the basis of morality." Morality guides us to not inflict harm, pain, or suffering upon others, and it is a central tenet of the peace movement. Indeed, an evolved society rises above the capacity to inflict harm, choosing instead the peaceful path, and it is essential on the path to becoming a healthy vegetarian.

There are the humanitarian concerns in relation to the cruelty to animals perpetuated in these factory farms, which we have also covered before, but not specifically regarding milking cows. The simple fact is that cows produce milk for the very same reasons human mothers do: to nourish their young. They give birth and are physically ready to raise their calves. Surely, there is a strong bond between a mother cow and its calf at birth and throughout the nursing period. Obviously, in many cases the bond is short lived due to the heartless practices of agribusiness, yet the heartbreaking emotions are still evident. Baby calves naturally suckle six to twelve months, but in the dairy industry, calves are separated from their mothers immediately after birth.[3] Female calves are carted away to be future milk pumps, and the males are raised and slaughtered for meat.

With her children robbed from her, a dairy cow will spend the majority of her milk-producing life—8 to 9 years of a cow's natural 25-year lifespan—standing, confined in over-crowded feed lots and living in her own filth. Not much of a life, and certainly not a life of natural order—where she would be grazing lush fields of green grass, soaking in the sun. According to a statement by the People for the Ethical Treatment of Animals, "The stress caused by the conditions in animal factories leads to disease, lameness, and reproductive problems that render cows worthless to the dairy-products industry by the time that they're 4 or 5 years old, at which time they are sent to be slaughtered."[4] So it's not just a horrific life, it's a short-lived one, too.

It is in knowledge of such realities that groups such as the Oxford Vegetarian Organization in the UK work, "To promote the vegetarian/vegan diet for the moral… benefit of humankind."[5] Such groups, beacons of hope, believe that only by ending the abuse of animals and ceasing the consumption of meat and dairy, will humans be able to drink the "milk of human kindness," which, as you know, is much sweeter than that which comes from a mistreated cow.

More about Conscious Consumption

These last two points touch deeply on ethical issues in relation to other humans. There are also moral questions that deserve consideration in connection to non-human animals. As will be shown below, the way animals are killed and treated before they are done away with in industrialized farms has caused many to turn to vegetarianism as a stand against cruelty. They can't tolerate the cruel, heartless destruction of these innocent creatures.

I have spent time doing health workshops with people with all diets, ranging from strict vegans to occasional meat-eaters. I've had people confess to me that though they see the value of vegetarianism, they just can't give up meat. They say, however, they will only eat free-range animals that have not been shot up with hormones or other drugs, or confined in pens.

While a purist vegetarian might look suspiciously at such people, I personally will congratulate them for at least acting on one all-important ethical goal, the refusal to support factory farming. In fact, one man, a free-range meat-eater who I've known for quite a while, said to me with total sincerity, that if no meat was available except from factory farms, he would become a vegetarian overnight, because he could never spend his dollars on such an implacably cruel system.

Unlike your average meat-eater, he acknowledged the merciless upraising and killing of animals associated with these industrialized slaughterhouses. Here are some startling statistics on global animal slaughter in a recent year: over 291 million cattle, over 504 million lambs and sheep, 1.276 billion pigs, and more than 46 billion chickens. In the United States alone, the numbers were almost 35 million cattle, 2.9 million lambs and sheep, 103 million pigs, and almost 9 billion chickens.[6] One other source notes that "fish and other sea creatures whose deaths are so great they are only measured in tons."[7]

And it's not just that so many die, because everything dies eventually, but it is how they are made to live up to their end point that is the issue. Food animals do not get to enjoy the sunshine, roam the fields, or smell the fresh grass after a gentle spring rain. How could they since they never go outside? They are locked up in dark cells, where they spend much of their miserable lives packed in so tightly they can barely move.

How do we know they are suffering? Because they demonstrate typical activities that reflect discomfort and pain, such as biting and gnawing on cages as well as themselves and other animals in close proximity. It is prudent to remember that we are animals, too, and experience damaging hormone responses when subjected to stress. Can you imagine the anxiety that you might feel if locked into a cage just slightly larger than your body's size and could not move around for the entire span of your life, sometimes many years? Yet, the majority of us are unaware that this is occurring in our country. Nor are they aware that when they consume these animals they are literally "eating" this stress.

Livestock raisers realized they could save money on feed if they kept the animals nearly immobile; this way the animals would use up less energy and therefore need less food. That's the bottom-line mentality adhered to by factory management constantly looking for ways to increase profit and reduce overhead. These are the people who make the life and death decisions over the fate of these poor creatures. For them, it apparently means nothing that hens are frequently crowded into tiny cages that they do not leave even once a year. Pregnant sows are tightly housed to control their movement. They can barely squeeze their bodies into the minute stalls that are their homes for three-month stints, and they "cry out" and demonstrate fighting behavior when their calves are dragged from them at birth.

In some of these animal factories, cattle and pigs do get to enjoy open-air feeding lots, minded by machines that feed and water them and remove their waste, never seeing a human tender. Although, perhaps, this is best, given the lack of compassion of many of those who are in charge of them. In my DVD *Chew on This*, I present footage of the physical cruelty administered to animals by uncaring workers; it is a heartbreaking reality. Yet, it *is* the reality, and the idea of small farms where animals roam in fields without much restraint is the small exception to this reality. Roughly 95% of hens, chickens, and turkeys, and more than half of beef cattle, dairy cows, and pigs are raised in the impersonal, high-tech environment of the agribusiness factory farm.[8]

And far from things getting better, it seems as if each year the stock raisers' already hardened hearts get become even more so. There is a recent trend in the US toward creating fewer and larger feedlots. The weekly agribusiness newspaper *Feedstuffs* reports that this trend is expected (on the upside for the agribusinesses) to mean big cuts in overhead costs for the animal industries. Oh, there's a downside but only for the animals —greater discomfort and more inhumane treatment. Chickens are now given only one-sixth the space that laying hens had in 1954, for instance. Overseas operations are not much better, as the Philippines government Department of Agriculture, Bureau of Animal Industry website attests to the necessity of giving anti-stress medications to growing chickens, "Birds are given anti-stress drugs, either in the feed or in the drinking water, 2 to 5 days before and after they are transferred to the growing houses," given that these buildings are so crowded and the birds so squeezed in.[9]

While it's rough being in these prisons, what's even rougher is that unlike, say, human prisoners in jails, many of these animals can't even turn around, let alone express other natural instincts. As to the former, confinement is so complete for chickens in many of these "farms," they don't even have the room to flap their wings. Regarding instincts, mating is so controlled and normal sexual activity so hampered, that male animals commonly become impotent and females cannot even menstruate regularly.

"Commercially extraneous behavior" is what meat and poultry producers call activities that may be natural to an animal but economically undesirable.[10] Hey, if a chicken is going to be allowed to flap his wings, we would have to give him more space and that's not in the budget, the raisers say. Methods are devised to inhibit natural "extraneous" behavior. Poultry are "de-beaked" so they will not peck when under stress, and pigs have their tails cut off because they tend to bite them. Not only is physical behavior controlled, but so are biochemical processes. Hormones are given to intervene in reproductive system activity, to produce an exceptionally large number of ova in the female, and to keep an animal's labor contractions and delivery time on schedule—on the animal factory's schedule, that is.[11]

But, wait a minute, is gnawing your tail off instinctive behavior? Not in a normal environment. But instead of displaying instinctive behavior, animals in these prisons act out with unusual aggression and hostility. If you spent every day in a walled-in area with no way out, no natural light, controlled central air rather than fresh air, shoulder to shoulder with other people, how do you think you would react? Predictably, animals living under such conditions become so highly aggressive and violent that normal interaction is rare. Subsequent depression lowers their will and ability to fight off disease, which can easily become epidemic.

Now, agribusiness has got a problem. Those in control were not batting an eyelash about the suffering and anguish their methods caused the animals they owned, but when the animals got sick, then they worried. If animals die, they generate no profits. What could they do? Improve their living conditions so they didn't constantly come down with illness? Or was it cheaper just to drug them up? A few calculations and the stock raisers came to the conclusion that pills and shots would be more inexpensive than reducing animal suffering, so they initiated "health programs" that are not actually designed to improve health at all, but merely to control sickness. Over half the cattle and nearly all calves, pigs, and poultry are fed a steady diet of antibiotics and related medications to keep infection and contagious disease at a controlled level.[12] One FDA official puts it bluntly, "Antibiotics are most effective in the early growing period and in warding off diseases in animals that are crowded or improperly housed or malnourished."[13] The official makes it clear that the drugs are a necessary supplement to keep alive animals living in foul conditions *as long as the growers have no intention of alleviating the* noxious *life situations.*

Okay," the stock raiser thinks, "I got rid of the disease problem, so what else could go wrong?"

But violating an animal's nature so basically cannot help but lead to unending difficulties. With the animal cramped in so little space, and with its physical activity restricted, it eats less and gains weight faster.[14] While overhead and feed costs drop, overweight animals pose a new problem. Chickens frequently gain so much weight that they can't even stand without intervention. Obese cattle may have fatty livers and abscesses that make them less desirable and marketable.[15]

It should go without saying that the animals raised in this way suffer unrelieved stress. And if this anxiety is rough in the factory farm, it peaks when they are transported to the slaughterhouse. On this journey, pigs' respiration and heart rate increase, and their blood vessels often constrict from muscular tension, causing insufficient circulation of blood and oxygen deficiency, sometimes followed by circulatory and respiratory collapse.[16] Many pigs cannot even stand during the trip to the slaughterhouse because of skeletal rigidity, while others drop dead long before they reach their destination. More than $1 billion is lost because of livestock injuries, stress, and death resulting from their mishandling and transport.[17]

Most cattlemen are not overly concerned with the comfort of animals being herded off to slaughter. What they are concerned about is that the color and quality of the meat be suitable for the marketplace. So here's another problem their violation of the animals' nature has created. Flesh is known to turn darker than desired in frightened cattle; the terror they experience creates chemical and physiological changes in their bodies.[18] And, of course, as I alluded to previously, when you eat the flesh, muscle, and organs of an animal that died in agony, you are ingesting the chemicals the animals released in these moments of terror and pain.

Is this what you intended to "nourish" your body with—stress chemicals from severely abused animals? Most of us do not, and there is some truth in that we cannot be held responsible until we know better. But once we know better, we owe it to ourselves—for our own happiness and health, and that of all living beings—to resist the urge to turn away, and make the necessary changes, straightaway. If you haven't embodied this sensibility yet, you will come to see in time that your dignity and self-respect depend on it. Trust me on this. In one study, conducted at the University of Birmingham in England, 108 participants were shown static images and film clips depicting painful events. Almost one-third of the group (31 participants) reported feeling pain in response to one or more of the images or clips. Furthermore, these people experienced not only the emotional component of pain, but also the sensory one.[19]

If all these animals are in a human-made hell, a special circle of it must be reserved for the calves slated for white veal, a delicacy for many. To ensure its meat is tender and white, the animal is allowed almost zero physical activity. The calf is squeezed into a small crate, where it remains for over three months. Its diet is mostly liquid, often leaving the animal gnawing at the side of the crate, trying to satisfy its natural craving for substance and roughage. By the time the confused calf is ready for slaughter, it is so lacking in normal muscle tissue, skeletal support, stamina, and vigor, it can barely stand without support.

And it shouldn't be thought that the dairy cow, which after all, is not slaughtered after she has been fattened up, but milked unnaturally throughout the year owing to artificial insemination, has an easy time. Once her milk dries up, she's chopped up and sold. Though her flesh, too old for prime cuts, is suitable only for export and hamburger.[20]

Roy Atkinson, president of the National Farmers' Union of Canada, has complained both about the inhumane treatment of animals and the deleterious effects of stopgap measures—shooting the animals full of antibiotics, for instance, to try and stave off the diseases that are the natural accompaniments of crowded, dirty living conditions. "We are living," he says, "in the midst of a social system gone mad, we are paying vast sums of money to sabotage public health."[21]

If you're wondering why this violence and abuse is allowed to continue, the leader of the Texas Cattle Feeders Association might give you a clue: "We, the cattle industry, are willing to produce any kind of animal the consumer wants."[22] In other words, the situation persists because we consumers support it with our dollars and our eating habits.

As remarked earlier, they support it because *they are either ignorant or in denial.* By ignorant, I mean some meat eaters don't have a clue how what they are eating was raised and killed. It is said that Leo Tolstoy, a vegetarian, once presented a woman who said she would like a chicken dinner with a live chicken. He asked her to decapitate it and prepare it for cooking, so she could have it for dinner. She turned down the opportunity.[23] I think most of those who are similarly naive would do the same if confronted with this stark reality.

Then, there's the dissonant person who holds two contradictory ideas in his or her mind without ever allowing them in contact. Think of how children are taught early to recognize all of their "barnyard friends"—their different sounds and habits. Yet, they think nothing of coming home from school, where they were learning about the animals, and eating a juicy hamburger or chicken leg. They don't make the association between the food and its source. That juicy hamburger is the friendly brown cow with the big, gentle eyes, and the chicken leg is the same one that was being used by a real chicken that might have been running in the yard a few days before.

But in America, we have what might be called mental illness made easy. It's not so hard to keep ideas about animals and meat separate if one has never seen dead cows hanging on hooks while the blood drips dry or heard the screams of the pig as it is hauled off to the slaughterhouse. Living in city apartments, shopping for neatly packaged, nicely colored prime cuts of meat, we've lost touch with the actual processes of food gathering and processing. Animal rights activist Dr. Michael Fox explains, "What the eye doesn't see, the consumer doesn't grieve [for]: a Styrofoam carton of impeccable eggs, neatly trimmed meat in plastic wrappers or a delicate slice of veal cordon bleu served on a silver platter does not tell the story."[24]

What would tell the story would be a trip to an animal factory or slaughterhouse. Author Richard Rhodes conveys a sense of what such an experience is like in describing his visit to the ID Packing Company, a meat producer for the Armour Meat Company:

> Down goes the tailgate and out run the pigs, enthusiastically, after their drive. Pigs are the most intelligent of all farm animals... They talk a lot to each other and to you if you care to listen... They do talk: Low grunts, quick squeals, a kind of hum sometimes, angry shrieks, high screams of fear... It was a frightening experience, seeing their fear, seeing so many of them go by. It had to remind me of things no one wants to be reminded of anymore, all mobs, all death marches, all mass murders and extinctions, the slaughter of the buffalo, the slaughter of the Indian, the Inferno, Judgment Day... [and] That we are the most expensive of races, able in our affluence to hire others of our kind to do this terrible work of killing another race.[25]

Trying to Alleviate the Pain

There's a good expression that used to be used for horses who were sick. A farmer might say, "He's off his feed." Well, if you are neither ignorant nor mentally ill and have learned about the mistreatment of animals (as well as the other downsides of meat and dairy consumption), you will probably be "off your feed" in terms of not being able to stomach this animal food any longer.

We've been talking about animal suffering, which has been a prime motivation behind some who were moved to vegetarianism. Isaac Bashevis Singer, author of *Yentl* and *The Family Moskat*, became a vegetarian when faced with the moral dilemma posed by eating meat. In doing so, he acknowledged that his faith, Judaism, has taught compassion for animals. Rabbis for millennia have taught their flocks to be humane and that even animal slaughter was to be performed as mercifully as possible by the *shochtim* (ritual slaughterers).[26] Still, Singer thought, it is difficult to reconcile compassion for animals with permission to eat meat. One may buy kosher meat, but does that ameliorate the suffering of animals?

Singer takes up the theme of the brutal and heartless treatment of animals in *Blood, The Slaughter,* and other works. He puts forth this question: "Don't animals have as much right to life as man, all being God's creatures." In a *New York Times* article titled "When Keeping Kosher Isn't Kosher Enough," he asks, "How can we speak of right and justice if we take an innocent creature and shed its blood?"[27]

Singer was interested in vegetarianism even as a child, but his parents discouraged it. As an adult, though, he championed the cause of vegetarianism and even adopted it as a basis for his belief system, for, as he said, he had serious reservations about adhering to any religion that could justify the practice of slaughtering animals.

Other activists, while not forgoing the vegetarian path and encouraging meat-eating, have asked another interesting question, which is whether or not using such cruel methods on animals being raised for meat is justified *even financially*. Dr. Fox notes that not all money-saving steps taken by animal producers result in bigger profits. In his opinion, happier, less stressed, more naturally raised animals would yield greater productivity while cutting deeply into the costly problems of infection, sickness, and untimely death. Even so, the key issue is relieving animal suffering, the concern uppermost in his mind, which he feels could only be accomplished if "husbandry conditions... allow the animal some opportunity to develop, explore and experience its purpose to some degree—its 'pigness,' 'chickness' or whatever." This would involve meeting basic animal needs:

- freedom of natural physical movement;
- association with other animals, where appropriate, of their own kind;
- facilities for comfort activities (rest, sleep, body care);
- provision of species-appropriate food and water to maintain full health;
- ability to perform daily, routine natural activities;
- opportunity for the activities of exploration and play, especially for young animals; and
- satisfaction of minimal spatial and territorial requirements including a visual field and "personal space."[28]

These are the conditions maintained in the few humane, animal-raising farms, but many feel that to encourage the generality of livestock raisers to switch to compassionate treatment is a rather futile endeavor in that they for many years have been deaf to pleas from the defenders of animals.

Others, expressing an equal reverence for life, believe the only way to derail animal abuse is for more people to give up meat and dairy. Among these people are the ethical vegans, who not only abstain from meat, but also shun dairy products and eggs, because, as they point out, animals suffer severely in the production of these foods just as they do in providing meat.

In *Radical Vegetarianism: Diet, Ethics and Dialectics,* Mark Braunstein writes of the creators of eggs and milk. The hapless hen is forced into endless labor throughout its life, producing more and more eggs while confined to tight quarters, hardly ever contacting the wider world. He notes, further, that dairy cows are grossly overworked in their meager quarters. They are even forced to surrender their young calves to meat producers trying to meet the demand for tender veal. A *Vegan Society* booklet, going into more detail, describes how dairy cows are scheduled by producers for annual pregnancies. At most, they are allowed to suckle their young for three days, though more often the calf, if it's not kept to be raised for veal, is taken for slaughter just after birth, to be processed as meat and have its stomach lining used as rennet for cheese.[29]

Braunstein explains that vegans' rationale for avoiding food that is rooted in animal suffering involves, "the vegetarian dialectic of diet and ethic [which holds]: that not coincidentally, but absolutely essentially, those foods which are the products of the least deprivation of life from others will contribute to the longest life in ourselves."[30] I see this as one of the most sane and helpful pro-life stances available to us today.

Ethical vegans not only eat in a green way to avoid causing pain to animals, but they don't use any products made possible by harming animals. This means they avoid fur, leather, silk, pearls, and animal-based soaps and cosmetics. Unlike the baby boomers—a group I spoke about early on—who took up vegetarianism mainly for health reasons, a survey done in England showed that 83% of vegans chose their lifestyle primarily for ethical reasons, their reverence for life combining with horror at the atrocities wrought on animals in the name of convenience and commercialism.[31]

There is no doubt that suffering affects every living thing, but to add so egregiously to animal suffering is so vehemently intolerable, and has deep ramifications. For one, as indicated by an organizer of a World Vegetarian Congress in India, vegetarianism is tied to international peace. He states:

> The demand for vegetarian food will increase our production for the right kind of plant foods. We shall cease to breed pigs and other animals for food, thereby ceasing to be responsible for the horror of slaughterhouses… If such concentration camps for slaughtering continue, can peace ever come to earth? Can we escape the responsibility for misery when we are practicing killing every day of our lives by consciously or unconsciously supporting this trade of slaughter? Peace cannot come where Peace is not given.[32]

Peter Singer, co-author of *Animal Factories*, likewise ties the implicit willingness of people to countenance animal abuse (even if ignorant or mentally ill) to the tendency to treat others with little respect. He puts it like this:

> The root of the problem is in our blithely taking power over the lives and deaths of other creatures, whose suffering is in no way necessary for our survival. If we so easily take the lives of animals who are only a few evolutionary steps removed from us, what is to prevent us from doing the same to humans who are physically very different from us—of a different color, or speaking an unintelligible language, or "primitive" in their customs?[33]

Thinking along these same lines, Fox shows that this willingness to exploit our brother and sister creatures arises from our belief that man is very different than animal, *and far superior*. This separation prevents us from respecting the animal as an equal—equal in terms of the basic rights that all living creatures share. Fox says, "Although it is an established biological and ecological fact that humans, other animals and nature are inseparable, it is clear that both culturally and philosophically humans are very separate, if not alienated, from the rest of creation." Denying animals basic rights because their intellectual level is beneath ours, he argues in a similar vein to Peter Singer, is only a small step away from denying rights to mentally disabled adults and "pre-verbal children."[34]

The question all this turns around is this: which takes precedence, a full soul and spirit *or* a satisfied ego and a full wallet? If it's ego (which is invested in a sense of personal power and separation) and money that's going to take precedence, then the degradation of animals and the human spirit will go hand in hand. As Michael Fox puts it, "Today, many animal rights and welfare concerns are flatly opposed by economic cost/benefit justifications to an extent and consistency that seem to indicate that we think only in terms of economics and this now takes precedence over ethics."[35] Surely, he continues, this is symptomatic of, "an unbalanced, if not distorted state of mind and of a growing atrophy of the human spirit."[36]

I cannot help but think that this growing atrophy of the human spirit that Dr. Fox speaks about is, in fact, *the* root cause of the illnesses that afflict so many of us today. If we were living in harmony with our spirit, we would simply not be capable of harming ourselves and others as we do through food, drink, drugs, violent, devious behavior, and more. And instead of behaving like voracious animals—as if that is the entire story of humankind—we would embrace our human nature fully and bring it courageously to the world without apology, uniting with any one and all of our brothers or sisters who desire the same.

I believe that recognizing and relinquishing the need for animal products is the only way to reverse this troublesome trend and the ongoing suffering we experience as a nation in disrepair. There is a quote that is frequently attributed to Mahatma Gandhi: "The greatness of a nation can be judged by the way its animals are treated." While it seems from my research that this attribution is in error, it hardly matters who has said this. But if we were to judge our society based on that criteria, we have to thank our vegetarians, many who are animal-rights advocates, for any shreds of greatness we as a nation still have left.

Respect for Human Life

The industry of killing animals for food on a mass scale is a disgusting one on all levels. According to Eric Schlosser in *Fast Food Nation*, the working conditions for US slaughterhouse employees are as unkind as the work itself. The workers are largely undocumented—and subject to the worst kind of working conditions. It seems that since that most basic law of legal employment has been violated, an environment is created wherein slaughterhouse supervisors and employees don't feel too compelled to follow other laws either. Eric Schlosser, author of *Chew on This: Everything You Don't Want to Know About Fast Food*, and *Fast Food Nation: The Dark Side of the All-American Meal* noted, "And workers who needed to go to the bathroom weren't allowed to take a break. They were forced to pee right on the slaughterhouse floor, near meat that people would soon be eating."[37]

It is an environment rife with sexual harassment and misconduct, to the point where women are often expected to provide sexual favors to supervisors in order to gain the privilege of less distasteful job duties, or indeed to get or keep their jobs. Sex is a common currency for women who want something different than what they currently have.

Since the workers are largely undocumented, they can't file claims for injuries that may occur on the job. Remember that these workers are working around large killing machines, and with product that will decay and spread bacteria fast if not properly attended to. Slaughterhouses are elaborate structures with huge machines and multiple floors of equipment that needs to be carefully maintained and cleaned. There is blood everywhere. It's easy to slip and fall on the floor or on a scaffold in the air, onto a hard floor or onto equipment. The risk of injury is high. It's easy for workers to injure themselves so gravely that they suffer permanent disability, crippling their earning potential for life. Since they are undocumented and the injury didn't officially occur, these people are left in an official void when it comes to getting any help.

Are these human rights violations?

Let me put that another way: *how are these NOT human rights violations?*

This ethic is what we are supporting when we buy meat at the grocery store and order it off of the menu. We are paying for these violations of basic human dignity and decency. We are supporting—and indeed encouraging—rape and brutal injury, harm to the body, the psyche, and the soul of our fellow human beings.

When we buy grocery store and restaurant meat, we might as well be the perpetrators ourselves of these evil and violent acts against our fellow men and women. We are not that far removed. When we knowingly partake in and support this industry, their innocent blood is on our hands as well.

Killing IS Killing

When we consider the implications on others of our choice to eat meat, the ripples are wide as well as deep. Let us think for a moment about what it means to kill another living, breathing, feeling being.

In order to kill, we must detach and desensitize ourselves from their suffering. This callousness enables us to engage in the most bestial and barbaric of all possible acts: murder, which is causing another being to cease its life at your hands.

Engaging in this omnipotent act—that of taking another's life from them—makes some of us feel powerful. There is no greater domination of another being than to take its breath and cease its heart from beating. But it makes most of us feel sick, for there is nothing on this earth more precious or valuable than life. Still, as a species, we are prolific killers.

The 20th century was one of the most violent periods in human history. It has been estimated that human beings have been responsible for the deaths of nearly 191 million other human beings in this span of 100 years.[38]

I've already related statistics about the number of animals that lose their lives to humans every year for food. Here are just some other realities related to our violent tendencies:[39]

- Violence causes more than 1.6 million deaths worldwide every year.[40]
- A World Health Organization report estimates the cost of interpersonal violence in the US at more than $300 billion per year.[41]
- US National violence containment costs are over $1.7 trillion.[42]

- 35% of women worldwide—more than one in three—said they had experienced violence in their lifetime, whether physical, sexual, or both.[43]
- The Bureau of Justice reported in 2010 that 25% of women have experienced domestic violence and 6 million children witness domestic violence annually.
- 38% of women who are murdered are killed by their partners.[44]
- On average, the cost of violence related only to paying for police, justice, corrections and the productivity effect of violent crime, homicide, and robbery is $3,257 for each US taxpayer or $460 billion for the United States economy.[45]
- The total cost of violence to the US was conservatively calculated to be over $460 billion, while the lost productivity from violence amounted to $318 billion. California was found to have the highest state burden of violence at over $22 billion per year while Vermont has the lowest at $188 million. For each state taxpayer, the total economic cost of violence varies greatly, from $7,166 per taxpayer in Washington D.C. to $1,281 for Maine taxpayers.[46]
- In the US, youth homicide rates are more than 10 times that of other leading industrialized nations, on par with the rates in developing countries and those experiencing rapid social and economic changes. The youth homicide rate in the US stood at 11.0 per 100,000 compared to France (0.6 per 100 000), Germany (0.8 per 100 000), the United Kingdom (0.9 per 100 000) and Japan (0.4 per 100 000).[47]
- Homicide disproportionately affects persons aged 10–24 years in the United States and consistently ranks in the top three leading causes of death in this age group, resulting in approximately 4,800 deaths and an estimated $9 billion in lost productivity and medical costs in 2010.[48]

If we are a society that kills, then we are a society that kills. This ethic will be reflected in all corners of society. It will manifest unexpectedly and in accordance with the society's cultural values. Thomas Jefferson spoke on this issue eloquently: "On the dogmas of religion, as distinguished from moral principles, all mankind, from the beginning of the world to this day, have been quarreling, fighting, burning and torturing one another, for abstractions unintelligible to themselves and to all others, and absolutely beyond the comprehension of the human mind."

If we stop killing animals, we also become a society that shuns and shames killing. Stopping the killing of animals paves the way to a social ethic reflecting less willingness and acceptance of killing our fellow humans. With the NRA currently spinning legislation for guns in schools in 14 states, our society is deeply in need of finding a way to stop the killing.

Stopping the killing of animals *is* the something we can do to help heal the mass murder-slash-gun violence in today's United States society. We can begin a cycle of nonviolence at the grocery store. We can protest mass killing of our children in their schools and our friends at the mall and the movies by not partaking in *any* mass killing of any creature. We can clear the path to a nonviolent world beginning at the grocery store and our favorite restaurants. We can generate a movement of nonviolence by stopping the violence against animals—which we will do if we stop eating their flesh.

Turning the Tide through Activism

Lest we think that efforts such as becoming vegetarian or investing in programs attending to the issue of violence remediation are for naught, consider these statistics:

- According to a recent report on the economic benefit of evidence-based prevention programs, the Botvin LifeSkills Training (LST) program produced a $50 benefit for every $1 invested in terms of reduced corrections costs, welfare and social services burden, drug and mental health treatment, and increased employment and tax revenue.[49]
- A major study by the non-partisan Washington State Institute for Public Policy found that for every dollar spent on county juvenile detention systems, $1.98 of "benefits" was achieved in terms of reduced crime and costs of crime to taxpayers. By contrast, diversion and mentoring programs produced $3.36 of benefits for every dollar spent, aggression replacement training produced $10 of benefits for every dollar spent, and multi-systemic therapy produced $13 of benefits for every dollar spent.[50]

- After the Longmont Community Justice Partnership (in Longmont Colorado) implemented its Community Restorative Justice Program, recidivism rates among youth dropped to less than 10% in its first three years.[51]
- In West Philadelphia High School, within two years of implementing a Restorative Discipline program, incidents of assault and disorderly conduct dropped more than 65%.[52]
- Up to 42% reduction in physical and verbal youth violence through Life Skills Training.[53]
- Meditation practices in schools have noticeable benefits. In a San Francisco School implementing transcendental meditation practices called "Quiet Time" saw suspensions decrease by 79% and attendance increase by over 98% as well as academic performance noticeably increased.[54]

It is well known that helping others increases happiness. Researchers at the London School of Economics examined the relationship between volunteering and measures of happiness in a large group of American adults and found the more people volunteered, the happier they were. Levels of happiness increased with frequency of volunteering: for those who volunteered monthly, the odds of being "very happy" rose 7% over those who never volunteered, rising 12% for people who volunteer every two to four weeks. Weekly volunteers were 16% happier—a hike in happiness comparable to having an income of $75,000–$100,000 versus $20,000, say the researchers.[55]

And the benefits carry over to health. An analysis of multiple studies by researchers at the University of Exeter Medical School indicated that people who volunteered seemed to live longer, healthier, and happier. In one study, older adults who volunteered at least 200 hours a year were 40% less likely to develop high blood pressure.[56] These same researchers discovered a 22% lower mortality among volunteers than those didn't volunteer, and noted that they were not only less likely to die earlier, but were also less likely to be depressed.

Most of the data prior to the Exeter Medical School release was anecdotal based on self-reporting. Still, the results are persuasive. One such study conducted by UnitedHealth Group (NYSE:UNH) and the Optum Institute revealed that 76% of

US adults who volunteer report feeling physically healthier, and 78% report lower stress levels, leading to feeling better than adults who do not volunteer. In addition to stress and health, volunteers reported to feel a deeper connection to their community and others, and were more engaged and involved in managing their health.[57]

As I spoke in the previous chapter, finding your "why" is crucial for leading a healthy life, and so is being social.[58] Humans are social animals; we need each other for our well-being. The company of others is so vital to humans that the worst-considered human punishment is the isolation from human contact, known in the prisons as solitary confinement. As for actual health benefits, research consistently shows that those with fewer social networks are 2.4 times more likely to suffer fatal heart attacks than those who suffer heart attacks but have larger social networks.[59] Further, emotional support and psychological health are supported by social ties, which may also reduce risks of unhealthy behaviors and poor physical health.[60] Finding and maintaining quality social relationships is vital to our mental and physical health.

Everyday Activism: What You Can Do

The word activist tends to get a bad rap today, as the word conjures images of protesters. While activism is an inherent aspect of protests, in and of itself it simply means being *active* toward a change that you wish to see. In this sense of the word, anyone who takes up exercise for the purposes of regaining or maintaining health is an activist—active in their efforts toward a goal. However, in this section, our intention is to highlight specific ways that you can become active toward the foundational principles of healthy vegetarian living.

Believe it or not, there is plenty you can do to help move society toward this. While this chapter presents some of these options for you, it is certainly not exhaustive. The point is to inspire you to contemplate of new ways of contribute your talents, skills and will in the world for the betterment of society. One thing to be certain of is this: as you incorporate these changes into your life, you will begin to see a ripple effect. Through your empowered actions, you will begin to experience a deep sense of personal satisfaction and be even more drawn to an activism-centered life, which is one of the tenets for happiness. Before long, you will find others inspired by your choices and your life.

Lifestyle Choices

1. **Teach by example**
   The first, best, and strongest thing you can do to contribute to this evolution in consciousness is to live the healthy vegetarian lifestyle through and through. If you are not ready to drop all animal products, then simply jump on board by consuming more plant-based foods and significantly reducing your consumption of animal products. Substituting a veggie burger for a turkey burger, a bean burrito for a beef burrito, or fresh guacamole for cheese and mayo is something that can easily be done. Over time, these small choices will add up, and before long, you will have significantly reduced your consumption of meat products.
2. **Avoid contributing to any exploitation of and harm to animals**
   In addition to not eating meat, you can help protect animals in multiple other ways. For starters, you can avoid the following events and activities that exploit and/or harm animals or humans. These are some of those circumstances:
   - Circuses
   - Zoos
   - Marine Parks (e.g., Sea World)
   - Horse-led carriage rides
   - Horse races
   - Dog races or dog fighting
   - Hunting with live ammunition; fishing with barbed hooks
   - Don't declaw your cats
   - Train your pets well so you have to punish them less
   - Avoid purchasing products tested on animals
   - Avoid purchasing leather and other animal skin goods when you can
   - Purchasing pets from pet stores who source their dogs from puppy mills; buy directly from individuals or breeders who you know treat their animals with care, or better yet, adopt a furry friend from your local shelter.

3. **Avoid contributing to human harm and stand for human rights**
Once we become aware of a human rights violation, we are pretty good about doing the right thing. As a nation, we rallied against apartheid in South Africa in the 1980s because of its race-based injustice. We are wary of and eschew inexpensive diamonds, for example, as we know that they may be so cheaply offered for sale to us because they are the result of bloodshed. We also get up in arms over sweatshops, targeting major corporations for boycotts when we become aware of their sweatshop manufacturing plants in other nations. These human rights violations include not only the things we purchase, but also how we dispose of our waste. Many of the world's people live in or near waste collection sites and are subjected to the water that runs through these spaces. When we dispose of batteries and other components comprised of acid or other harmful chemical products, we are subjecting these people to contaminated living conditions that lead to birth defects and physical deformity. But such human atrocities don't only occur overseas. Human rights violations occur on US soil as well, to no less a degree than they may occur in other parts of the globe. They are happening in our slaughterhouses every day.

Believe it or not, there is something we can do. Recall the Nike debacle in 2001 when people found out that they were using sweatshop labor? It was all over the news. The nation was upset, and lots of people were up in arms about it. Overnight, one of America's darling companies had become a bad guy, and people were lamenting that they'd been inadvertently supporting human rights violations by buying Nike products. I bring this up because that entire calling-out was initiated by one person. One person! A grad student started that whole thing by first emailing the company (ordering a pair of personalized shoes with "sweatshop" embroidered on them), then sharing that email with a few friends. It snowballed, and before you knew it, Phil Knight and the company he created was buckling under the growing wall of severe criticism—it had to. My point in bringing this up is to illustrate how one person does make a difference. One person. And it doesn't always take a whole lot of effort to foster significant change. These are some of the actions you can take to protect human beings and reduce the suffering of our fellow humans:

- Do not purchase animal products.
- Help prevent starvation in your community and in your neighboring communities. One way to do this is to find ways to connect those with extra food (e.g., restaurants, grocery stores, and farmers) with those who need it. Another is to create a volunteer community garden, with food and proceeds from food sales going toward those who need it.
- Participate in peaceful demonstrations that support human rights.
- Create and participate in social media campaigns supporting initiatives that protect the health and rights of humans.
- Conduct protests and wage campaigns against ordinances that outlaw feeding the poor.
- Join and support organizations like Amnesty International, Human Rights Watch, etc.
- Make personal evaluations absent skin color considerations (e.g., when serving on a jury or otherwise assigning guilt, innocence, or any character trait).
- Support minorities in assuming and retaining leadership positions in an effort to achieve leadership demographics that accurately reflect our society's demographics.
- Defend those being bullied, regardless of the cause, skin colors, or participant ages.
- Support referenda that raise the minimum wage to an actual living wage, such that someone working 40 hours a week on the minimum wage can adequately support themselves and their family.
- Stand up against criminalizing the homeless.
- Support immigration policies that are fair and equitable to those wishing to immigrate, as our own fore-parents enjoyed.
- Recycle batteries in city-designated areas.
- Recycle all chemicals, including paint and vehicle liquids such as motor oil, in city-designated areas.
- Blow the whistle on companies that improperly dispose of their waste; e.g., into our air, ground, and/or water systems. If you see strange behavior, especially during night-time hours, raise suspicion and alert the authorities.

- Write companies and urge them to improve their human rights practices. This might involve some creative approach to the problem, such as that undertaken by our grad student friend who rocked Nike's world.
- Support companies that stand for the equitable and fair treatment of farmers and manufacturers from which they source their products, i.e., *fair trade.* Pay a little more for *fair trade* products to ensure growers and manufacturers are properly treated and compensated.

4. **Seek out a community of healthy vegetarians/vegans**

   The main reason people don't stick with a healthy vegetarian diet is because it's difficult to fight the status quo on a regular basis. If you surround yourself with a community of like-minded souls looking to improve the quality of their lives and their worlds through healthy vegetarianism, your chances of success will also improve.

   - Search out vegetarian groups and societies.
   - Join a yoga class. You will likely find a group of vegetarians there.
   - Observe organizations and gatherings advertised on message boards in places where vegetarians go, such as Whole Foods or the grocery co-op.
   - Attend meditation sessions offered in your community.
   - Attend vegetarian events.
   - Attend health lectures in your local community.
   - Hold pot-lucks with interested, like-minded people.
   - Share articles, resources, and recipes.

5. **Support social movements and organizations that promote a healthy vegetarian lifestyle**

   Healthy vegetarianism is in the minority within society at large, but these organizations do exist. Join forces with these and other environmental groups for the support you need. The individuals in these groups are typically interested in both personal and societal health. Here are some types of movements and organizations that are on this track. These groups include those who aim:

   - to reduce and eliminate use of harmful pesticides—on any species
   - to go organic

- to preserve and protect our natural world; e.g., Nature Conservancy, Ocean Conservancy
- to reduce our reliance on fossil fuels
- to provide refuge for animals; e.g., shelters, sanctuaries, preservations, etc.
- to protect human rights; e.g., Amnesty International, Human Rights Watch, Freedom House, etc.
- to protect consumers' right to know; e.g., Democracy Now, Organic Consumer's Association
- to protect food quality; e.g., Non-GMO Project, NSF International
- to promote consciousness e.g., Chopra Center for Health, Institute of Noetic Studies.

6. **Help protect our children from the dangers of an omnivorous lifestyle and guide them to a healthy vegetarian lifestyle**
   It's not trite to say that our children are our future. What they learn as right and correct is what they will also live and teach as right and correct. They (and we) learn implicitly, by example, as well as explicitly, through direct instruction. Whether or not you're a parent, you can help guide our future onto a healthier path. You can:

   - Attend School Board meetings (even if you're not a parent) and PTA meetings (if you are a parent) in your area. Speak out for healthy vegetarian options and help condemn unhealthy omnivorous and processed food choices in your area's schools;
   - Contact the USDA and urge them to move toward healthier school food options
   - Become active in local government to work toward ongoing community health.

7. **Host vegetarian dinner parties, lunches, or other social events**
   Food brings people together. This is no secret. One reason so many people eschew the vegetarian lifestyle is because they can't imagine that vegetarian and vegan food actually tastes good. So show them it does! You can either do all of the food preparation for your omnivorous friends, or you can assign them each a dish to

prepare and bring (or just have them bring the ingredients and chop vegetables together!). Most people are happy to bring an appetizer, salad, or dessert, even if the request is to prepare it with no animal products. You may have to provide some recipes and a little guidance, but those who are interested in the lifestyle will appreciate this. Expose your omnivorous friends to the beauties and delicacies of the healthy vegetarian diet.

8. **Attend the religious service of a healthy vegetarian culture**
   A main source of our values is the religious institution to which we adhere. Attend the religious service of a healthy vegetarian culture to expose yourself to some of the values bases of the healthy vegetarian lifestyle. If you enjoy the service and decide to participate more regularly, you can also find a wonderful healthy vegetarian community in them. In particular, try the services of:

   - Hinduism
   - Buddhism
   - Sufiism
   - Judaism
   - Seventh-day Adventism

9. **Solicit your omnivorous friends to help support your lifestyle**
   Invite your omnivorous friends, or as yet not quite healthy vegetarian friends, to join you in your practices of your healthy vegetarian lifestyle. Invite them to join you in:

   - a meditation group;
   - a visit to a local organic farm or farmer's market;
   - local protests against unhealthy habits and companies;
   - to attend a movie premier or showing of an important topic.

10. **Question authority**
    When evaluating information, remember that you are being told what others want you to hear. Become a healthy skeptic. Consider who benefits when you buy the information you're being sold, and then consider if that's something you want to support. *Think.*

11. Recycle, reuse, repurpose... and compost

This seems like such a no-brainer, but it really isn't. The US makes about one third of all the trash in the world, even though it accounts for only 5% of the global population, and of the 250 million tons of trash generated in 2011, less than 35% of it was recycled.[61] In reality, after 20+ years of curbside recycling programs, only about 34% of US residents recycle compared to Germany's 70%.[62] By adopting an R-R-R mentality, you will gradually shift the way you think about *everything* you use and purchase. Spending time to find the "right" home for products, items and containers that have lost their usefulness to you is an essential quality of sustainable living.

Moreover, if you have the means to compost vegetable matter, please do. This not only returns to us (over time), nutrient rich soil, but it prevents organic matter from rotting in our landfills, which releases the potent greenhouse gas, methane, and contributes to global warming.

- Use Internet services to find new owners for things you don't want (Craig's List and Free Cycle are excellent for connecting people).
- Donate items to charities whose fundraising goes to supply food and medical services to animals and people.
- Visit a local recycling plant; or call your local waste services department to find out what recycling services are available.
- Become involved in local government to improve recycling efforts.
- Create or participate in community tag/yard sales.
- Create a community compost initiative.
- Write editorial pieces for the local newspaper promoting these ideas.
- Call local churches and other similar organizations and ask them if they are in need of the things you are giving away.

Food Choices

When you make healthy food choices at the grocery store, you "vote with your wallet." That is, you make your choices known through your purchasing decisions. Think about this for a second—the grocery stores now have ever-growing organic and gluten-free sections because their clientele is demanding it. Their clientele is *you.*

Whether you buy fresh organic or canned vegetables matters to the company whose name is on the product you're purchasing. When it comes to *voting with your wallet*, there is a LOT you can do:

12. **Boycott companies that process our food from its natural state and turn it into the equivalent of poison to our bodies**
    This is the processed food industry. Avoid purchasing foods from major food processing companies, including especially the following:
    - Monsanto (which means you will essentially have to buy either non-GMO or organic foods)
    - Mondēlez (formerly Kraft/General Foods. (Remember these are owned by tobacco giant Philip Morris)
    - PepsiCo
    - Nabisco (also owned by Philip Morris)
    - General Mills, which in 2014 was ranked the lowest of the big 10 food producers by OxFam America's "Behind the Brand's" campaign, rating seven themes from battling climate change to equal rights for women. Analysis noted "specific issues faced by female workers" and "one big no" for not taking action on farmland being used to grow fuel crops."[63]

13. **Support companies who are committed to retaining foods' original nutritional value, such as organic brands**
    We can work to turn the tide of food available to us in the grocery stores away from the junk processed foods and toward healthy options. Support organic brands such as:
    - Newman's Own
    - Hain Celestial Group (Earth's Best, Health Valley, Arrowhead Mills, Garden of Eatin')
    - Frontier Natural Products
    - Lundberg Family Farms
    - Numi Teas
    - Nature's Path
    - Amy's Kitchen
    - Eden Organic

14. Buy organic

I know we've spoken about this before, but it bears repeating. The only way to really vote with your wallet against food modification (GMOs) and toxic chemicals (including pesticides, herbicides, etc.) is to buy all organic foods, or purchase locally from farmers who do not use conventional pesticides or GMO seeds. On top of it, organic foods are better for you. As mentioned earlier, a study published in the prestigious *British Journal of Nutrition* in July of 2014 by an international team led by Newcastle University in the UK showed that organic crops are between 19% and 69% higher in a number of key antioxidants than conventionally-grown crops.[64] This is the equivalent to eating between one to two extra portions of fruit and vegetables a day. Unsurprisingly, the study also showed significantly lower levels of toxic heavy metals in organic crops. Cadmium, a metal contaminant regulated by the European Commission was found to be almost 50% lower in organic crops than those conventionally-grown.[65]

Further, if you do not buy organic, your food has a chance that is genetically modified such as with zucchini, yellow squash papaya, and milk.[66] Non-organic processed foods have a very high likelihood of containing foods that are GMO (such as soy, corn, canola oil, milk and sugar), in particular because so many products contain these substances. For example, 90% of all soy is genetically modified, and you can find soy in hidden place—in meats[67] (yes, meats—as a filler), salad dressings, low-carb versions of high-carb foods, and cereals. If you want to be healthier, buy organic and local whenever possible. You are also not supporting power-hungry food giants Monsanto when you buy organic.

Although the US does not require GMO foods to be labeled, you may still find out whether or not your produce is genetically engineered by looking at its PLU[68] (price lookup) code:

Conventionally Grown: 4-digit code: E.g., Conventionally grown banana: 4011

Organically Grown: 5-digits starting with #9: E.g., Organically grown banana: 94011

Genetically Modified: 5-digits starting with #8: E.g., GMO or GE banana: 84011

15. Support local growers when possible rather than large box-store brands

When you buy local, you not only support your own community and keep your cash local, but you cut out most of the middle people between the plant and your refrigerator. This also means that your purchasing dollars are actually going toward the costs of tending and harvesting the food rather than to a long list of business people who each get a bite out of that apple before it gets to you. Pay for your *food* rather than *corporate profit*. An added advantage is that you save on fuel costs, thus decreasing your carbon footprint.

16. Plant a garden; teach your children to grow a garden

Even if you plant some herbs on the window sill, or in a pot on the porch, gardening teaches self-reliance. If you're a parent, also teach your children to grow a garden so that they not only see and understand where food comes from, but they gain a sense of dietary independence as they learn that they don't have to rely on Safeway to eat. They can grow and make their own food! Kids who are exposed to gardening have a greater understanding of their bodies, health, and the environment; they are also more likely to try what they've grown *and like it.*[69]

17. Expand your food repertoire

This may not seem much like activism, but it actually can be considered as such. Whatever you do to help further the healthy vegetarian lifestyle can be considered activism. By expanding your food repertoire, you learn new and exciting ways to prepare healthy foods. When the food you make and eat is delicious, it's much easier to stay on the healthy vegetarian path—and get others to join you. Here are some ideas:

- Learn some new recipes incorporating different foods.
- Support vegetarian, vegan, and organic restaurants.
- Ask kindly, but repeatedly, for your favorite restaurants to include more vegetarian and vegan options.
- Try more of other cultures' foods, such as Thai, Korean, Vietnamese, and Indian restaurants in addition to Chinese and Japanese, but be aware that Chinese food typically contains a fair amount of MSG, which is a known food toxin. Discover the vast variety of ways the vegetarian diet can be enjoyed.

Change is slow, but evolution is possible. We as a society have come quite a ways since our inception, and have grown together into a nation of greater mental, emotional, spiritual, and physical health over the last few centuries. We can continue this evolution toward greater health in all of these areas by embracing a healthy vegetarian lifestyle and encouraging others to do the same.

The single-most important thing you can do to contribute to this evolution is to *lead by example*. Hold fast to your dedication to a vegetarian lifestyle. Your omnivorous friends may mock you, but they will also likely respect you. They know it's healthier; they just can't be bothered. Stick to your vegetarian lifestyle and inspire others through example. Some of them will follow.

But no matter what, live your truth.

Chapter 10

Natural Resources

"Earth provides enough to satisfy every man's needs, but not every man's greed."

– Mahatma Gandhi, Spiritual and Political Leader

Of course this high-tech, high-cost meat production is very demanding on resources and consumes an inordinate amount of land, water, energy, and raw materials. In underdeveloped countries such as Brazil, where US agricultural corporations have taken over huge domains to raise cattle, they have pushed peasants off their small plots and, most devastatingly, chopped down huge swathes of rain forest for grazing land. I don't have to tell you that the Amazon rain forest is the lungs of the earth, pumping oxygen produced by the plants into the atmosphere. The cattle ranching that is invading and eliminating the forest's trees is choking our planet, not to mention disrupting all of life.

Natural Resources: In Search of Ecological Harmony

I've said that full-scale vegetarianism is not simply a way of eating but a world view, an all-encompassing one that takes in both the health and monetary considerations we have already surveyed, but also plays a part in how we live in relation to our fellow humans, our fellow creatures, and, if I can put it this way, our fellow planet. The fundamental driving force of vegetarianism is toward balance, a give and take with our partners. By sharp contrast, the philosophy of meat eating pivots around dominance, denial and usurpation. From this foundation, the human doesn't share with animals, for example, but removes their rights and objectifies them. And US inhabitants don't typically work together as brothers and sisters in partnership with our global community, but rather, it's every person for him- or herself, with no regrets for those who, like the poor or elderly in our society, are left behind. This is a way of thinking totally out of sync with the principles of healthy vegetarianism… and humanitarianism, for that matter.

Now it's hardly difficult to see the positive aspects of vegetarianism, but it's also necessary to realize that those who accept the beliefs central to this way of living did not usually arrive at it strictly for sentimental reasons but after serious, logical, and heartfelt thinking about the quality of life for all beings right now as well as the future of our world. The manner of a shallow and selfish businessperson who thinks *solely* about the profits and losses of the next quarter or, at best, the next few years is in direct contrast to the healthy vegetarian who cannot think about profits alone. Healthy vegetarians generally only think of profits *in relation to* the health, financial, physical, psychological implications—for themselves, their family and community units, the world and all its inhabitants (human or otherwise), and the Earth upon which we live and depend for sustenance and survival. They *also* think about the implications of any one action on the next generation, and their children and grandchildren, for they realize that the future is *created* by decisions made *right now*, not in some illusory future. There seems to be a pervasive way of thinking in our world—propagated by many in mainstream business today—that is founded on the fundamental delusion that the future can be somehow different than the quality of the decisions we are making today. If we insist on continuing to promulgate destruction and violence toward animals and fellow human beings, practicing harmful decisions now while expecting that somehow our "future" will be better, we are in for a big surprise. Albeit typical, this type of thinking is what has us presently on this very slippery slope. If it continues, what else could we possibly expect but complete self-annihilation?

Considering outcomes consciously and realistically will result in a society that puts more profound concerns at the forefront, such as preserving our natural resources and the quality of these resources, which are being deeply taxed by the actions of meat eaters, among others interested in exploiting. This type of thinking—which is deeply entrenched in the traditional vegetarian lifestyle—is essential for our survival as a species. Albert Einstein said this about vegetarianism: "Nothing will benefit human health and increase chances for survival of life on Earth as much as the evolution to a vegetarian diet."

I dare say, because of his great intelligence, that Einstein not only understood the health implications of the diet, but the governing values behind it and the larger implications for the adoption of those values in society. This, in large part, is what I aim to reinforce in this part of the book—healthy vegetarianism as a gateway and path to a truly fulfilling life that promotes sustainability, health, and happiness, while tapping into the vast human potential available through a life in service to one another and all living things.

As I say this, I am aware that in spite of its vast benefits, vegetarianism itself must continue to evolve. Because of widespread (worldwide) water shortages (which we will discuss in more detail a little later), we are at a point where we must rethink soil agriculture altogether. It is not the feasible option in the long run, for any number of reasons, in addition to the all-important fact of rapidly decreasing water supplies. In reality, more effective processes for growing using less space and fewer resources, is already being done successfully today with hydroponic and aeroponic technologies; and we've just begun to scratch the potential of these technologies here in the US. Further, transport times, which are a huge problem in the US, are currently resulting in food spoilage and waste as high as 30%; so growing solutions also must be near to where people live.

This is why I am going to such great lengths in this book to prove the local, regional, and global viability of the vegetarian diet as a necessary aspect to life on this planet as we know it, and to provide instruction and resources so that ultimately you will be successful at it. Regardless of whether our collective actions to adopt a vegetarian diet and lifestyle change the world, you can rest assured that it will change the quality of your life (and the life of those whom you influence) right now, and that—as they say in the commercials—*is priceless!*

The Breadth of the Challenges We Face

One thing green eaters know is that wearing out the soil and other resources and using a substantial portion of plant foods for livestock feed for the sole purpose of cultivating animals for food is simply wasteful and unjustifiable. Those of us who have been exposed to this information know that cultivating vegetables and grains rather than livestock makes much more sense and is a far greater and efficient use of our soil at this point. However, land, water, and other environmental stores have become polluted and depleted because of this current focus, and there is currently not enough of a movement away from cattle raising that these resources will become reinvigorated any time soon. Further, cultivating food the way we used to in the past is not effective; there are better ways, as I've mentioned above.

So not only must we be open to changing our ways, but we have to want to change them in order to allow the planet to heal. We must also expose ourselves to innovators for the purpose of spawning truly helpful and advanced concepts. If we continue to think the way we have thought and remain stagnant in terms of our imaginations and the inventions they produce, we will be unable to discover the new possibilities that are available to us now.

One aspect of the transition to a new way of thinking is to remember that the resources these industries are depleting really don't belong to "someone," even though some people think that they do. A cattle farmer buys land that has been on the earth for millions of years and will be there, if we are lucky, for many more years after he or she is dead. What gives this individual the right to bury toxic waste, for example, on the land that will make it unusable for thousands of years? From any ecological or religious or even fully human perspective, nobody can own the air, water, or soil.

This thought leads us to an idea held by many in the field of vegetarianism, health, environment, etc., which is that, just as no one has a right to waste natural resources, even if he or she nominally owns them, no one has the right to throw the relation between man and animal, man and man, and animal and animal out of balance.

The last category, animal and animal, might seem surprising, but I'm thinking of what might be called the competition between livestock and wildlife. You see mass meat production eats up land resources on a large scale as poultry and other livestock farmers tend to house tens of thousands of animals on one site. Two years ago, pig farms in America held over 24 million animals. The 18.1 *billion* animals that make up our livestock herds use almost 80% of the land that could be used to grow crops. And it's not just that livestock farms are dotting the landscape and crowding out other uses. That's a small disturbance compared to the great amount of land that must be used to grow feed crops for all this livestock. In the United States, 26% of our land is used for animal grazing and pasture,[1]*and almost 80% of our grain is livestock feed.*[2]

To make matters worse, the land upon which livestock-feed grain is grown is typically worked without regard for the essential principles of crop rotation. The crops grown for the animals, primarily corn, soybean, and alfalfa, have the downside that they tend to promote soil erosion. These annual crops, in contrast to perennials such as grasses, take more than they give back and have to be rotated with these others in order to keep the soil healthy. However, when profits are in the balance, weighed against the depletion of resources, it's hardly newsworthy that agribusiness shows little concern for anything but the almighty buck. As one well-informed researcher notes, "The most erosive production system— continuous [i.e., not rotated with grasses] corn—produces the highest net income."[3] So that's the crop feed growers prefer. (I'll talk more about soil erosion below.)

Land used for meat and dairy production provides food for fewer people than land used only for plant foods. According to one estimate, up to 14 times as many people could be fed using the same land exclusively for plant foods as is fed by the animal food provided when that land grows livestock food.[4]

Like it or not, there are a lot of people in the world today. Estimates put the global population at about 7 billion, 300 million + (in early 2015), with China and India each accounting for more than 2.7 billion. The third most populated country, the US, only tips the scales at the much smaller 324 million mark.[5] Obviously, then, in such a world where malnutrition and starvation are prevalent, land use is a critical, but so are more innovative ways of raising healthy plant foods.

There is now approximately one acre of fertile land in the world per person. Perhaps, not so bad, given that a third of an acre can supply a person's annual protein needs. But the one third acre estimate is based on the assumption that the person's protein needs are being filled by grains, fruits or other vegetarian sources. Once we begin using animals as our source of protein, a full three and a half acres per person are required![6] If eating meat is the way many eaters go, then other people will go hungry. The math is simple: there just isn't enough land or water to support an omnivore diet and feed all of the world's people.

Such extravagant land usage is not only seen in our own land but in that of underdeveloped countries, where the land is used to grow export crops, including food for animals, or fodder for the richer nations. But again, the exporting nation's population does not benefit; only the business owners do. Here's another extremely salient point, the clearing of vast tracts of forest land and the appropriation of grasslands for use as livestock grazing grounds necessitated by this large-scale production leave large numbers of wildlife homeless. As they scatter in search of new shelter and hunting grounds, many are trapped or poisoned.

One result of the growth of the meat industry has been to push out and even drive into extinction much of our wildlife. This is not to mention the widespread destruction of entire rain forests to make way for cattle. Let's just present this reality one more time so that it really sinks in: more than *20% of the world's oxygen* is produced in the Amazon Rainforest, and it provides *20% of all fresh water* on Earth.[7] The rainforests now occupy a mere 6% of the Earth's land surface, which is less than one-half than previous recordings. Furthermore, a large number of the medicines that doctors prescribe originally come from plants and animals found in the Amazon Rainforest. Experts estimate at this current rate our world's rainforests could be consumed completely in less than 40 years; they also estimate that we are losing 137 plant, animal, and insect species every single day due to this deforestation,[8] which equates to 50,000 species a year. Sadly, in March of this year, *Newsweek* reported that after a remarkable 39% decline in greenhouse gases due to reduced deforestation between the years of 2005 and 2010, the pace of deforestation in Brazil has more than doubled in the past six months.[9]

As I said previously, our rain forests are not just the "lungs" of our planet; without these precious life sustaining tropical forests, human life itself is in danger. The Amazon rainforest contains the largest collection of living plant and animal species in the world, and the diversity of plant species in the Amazon rainforest is the highest on Earth.[10] So not only are we putting the world's population at risk—by suffocating ourselves for lack of clean breathing air in favor of making space for cows that we don't even need to live or to remain viable as a species—but we are affecting the ecological balance, significantly. This, simply, does not make good sense.

Raintree.com notes:

> Massive deforestation brings with it many ugly consequences-air and water pollution, soil erosion, malaria epidemics, the release of carbon dioxide into the atmosphere, the eviction and decimation of indigenous Indian tribes, and the loss of biodiversity through extinction of plants and animals. Fewer rainforests mean less rain, less oxygen for us to breathe, and an increased threat from global warming.[11]

Because we tend to think in terms of separation, it is easy (and unwise) to disconnect from the idea that the loss of anything from an ecosystem—whether a rainforest, a reef, a species, or even the loss of purity of air, water, soil, etc.—may, indeed, lead to the destruction of our own species. We may, mistakenly, not give credence to the reality that a loss of rainforest could cause extreme and potentially catastrophic weather patterns, in addition to a number of other grave occurrences. But when you look at basic, naturally-occurring examples of interdependence, the possible peril becomes abundantly clear. According to the US Department of Agriculture (USDA), for example, more than a quarter of America's diet relies on pollination by honeybees.[12] There are specific cultivars, according to the American Beekeeping Federation—apples, cherries, onions, celery, cabbage, almonds and blueberries, plus a long list of others—that are 90% dependent on bees for pollination. But that's only the start. Bees pollinate 71 of the around 100 crop species that feed 90% of the world. According to a *BBC* article, "If we lose bees, we may also lose all the plants that bees pollinate, all of the animals that eat those plants and so on *up the food chain*. Which means a world without bees would struggle to sustain the global human population of 7 billion."[13]

An article titled, "GMOs Are Killing the Bees, Butterflies, Birds and . . . ?" posted by the Organic Consumers Association, notes that scientists now believe at least some of these pesticides play a major role in Colony Collapse Disorder (CCD), the ongoing death of honeybee colonies; the increased use of a class of pesticides known as neonicotinoids, in particular. Science writer George Monbiot notes, "The quantities [of neonicotinoids] required to destroy insect life are astonishingly small: by volume these poisons are 10,000 times as powerful as DDT, let's reiterate *ten thousand times more powerful.* When honeybees are exposed to just 5 nanogrammes of neonicotinoids, half of them will die."[14] The danger doesn't stop there; these pesticides are highly persistent, lasting up to 19 years, and are water-soluble.[15] One study conducted in the Netherlands showed that this pesticide at much lower concentrations than the limits set by the European Union wiped out half the invertebrate species they expected to find.[16] With 90% of them entering the soils, there is no telling the damage that will continue to occur. So it's not just the bees that are dying; the butterflies and birds are dying, too, and so are fish and other wildlife. As an important note, these pesticides, which are made by Bayer and Syngenta, were licensed prior to sufficient testing (as was DDT in its time) and are now the most widely utilized pesticides in the world,[17] and being offered for sale for home use by both Home Depot and Loews in America.

In her book *Silent Spring*, celebrated environmental activist Rachel Carson said, "It is ironic to think that man might determine his own future by something so seemingly trivial as the choice of an insect spray." The name for the biological relationship between two species that live in close proximity to each other and interact regularly in such a way as to benefit one or both of the organisms is *symbiosis*, which comes from two Greek words meaning "with" and "living." We seem to forget in our use or consumption of any product that we are *living with* a host of other living organisms, as well as nonliving components such as air, rocks and water) in this wondrous and diverse yet interconnected ecosystem.

This, of course, applies to eating meat as well. As livestock is pitted against wildlife, so is human pitted against human. The raising of animals for slaughter serves to feed those wealthy enough to buy meat, but it also both damages and wastes natural resources and increases the price of farmland. The result is that in two ways the poorer classes are hurt. For one, when the developers need more land to graze cattle or build factory farms, they drive the poorer farmers off the land (a point mentioned previously) and also bid up the price of land in that there is more profit in animal foods than plant products. And when this is done in an underdeveloped nation, to make a point I raised before, the cattle are not even being eaten in the land where they are raised, but their meat is sent to "richer" countries. As Frances Moore

Lappé, an authority on food and hunger, illustrates, "Two-thirds of the agriculturally productive land in Central America is devoted to livestock production, yet the poor majority cannot afford the meat, which is eaten by the well-to-do or exported."[18]

The president of the Worldwatch Institute, an organization that works on developing a sustainable world, says that such things as the rise in meat exports from poorer countries is "creating an illusion of progress [since some in the exporting countries may be increasing their wealth] and a false sense of security."[19] Long term, however, such an arrangement is not only putting more people, from displaced farmers to impoverished city dwellers, under stress, but is selling short the next generation that will no longer be able to depend on what was once a very large reservoir of natural resources.

Dead Zones

Dead zones are areas of low oxygen (hypoxia) found in the world's oceans and lakes. Without oxygen, the marine plant and animal life in the area suffocates and dies (or in the case of fish that are more mobile, leave the area) hence the term "dead zones." Such dead zones are caused by excessive nutrients, particularly nitrogen and phosphorus, polluting the water, and are predominantly linked to human activities such as the leakage of sewage or industrial pollution into waterways. One major source of excessive nutrients is agriculture. When farmers fertilize their lands, rain and irrigation washes the fertilizer into streams and rivers, known as run-off.

The high concentrations of nutrients in the water, or eutrophication, can stimulate the rapid growth of algae, phytoplankton, and seaweed on the water's surface, a phenomenon known as algal bloom. The bloom blocks both sunlight and oxygen from the marine life beneath causing hypoxia. Furthermore, the bloom itself soon dies and its decomposition consumes oxygen, further depleting the supply available to marine life. Lack of fish can lead to the death of marine mammals and shore birds that rely on fish for survival. What's more, some of the algae produce toxic by-products, which can be dangerous to marine life and humans. One study published in *Nature* linked the death of more than 400 California sea lions in Monterey Bay in spring 1998 to an algal bloom.[20] People can become sick from consuming shellfish that have absorbed some of the toxins, or by drinking contaminated water.

In developed countries such as the United States and nations in the European Union, heavy use of animal manure and commercial fertilizers in agriculture are the main contributors to eutrophication. In fact, according to a growing body of scientific evidence, algal blooms and dead zones are growing in both size and number. A 2008 study counted 405 dead zones worldwide[21] and the second largest dead zone in the world is located in the US, in the northern Gulf of Mexico, largely caused by agriculture fertilizer being washed down the Mississippi River.

In August, the drinking water supply for Toledo, Ohio shut down due to an algal bloom in Lake Erie, which supplies the city's water. The bloom has been linked to fertilizer run-off from the corn and soy crops growing in the area.[22] According to an article in the *Wall Street Journal,* "More than 80% of the Maumee River watershed is devoted to agriculture, mainly the corn-soy duopoly that carpets the MidWest,"[23] and a study carried out by scientists from the US Geological Survey found that 66% of the nitrogen delivered to the Gulf of Mexico originates from cultivated crops, mostly corn and soybean,[24] 60% and 47% of which are used for livestock consumption,[25] respectively.

Soil Erosion

I wanted to say a little more about soil erosion as a way to make concrete my previous comments on the depletion of our resources. I will follow this with sections on water and of course energy, two other elements of the earth's architecture that are being sadly overstressed by the animal products industry.

In addition to its mixture of minerals contributed by clay and sand, healthy soil contains organic matter (humus) and a diverse and complex living system of bacteria, fungi, microorganisms, worms, and insects, which act together as a medium for plant growth and also, importantly, as a water store. The ability of land to provide food and sustain life is primarily affected by soil health. Soil is a basic resource, and as I've already mentioned, soil erosion is a grave problem affecting the productivity of the land for agricultural use.

The United States is losing soil 10 times faster than it can be replaced through natural processes,[26] let alone unnatural ones, costing an estimated $44 billion each year in loss of productivity.[27] Degraded soil will mean that we will produce 30% less food over the next 20-50 years against a projected increase in demand to grow

50% more food for the increasing world population. Further, as wealthier people in countries like China and India eat more meat, which takes more land to produce weight-for-weight than, say, rice, the problem will compound.[28]

Soil can be eroded by both rain and wind leading to the gradual loss of soil productivity and degradation of land, a process known as desertification. In addition to erosion, soil quality is affected by other aspects of agriculture and human activities, including compaction, overgrazing and, as previously mentioned, the use of pesticides and deforestation. Some 70% of the land cultivated for agriculture is already threatened by desertification, thereby challenging the livelihood of over 1 billion people in more than 110 countries around the world.[29] For example, with the clearing of tropical rainforests in Costa Rica and Brazil for land to grow crops, the washing away of the bare topsoil by the heavy rains and the loss of soil fertility has become a very serious problem for farmers in that region.

To my mind, of the three, soil erosion is the least appreciated of all of the dangers facing us. The few feet of earth that comprise topsoil is where the action is. This is where there is found a great deal of organic material (such as decaying plant matter) and an abundance of micro-organisms that sustain plant growth. It is crucial to take note of this: *without topsoil almost no plant life is possible, and without plant life…* well you know where I'm going with this.

I noted above that certain practices of animal-oriented agribusinesses, such as failure to rotate crops and the growing for feed grains of the most soil-depleting plants, has caused unprecedented erosion. One Iowa conservation official, William Brune, put the results in chilling terms. He began by noting that, "it can take 100 to 500 years to create an inch of topsoil," but, he continued, because of current agricultural practices, this small amount "can wash away in a single heavy rainstorm."[30]
Here are a few more statistics on the problem that should indicate that this is not something to be taken lightly.

- The harvest of 1 bushel of Iowa corn results in the loss of 2 bushels of topsoil.[31]
- Only 6 inches of topsoil remain on some Iowa farmlands.[32]
- Our present erosive conditions have been compared to those experienced in the Dust Bowl during the Depression of the 1930s, when millions of acres of farmland were rendered useless for crop raising.[33]

- A third of our topsoil is completely gone in the major farming states.[34]
- Corn is responsible for a quarter of our national soil-erosion problem.[35]
- Water erosion is now a serious issue.[36]
- Indirect costs of soil erosion, such as the need to use chemical fertilizers to replace the nutrients lacking in the rundown land, amount to nearly $1 billion a year. Overall costs due to continual erosion of the soil are estimated to be nearly $2 billion a year.[37]
- In the US, 1.7 billion tons of topsoil are lost to erosion every year.[38]
- Worldwide, over 25 billion tons of farmland topsoil are lost annually.[39]
- The global loss of topsoil closely parallels what is happening to our depleted oil supplies.[40]
- For every inch of topsoil lost, we produce 6% fewer crops.[41]

This situation is so threatening that you may wonder why you (probably) haven't heard of it before. Certainly, the pro-corporate news is not going to touch it, even while it impacts us at home and affects others globally where, "*a quiet crisis that could lead to famines in some parts of the world*" is brewing.[42] Here, we have some 30 regions in the US that have been classified as high-risk in loss of topsoil, mostly in areas of extensive soybean and corn production, where crops being grown for feed are denuding the farms of their most vital earth.

The Depletion of Our Water Supply

Water is essential for all life and safe, affordable, and accessible water is a fundamental human right. "The human right to water is indispensable for leading a life in human dignity. It is a prerequisite for the realization of other human rights."[43]

The critical need for clean water is already an issue for millions of families across Asia, Africa, and Latin America. Today, half of the world's population lives in towns and cities and one-third of this urban population live without clean drinking water.[44] By 2020, increases in temperatures due to climate change will expose between 75 and 250 million people in Africa to increased water stress[45] and China alone has 300 cities currently facing serious water shortages.[46]

Closer to home, I've previously mentioned the issues of the overuse and contamination of water, but with global temperatures already on the rise, extreme weather events, including flooding and droughts, are an ever increasing issue for all of us. Many states are already experiencing drought, and states such as Colorado, New Mexico, Nevada, Oklahoma, Utah, Kansas, and most of Texas and California, are likely to be uninhabitable in the future due to lack of water for the increasing human populations, in addition to the requirements of industries, livestock, and crops. By 2020, yields from rain-fed agriculture could be reduced by up to 50% in some areas.[47] In fact, in California's Central Valley—by far the most productive area of the United States and arguably the world—there is no longer enough water to sustain it, and about two million acres of agricultural land has already been taken out of production from insufficient water supplies. This is also due in part to the reduced snow melt from the mountains of the Sierra Nevada caused by global warming and has had a huge effect on the farms and dozens of small communities. For example, Mendota, the cantaloupe capital of the world, no longer has water supplied to it and is facing a 35% unemployment rate. In February 2009, Robert Silva, the mayor of the Central Valley town said, "… my community is dying on the vine." At the University of California, Davis, Professor Richard Howitt estimates a crop loss of over $2 billion and job loss for 60,000 to 80,000 workers.[48]

There is much more awareness in our nation about our problems with water. However, ask the average person where these problems lie, and they will most likely say with pollution. Water *is* becoming more and more unusable, transformed from a health-giving life sustaining liquid into a poison. Question the person further as to what is behind the situation and you will probably get the answer that it can be attributed to chemical wastes being dumped in our lakes and streams by industries.

While they would of course be correct in several instances I imagine that they would be surprised to learn there is another different, pressing problem, and, with it, a different culprit. The problem is *overuse*, an extravagant consumption of water so great it is outrunning the ecosystem's ability to replenish the supply.

In the beginning, farmers were dependent on nature to water their fields, either through rain or annual flooding. When irrigation was introduced, it increased the amount of arable farmland. By siphoning off water from rivers and channeling it to where it was needed, farmers could grow crops even in arid regions or during dry seasons.

While this has helped us increase crop production significantly, over the past two decades agribusiness has been irrigating land almost exclusively for the purpose of growing food for livestock. In plain figures, this translates into 8% of the world's water going for livestock production, with 7% going into livestock feed production.[49] In fact, the agriculture sector is responsible for 93% of the world's water depletion.[50] According to the US FAO (Food and Agriculture Organization), non-agricultural water usage is expected to increase by 62% between 1995 and 2025, while irrigation water will rise by only 4% in that time period.[51] But let's look at more sophisticated figures. A researcher has translated this water usage into the actual relationship between a meal and water loss. It takes 12,000 gallons of water to produce beef to get a 16-ounce T-bone steak[52]—that is a remarkable 15 times more than a vegetarian alternative with the same protein content. Let's put this another way: "The water that goes into a 1,000 pound steer would float a small boat."[53] If the average American meat consumer were only eating an occasional steak, things wouldn't be so bad, but for the average eater, it's "water, water, everywhere" in terms of consumption. It's been found that the average American's *daily* food intake represents over a 1,000 gallons of water, of which nearly two-thirds went into the animal products being consumed?[54]

You may think, "Well, even if agribusiness is using up an awful lot of water, and drying up some streams to do so, it will be replenished by rainfall." But, it's not just rivers that are giving up their water. The water is now being pumped out of aquifers, underground areas where water has collected in the rock, for irrigation. This is why in California, where nearly 50% of the irrigated water is used for animal production, land is drying out and actually starting to sink as the aquifer is being drained to the point of collapse. Texas may soon follow as 25% of its underground water has been used in the last 20 years. There is no way rainfall can keep up with this unheeding desertification of our country. So if you want to save and conserve clean drinking water for yourself and future generations, eat your vegetables.

Clean Air

Trees are a vital component of the clean air equation; they turn carbon dioxide, which is poisonous to humans in mass quantities, into oxygen, which we need for life. When you cut down the trees to make room for growing cattle, guess what happens to the air. Everyone around the globe pays for these unconscious decisions that large and small property owners are making daily.

The most obvious and well-known effects related to air quality are the environmental effects of carbon dioxide on climate change due to greenhouse effect so when it comes to trees we need to cut down less and grow more. The oceans also take up carbon dioxide from the atmosphere, leading to their acidification.[55] In fact, an estimated 30–40% of the carbon dioxide released by humans into the atmosphere dissolves into oceans, rivers, and lakes, forming carbonic acid.[56] This ocean acidification is a real threat to the marine ecosystem as it inhibits shell growth in marine animals and is a suspected cause of reproductive disorders in some fish.[57] And let's not forget acid rain, caused by atmospheric pollutants—particularly oxides of sulfur and nitrogen—that react with water in the atmosphere to form sulfuric and nitric acid, and which can damage property, vegetation, and aquatic life in lakes and streams.

The levels of air pollutants, including ozone, carbon monoxide, nitrogen and sulfur oxides, lead, and airborne particulates—an effect of wind erosion—are a real threat to human health. The WHO estimates that in 2012 there were 3.7 million deaths in 2012 from urban and rural sources worldwide as a result of air pollution exposure.[58] A study found that people who live near polluted cities or major highways are at a higher short-term risk of having a heart attack due to air pollution.[59] In addition to the harmful effects on the cardiovascular system, air pollutants can lead to an array of respiratory problems, particularly amongst the young and elderly.[60] Airborne dust has been linked to asthma and an increased risk of lung cancer, and ozone can increase the frequency of asthma attacks, cause shortness of breath, aggravate lung diseases, and cause permanent damage to lungs through long-term exposure.[61, 62]

"Few risks have a greater impact on global health today than air pollution; the evidence signals the need for concerted action to clean up the air we all breathe," said Dr. Maria Neira, Director of Department for Public Health, Environmental and Social Determinants of Health, WHO.[63]

Air pollution is now the world's largest single environmental health risk, not to mention regional haze that impairs visibility in national parks and other recreational areas. Beijing is one of the most polluted cities in the world. The severe air contamination—at least two to three times higher than levels deemed safe by the World Health Organization—was brought to the media's attention by of the 2008 Olympic Games, especially when several athletes withdrew due to fears for their health.[64,65] What has been the response to the bad air in China? It's not to get to the root of the matter, not to become radical about it, not to try to reduce the pollution, but instead, for corporations to monetize the situation and sell clean air. You can buy clean air in cans and bottles in China now, such as "Fresh Air," which sells for 5 yuan (80 cents) a can.

However, it is encouraging to know that the Clean Air Act has successfully lowered levels of the six common pollutants in the US by 72% since its introduction in 1970, showing that concerted efforts by the governing bodies and private sector companies can be effective.[66] An ongoing project that aims to reduce emissions and improve air quality is being undertaken in British Columbia's Georgia Basin and Washington's Puget Sound as a joint Canada-US venture. The priority is the reduction of fine particulate matter and toxic emissions from diesel fuel in the area. To do so, they are introducing cleaner vehicles and fuels in the region, actively performing on-road testing of heavy duty vehicle (truck and bus) emissions, introducing cleaner motor vehicle fuels, and reducing marine vessel emissions in and near ports.[67]

Still, we are a long way away from taking formidable steps to resolve this issue. A US Geological Survey noted: "Nearly every pesticide that has been investigated has been detected in air, rain, snow, or fog across the nation at different times of year."[68] An article in *Earth Island Journal* said this about the issue:

> A seemingly innocuous spraying or fumigation of a rural farm field can let pesticides drift through air currents for hours, even days, ending up as residue in nearby towns, ruining organic crops downwind and further polluting waterways. Diazinon, a highly volatile agent sprayed widely on nuts and stone fruit, actually increases its drift concentrations as time passes, the greatest amount of drift showing up two to three days after spraying… More than 90 percent of pesticides used in California (including non-agricultural pesticides) are likely to drift, and roughly a third of those are highly toxic to humans, according to a 2003 study by Californians for Pesticide Reform.[69]

Unsurprisingly, air pollution is directly related to health, and not just lung health. A study sponsored by National Institute of Environmental Health Sciences (NIEHS) and conducted by University of Medicine and Dentistry of New Jersey (UMDNJ) researchers and colleagues used the 2008 Beijing Olympics as their laboratory.[70] The results, appearing in the *Journal of the American Medical Association*, found biological evidence that even a short-term reduction in air pollution improved one's cardiovascular health.[71] "The study underscores the fact that people's health and the environment are indelibly linked....When air pollution levels are lowered, the health benefits can be immediate," said program administrator Dr. Caroline Dilworth of the NIEHS.[72]

Our Dwindling Energy Supply

The next resource to look at is energy. The United States gets a large part of its energy from oil, about 40%, with another 25% each coming from coal and gas. This leaves a smaller percent for nuclear and renewable energy sources. These renewable ones, such as energy captured from the sun or wind, amount to around 7%, and they are the only ones that once used are not lost forever.

Our concern here is the energy used in raising animals for human consumption, which I figure adds up to nearly 15% of our country's annual energy budget, equal to the energy needed to run *all our cars*. Why so high? Well, there are many steps and stages—hardly efficient or optimal in terms of energy and sustainability—to get a product to your supermarket shelves. This is especially true if the product is sold by a multinational conglomerate as opposed to one made and distributed by small, local producers. The simple example is purchasing from a local farmer rather than from a grocery store, which houses products from across our nation and oftentimes beyond. I also compared the work that is required for raising, killing, rendering, packaging, and distributing animals used for food as contrasted to the fewer steps and manipulations vegetable products faced before being available at the market. Now, combine these two (multinational dimensions of animal production) and you have a real doozy of an expensive, energy-gorging routine—to go from, say, the hatching of a chicken egg to the fowl's legs being displayed shrink-wrapped in the meat section of the grocery store. Because there are many more stages of processing, each with its own energy requirements, so the energy bill keeps going up.

A book titled *Food And Energy Resources*, edited by David Pimentel, former professor at Cornell University and long outspoken adversary of the inefficiencies of meat-based agriculture stated:

> …the complete vegetarian diet [vegan diet] is more economical in terms of fossil energy than either of the other two types of diets [lacto-ovo vegetarian diet and a high animal-protein diet]. Nearly twice as much fossil energy is expended to produce the food in the lacto-ovo vegetarian diet than is expended for the complete vegetarian diet. For the non-vegetarian diet, the fossil energy input is more than threefold that of the complete vegetarian diet.[73]

This long and somewhat circuitous route is the reason why every calorie of animal protein eaten requires on average 78 calories of fuel to produce. Wheat and corn, in comparison, require only 3.5 calories of energy per calorie of protein; soybeans need 40 times less than beef.[74]

Moreover, each stage, each unit of energy used in prepping the animal and its meat, also needs its requisite, supplementary raw materials. A Department of Interior and Commerce study indicates that the livestock industry uses one-third of the value of all raw materials consumed in the US, just for feed. Plastic wrap, aluminum foil, Styrofoam and cardboard containers, paper labels, ink, preservatives, artificial flavors and color additives—all used by the meat-packing industry—further deplete our raw material supplies. These raw materials include aluminum, copper, iron, steel, tin, zinc, rubber, wood, and petroleum products.

As part of the conclusion to one of the largest international assessments of animal agriculture ever undertaken, the Food and Agriculture Organization of the United Nations said:

> The livestock sector is a major stressor on many ecosystems and on the planet as a whole. Globally it is one of the largest sources of greenhouse gasses and one of the leading causal factors in the loss of biodiversity, while in developed and emerging countries it is perhaps the leading source of water pollution.[75]

The UN even reported in 2010 that a shift to a vegan diet was vital for saving the world from hunger, fuel poverty and the worst impacts of climate change. The report noted:

> Impacts from agriculture are expected to increase substantially due to population growth increasing consumption of animal products. Unlike fossil fuels, it is difficult to look for alternatives: people have to eat. A substantial reduction of impacts would only be possible with a substantial worldwide diet change, away from animal products.[76]

A slow growing number of valiant souls are standing up against the insanity and tapping into a larger sense of responsibility by switching to vegetarian eating and to green living, which includes the possibility of either sourcing or growing food and other items locally, and conserving water and energy resources through the use of solar or wind power. As I have mentioned before, the time is now *mission critical* for this evolution. While multinational and multi-pronged agribusinesses continue to experience competitive pressures due to globalization, trade liberalization, and environmental regulation, as well as increased consumer awareness related to animal welfare and food safety issues, they are hardly scaling back. On the contrary, they are charging ahead.

For certain, the average person, here and abroad, is bearing the greatest costs from the policies and initiatives of these companies—either through the forfeiting of natural resources for themselves and future generations or, more immediately, by losing land that they, and perhaps their families, have occupied and developed for generations. Ironically, meat companies themselves are also paying an unexpected price. As they devastate and pollute land, water, and other natural resources in the production of farm animals, the value of any remaining natural resources rises. That is basic supply and demand economics; when less available, the price goes up. Hence, these large agribusinesses end up driving up the costs of their own production through the abuse of our natural resources. Faced by increased costs, not all of which can be passed along to the consumer, what do these companies do? They certainly do not diversify into raising vegetables, for, after all, the profits in that trade are much less than in selling meat. No, their solution is to raise more animals for slaughter, while increasing advertising campaigns and industry-sponsored "science" to convince the beleaguered consumer to purchase even more of its products.

However, we can all do our part to stop this madness, with a simple determination to choose an organically grown plant-based diet. We might say this is crunch time—for all of us and most importantly for our children. Without being an alarmist, it's hard to see how humanity will survive if we continue to consume meat and the meat producers keep upping the ante. If we don't find suitable ways for growing food that is resourceful in terms of water, soil and energy use, and does not destroy other irreplaceable resources, drive farmers off their land, and poison a willing but misinformed customer group, there is very little hope.

While consuming a locally-grown vegan vegetarian diet will do quite a bit to reduce our reliance on fossil fuels, the reality remains that we are running out. According to Carbon Counted, experts believe that we have about a 50-year supply of natural gas left, that we have anywhere from 10-65 years left of oil,[77] a plentiful supply of coal (but it is the most hazardous fuel source from a health standpoint), and shale, which is extracted by the controversial process called hydraulic fracturing, or more commonly referred to as fracking.

The point is that these are non-renewable sources; once they are used they are gone forever, as I said at the top of this section. But renewable sources are not yet well developed or distributed. In 2013, only 9.5% of all energy consumed in the US was from renewable sources.[78] A more recent report noted that total renewable energy production and consumption—particularly from wind and solar—reached record highs in the US at 11%.[79] Samantha Smith, WWF leader of the Global Climate & Energy Initiative stated, "With a fast global shift to renewable energy and supported by strong energy efficiency measures, we can drastically reduce CO_2 emissions, which eventually will also stabilize and reduce atmospheric CO_2 concentrations."[80] She also noted that costs of renewable electricity have dropped radically, and in 2011, investments in renewables outstripped investments in fossil fuel power for the first time. So renewable energy can become "the new normal," but it requires constant pressure from the public, advocacy organizations, and commitments from governments if it is to happen quickly enough and at scale. We can only hope that those with the power to shift this take Smith's words to heart and, better yet, take immediate action.

Agriculture's Role in Global Warming

In addition to the strain on our natural resources due to housing and feeding these expansive bovine populations, we cannot overlook the issue of the methane gas excretions from cows—major contributors to global warming. In fact, according to the US Environmental Protection Agency, the agriculture sector is the number one producer of methane gas (CH_4) worldwide,[81] and human activities are responsible for 60% of all emissions.[82] Why is methane so dangerous? Unlike carbon dioxide (CO_2), which also affects global warming, methane gas is much more likely to trap radiation than CO_2. Pound for pound, methane gas has a 25 times greater impact on global warming than CO_2 over a 100-year period.[83] Experts predict that the worldwide consumption of pork, beef, poultry and other livestock will continue to increase as wealth in developing nations increases. As you may recall, this trend of consuming more meat as wealth increases is a reflection of the Western views and traditions.

Animal agriculture accounts for 18% of total greenhouse gas emissions,[84] with some studies indicating up to 25% if you count emissions from deforestation initiatives to make room for livestock-raising.[85-87] This is at least equal to emission from transportation, which log at around 27%. And methane gas is not the only culprit; livestock is responsible for 65% of all emissions of nitrous oxide—a greenhouse gas that is 296 times more destructive than carbon dioxide and stays in the atmosphere for 150 years.[88] All told, emissions from livestock constitute nearly 80% of all agricultural emissions.[89-93] Further, emissions for agriculture are projected to increase 80% by 2050.[94] A particularly bothersome side note, given the water supply challenges now facing the US and the world, is that agriculture is responsible for 80-90% of US water consumption,[95] with 56% of water in the US going toward growing feed crops for livestock.[96] Feed crops comprise 70% of all crops in the US,[97] which according to Cornell ecologist David Pimentel would feed nearly 800 million people globally. Are we insane? Based on these numbers, I'd say so.

The plant-based diet is far more efficient in terms of consumption of natural resources. The land that is required to feed 1 vegan for 1 year is one-sixth of an acre; contrast this with the vegetarian, which is 3 times as much as a vegan, and the meat eater, which is 18 times as much as the vegan.[98] Big Difference. Perhaps the biggest question now is: "What are any of us willing to do about it?" Yes, the situation is dire, which might cause people to say, "*What impact can I really have? Why would I want to go through the challenging exercise of converting my diet, when so many others aren't going to?*" The answer comes back to your *Why* for being here. Is your why to continue to participate in rituals that make no logical sense regarding health and sustainability, or to choose the path of sanity? Only you know the answer to this question.

For those who do choose a new path, know that it will be difficult at times—not only with your discipline but regarding the social effects of taking a stand. But numerous gains in terms of life and vitality will be made, when simply shifting our focus away from animal agriculture toward an energy-efficient solution for cultivating plant-based foods. Other things, besides abandoning animal agriculture, are needed to reverse global warming. Our planet still holds vast reserves of fossil fuel that could be extracted economically. But a new analysis notes that a third of the world's oil, half of its gas, and 80% of its coal reserves must remain *unused* if we are to have a good chance of avoiding potentially devastating climate change.[99] The study, authored by researchers at the University College of London and published in MIT Technology review in January of 2015, is the first to suggest which specific resources, and where, should be left in the ground.

While it is unlikely that industrialists will heed the call, we can help cause the shift through our purchasing power. Attention to how we use natural resources in every area of life is a good start.

Energy "Resources" That Promote Food Shortages

The argument of diverting grain to human consumption rather than to cattle assumes that the potential benefit of the provision of more grain and other vegetarian foodstuffs to the poor will not be stolen by treacherous governments or businesses. Indeed, in Lester R. Brown's book, *By Bread Alone*, which I mentioned earlier, he alludes to this type of problematic situation in which crops are being shifted away from being used as feed for livestock, but not turned in *the positive* direction of generating low cost human food. Instead, excess grain is being used to produce ethanol for cars. As he states, "We're putting the supermarket in competition with the corner filling station for the output of the farm."[100] If the use of ethanol takes off, he believes the result will simply be more hunger.[101] The reason is—unsurprisingly—money. As we saw wealthy farmers in underdeveloped countries preferred to sell their crops for livestock feed rather than to market it as food for their countries' people since animal feed earned bigger bucks. In a similar way, according to Brown, as the price of oil goes up, the price of corn ethanol used to replace it will also skyrocket, increasing the upward price pressure on corn and grain generally, making it even more unaffordable to poorer people.[102]

This is another topic seldom or never covered by the corporate media, but if you look into it, you'll find the embrace of biofuels in the US and Europe is already having serious global and local consequences. A World Bank study holds biofuels responsible for up to 75% of the rise in global food prices since 2002, causing growing hunger and even rioting in some countries.[103] Here at home, close to a third of the corn grown in the Midwest currently goes to ethanol production, kicking food prices up 6.8% in the first half of 2008 alone.[104]

This was the effect in 2008, when refiners blended over 9 billion gallons of biofuels into the nation's fuel supply. Worse was in 2009, when the law mandated a 23% increase to 11.1 billion gallons of biofuels, worsening the problem. And what of 14 years hence, in 2022, when the same law mandates a 400% increase to 36 billion gallons of biofuels?[105] It's not hard to see that the pressure on grain stocks and the land employed to raise them, which is already largely devoted to raising animal feed, will be all the greater, pushing prices for human food even higher.

The Environmental Impact of GM Crops

As nations take a step back and reconsider the threats of climate change and global warming to future food supplies, GMOs are steadily failing to hold up to their promises of higher yields and drought resistance. To the contrary, study after study lean towards the conclusion that GMO-based agriculture may be the most dismal failure since humans first started sowing seeds and harvesting crops. In June, the *Guardian* reported that the introduction of Monsanto's Roundup Bt brinjal eggplant into Bangladesh is facing widespread collapse, with a failure rate of four out of five farms.[106] GMO soy and corn are rapidly losing their pest resistance. Bugs and weeds are turning into mega-threats to the future of yields of staple crops, which the industrial makers of processed foods depend on. Farmers in Latin America are demanding compensation from Big AG companies such as Monsanto, DuPont, Syngenta, and Dow for unexpected financial duress and being forced to purchase larger quantities of pesticides in order to sustain their harvests. In Brazil, after only three years of GM Bt cultivation, pest resistance has been observed. Similar observations are being reported in Bt maize in Puerto Rico, Brazil, Philippines, South Africa, and the US, and in Bt cotton in Australia, China, India, and the US. Last month American scientists confirmed that rootworms destroying corn fields are no longer resistant to GMO corn.[107]

An article in India's *Hindustani Times* states that "There are over 500 research publications by scientists of indisputable integrity, who have no conflict of interest, that establish harmful effects of GMO crops to human, animal, and plant health, and on the environment and biodiversity… On the other hand, virtually every paper supporting GM crops is by scientists who have declared conflict of interest or whose credibility and integrity can be doubted."[108] Monsanto's Bt cotton in India has been particularly disastrous to hundreds of thousands of farmers. Aside from the oft-reported epidemic of farmer suicides who fall into debt and poverty after buying into Monsanto's GM cotton—farmer suicides have now reached over 270,000—pest resistance is rampant, further weakening the natural immunity of GM plants and predisposing them to less serious pests. India is also witnessing record numbers of cattle die-offs after grazing on post-harvest cotton plants. Regions with higher proportions of Bt cotton farming are confronting grim water futures because GM agriculture requires more irrigation than traditional farming methods. Last March the Indian state of Karnataka banned Bt cotton seeds following pervasive crop failures.[109]

One of the most massive GMO failures, spanning a decade, has been the deplorable collapse of the introduction of GM corn in the Philippines. The decimation of Filipino corn farmers came to world attention following the release of the film "Ten Years of Failure" which follows the lives of farmers whose families fell into debt and poverty after the introduction of GM corn by the Philippine government in cooperation with the US government and Monsanto.[110] Intent on avoiding a similar fate to Brazilian corn farmers, a Brazilian court banned the release of Bayer's GM corn. The ruling now establishes a new precedent that will make the approval of future GMOs in that country more difficult.[111] And China's recent rejection of GMO corn importation has agro-giants further worried as one of their largest potential markets takes a step back to reevaluate the safety and environmental impact of GMOs.

Big Ag's only response to the failures of its genetic experimentation has been to increase the development of new GM seeds to compensate for the failures of the old ones. In addition to genetically engineering seeds to withstand every higher levels of pesticides, new traits are being genetically engineered to withstand other toxic chemicals. In the US, millions of acres of farmland growing GM corn, cotton, and soy are experiencing invasions of super weeds resistant to over-pesticide use. As pesticide use increases, soil quality is further depleted and yield per acre drops dramatically. The economic costs to farmers are becoming unsustainable as expenditures to fight pests and weeds increase and harvests diminish. A recent trend among farmers to revert back to traditional or organic methods is gradually taking hold. This aligns well with the last UN Commission on Trade and Development report warning against corporate dominated monoculture farming methods and promoting farm diversity and small scale organic farming as the most sustainable way to feed to the world's population.[112]

Aside from glyphosate, other pesticides are being genetically engineered into new lines of GM seeds. New varieties of GM cotton and soy are in Monsanto's pipeline and will likely pass with minimal review through the USDA and FDA. These new GM strains now include resistant genes to the pesticide dicamba. In addition to glyphosate's long list of human health risks, dicamba, a known neurotoxin, has been linked to adverse reproductive and mental development effects. Against strong public opposition, the US government will also likely approve Dow Agroscience's new Enlist corn and soy strains, a toxic cocktail of glyphosate and the herbicide 2-4 D, best known as a major toxic ingredient in Agent Orange that "has been linked to cancer, reproductive effects, neurotoxicity, kidney/liver damage, and birth and developmental effects."[113] Agent Orange contamination has resulted in genetic abnormalities and the deaths of hundreds of thousands of people. Its use as a bioweapon in Vietnam, Cambodia, and Laos is a sad reminder of the extremes the US is willing to take at the cost of innocent lives to reach its foreign policy objectives. And now, out of desperation to preserve agro-chemical agriculture and the GM corporations' revenues, the US government will resurrect one of the most toxic agrochemicals known and introduce it into America's food and, therefore, water supply.

I could go on about the destructive effects of GM crops. The good news is that GMO propaganda is increasingly being exposed as erroneous. As time passes, more and more research will inevitably emerge to further damn Monsanto and the GM experiment. It is only a matter of time before the false promises of GMOs will be exposed as orchestrated by Big Ag and the US government to control the world's food supply. Let's hope it's not too late.

Other Human Impacts on Natural Resources

In addition to agriculture, there are other human activities that contribute to air pollution, global warming, and the depletion of natural resources. I wanted to give you a synopsis of these as a way of reinforcing the imperative need to move forward to the healthy vegetarian lifestyle for increasing practices that can help reverse these deleterious trends, and for you to encourage and support others in doing the same. I will finish up by providing a brief overview of the hazardous household products, including air pollutants and other potentially harmful chemicals that warrant our attention.

However, the human activity that is by far the biggest source of greenhouse gas emissions, both in the United States and globally, is the combustion of fossil fuels for energy.

According to the EPA's *Greenhouse Gas Inventory Report*, more than 40% of carbon dioxide emissions in the United States in 2013 came from electric power generation.[114] Some 39% of the electricity generated in the US is produced by the combustion of coal, 27% by the combustion of natural gas, and a further 19% is generated from nuclear power.[115] Unlike fossil fuel combusting power plants, nuclear reactors do not emit greenhouse gases. However, the mining and refining of uranium ore require large amounts of energy, as does running the reactor. The main environmental concern related to nuclear power is the creation of radioactive waste, the majority of which is buried in the ground near the processing facility and covered with clay and then a layer of soil, rocks, or other materials,[116] and can remain dangerous to human health for thousands of years. Given this reality, what happened in places like Chernobyl and Fukushima, the latter of which, of course is still unresolved as of this writing, more than four years after the accident? The contaminated water is still being dumped into the Pacific Ocean every day; in fact, *Global Research News* reported as recently as March 1, 2015 that radiation levels were up to 70 times, or 7,000 percent, higher than normal, which prompted an immediate shutdown of the drainage instrument.[117]

In addition to human error, the increasing incidence of extreme weather patterns—tornadoes, hurricanes, earthquakes, tsunamis, and, of course as in the case of Fukushima, tidal waves—is a further reason that nuclear power is not a viable solution for energy in terms of health or sustainability.

Burning fossil fuels to power our cars, trucks, ships, trains, and planes accounted for a further 27% of our greenhouse gas emissions in 2013, while industry other than agriculture accounts for 21% of the 2013 greenhouse gas emissions.[118] Many industries require the burning of fossil fuels for energy, such as the production of metals like iron and steel, and certain industries that rely on chemical reactions to produce goods from raw materials, such as the production of cement and chemicals. And since industrial processes rely on electricity, they also contribute to emissions from electricity production.

Additional sources of greenhouse gas emissions besides residential buildings are landfill waste and the treatment of wastewater, both of which are significant contributors to global emissions of methane and nitrous oxide. Emissions from wastewater are projected to increase, driven by population growth and poor sanitation conditions in the developing world.

The major greenhouse gas released by human activities is carbon dioxide, about 30 billion tons of CO_2 per person every year.[119] One ray of hope is the fact that in the United States, improved forest management and strategies introduced to minimize soil erosion led to an increase of about 14% of the total carbon sequestration by this sector since 1990, both by reducing emissions caused by deforestation and by removing carbon dioxide from the atmosphere. CO_2 stays in the atmosphere anywhere between 20-200 years, so reducing your carbon footprint, including planting trees, is a worthwhile practice. Non-CO_2 greenhouse gases such as methane, nitrous oxide, and fluorinated greenhouse gases contribute more significantly to climate change. These greenhouse gases have a higher heat-trapping ability and therefore more significant climate change effect than carbon dioxide, but are thankfully far less abundant in the atmosphere.

Methane is the second most prevalent greenhouse gas emitted in the United States from human activities, and over 60% of total CH_4 emissions come from human activities.[120] Major sources of methane are landfills (794 million metric tons of carbon dioxide equivalent, MtCO2e)[121] due to the decomposition of solid organic waste, the treatment of wastewater (477 MtCO2e), and coal mining (522 MtCO2e),[122] as well as some industrial processes such as iron and steel production and silicon carbide production.[123] For comparison, livestock contributed to 1894 MtCO2e, more than these three sources combined. Therefore, by far our biggest contribution to the reduction of methane emission is through maintaining a vegetarian lifestyle.

Nitrous oxide is naturally present in the atmosphere as part of the Earth's nitrogen cycle and has a variety of natural sources. However, some 40% of global N_2O emissions come from human activities,[124] and agricultural activities such as fertilizer use, are the primary source of N_2O emissions. Nitrous oxide is a byproduct of fuel combustion and emitted by car exhausts, although its levels can be reduced by the use of a catalytic converter. In addition, nitrous oxide can be released from certain industrial activities including wastewater treatment, metal production, and the production of synthetic fibers like nylon. Nitrous oxide molecules stay in the atmosphere for an average of 114 years and have almost 300 times the warming capacity of carbon dioxide.[125]

The fluorinated gases—hydrofluorocarbons (HFCs), perfluorocarbons (PFCs), sulfur hexafluoride (SF_6), and nitrogen trifluoride (NF_3)—are also potent greenhouse gases, with a high global warming potential, up to 23,000 times greater than carbon dioxide in the case of SF6. Fluorinated gases are synthetic and originate solely from human-related activities. They are often used as substitutes for ozone-depleting substances, such as the chlorofluorocarbons (CFCs) that received so much media attention in the 1990s, as they do not damage the atmospheric ozone layer. However, they have the longest atmospheric lifetime of the greenhouse gases emitted by human activities and can affect the climate for tens to thousands of years. HFCs are emitted from a variety of industrial processes where they are often used as coolants in refrigerators, freezers, tumble dryers, and air-conditioning; foaming agents; solvents, and as propellants in fire extinguishers and aerosols. All the fluorinated gases are emitted by the manufacture of flat panel displays; PFCs and SF6 are also typically used in the electronics sector, as well as in the cosmetic and pharmaceutical industry.

The air conditioning units included in vehicles are responsible for the largest amount of HFC emissions due to their high rate of coolant loss,[126] another reason to look for alternative transport methods. We should make sure our refrigerators and freezers at home are serviced regularly, as HFCs can be released into the atmosphere through leaks, so it is important that old appliances are properly disposed of. And to avoid the use of air conditioning, why not try a solar fan (I mention these in Chapter 12), which emit no polluting fluorinated gases and will help lower the energy burden of our household. Finally, it's worth mentioning the variety of consumer products that can contribute to fluorinated gas emissions, such as spray deodorants, hair sprays, metered dose inhalers (such as those commonly used by asthmatics), insecticide sprays, spray paint, signal horns, decorative snow spray, and pepper sprays used for self-defense, which release these highly polluting gases directly into the atmosphere every time they are sprayed.

Chemical Assaults at Home That Stress the Environment

I'd like to shift our discussion before we end this section on the number of chemical assaults within our home that we are confronted with daily that affect our health and that of the environment. Few of us think about the onslaught of indoor pollution as a byproduct of the products we purchase and use. Sadly, these chemical products not only affect us but our environment's natural resources, through both production and use in terms of poisoning our water supplies and land, in particular. Thankfully this topic has received quite a bit of attention over the years. However, because so many products are petroleum based today, it bears repeating.

Hazardous Chemicals Contained in Household Items

Some recent research found that the average American home contains more than 1,000 different chemicals and over 150 of them have been linked to allergies, birth defects, cancer, and psychological abnormalities.[127] For example, a study published in 2013 found alarming amounts of volatile organic compounds (VOCs) released by 25 common brands of scented laundry products.[128] By alarming, we're talking over 600 VOCs—two of which are considered by the EPA to be carcinogenic, and seven of which are classified as hazardous air pollutants—yet none of the detected VOCs were listed on the product labels. VOCs can contribute to respiratory problems and aggravate allergies, asthma, and other respiratory illnesses. Many other fragranced consumer products, including air fresheners and aerosol sprays, skin-care products and shampoos, upholstery cleaners and oven cleaners, may also contain VOCs. Furthermore, in the case of air fresheners and cleaning products, many of them also contain significant levels of ethylene-based glycol ethers,[129] which are classified as hazardous air pollutants[130] and known to cause neurological and blood effects, including fatigue, nausea, tremor, and anemia.[130]

It is not only generally accepted that consumer products may contribute to indoor pollution, but *the EPA actually states that toxic chemicals in household cleaners are three times more likely to cause cancer than air pollution.* To protect your family from the potentially harmful effects of fragranced consumer products, we recommend you always keep air circulating when using cleaning products or choose unfragranced, natural cleaners wherever possible. Method, Seventh Generation, and Bon Ami are some commonly available alternatives, or you could try making your own cleaning products out of common household items—the Internet is a wonderful resource for these types of projects. In the place of air fresheners, achieve your favorite aromas by simmering lemon, orange, ginger, rosemary, cinnamon, or cloves in water and allowing the natural scent to fill your home.

Skin care products, shampoos, and cosmetics, in addition to the wide use of non-vegetarian ingredients, often contain other nasties such as BHT and BHA, whose health risks we've already mentioned, and parabens, which have been found to be endocrine disruptors[131] and allergens linked to dermatitis.[132] Check the list of ingredients for these chemicals; choose paraben-free, or natural or mineral makeup options.

Nowadays, many skin-care products contain antibacterial ingredients, most commonly Triclosan. Triclosan has been shown to be toxic to some aquatic organisms, has been connected to endocrine disruption, particularly of the thyroid, and a study by the Environmental Working Group found that 97% of breast feeding mothers had triclosan in their milk.[133] For these reasons, the FDA is currently, "reviewing all of the available evidence on this ingredient's safety in consumer products,"[134] although some states, such as Minnesota, are planning to ban the component as of the year 2017. Check the label for triclosan or microban or avoid antibacterial products if in doubt. Alternatively, try plant-oil based natural anti-bacterials such as thyme oil or tea tree oil.

Another group of chemical additives you should avoid in bathroom products such as shampoo, deodorant, and hair spray, are phthalates, which are suspected endocrine disruptors.[135] Phthalates are used to bind the color and fragrance in cosmetic products, but they are also commonly added to plastics to increase the material's flexibility and durability. You may have heard of them in the media since some were banned in the EU for use in children's toys in 2005,[136] and states such as California, Washington, and Vermont have banned the use of phthalates in toys for younger children. In 1998, the U.S. Consumer Product Safety Commission reached a voluntary agreement with manufacturers to remove two phthalates from plastic rattles, teethers, pacifiers, and baby bottle nipples.[137] Nevertheless, these toxic chemicals are still found in many beauty products. Be particularly vigilant when reading the labels of your cosmetics and body-care products in order to avoid these hormone affecting chemicals.

To finish this brief section on hazardous chemicals found in household products, I'd like to finish with clothing, because Greenpeace has recently launched its Detox Campaign. As part of this campaign, laboratories carried out a series of tests on major clothing brands, including Disney, Adidas, Zara, Primark, GAP, and Nike, as well as luxury brands such as Levi's, Giorgio Armani, Burberry, Dior, Dolce & Gabbana, Louis Vuitton, Valentino, and Versace. Practically all of the clothing tested was found to contain toxic chemicals, such as PFCs, phthalates, and many others as a result of their use during manufacture.[138] For example, in one such test, 141 items of clothing were purchased in April 2012 from 29 different countries and retailers: High levels of phthalates were found in four of the garments, and cancer-causing amines from the use of certain dyes were found in two of the garments. In another study of 27 children's clothing products, 16 of them tested positive for one or more of these hazardous chemicals, evidence that all but one of the brands studied was selling children's products, including baby booties, containing hazardous chemicals.[139] These chemicals pose a threat to human health and also to marine life since they can seep into the environment from the factory where the clothes are made and thus affect water sources.

Some brands, such as Zara, H&M, Valentino, Mango, Victoria's Secret, Levis, Burberry, and Primark have signed Greenpeace's Detox commitment to stop using hazardous chemicals. However, some companies, such as Disney and GAP, continue to refuse to sign up. You should wash all new clothes before wearing them (although washing doesn't remove all types of chemicals), choose eco-friendly brands, and look for natural fibers—particularly for children—for example by choosing organic cotton garments.

As a healthy vegetarian, our shopping decisions are based on more than just whether an item contains animal-based products or not. I have included some suggestions in Chapter 9, as well as Chapter 12. We increasingly make ethical choices based on safety, fair trade, and workers conditions. But we should also include necessity in this list when considering whether to buy an item as part of our efforts to reduce our consumption while being mindful of our larger home, planet Earth.

Chapter 11

Global Food Resources

> "The question is whether any civilization can wage relentless war on life without destroying itself, and without losing the right to be called civilized."
>
> – *Rachel Carson, Author of* Silent Spring

On this same topic of how earth resources are squandered, let me mention the equation brought up earlier. In the world's non-industrialized countries, where the vast majority of the planet's citizens live, a lacto-ovo vegetarian diet or a pesco-vegetarian one is the norm. As will be described fully below, with the world population pressing on food stocks, it has become critically dangerous that overmuch land and resources are being given to animal raising and the growing of grain for animal feed instead of using this land to grow grain, vegetables, and other plants for people to eat.

Land is capable of supplying food for nearly 14 times as many people when used to grow food for them as it would if it is used to grow crops for livestock, whose animal products eventually supply food for people. We took a look at some of these realities in the previous chapter. If you remember, cows, for instance, eat approximately 16 pounds of grain to yield just one pound of flesh. It is estimated that farm animals use more than one-thirteenth of all water used by people.

On the other hand, if meat-consuming societies curtailed their meat demand and freed up grazing land for the more efficient growing of human food crops in controlled venues like greenhouses, it's been estimated that the resulting yield of plant foods could feed more than double the world's population, likely solving the growing world hunger problem.

Current Food Resources

How Big a Problem Is World Hunger?

I am not an expert on global economics, but I can see all too clearly that the expectations held for the poorer countries—such as India, the Philippines, Brazil, and Argentina, for example—after World War II were never fulfilled. If they were engaged in more egalitarian societies and would have been encouraged toward farming, these nations could have become more self-sufficient in terms of providing food for their people. Fewer would have had to move from the country to the city, where ghettos were formed, and they could have grown some of their own food. They would have still been poor, but they would not have been engaged in the chronic famine, as they were, and continue to be in certain parts of these nations still today.

Fifty years on, and the same famines and lack of adequate nutrition are still prevalent, and even more so. One thing that has stifled their advance is *the terms of trade*, the fact that these countries sell low in export (marketing raw materials that fetch low prices) and buy high in import (paying top dollar for manufactures from the well-off countries). Due to this imbalance, and other factors we will pinpoint in a minute, a significant percentage of the world's population—around a fourth—has been condemned to a life of hunger and eventual starvation. It is estimated as of 2011-2013 that 12% of the world's population[1] suffers from malnutrition and that at least a billion people suffer from malnutrition, receiving such inadequate amounts of nutrients that even their basic physiological functions are impaired.[2]

When we think of haves and have-nots, the most common perspective is to see this in terms of some people having good housing and modern conveniences, and others not having these possessions. But, it would be more accurate to think of the world's peoples as divided between those that *have and those that have not enough food to eat or clean water to drink.* In fact, 30% of the food we grow is never even eaten.[3] Isn't it strange that with 50 million Americans (including 17 million children) experiencing food scarcity that we haven't found a better way of dealing with this. This is leaving aside the number of people in the US that *do* have plenty to eat but that routinely throw away food that children in Ethiopia, the Sudan, Somalia, India, or Southeast Asia pray for, but seldom receive. In drought-ridden northeastern Brazil, where some 350,000 refugees, known as *flagellados,* have starved to death,[4] children suffer severe growth abnormalities and irreversible brain damage for the kind of nutrients that could be collected in our garbage pails. Infant brain damage is a very serious problem in this region of Brazil because of chronic dietary protein deficiencies. "There seems to be little disagreement among scientists," according to an *American Scientist* article, "that a continuous protein-deficient diet produces irreversible damage to the brain."[5]

Media pundits in the US, at least those beholden to corporate advertisers, are hardly going to condemn the global neo-liberal, international-based, and balkanized business structure, which pivots on unequal terms of trade for world hunger, so they look for other (and relatively plausible) explanations. One of these is that overpopulation in these poor countries places an undue strain on the already tenuous food supply. A second explanation offered is that these nations are technologically "backward." They don't have the latest in machinery, fertilizer, and so on to keep pace with food demands generated by modern population growth rates. It is also assumed that there is ignorance in these countries of those modern agricultural techniques that help farmers increase yields. This last point overlooks the glaring fact that modern agricultural techniques have been created for mass production agriculture and are of use *only* on giant farms, which employ few people. So, if they were even affordable, and instituted in poor countries, they would certainly increase food production but throw all the small farmers out of work and hence create more problems than they solved.

I'm not saying there is absolutely no truth whatsoever in these explanations. However, assuming that modern ways of doing things are always superior to centuries-old traditional methods employed in many of these societies is simply arrogant. They are also often couched in a way that is culturally prejudiced. The same prejudice I've encountered from people when I've said, for example, that a Native American or traditional Chinese remedy for a common ailment may be superior to a modern pharmaceutical. But the most basic mistake in these sorts of explanations is that they assume that world hunger can be overcome by increased agricultural production, coupled with stringent birth control measures.

Those who advocate this view often get people's attention by citing startling facts about population growth. They might bring up the "fact" that at the present rate of increase, "700 years from now people would be standing shoulder to shoulder on every foot of the earth's land surface ... In 7,000 years, our population would be expanding outward into space at the speed of light."[6] This overlooks the idea that population growth can shift. After all, China has been controlling its birth rate, one child per family, for decades. Yet, even while such reductions would be helpful, this cannot be the only solution to world hunger.

What we need to understand is that *starvation is essentially human-made.* It's not just an artifact of the terms of trade, but also of (in the more well-off countries) using animal products for food. Certainly, population increases coupled with production decreases caused by droughts or floods or other natural or man-made phenomena are decisive factors. Still, as Frances Moore Lappé writes, famine is not a necessary part of national experience, even in notoriously poor countries. "Bangladesh," she points out, which suffered a devastating famine in 1973/'74, "is by no means a hopeless basket case."[7] Yes, this small country does have an extremely dense population. Yet in Taiwan, with twice the number of people per cultivated acre, the people are far from starving. Population density may be a variable in the question of whether a country's food supply is sufficient to support its people, but *considerably more significant* is how efficiently a country's land and food supply are used, and more critically, the priorities and motivations of a society. (We will return to a discussion of Bangladesh in a moment.)

I won't cover the same ground I've already crossed by noting how the animal industry is based on gross misuse of the land, which would be better employed to feed people rather than cattle, or on how inefficient animal consumption is in terms of nutritional return to the consumer. And we've already seen that the ill effects of meat production come not only to those losing their lands in the underdeveloped nations, but to meat eaters themselves, privileged yet ironically suffering the detrimental health effects that accompany such a diet. (For example, in a large cohort study in the UK, body-mass indexes were significantly higher in meat eaters than in vegetarians, and higher scores, generally associated with being overweight, correlated to high-protein and low-fiber intake.[8] This is to say, overweight conditions, strongly associated with diminished health, are the normal accompaniers of meat-centered diets.)

What is important to recognize is that the recurrent difficulty of poorer people in underdeveloped countries finding sufficient food is not an inevitable fate, but created by human circumstances. As to the danger of population growth, it is true that if the current population explosion continues, the world will eventually reach a saturation point for its traditional food resources.[9] Of course, one company in American named *Soylent* has created a food product designed for use as a staple meal by all adults. One scoop of Soylent and one scoop of water make one meal, which they claim provides maximum nutrition value. It was created after the owners recognized the disproportionate amount of time and money they spent creating nutritionally complete meals.

I wonder: could we be approaching the end of food as we know it? More so, what are *you* willing to do for the benefit of enjoying a crisp green lettuce salad with a plethora of rainbow-colored fresh-picked fixings? Likewise, what are we willing to do so that juice-filled oranges and apples remain in our grocers? Please also contemplate this: What would life be like without fresh broccoli, spinach, tomatoes or almonds? In a sense, I believe the old adage *plan for the worst but expect the best* is our imperative here. This will allow us to go about the work that is needed steadfastly and joyfully.

While estimates predict that our present world population of 7.3 billion must increase twofold before we actually face this situation, this does give us time, albeit not a lot, to begin working constructively toward a solution. One characteristic in humans that prevents us from moving forward is that we take what we see with our eyes as evidence of the truth (even when it may not be) and, as I said before, because most of us don't have evidence of the hardship I pointed out in this chapter, we don't take formidable action. This does not make us "bad," per se, it makes us human. So I'd invite you to ask yourself: what is needed, overall, and what actions do I wish to take starting now? In that world hunger has been created by us and our structures, it is up to us to change those structures, starting with ourselves.

Raising Food without Feeding People

Attempts to Lower Food Intakes

Lack of adequate food has plagued the poorer countries from the time they have been invaded and colonized, so there has been plenty of time to devise what looked like solutions to this tragedy.

Not every tentative attempt to reduce the grain going to livestock, as an example, was targeted at world hunger, however. Some of these moves were simply made in relation to the bottom line. For instance, recognizing that cattle must consume 16 pounds of feed to produce a single pound of flesh, agribusiness saw the need to lower the grain consumption of their cows to slash costs. Their egregious and cruel solution was to build facilities where the animals' movement was severely restricted, thus dropping their feeding requirements. The "beasts of burden" are now lined up in crowded and squalid "feedlots." While the cattle endure this unnatural, painful life, the corporate executives are too busy counting their money to give them a thought, in that livestock are fed in these mechanized feedlots now reach their target weight and are delivered to the slaughterhouse in roughly one-third the normal time and with lower grain consumption.[10]

Cattle and other livestock still eat a lot, nonetheless, because feedlot operations speed weight gain—a desired effect to get animals to market sooner—by feeding cattle an unnatural diet of grain and by-product feedstuffs (waste products from the manufacture of human food, including sterilized city garbage, candy, bubble gum, and floor sweepings from plants that manufacture animal food, bakery goods, and potato wastes, and in some cases even dead cows,[11] as an example). In addition, the cattle are treated with synthetic hormones, and their food is doctored with antibiotics. Incessant propaganda by the meat industry coupled with the mistaken belief that consuming animal products delivers good nutrition and conscientious weight loss have brought about a rising lust for meat, globally, but also among American consumers. This translates into an uptick in overall feed requirement as more animals make their way to the slaughterhouse. So, the two contrary pressures here did not balance out: the meat makers' desire to reduce their animals' grain consumption among rising levels of meat-eating in the US through 2007 demanded more livestock be raised for slaughter. Since meat consumption has been falling steadily (albeit slightly) since 2007, this eases the pressures. However, there is still an enormous amount of strain on humans and the environment.

Use of livestock feed in the United States is now averaging about 200 million tons annually, compared to 100 million tons on the eve of World War II. Although this figure accounts only for grain given to animals in the US, it is equivalent to all the grain that is currently imported by every nation in the world. Corn grown for grain constitutes about one-fourth of this country's harvested crop acres,[12] and 80% of all corn grown in the US goes to livestock, poultry, and fish production at home and overseas.

The number of poultry as well as livestock that are fed grain has doubled over the last 30 years, with 75% of all livestock currently grain fed. Pigs consume as much grain as do cattle, each animal requiring an average 5,000 pounds of grain, soy, and additional crops annually.[13] Remember that in the days of family farms, when cattle might eat whatever grass or scrubs they chanced upon, there was no such drain on grain resources, but now such free ranging animals are a rarity, and so the overtaxing of the environment is the norm.

The largely selfish move by the livestock interests to cut animal grain consumption by restricting their lives failed. But the agribusinesses succeeded, in that they hadn't reduced overall feed use, but had reduced the amount of feed per cow and were enjoying mega-profits thanks to consumers upping their meat intake.

Attempts to Increase Grain Yields

While the program to reduce feed intake per individual cow, cruel as it was, might have done a little to alleviate the strain on the ecosystem of massive grain production for livestock, there were concurrent and decidedly more humane programs that might have eliminated some of this strain by making land more productive. That is, if they would have been better supported. I'm referring, of course, to the Green Revolution, which was already referenced when I noted that such programs went wrong by relying too much on large investments in machinery and other agricultural inputs. But there is more to be said about this program.

The Green Revolution program, which was initiated around 1940 but started to pick up steam in the late 1960s, aimed to end world hunger by introducing new crops bred specifically for rapid growth and high-yield performance. But the crops were very expensive to grow because of the uncommonly large amounts of fertilizer they required. Again, a program was planned and funded that wouldn't benefit the poor farmers, who made up the majority of crop raisers. Only the elite agriculturalists, who could come up with the capital to buy the fertilizers and who often had the political ties to achieve subsidies to buy more land and displace more poor households, benefitted. The displaced small farmers had to leave their land and make the trek to the cities.

Another weakness of the Green Revolution was its overemphasis on grain production. Grains largely replaced many varieties of legumes, vegetables and other plants, ones that gave the native diet variety and different nutritional elements. With the Green Revolution, the focus was on foods whose surplus, over the farmers' needs, could be sold in the market. In other words, the watchword here was commerce, and not fulfilling the eating needs of the country's populace. Nutrition was seldom considered. Dr. R. S. Harris, professor of biochemistry and nutrition at M.I.T., found that the indigenous strains of crops being replaced by the new high-yield varieties of the Green Revolution were actually superior in nutrition.[14]

In *Food for Naught*, Ross Hume Hall talks about the shortsightedness of the project: "'The Green Revolution' devised in Western countries as a solution to the nutritional problems of other cultures, is based on the fully mechanized technology of Western countries. It is not just a matter of planting new strains of rice or wheat, it is also a matter of applying fertilizer at the right time, irrigating at the right time, applying insecticides, herbicides and using new types of machines—the whole complex of business."[15]

I don't believe there was a nefarious plot involved in this but it was, instead, simply another instance of the law of unintended consequences or not having enough foresight to see the end results—like many government programs that were purportedly targeted at uplifting the poor and did not, such as welfare programs that resulted in the breaking up families. The Green Revolution program disenfranchised the people it was purporting to help. A program that pretended to have the capability of ending third world hunger, drove peasants from the land, where they could have, at worst, been able to raise food to live at a subsistence level. In the cities, where their agricultural skills were valueless, they often starved. They couldn't afford to buy the grain that was raised on the land from which they were evicted, so most of the increased food supply went to livestock for the meat and dairy industries. It would be almost *comical if it wasn't so tragic*.

Eating Meat Is Wasting Food

Much of what I have said and will say on the wasteful use of resources going into meat and dairy production is being made with an assumption, which needs to be laid bare, particularly as many advocates of vegetarianism gloss over it. The assumption goes like this: First, we have so much hunger in the world and meanwhile have vast amount of food going to feed livestock. (This colossal waste is enough to provide one cup of grain daily for every person in the world for an entire year;[16] the combined surplus of both grain and legumes eaten by these animals could be eaten by 800 million hungry people.[17]) Second, if livestock-raising was eliminated, hungry people would have a good chance to be fed. Now, do you see the weakness in the so-called logic?

If authoritarian governments and greedy businesses are allowed to rule the world without strong opposition, sucking people dry, throwing them off their lands and out of work, and leaving them for dead, little can be done or hoped for in terms of ending starvation. I sincerely hope and trust that will not be the case for much longer. However, long before there is any seismic shift in the political climate in a country, there are lengthy and protracted frustrations of the endemic corruption, cronyism, nepotism, and inequalities. Then, one day, a seemingly insignificant event serves as a catalyst to mobilize a mass social movement among a nation's people; along with this, there may be a challenge to those in power. These events used to be triggered mostly by younger people but today we see older people involved—and in countries like Greece, Italy, Spain, Ireland, Portugal, and France, where entitlements, pensions, and social services are being reduced or eliminated through austerity programs. Now they are in the streets by the hundreds of thousands throwing out more conservative governments and instating more populist governments. This is happening, as I said, right now in other parts of the world but not in the US.

Nevertheless, if we assume the more pessimistic scenario does *not* take place and it is possible that individuals, groups, and organizations that want to end this misery will keep rising up, then my argument becomes more modest. In this more optimistic world arrangement, my belief is that for world hunger to end, the lopsided use of global resources to feed and consume livestock has to cease.

Look at how much is taken by the meat and dairy industries, and how warped the situation has become. In a recent year, our livestock used up 145 million tons of grain and soy to produce a meager 21 million tons of animal products—not a very good ratio. Would you buy 145 gallons of gas for your car if you could only use 21?

Certainly, not every animal consumes the same amount. As noted, cattle must be fed 16 pounds of grain to produce a single pound of flesh. By contrast, to yield that same pound of flesh, pigs consume about 6 pounds of feed, cows requires approximately 7 pounds of grain for each gallon of milk we drink and poultry only need 3 to 4 pounds.[18]

Let's contrast the animals' consumption to what yield it would bring if the grain had been given to humans. If the 16 pounds of grain used to put 1 pound on a cow was given to a human, he or she would net 20 times the calories and 10 times the protein that the individual would have gotten from the pound of beef. As I have been stressing, the body cannot take full advantage of the protein available in meat and dairy. If we look at the protein in the whole cycle, from another vantage point, counting that which the animals drew from plants and how much of that we ultimately got if we ate the animal, we see gross inefficiency. We get to use only 25, 12, and 10% of the protein that goes into producing milk, pork, and beef, respectively.[19]

In other words, it's not as if by eating animals that took in proteins from plants, you are somehow getting a condensed version of the plant protein. Most of that protein has been used to maintain the animal and is lost to human meat eaters. In terms of land use, a single acre of farmland can yield 800,000 calories to human eaters by growing vegetable food. If we feed the same vegetables to animals first, though, the meat and dairy produced by that acre of farmland comes to only 200,000 calories, a 75% loss in terms of nutrition. Can you see the insanity of this? I hope so, and more importantly, I hope you will help others see also.

To go back to my opening thought, if we imagine we could get a consensus of people to agree to fight world hunger (and preclude from our consideration the possibility that a greedy elite will run the world as they like with no pretensions of justice or equality), then the first thing we have to do to address the problem is stop allowing meat eating to rob us of millions of tons of calories and proteins, millions in our tax dollars, and the distress associated with being aware that our choices are creating suffering—not only for animals, but for humans and our planet at large. This is truly something that is very much within our reach.

Land for Food

I talked a few pages back about those who have and those who have not with respect to food, discussing how the interventions of advanced countries into developing countries, as in the fomenting of the Green Revolution, usually ended up being a disaster for the latter. However, I still don't think I have said enough. For one, while such interventions often come with excuse of being well intentioned or at least neutral toward the impoverished, this is not the case.

One such example of this is the US's coaxing (starting in the Reagan-Bush years, and culminating with the Clinton administration) of Haiti to liberalize trade arrangements, including the reduction of tariffs on imports. In short, with US rice selling for 30-50% less than local rice, these efforts caused Haiti to go from raising and providing 100% of its rice in 1987 to less than 20% by 2003. Needless to say, this resulted in the decimation of Haiti's once viable farming industry and the impoverishment of many—a situation lamented by former president Bill Clinton when he said, "It [Haitian trade policies that cut tariffs on imported U.S. rice] may have been good for some of my farmers in Arkansas, but it has not worked. It was a mistake." He further lamented his persistent championing of such trade policies: "I had to live everyday with the consequences of the loss of capacity to produce a rice crop in Haiti to feed those people because of what I did; nobody else."[20] However, when you take a closer look, it really doesn't require a whole lot of foresight or intelligence to see the likely backlash of these trade policies.

There are other actions that are almost hostile toward impoverished people insofar as those who perpetuated them allowed their lust for riches to override any humanitarian considerations. This is most certainly the case in this country.

As established so far, the subsidies and expenses needed for the Green Revolution or any Western-led agricultural production tend to favor the well off and end up displacing the small peasants. What has not been mentioned, yet, is what is done with the land—which is, it is very often assembled into larger farms, by the better-off agriculturalists. In *Food First: Beyond the Myth of Scarcity* Frances Moore Lappé and Joseph Collins take up this thread of the argument when they point to the activities of small but powerful groups of wealthy landowners, who typically use their large land holdings in underdeveloped countries to turn profits.[21] Instead of growing grain, legumes, vegetables, and fruits for the people all around them, such as those they have displaced from their small plots of land, these landowners raise crops grown for dollar profit. The concentration is on such commodities as coffee beans, sugarcane, tobacco, and beef, quite often destined for overseas consumers who will pay dearly for them. As mentioned before, the poor farmers, no longer tilling their own plots, but now paid even poorer wages as agricultural laborers on the big plantations, can't afford to buy these products. Look at beef production, which rose over 90% in some areas of Latin America in the last few decades. At the same time, it has been shown that this beef was being shipped off to foreign parts while beef consumption in the countries where the cattle were being raised dropped over 30%. Alan Berg, an authority in the field of nutrition, lays it on the line, "The meat is ending up not in Latin American stomachs, but in franchised restaurant hamburgers in the U.S."[22]

It's not that no staple crops, such as corn or wheat, are being raised in these nations. Yet, even the prices of these non-luxury items, in country, are often too high to be in reach of the have-nots because they have been bid up by those buying the grain for animal food. The steeper prices are not affordable to any but the affluent minority. Doesn't that mean some of this high-priced food will go unsold? No, the balance is shipped out of the country.

I alluded to Bangladesh previously, but only to say that this small country, with 80 million inhabitants at the time of the Lappé and Collins study, did not necessarily have too many people for its resources. But I didn't explain why, if it theoretically had enough resources—the land yielded enough grain to provide each person with 2,600 calories daily—it turns out two-thirds of the people are protein- and vitamin-deficient. A glance at *Food First* tells the story.

Lappé and Collins found that the problem was not with food production, but with the manipulation of land and produce by the small minority (the ill-intentioned) that owns the majority of land in Bangladesh. These landowners continually bleed the poor tenant farmer by constantly raising their rent. And many landlords, not content with monopolizing the market, go on to become "moneylender-merchants," hoarding grain, causing food shortages, and driving up prices. When grain is abundant and prices low, they stockpile their produce, waiting for the right moment. Then, for example, when a drought causes a shortfall of food and desperately hungry people are ready to pay almost anything, they open their hoards and offer to sell at jacked-up prices, which means either the poor can't buy any or don't buy enough to stave off malnutrition. It's as if these people care nothing of the lives of others save themselves and their families. Sadly, this lack of consciousness is the root cause of these issues, and they will not clear up until each of us is able to take responsibility for eliminating the lack of consciousness in our own lives.

As Lappé and Collins explain, "Landless laborers, dependent on meager wages, are particularly vulnerable. Precisely when floods and droughts deprive them of work altogether, speculative food prices … shoot up 200 to 500 percent. Once we became aware of these realities, we were not surprised to learn that, while many starved after the 1974 floods, hoarders stocked up an estimated 4 million tons of rice because the vast majority … was too poor to buy it."[23]

In other words, the situation was no different from the others we've been describing in which the country has the natural resources to feed its people, but the power structure stops this from happening. A committee of the US Congress reported this on the Bangladesh situation: "The country is rich enough in fertile land, water, manpower and natural gas for fertilizer not only to be self-sufficient in food, but a food exporter."[24]

Let's look at another down side. Having lost their holdings, the people are working as sharecroppers, and this means they have to turn in a large "share" of their crop to the owner of their land for rent. This turned-in produce is subject to the same conditions, meaning they often can't afford to buy at the market when they are in need. It doesn't make good economic sense for these renters to do anything that would substantially improve their plots, because it would only raise the value of the land. When the next time to negotiate a contract came around, the landowner would take note of any improvements and increase the rental price.

As *Food First* documents, it is discouraging to see that such calculations even affect small landowners, not just renters. Some see that building small scale irrigation systems would allow them to use conserved monsoon waters to irrigate their fields during droughts and dry seasons. What holds them back from making these small but crucial improvements is their well-justified fear that by increasing the value of their lands, they will make them tempting prizes for wealthy farmers, who will use their money or power to grab these lands for themselves out from under the improving owners.[25] So they would rather remain nominal than draw attention. On the flip side, and even more perversely, some landowners are so power-hungry that rather than let their sharecroppers benefit from whatever improvements they have made on the rented land—such as irrigation systems—they will remove and destroy these additions each time the land's lease is to be renewed. The demented logic at work here is that if the land grew more fruitful and profitable, the laboring farmer might begin to gain some independence from the landlord.

I mentioned the greedy landlords of Bangladesh taking advantage of their tenants and laborers. This is not an isolated case. Rather such warped situations are widespread in the underdeveloped world. In the semi-desert of northeastern Brazil, for instance, where a serious drought has persisted since 1978, similar land abuse has caused tremendous suffering. The wealthy landlords reserve the vast majority of the land for cash crops and for raising cattle for the beef industry. The cash crops and beef use up all the water and hog the land, leaving millions of local Brazilians land poor, dying of thirst, and, since they can't afford the cash crops or find adequate work, they are displaced from their farms, starving. Jose Matias Filho of Caera State University's Department of Agriculture explains, with "our present water resources and technology, we could produce five times as much food."[26] But landowners prefer to raise animals for slaughter rather than raise grain. Again, it's all bottom line: Meat can be sold to the American and European markets for far more money than would be made selling food to poor peasants. The result: America is awash in hamburgers (and its associated health problems) supplied by an area, which, as one leading nutritional expert, notes, surpasses every other region of the world in its "low living standards."[27]

I've already inundated you with statistics, but needed to add one additional one before moving into a cost analysis: if we took the 170 million tons of grain a year we feed to animals, and ate it directly, we could alleviate the world's caloric deficiency four times over.[28] It comes down, simply, to a question of responsibility and priority.

We All Pay for the Meat Any of Us Eat

By the way, I'm not saying meats' high prices are not justified. On the contrary, the nutrients needed to sustain life ultimately come from plant foods. You get these nutrients in one of two ways: either directly by eating the plant, or indirectly by eating the animal that was fed on the plant. When you consume meat, poultry, and dairy products, you are eating higher on the food chain than when you consume grains and vegetables directly, because you are in essence getting plant proteins secondhand, as such since it is filtered through an animal.

The simplest notion of the expense of this secondhand consumption is that over its lifespan the animal has eaten a lot of plants, so you are paying for the fields of grain or other materials that have gone through its system. That would be all there is to it if you, say, shot a deer in the wild and ate it. But for meat processed through the food industry, you also have to foot the bill for the rancher's overhead, for the high cost of the animal husbandry (including, as we saw before, pharmaceuticals and other chemicals), as well as the animals' slaughter, processing, packaging, and transport to the market and the percentage associated with the retailers' sales. Come to think of it, in a roundabout way, you also pay for the meat-purveyors propaganda in the form of insipid advertisements and the studies of coddled scientists.

Unfortunately—and this goes way beyond the animal products industry—with the gargantuan nature of the business enterprises in our multinational capitalist world, outsourcing and over packaging is the order of the day, and it has largely stamped out small producers in farming and other areas.

Let me give you an example of what I'm talking about. In the not-too-distant past, if you wanted to buy a sweater and lived in a region where sheep were found, you could procure one made by a loom in your hometown. Now, even if you live on a sheep farm, chances are you can't go to town and get a locally-made sweater. Why? Because all the wool on surrounding farms is sent to a distant factory to be combined, more than likely, with synthetic fabrics, designed, sent through an assembly line, folded, pinned, transported to a wholesale distributor in yet another distant city, and finally bought by and shipped to a retail outlet right back in your hometown. This was all done under the rationale of cost savings, but is anyone going to tell me this wool sweater feels as good or was made with as much care or is as safe, given it is probably coated with chemicals, as the one my grandmother could have bought from her neighbor? This sweater is about as close to the sheep as ground beef is to hay, the hay that originally nourished the cow that was slaughtered for the beef.

This is not the place to get into international economics. And I admit I am not well versed in the details of this field. But I know enough to realize that a truckload of money is spent on importing meat and dairy products, farm equipment, fertilizers, and petroleum. There are seemingly endless complaints in the business news about America's trade deficit, the fact that it spends more money on imports than it gets back on its exports. Certainly, this imbalance would be partly healed if our country's citizens shifted away from their meat-fixated diets. As I explored in the previous chapter, this shift would free up more resources to tackle the critical global issues of starvation and peace, and give us the opportunity to support current more sustainable industries like organic farming as well as create new truly valuable and sustainable industries.

The Cost Factor

We have looked at some of the good things waiting for anyone who takes up a vegetarian diet. Now let's switch to a final survey of what a meat- and dairy-oriented eating is doing to America's health and pocketbooks.

Is the Vegetarian Diet Less Expensive Than the Meat-Based Diet?

If you factor in costs associated with illness related to consuming an animal-based diet, which we will discuss in a moment, and the fact that the meat and dairy industries are highly subsidized—to the tune of 63% of all agriculture subsidies, with another 20% going toward soy and corn to feed livestock, with a mere 3% of farming subsidies going to fruits, vegetables, nuts and legumes (the foods that are actually proven to aid in health)—according to 2011 figures forwarded by the Physicians Committee for Responsible Medicine,[29] the answer is unequivocally yes. As I've shown in other places in the book, vegetarians across the board have consistently demonstrated lower rates of lifestyle diseases such as heart disease, diabetes, obesity, and cancer.

On the basis solely of money-out-of-your-wallet, the answer is less clear. At the time of this writing, the average cost per pound of ground chuck was $4.40, a Boneless New York Strip Steak $8.35:[30] Filet Mignon rested comfortably around $15.39 per pound. Fresh whole chicken is at $1.55 and chicken breasts at $3.51 per pound. Eggs are at $2.08 per pound; ham and pork is anywhere from $2.48 to $5.47 per pound; and dairy (milk) starts at $3.60 per pound,[31] increasing substantially for cheese.

These are all non-organic prices; organic prices will be on average 50% more.[32] Chicken is the most widely available and utilized organic meat; it is purchased by more than seven in ten shoppers[33] (73%). Prices range as low as organic chicken is $2.69 a pound at Trader Joe's, the US grocery chain, and $4.99 per pound from online grocer Fresh Direct. Whole Foods sells boneless, skinless organic chicken breasts for $8.99+ per pound. And it's not unusual to pay more than $10 per pound for similar organic chicken breasts at upscale butcher shops.[34] Because the demand for chicken continues to increase, its price will increase too. An article in the *Wall Street Journal* noted that large-scale US chicken producer Tyson projects US chicken demand to rise 3% to 4% in 2015, potentially outpacing an anticipated 2% to 3% increase in domestic production, studies predict.[35] So, don't be surprised to see an increase here.

Meanwhile, the majority of non-organic fruits and vegetables with the exception of grapes, berries, Romaine lettuce, and peppers are averaging under $2/pound;[36] beans and legumes (a primary source of protein) ring in around $1.48 per pound, with organics running as low as $2.40/lb.; tofu sits at around $2-$2.50 per pound; brown rice at $1.99 per pound (you can even get organic Brown rice for as low as $2.56 per pound on Amazon today[37]); and tubers (potatoes, yams, etc.), as low as $.73/pound.

Additionally, several organic fruits and vegetables are currently available for under $2/pound: apples, avocados, bananas, mangoes, oranges, pears, tangelos, onions, potatoes, broccoli, cabbage, carrots, cauliflower, celery, cucumbers, green onions, sweet potatoes, and tomatoes.[38] Plus, as I mention in Chapter 2, you can save even more by buying in bulk, at your local food coop or famer's market.

Per pound, nuts and nut butters are as or more expensive than meat, but only because meat and dairy is heavily subsidized—to the tune of about 60%.[39] So, without subsidies, you would be paying at least twice retail prices, right in the same ballpark as nuts. But since nuts and nut butters constitute a low percentage of the basic vegetarian diet, because of their fat content, and are consumed at lower volumes—think about eating a 16 oz. steak vs. consuming a one-pound bag of walnuts, almonds or cashews in one sitting—per pound pricing is not nearly as relevant.

Still, an average chicken breast weighs 6-8 ounces; 6-8 ounces of nuts by weight would translate into 1½ -2 cups by volume,[40] which would be an extraordinary amount of nut product to consume in any one meal, let alone consuming a pound of nuts. In terms of protein content, nuts and seeds can have much more protein than some legumes or grains (see chart in back of the book), but the amount of fat in nuts acts as a counterbalance, making legumes and grains a more viable source of vegetarian protein. As an example, a 6 oz. serving of walnuts contains 144g of fat and approximately 30 grams of protein,[41] while a 6 oz. serving of lentils contains approximately 2 grams of fat and 18 grams of protein. Big disparity.

Bottom line, good nutrition through the basic vegetarian diet featuring fresh vegetables, starchy grains, legumes and beans, is less expensive pound per pound than a meat-based diet. When you count other costs, including health and environmental, the vegetarian diet blows the meat diet away. Raj Patel, author of *The Value of Nothing: How to Reshape Market Society and Redefine Democracy* argues that the cost to society is so high that the real cost of a hamburger should be about $200.[42]

Personally, I have counseled thousands of people to switch to a vegetarian diet, and they have saved anywhere from 30-50% by eliminating meat and dairy products, as well as packaged foods, which brings me to my next point.

Less Production is the Key

If you want to save money, switch to a vegetarian diet that does *not* include processed foods. Processing adds to the cost of everything. Instead of buying a bag of popcorn for $3-$4 in the health food store, pop your own; it takes minutes and you control the amount of salt and oil that you use, making this an obvious healthier and more cost effective option. Same goes for bread (with the convenience of bread-making machines today), and potato chips, for example—you can slice an organic potato within minutes and place the rounds on a lightly greased baking tray with seasoning and have homemade potato chips in no time. And you most likely save a fortune by not getting as sick as often as your meat eating counterparts.

Obviously, the issue of time related to food preparation is something that you must consider as well, since we pay for convenience. Dried beans, which are healthier than canned beans, cost less, for example, but they don't offer the same convenience, since dried beans are optimally soaked for four hours or overnight prior to cooking, and then you have the cooking time. Some consider it wise to keep a stock of both in your pantry; this way, you can opt for the lower cost items when your planning allows for it. However as an important side note, the lining of cans used in food production typically contains hazardous chemicals. One that is getting broad attention now is Bisphenol-A—better known as BPA—an industrial chemical used in numerous household plastics and food packages. BPAs are long-proven endocrine disruptors, and at lower dosage levels than scientists suspected.

BPAs lead to abnormal cell changes and cell growth and are implicated in cancer, early puberty, infertility, prostate enlargement and other reproductive system disorders, obesity, cardiovascular damage, brain function, and many other ills.[43] While they are especially dangerous for developing fetuses and young children, they are affecting people at any age. A study, published in the journal *Hypertension,* found that the chemical not only made it into the body but registered at a 16 times greater level than for subjects who did not drink from the BPA-lined vessels; further, it seems to have caused a significant increase in blood pressure.[44] In spite of overwhelming evidence of the dangers of BPA, in January of 2015, the FDA quietly affirmed its position that Americans are not being harmed.[45] Some companies like Eden Organics are using BPA-free cans now, but some watchdog organizations say that replacing BPA often requires the use of equally deleterious and hazardous chemicals. Until this gets sorted out on the national and industry level, it is best to soak dried beans, and cook them. Use freezing to help with convenience.

Now, let's get back to the subject of the time and convenience tradeoff in food preparation: Not as clear in terms of savings are items like veggie burgers, which take time and effort for planning and preparation. But you must look at the tradeoff in terms of the purity of ingredients. Soups, on the other hand, are typically simple in terms of the number of ingredients and easy to make, requiring little prep time. However, as I've noted throughout this text, making food in bulk and freezing it is an excellent way of enjoying the benefits of your highly nutritious creations without much effort and fuss. You can easily freeze most soups, juices, smoothies, and a host of other entrée dishes, such as burgers, stews, and more.

A key in succeeding at the plant-based lifestyle while keeping your costs low is to go back to handling as much food as you can while devising creative ways of simplifying the process. I suggest to people that they select recipes during the week, do all their shopping on Saturday, and prepare and cook as many of those foods for the week on Sunday. It is much easier, for example, to make a great big salad, or humus and fresh-cut veggies, one day of the week and store them in air-tight containers so you don't have to prepare a salad every day of the week. Plus, as your palette shifts, you will enjoy foods in their simpler forms; a bunch of lightly steamed broccoli rabe with a drizzle of olive oil and sprinkle of dried herbs and pignolia nuts is quick, easy, and delicious; and, it's the kind of highly nutritious "fast food" upon which a healthy vegetarian thrives.

The Medical Costs Associated with Poor Eating

At the grocery store, eating a healthy vegetarian diet, especially if you buy all organic, prepared foods may not carry a low price tag respective to typical American fare. In the long run, however, and on the personal and societal level, not eating a healthy vegetarian diet is gravely expensive. Unhealthy eating imposes a substantial burden on society.

In these days of increased attention to the national costs of health care, an article in *Preventive Medicine* approached vegetarianism from this perspective. Specifically, the authors ask this question: "How much does meat-eating cost our society in terms of increased medical bills?" The results are staggering: the consumption of meat adds somewhere between 28 billion and 61 billion dollars annually to Americans' health care costs.

Cost-of-illness studies have been done for tobacco use. But medical cost estimates related to meat consumption are relatively new. So the authors of the *Preventive Medicine* article had to work out the proper methodology to assess this price tag. They examined the differences in the prevalence of a variety of diet-related illnesses between omnivore and vegetarian populations, using studies that controlled for other lifestyle factors. The diseases considered were those of the heart, hypertension, cancer, diabetes, gallstones, obesity-related problems, and food-borne illness. Their final estimate, then, compared the probable appearance of these diseases between a green-eating and meat-eating population. The differences of the costs of the increased incidences of all these that would occur if everyone ate meat as opposed to if everyone ate green diets gave them the final tallies.

Even though the majority of modern countries recognized that Americans are unhealthy, we are in deep denial about it. A June 2014 article in the *Huffington Post* noted that 55% of all Americans said, "they don't think they are overweight and aren't making an effort to shed pounds."[46] Remember also the study I noted earlier in the book where 9 out of 10 Americans think they eat a healthy diet. This, of course, is in direct contrast to the realities. Currently 67% of all Americans are overweight. In 2008, nearly half of US adults, 107 million people, reported having at least one of six chronic diseases, all of which are diet-related: cardiovascular disease, cancer, chronic diabetes, arthritis, obstructive pulmonary disease, and asthma. 70% of US deaths result from chronic diseases each year. 50% of all annual deaths can be traced to heart disease, cancer, and stroke. Diabetes is the leading cause of kidney failure, blindness, and non-injury lower-limb amputations. One-third of the population, 63 million people, have hypertension or high blood pressure, which accompanies 70% of first heart attacks and 77% of first strokes.

Obesity can lead to heart disease, type 2 diabetes, and cancer. Obesity costs the US $147 billion annually in 2008 dollars. By 2030, annual obesity-related medical costs are expected to soar to $390 to $580 billion. The five most expensive and preventable chronic conditions cost the US nearly $347 billion in 2010—30% of all health spending.

Including costs of health care and lost productivity, the economic costs of heart conditions totaled $202 billion in 2008 data, cancer totaled $217 billion in 2010, diabetes, $120 billion in 2012, and hypertension cost $68 billion in 2010 dollars.

We can do something about this.

Preventing disease is more desirable than treating it for two reasons. First, if the disease isn't there in the first place, there's nothing to treat. The disease doesn't enter the sacred space of your body. Second, not treating is cheaper than treating. So it costs less to not have to treat something than to have to treat something. The figures associated with prevention are breathtaking.

The anti-smoking campaign decreased youth smoking by 22% from 1999 to 2002 and saved $1.9 billion in future health care costs. Such are the economic impacts of improved health and effective marketing campaigns that have the public's best interest in mind. Prevention and early treatment of colorectal cancer alone could save $26 billion annually from lost productivity costs resulting from premature death due to colorectal cancer. Investing in prevention and treatment of the most common chronic illnesses could save the US $218 billion annually, and reduce the economic impact of disease by $1.1 trillion each year. But in order for this to occur, each of us i*ndividually* must become invested in prevention and health creation; this will assist the migration of big business' attention away from "disease" management, a highly lucrative business.

Disease is expensive; real health is cost effective. As such, it is time for us, as a nation, to rethink its values and its spending priorities regarding health.

Conclusion

In Part II, we took a closer look at our moral responsibility individually and collectively. We now understand that when we say "yes" to consuming animal products, we are also saying "yes" to violence and killing as well as the continued propagation of suffering—for animals and humans both. This is a fact. And there are consequences to this. By saying yes to any kind of violence, we are participating in creating a violent and fearful society. When we choose to eat meat, we are also saying "yes" to a way of living that condones any number of unhealthy behaviors, including the abuse of animal and human life and the environment, or supporting organizations that only care about their bottom line. For some of you, it may have been dismaying to learn that your hard-earned tax contributions are going to support the killing of animals and the poor treatment of human beings through government subsidies to already wealthy agriculture companies. Sadly, this is a reality; but you can do something about it starting now.

In terms of the costs, we also saw how a basic vegetarian diet is less costly, pound per pound of protein, than an animal-based diet, learned about the enormous costs associated with ill-health that the animal-based diet presents to our country, and learned about the enormous benefits to health costs that the green diet provides. And there are more costs: when we don't put an end to poverty through viable plant-based initiatives or to the continued destruction of our rainforests and the desertification of our lands due to cattle-raising, we harm ourselves. When it comes to feeding the world's people, the price to some of us is a very heavy heart, in that we recognize there is a solution, were it not for our nation's and other's steadfast attachment to power and a meat-centered diet, as well as the political barriers to getting the food to the people who need it most. When it comes to natural resources, we now know how depleted these are becoming. The very aspects that are fundamental to life on Earth—clean air and water to name two—are, today, seriously compromised and threatened. For most reading this book there will be sadness in this recognition.

It is easy to think that there is a lot to do by the number of possibilities that we outlined in the 36 section on living an active life, but in reality, there is only *one* thing to do—to take full responsibility for our hand in this, which means to be in action to correcting it. Pointing fingers will only keep us where we are. Once we do this, there is a chance for the tide to turn. Taking full responsibility does not mean that you need to do everything that we've delineated here. But the process of becoming responsible means also that we become more honest with ourselves about what we are willing to do or not; this is better than ignoring the facts. Once you do this, you have the opportunity for a brighter life now and into the future, regardless of outcomes, which is what we will be discussing next in Section III.

Part 3:

Future Directions

If I were to wish for anything, I should not wish for wealth and power, but for the passionate sense of the potential, for the eye which, ever young and ardent, sees the possible. Pleasure disappoints, possibility never.

— *Kierkegaard, philosopher*

Chapter 12

What the Future Holds

A Vision of the Future

Americans are a resilient and innovative people, and our weak ties to traditional ways of doing things allow us the freedom to solve problems differently than before. However, we are hindered in that our tradition, as explained in Chapter 7, does not involve a close relationship with nature and to our Earth. If we don't change this and our current trajectory, there will be further deterioration along with an untold amount of suffering.

The good news is that with our creativity and genuine desire to contribute to a better world by the common person, change is not only possible, but inevitable.

In a world where we are conscious of where our food comes from and want to ensure it comes from ethical and healthy sources, we have some creative choices. Soon enough, we're going to have a large group of people doing hydroponics, aquaponics, greenhouses, sprouting, indoor gardening, rooftop gardening, and community gardening, *out of necessity*. Some will follow this path out of desire and others because they, potentially, won't be able to afford fresh produce and can get fresher, less expensive produce when they grow their own.

Owing to their dedication to doing the right thing, I believe that in the near future you're going to see more people turning to food co-ops. The largest food co-op I know of on the east side of America is the Flatbush Food Co-op in New York City; it has 16,000 members from all walks of life. One of the reasons that these people are members is that they get fresh and organic produce at a reasonable price, much less than what you would buy if you went to the health food store.

We also have a growing number of farmers markets. In fact, I saw the farmers market in Naples, Florida, start with about ten little booths, and today, it has over a hundred with another hundred that want to get in but can't because there's no room. They have wonderful hand-crafted products, herbs, foods, microgreens, and sprouts, at very reasonable prices. And now there are over ten farmers markets in this one town. The largest farmers market in America is in Dallas, Texas; it's huge. It's the size of three football fields, and growing. So with farmers markets, growing on your own, homesteading projects, and cooperative community projects, people who have restricted or limited means are going to get healthier foods.

The Future of Food

Permaculture: Present and Future opportunities for Enhanced Sustainability

Our lifestyles and behaviors have a direct impact on the environment and can contribute to climate change. Although it may seem daunting, it *is* possible to take action at home, at work, and within the community to help prevent environmental crisis. In this chapter, we will review some current strategies that are making a positive difference and offer some ideas of simple changes that can be made to live in a more ecological fashion. I sincerely hope this inspires you to make some active changes to live a more sustainable and enjoyable lifestyle.

Start by Reconnecting

Many people are disconnected from where their food comes from. The same can be said for clean water and energy; we just turn on the tap or flick the switch, and it's there at our disposable. The human race—and Americans in particular—must get back to basics and learn from indigenous populations past and present to live in harmony with nature; they know not to take too much and to always give back. With the acquired knowledge base in relation to the earth's ecosystem and environment and the huge advances of modern technology, we must develop modern sustainable systems that can support human life by incorporating traditional agricultural methods, respecting Mother Earth and working with, rather than against, nature.

Such a philosophy is known as permaculture, from the contraction of the words "permanent," and "agriculture," and was first coined in 1978 by Bill Mollison, an Australian ecologist and University of Tasmania professor. Bill had spent the greater part of his life observing how natural systems work—such as forests, grasslands, and wetlands—and the destruction caused to such natural systems by human impact. "It is the harmonious integration of landscape and people providing their food, energy, shelter, and other material and non-material needs in a sustainable way. Without permanent agriculture, there is no possibility of a stable social order."[1] Bill Mollison.

Permaculture is more than just self-sustaining agriculture; it is a self-reliant, living philosophy and one that can be incorporated into all aspects of life and modern society. Through learning the principles of permaculture (beautifully explained on the Permaculture Principles website,[2]) and applying them to our daily lives—scaling from small changes for the better use of local resources to the complete reform of governmental policies—we can help ourselves, our communities, and future generations live sustainably on the planet and be better prepared for imminent changes in the dawning global warming era.

A Better, Sustainable Use of Resources

There are opportunities to make positive changes in all aspects of our everyday lives to minimize our negative impacts on the planet. In reality, we must get involved now if we want to see changes. By taking positive actions, no matter how trivial they may seem to you today, you will be contributing to the wellbeing of your community and the environment. The permaculture philosophy offers alternative solutions, and more importantly, hope to combat our society's increasing environmental and sociological problems. In exchange, you will most certainly begin to feel better about yourself.

"We need a vision of what that new world would look like and a set of strategies for getting there. The international permaculture movement offers both."[3] Starhawk (starhawk.org).

In the following sections, we will offer practical guidance on how you can start making changes to live more ethically, sustainably, and healthily—in relation to water, soil, land use, air quality, sanitation, recycling initiatives, and in particular community resources—and consequently, contribute to the support of the stability and biodiversity of the planet as a whole.

Growing Your Own Food Outside and/or Indoors

Strange as it seems, the small plot doesn't even have to be outside, even though many people are now developing small gardens. Urban apartment dwellers can grow fresh produce, at least in the forms of sprouts, right indoors. Sprouts are high in nutrients and easy to grow anywhere. Please see Appendix B for details on how to sprout your own food indoors. I'd like to make mention here of some other technologies that you will hear more about in the very near future.

Of considerable interest, considering the dire state of the world's soil, is the emergence of "alternative" cultivation methods that do not rely on soil for plant growth. Hydroponics is a method of growing plants in a nutrient-rich liquid medium, rather than soil, which has been around since the 1970s. More and more people are being introduced to hydroponics, aquaponics, and aeroponics at the Disney World Epcot theme park in Orlando, Florida. There they take you through a 30-minute boat ride showing a multitude of functioning hydroponic and aquaponics systems; they do a decent job of covering the basics and show you a variety of different fruits and vegetable as well as seafoods that are grown there and used daily in their restaurants.

Essentially, hydroponic has the advantage of being a controlled system, where optimal nutrients are directly supplied to the roots, and allows you to grow crops otherwise not possible to grow in certain regions and environments. You're not going to have to worry about soil, weather, or water, because you're controlling all of that," says Matthew Stein, author, engineer, designer, and green builder.

Aquaponics is a very intensive and efficient method of food production, where plants are grown together in a re-circulating closed loop ecosystem with fish, snails, crabs, prawns, or other aquatic animals. This system follows closely the permaculture ethics, since the waste produced by the fish (typically ammonia, which is a byproduct of their metabolism) gets converted by microbial activity into nitrate, which is a form of nitrogen that is readily usable by plants. Nitrogen is actually a major nutrient requirement for plant growth and within soil; it is often times a major limiting factor to plant growth. This method is particularly lucrative since plant crops can be harvested in addition to the fish—under current huge demand due to overfishing—and the water is re-circulated. However, the disadvantage to aquaponics and indeed hydroponics, is their reliance on electricity to circulate the water.

Another "new" method of soil-free agriculture is aeroponics, which first gained attention following interest in this technique by NASA.[4] Aeroponics is similar to hydroponics, yet, in aeroponics, no growing medium is used. Instead, plants are suspended, and the covered roots are fed using a nutrient-rich mist. This method is particularly suitable for growing plants indoors and requires little space, making it a good option for urban agriculture.

Another agricultural method that is particularly well-suited to the urban environment are vertical gardens, also known as green walls. Any unused walls can be optimized to grow vegetation, although this method does rely on soil, and most rely on an integrated water delivery system. As of 2015, the largest green wall is located at the Los Cabos International Convention Center, Mexico, covering some 2,700 square meters (29,000 square feet).[5] Green walls are becoming increasingly commonplace in public places such as airports and in city gardens as a way to take advantage of space for growing plants and making concrete areas more attractive. They also have the benefit of reducing the overall temperature of the building.[6] The Woolly Pocket website has some great ideas and information for making your own green wall (http://www.woollypocket.com/).

What Is Being Done and What Can We Do to Help?

Water

Desalination—the removal of salt from seawater to produce fresh water suitable for human consumption or irrigation—is receiving renewed interest due to the critical shortage of water in some areas of the world. Traditionally, desalination has not been viewed as cost effective because of the high energy consumption required; hence its popularity in the oil-rich Gulf countries. In fact, in Israel some 40% of all drinking water comes from desalination[7] and some 70% in Saudi Arabia.[8]

"At the moment, around 1% of the world's population is dependent on desalinated water to meet their daily needs, but by 2025, the UN expects 14% of the world's population to be encountering water scarcity," said Christopher Gasson, publisher of Global Water Intelligence.

In recent years, desalination technologies have made the process more energy efficient than before, with reverse osmosis currently offering the most energy-efficient technology.[9] In 1977, Cape Coral, Florida became the first municipality in the United States to use reverse osmosis for large scale desalination, and by 1985, the city had the largest low pressure reverse osmosis plant in the world.[10] Currently, the largest desalination project is the Ras Al Khair Desalination Plant in Saudi Arabia, which is capable of serving all of Saudi Arabia's water needs.

Many large-scale seawater reverse osmosis desalination plants are under construction in water-stressed countries as desalination is the only additional source of freshwater available on the planet. "The ocean is the one source of water that's truly drought-proof. And it will always be there," Peter MacLaggan, vice president of Poseidon Water.

Some 15 desalination projects have been proposed along the California coast, and the state has plans to construct the largest ocean desalination plant in the Western Hemisphere in Carlsbad, San Diego County. The project is expected to provide 50 million gallons of drinking water a day.[11] However, two gallons of seawater will be needed to produce every gallon of drinkable water at the site, and the energy equivalent of powering 28,500 homes will be required to purify it,[12] leading to huge concerns about the potential environmental impacts of large-scale seawater desalination plants. Other methods of obtaining water are less expensive—building a new reservoir is half the price, and conservation methods, such as paying farmers to install drip irrigation or offering grants for people to install water-efficient toilets, cost just a quarter of the price—according to a 2013 study from the state Department of Water Resources; not to mention the harm done to marine life from the sucking up of the seawater. But desperate times call for desperate measures, and California, with its long-running drought, is certainly in desperate need of more water.

In addition to the already present and increasingly threatening water shortages, we also face a crisis of water quality.[13] Urban runoff is a major source of water pollution in urban communities worldwide. Rainwater can pick up pollutants including heavy metals, trash, and oil and gasoline as it runs over impervious, generally paved surfaces, in addition to fertilizers and pesticides from heavily-maintained lawns.

Well managed natural forests are crucial to the provision of high-quality water, which is why we need to shift from clearing forests to supporting their growth, instead. In fact, forest watersheds play an important role in safeguarding the drinking supplies for 33 of 105 of the world's major cities; for example, half of all the drinking water in Puerto Rico comes from the rainforest in the Puerto Rico National Park, and the

Gunung Ged-Pangrango National Park in Indonesia supplies the drinking water for Jakarta and two other major cities, in addition to agricultural use.[14] For a better use of resources, our governments and city councils should be rallied to maintain quality urban water supplies through the management of natural resources, particularly forests and wetlands, a simple but effective measure that would benefit the wellbeing of all living creatures. The Government of Spain has taken this necessity on board and has started a huge project for the reforestation of the Pyrenees to improve the quality of its downstream water resources. Closer to home, in Utah, the Upper Sevier River Community Watershed Project (USRCWP) aims to improve natural resource conditions within the 1.2 million acre Upper Sevier River Watershed through a range of restoration activities, including increasing the presence of aspen, grasses, and forbs, to reduce erosion within the watershed.[15] Check out the US Forest Service website (http://www.fs.fed.us/) for more details about ongoing projects across America.

As a culture, we need to reduce global agriculture's water consumption. Shifting to a plant-based diet is a big first essential step, but with the way water continues to disappear, we need to find innovative ways of growing food with less water and of conserving water in our daily lives. We need to consider every behavior—from how often we water our lawns, and what time of day to how frequently we shower or flush our toilets to how we clean our dishes. When you multiply these simple water-saving actions by the over 115 million households in the US, you can begin to grasp the impact that each one of us makes respect to water conservation.

The harvesting of water fog or mist—once a common technique in ancient Egypt and in use in Chile for the last 30 years—is being revived. Inexpensive and readily available mesh nets are hung in mountainous regions or in foggy areas, and water droplets that attach to the netting are caught and collected. One square meter of netting can provide five liters of water per day using this method.[16] Other water-efficient methods include the use of Mycorrhiza, a root fungus that grows symbiotically with plant roots, acting to increase the surface area of the root that comes into contact with the soil. Thus, the fungus enhances nutrient uptake and can reduce the plant's water requirement by 25% among a plethora of other advantages. You can purchase Mycorrhizal fungi to add directly to poor soil to improve cultivation.[17] Ben Falk, founder of Whole Systems Design, who designs and implements regenerative food, fuel, and shelter systems (http://www.wholesystemsdesign.com/), has recently had success tending small rice paddies on their New England farm without utilizing the common inundation method. Rice doesn't require high-quality soil to grow, unlike some other soil intensive grains, and they were able to produce a good crop of rice without any fertilizer, just on rainfall alone. These examples show that by using simple, non-technological methods and forethought, the cultivation of crops with less water is possible.

"Rice is basically a fertility-free crop: all you need is the rainfall that falls on the area," said Ben Falk, founder of Whole Systems Design.

On an individual basis, we can participate at home by buying more water-efficient appliances, such as WaterSense endorsed washing machines and dishwashers that are approximately 20% more efficient than their standard counterparts (http://www.epa.gov/watersense/), and implementing simple water saving strategies, such as catching roof water and water from laundry and showers, and storing it in tanks for use in the garden to water the plants and the lawn. Many more water saving tips can be found on the EPA's website.

It's important that communities maintain the control of their own water systems, and the privatization of water should always be discouraged. We as consumers can source responsible water suppliers, many of whom are picking up their game and contributing to the sustainability of water by investing in sustainable infrastructures or playing an active role in protecting local watersheds, such as the San Francisco Public Utilities Commission that has developed an urban watershed management plan. Other state suppliers are focusing on the treatment of wastewater, including The Orange County Water District that won the US EPA's Water Efficiency Leader Award for its efforts to reuse wastewater for drinking, and East Bay Municipal Utility District, which is using food scraps from local restaurants to provide the energy for its wastewater treatment plant. The Green City, Clean Waters 25-year plan of The Philadelphia Water Department aims to protect watersheds and improve storm water management with an innovative green infrastructure.

Soil

Protecting existing forests and replacing vegetative cover is the pivotal strategy against desertification. Vegetation protects vulnerable bare soil from wind and water erosion, with trees and shrubs providing an extensive root network that helps anchor soil in place, act as natural windbreaks, and are effective in preventing soil erosion by absorbing rainwater and preventing run-off.

On an agricultural level, no till farming keeps the soil anchored in place and prevents the carbon in the soil from becoming oxidized and forming carbon dioxide in the atmosphere. Traditional terrace farming, as well as microbasins and bunds—commonly used throughout Africa and reported to have been responsible for yield increases for sorghum of up to 80% in Somalia[18]—slow down water flow, allowing higher amounts to be absorbed, preventing runoff, and acting as windbreaks to prevent further soil erosion. On a much larger scale, a "great green wall of China" of more than 5700 kilometers in length (that's 3,542 miles long) is being built in northeastern China to help combat soil erosion.

Incorporating organic matter back into fields is another important strategy, as organic matter acts like a sponge, and mulching, by acting as a protective cover, are two cheap and simple strategies to prevent water loss and soil erosion. Biochar, a charcoal produced from forest and cardboard waste, can also be used for mulching, which has the added value of preserving the carbon in its source.[19]

Through careful management and a combination of tactics, the heavily degraded Machakos Reserve in Kenya, which was described in the 1930s as "an example of a large area of land that through misuse and mismanagement became a parching desert of rocks, stones and sand" (Colin Maher, senior soil conservation officer, 1937), has been restored, and agricultural output (food and cash crops, horticulture, and livestock) increased from less than 0.4 tons per capita in 1932 to nearly 1.2 tons per capita in 1989, and from 10 to 110 tons per km^2.[20] Promoted by the Machakos Integrated Development Program, the planting of trees became universal practice as did the construction of terraces, mulching, and composting among other initiatives.

One example of the US Government's effort to establish land reclamation programs for degraded land is the USDA Farm Service Agency's Conservation Reserve Program. The purpose of the program is to assist land owners in the restoration of grass or trees on highly erodible or fragile cropland. In exchange for removing environmentally sensitive land from production and introducing conservation practices, farmers, ranchers, and agricultural land owners are paid an annual rental rate.[21]

Taking steps to preserve soil is an important part of following an environmentally responsible lifestyle. We can all make a huge difference by simply composting our household's organic matter from the garbage, providing our own much needed compost to feed the garden. What's more, the humus in healthy soil is a form of organic carbon, making soil an important carbon sink. In fact, soil constitutes the third largest carbon pool[22] and the sequestering of carbon by soil by the return of organic matter has the potential to reduce carbon dioxide induced global warming and thus further desertification. Or why not take the composting step further and organize a community composting scheme, such as the set up Community Compost Initiative in Albany, New York (visit http://radixcenter.org for more details), to collect organic waste from your local area for composting?

Air Quality

Compared to 1970, vehicles are roughly 99% cleaner for common pollutants, although transport remains a major source of greenhouse gases, with over a quarter of domestic carbon dioxide and other greenhouse gas emissions coming from transport. We can contribute to reducing emissions and air pollution by taking measures as simple as making sure our car's tires are inflated to the recommended pressure, which alone can save up to 10% on fuel consumption.

If you happen to live, like many people, a fair distance away from where you work, then a good deal of the energy that you're using is spent on the commute. As such, a lot of people are beginning to think carefully about how much energy they use for their transport and are looking at a number of alternatives. As individuals, we take action by choosing lower- and zero-emission modes of transportation more often, such as public transport, walking, and cycling. Encourage your workplace to provide bikes at the office for business travel (see British Colombia's "Work-Bike Policy: Use of Bicycles for Business Travel" for inspiration).

Car pooling and car sharing are easy options and will save you money too; check out services such as LyftLine and UberPool. Companies like Zipcar, Citycarshare, and Getaround, allow you to rent a car for a few hours, helping many people who live in urban areas to live without a car at all. Low emission vehicles, such as hybrids, hydrogen-powered and electric plug-in cars, are becoming increasingly popular, and more and more recharging stations are available at many locations, so that's another real potential to better the air you breath and better visibility, not to mention save money.

Another option would be to ask your employer to consider switching to alternative work patterns, such as remote working using the telephone and email. It's easier than ever to work remotely. Remote working and video conferencing is the future. The old jobs that we used to go to, those are in the past and are not coming back; not in our lifetime.

The London Borough of Sutton increased cycling rates by 50% and public transport usage by 13% in just two years through its "Smarter Travel Sutton" initiative. Trained advisors helped every school to put in place a Travel Plan to encourage parents and pupils to travel more sustainably, and knocked on the door of every resident in Sutton to offer free support and advice about transport alternatives. So encourage your local schools to introduce school buses, or even better, a walking school bus, where adults organize groups of children to walk to school[23] or similar bicycle train.

In terms of energy expenditure, the third biggest culprit, after industry and transportation, is the home. Most of our household energy is used for heating, but a lot is wasted because of inefficient house construction and poor heating methods. In addition to investing in proper insulation, and energy saving light bulbs and appliances, the best way to use money on energy efficiency is getting what's known as an energy audit: A team will come and take a very careful, detailed look at your home and suggest a wide range of possible energy efficiency retrofit strategies such as energy efficient windows and many others. A number of studies have shown that that type of investment in energy efficiency probably has the quickest pay back in terms of the money that you spend versus the money that you save after having made those retrofits.

We might consider introducing some renewable energy systems into our homes, including solar panels, solar water heaters, or solar fans that only cost about $100–150. You put it on the roof—it's a relatively small panel—and then in the attic, you have the fan itself with an exhaust. One fan can bring the temperature down by about 50°F in an area of up to 1500 square feet and can reduce our reliance on energy hungry air conditioning systems, even during brownouts and power cuts.

When people are planning to buy or construct a new home, many choose the location and orientation in terms of the best view, but ideally, the home should be designed to maximize the available solar energy, a concept known as passive solar home design. Passive solar homes catch the natural sunlight that comes through the windows provide light for free and offer warmth in the winter yet prevent overheating in the summer. An energy-efficient house that traps passive solar energy and retains it by minimizing air currents can reduce annual energy consumption by over half that of a conventional home and can create substantial benefits for both the atmosphere and our energy bills (Matthew Stein's book, *When Technology Fails: A Manual for Self-Reliance, Sustainability, and Surviving the Long Emergency* contains useful information on renewable energy systems, passive solar homes, and home retrofitting for increased energy efficiency).

For those of you who may live in urban areas where your home isn't oriented properly for the sun or is shaded by adjacent buildings, or perhaps you live in an apartment that doesn't have access to the roof to install your own solar panels, solar gardens or solar farms are a fairly recent and exciting development. Basically, a group of neighbors or businesses come together in a community-owned project to collaborate together and design and build a large-scale solar project to be located somewhere in the general area. Each of the participants in the project can lease or buy a number of solar panels as part of the project and the electricity that's generated by the panels that they own or lease is credited to their electric bill by the electric utility every month, thereby reducing the amount of money that they pay for their electric bill. The One Block Off the Grid campaign is enabling communities across the United States to collaborate in bringing solar power to their homes by providing an additional 15% discount on top of government rebates through the collective bulk purchases of solar panels (http://pureenergies.com/), helping to improve the accessibility of solar power to all.

Land Use

After decades of abusing Mother Earth, we must learn from nature in how we plan our future land use, particularly for any new urban developments, in order to best harness renewable energy and food while respecting the natural ecosystems. Above all else, we must make a global effort to reforest (and of course, to stop any further deforestation), as healthy soil and clean air and water are intricately linked to sustainable forests.

Some 20% of the world's greenhouse gas emissions are caused by deforestation and land use changes globally, and if current rates of deforestation in Indonesia remain the same, the emissions from this deforestation would equal almost 40% of the annual emission reduction targets set for Annex 1 countries under the Kyoto Protocol.[24]

We should fund tree planting in the form of diverse forest systems, not as current monospecies currently favored by logging companies, and favor traditional forest management tactics such as coppicing, which is more beneficial for biodiversity and provides wood without the associated soil erosion problems.

Cities and urban areas can also do their bit by planting more vegetation, including grass, trees, and shrubs. As little as one square meter of green roof can offset the annual particulate matter emissions of a car.[25] Trees can provide much needed shade in residential areas, in addition to fruit, and well provide clean air for our communities. On March 4, 2015, Matthew Pencharz, the Mayor of London's Environment Advisor, planted the 10,000th street tree of the Street Tree Initiative aimed to improve areas of poor air quality and improve local neighborhoods.[26] A recent study found that the trees in the Greater London area remove somewhere between 850 and 2000 tons of particulate pollution from the air every year.[27] The use of evergreen trees was found to be particularly effective since "Trees which have leaves the whole year are exposed to more pollution and so they take up more," Professor Gail Taylor, University of Southampton. Closer to home, cities including Los Angeles and New York have ambitious "Million Trees" initiatives to increase the number and diversity of urban trees while in Adelaide, Australia, an initiative to help cool the city, improve air and water quality, reduce carbon dioxide emissions, and make the city more attractive was set up with the aim to plant 3 million native trees and shrubs.[28]

Xeriscaping is a method of landscaping that favors the use of native plants, which are better adapted to the local growing season, climate, and soil, and often require less water—the key objective of xeriscaping. Incorporating plants appropriate to arid conditions, such as drought-resistant desert willow trees and juniper bushes, in addition to grading and mulching—to prevent evaporation and run-off—xeriscaped gardens can be particularly useful in regions without a reliable water supply and have the added benefit of being of low maintenance. Some native grasses for lawns, such as buffalo grass and blue grama, can survive with a quarter of the water that bluegrass varieties need,[29] and according to Scott Varner, the late executive director of the Xeriscape Council of New Mexico, water use can be cut by about 50% through xeriscaping.

By careful consideration of which species we plant in our own gardens and indeed in towns and cities, we can contribute to a reduction in our water consumption. Indeed, the increasing understanding of the need to optimize our natural resources such as water, and the sun, for example by building passive solar homes, and the acceptance of most policy-makers that we must start to live in a more sustainable fashion, has led to a new phenomenon in urban development—the so called green city or eco-city. The first round of eco-city initiatives, including Curitiba (Brazil), Waitakere (New Zealand), and Schwabach (Germany), emerged following The United Nations Earth Summit (Rio de Janeiro, 1992) and the resulting sustainable development program (Agenda 21).

For example, a new suburb located in Dublin, Ireland, called Clonburris, was conceived in 2007 with the plan consisting of 15,000 newly built homes following the highest sustainable standards, including: "the use of recycled and sustainable building materials, a district heating system for distributing heat, the provision of allotments for growing food, and even the banning of tumble driers, with natural drying areas being provided instead."[30] Unfortunately, completion of the project is taking longer than expected due to the current economic downturn.

However, more and more eco-cities are being planned or are under development in China, India, Kenya, and the United Arab Emirates, to name just a few countries. All these projects have the common motivation of revising land use priorities to create cities optimizing renewable energy sources, such as wind turbines and solar panels; creating sustainable and economical housing and supporting local urban agriculture.[31]

Similar smaller-scale projects are planned for Denver's Lower Downtown (Living City DC 14th & U) and Seattle's 2030 District, which has introduced a set of targets to incrementally reduce carbon emission to reach zero emissions by the year 2030. For example, the Seattle US courthouse building has incorporated a displacement ventilation system to reduce energy expenditure, waterless urinals, to lower water consumption, and offers electric vehicle charging facilities.[32]

Local agricultural systems, such as vegetable plots within city centers, mean a reduction in food miles and help contribute to the creation of more green spaces. Like tree cover, green spaces help counter the "heat island effect" caused by large areas of tarmac and asphalt, which can make urban areas as much as 42°F warmer than surrounding rural areas,[33] and thus help to reduce the need for air conditioning. In fact, so-called urban agriculture is on the increase. In Havana, for example, 90% of the city's fresh produce now originates from local urban farms and gardens using organic methods.[34] Todmorden, a town in Yorkshire, England, is another example of the success of urban agriculture. Food crops have been planted across the town at 40 different locations by volunteers, including at the police station, railway station, schools, and even the cemetery.[35] Locals may pick the produce in an initiative for residents to consider the importance of eating locally grown and seasonal food.

Urban agriculture has the added benefits of saving energy from food miles and the resulting waste of produce that can occur during its transportation and storage whilst improving the quality of life for urban residents and the planet as a whole. Community gardening projects are helping to shift food production back to local areas while creating social ties, and can provide an important source of organic locally produced food, minimizing food miles and packaging. As early as 1893, citizens of a depression-struck Detroit were asked to use any vacant lots to grow vegetables. The gardens produced income, supplied food, and boosted independence during times of hardship. And as many as 5.5 million Americans took part in the victory garden movement for food growth during the Second World War to reduce pressure on food production to support the war effort.

In urban areas, and particularly in abandoned inner-city locations, local residents can transform vacant sites—often victim to illegal dumping—into green sustainable plots for growing fresh fruit and vegetables, in addition to providing a space for wildlife to thrive, and offer our communities a valuable resources as safe areas for recreation and education. The gardens offer the opportunity to learn sustainable environmental practices, such as composting and recycling, and the organic production of our own food. With increasing concerns about obesity and associated diabetes and heart disease problems, linked to low levels of physical activity and poor eating habits, community gardens offer health benefits from regular physical exercise and access to fresh, cheap produce on a daily basis. In addition, they help to reduce air contamination and plants can help absorb urban noise, rather than hard flat surfaces that reflect sound waves, helping reduce noise pollution and improving quality of life.[36]

There are many social benefits that have emerged from urban agricultural practices: Individuals involved in community urban agriculture have reported lower stress levels as they offer a space for retreat and relax in densely populated urban areas.[37] Community gardens can play a significant role in enhancing the physical and spiritual well-being, and serve to unite communities, offering a way to socialize with neighbors in a sustainable community. Community gardens can take things a step further and set up systems for composting and rainwater collection, they can raise chickens for egg collection, or even set up beehives to help pollinate their gardens (For more inspiration see Scott Kellogg's book, *Toolbox for Sustainable City Living: A Do-it-Ourselves Guide*).

> "Work with members of your human community to do those things that don't support the corporations and the corporate government, and that do support life, including human life, in your own community and your own place." Guy McPherson, University of Arizona.

There are hundreds of empty spaces available in cities, the majority with no plans for development. Speak to your city or county; most are happy to actually donate a parcel to a non-profit or charity organization. 596 Acres is an NGO that has catalogued all the vacant parcels in New York City and has come up with a guide to instruct people on the process for acquiring access to these spaces (596acres.org) and the EPA has published a number of really helpful guides for accessing the potential for reusing vacant lot properties for urban agriculture (http://www.epa.gov/landrevitalization/). Even vacant lots that may not be suitable for vegetable production because they're shaded by trees or buildings and may not get enough light to grow vegetables can be put to good use as places to make compost or even cultivate edible mushrooms.

Sanitation

Sanitation is described as the facilities for the safe disposal of human waste (feces and urine), as well as services such as garbage collection and wastewater treatment.[38] In Western countries, we take for granted our sanitation facilities, particularly access to a flushing toilet; but despite access to sanitation being considered a fundamental human right,[39] some 2.6 billion people around the world live without access to a toilet at home.[40]

"Sanitation is a cornerstone of public health. Improved sanitation contributes enormously to human health and well-being, especially for girls and women. We know that simple, achievable interventions can reduce the risk of contracting diarrheal disease by a third," notes Dr. Margaret Chan, WHO Director-General.

Ninety-five 80% of all human waste is discharged completely untreated into surface waters,[41] and many major cities in developing countries do not have any sewage treatment system at all. All over the world, we can find examples of natural ecosystems destroyed by the discharge of untreated or partly treated sewage and fecal contamination of groundwater, lakes, and the sea is a problem. Sanitation is an often forgotten but ever increasing problem that is reaching crisis proportions as the world's population continues to grow at an alarming rate, particularly in urban areas. The World Health Organization estimates that currently 80% of all diseases are related to inadequate sanitation and polluted water.[42]

But introducing more flushing toilets is not the answer. Flushing systems do not work without water and approximately 15,000 liters of pure water are required per person per year for flushing. Nearly 3000 million people do not even have access to a water supply in their home,[43] and global warming induced water shortages make flushing toilets an unfeasible option. There is an urgent need for the shift away from non-ecological flushing toilets and an increased need for more sustainable toilet systems; we call this new paradigm ecological sanitation.[44]

Dry toilets and composting toilet schemes—which use no water—are being introduced throughout the third world to try to deal with the urgent need for improved sanitation conditions, and are being driven by the WHO and a number of NGOs, such as theEcoSanRes (Ecological Sanitation Research) Program. In addition, in many sites across the US, such as national parks, ecological toilets are being introduced (for example, at the Rocky Mountain and Mount Rainier National Parks).

Ecological toilet systems not only help to relieve the enormous problem of the safe disposal of human waste—with its associated consequences for human health and pollution caused by sewage discharge into water resources and ecosystems—but in addition, human waste can be collected and returned back to the soil as a natural fertilizer. Urine acts as a wonderful fertilizer and certainly is one of the most natural ones! Both urine and feces contain significant amounts of nitrogen, potassium, and phosphorous in a form that plants can absorb easily. A pioneering project was launched in the slums of in Mexico city in 1988 by the NGO network ANADEGES to grow vegetables in containers for rooftop cultivation using human urine as a fertilizer (and had the added benefit of utilizing old car tires as planting containers). The fact that the project is still running and more than 1,200 urban households are currently participating[45] just goes to show its overwhelming success and results from the study have revealed that plants fertilized with human urine grew more rapidly, larger, and healthier than those grown with conventional agricultural techniques and critically, less water was needed.

The use of human excreta or humanure for crop fertilization is widely practiced in many regions of the world and has been for many years. The Chinese have been composting human waste for thousands of years[46] and Japan introduced the practice of recycling human feces and urine for fertilizer in the twelfth century.[47] In the Western world, the use of "humanure" is gradually gaining popularity among the more ecologically minded and less squeamish, Taking advantage of human waste as a resource to be recycled rather than as waste to be disposed of is therefore not only an option for the poor.

Urine can be diluted with water and is safe to use directly. The 400,500 liters of urine produced by each person during a year contains enough plant nutrients to grow 250 kilograms of grain, enough to feed one person for one year. This important resource is much easier and safer to handle in the form of pure urine than it is in a mix of urine and feces. In fact, urine diversion is big business In Sweden, where farmers collect urine from underground tanks for a fee, to apply as a natural fertilizer to their crops.[48] For those of you worried about the health aspect, urine from healthy individuals is virtually sterile, and free of bacteria or viruses.[49] For the safe use of human feces, humanure should always be composted before application. Proper composting destroys possible pathogens and removes any odor.

Many human pathogens have only a limited period of viability in the soil, and the longer they are subjected to the microbiological competition of the compost pile, the more likely they are to die.[50] But knowing that many people will use a composting toilet only if they do not need to have anything to do with the toilet contents, most commercial composting toilets are comprised of a large composting chamber underneath and the contents only need to be emptied occasionally.

The recycling of human waste has the benefit of returning nutrients to soil and plants and helps to restore the natural cycling of materials that our present-day sanitation procedures interrupt. Schemes for the use of humanure on a local scale would help to significantly lower water consumption and save energy in the process due to the reduced strain on sewage treatment plants and would reduce the need for chemical fertilizers. Perhaps in the future, composting toilets will be more common place across America.

Recycling Initiatives

As we've discovered, the choices that we make in our everyday life have a significant impact on the Earth's natural environment. Within the doctrine of the six Rs—refuse, reduce, reuse, repair, recycle, and re-think—re-thinking is probably the key. We cannot simply shop our way out of climate change; the needed changes are too big, and the destruction is too vast for us to simply "buy green" and assume that will be enough. That's not to say that we shouldn't continue the practice of buying wisely and sourcing responsible suppliers, but we need to urge an overall reduction in consumption, and we urgently need to think of ways that the "waste" of one industry can become the raw material for another, in order to recycle the earth's natural energy, nutrients and resources.

To reduce our carbon footprint we should buy locally, with minimal packaging, and second-hand wherever possible. Investing in good quality, long-lasting products and looking after them with careful maintenance can also help reduce waste and overall consumption levels. The Swiss have to pay for their rubbish per bag thrown, a strong financial incentive to recycle everything possible and to cut down on consumption, which certainly would help some people to be more responsible.

Take bottled water for example, where global companies are profiting by taking a natural and essential resource, then selling it back to us—causing a 300 fold increase in the water's carbon footprint per liter compared to tap water in the process! A comprehensive American study found the total energy required for bottled water production was as much as 2,000 times the energy cost of producing tap water.[51] However, it's not just the costs to the environment of bottled water that causes a problem; 70% of the plastic water bottles, weighing a massive 75,000 tons, are not recycled and find their way into landfill or waterways every year.

Taking the concept of "refuse" to a community level, the residents of Bundanoon, a rural Australian town, were the first community in the world to ban the sale of bottled water. "It's time for people to realize they're being conned by the bottled water industry," said Jon Dee, 'Bundy on Tap' campaign.[52] The good news is that more and more cities, schools, businesses, and everyday citizens are saying no to bottled water. For example, Greg Nickels, the mayor of Seattle, has phased out the purchase of bottled water for city-owned facilities and city-sponsored events, and the city council of Chicago has placed a landmark tax of 5 cents on every bottle of water sold in the city to discourage consumption.

In your own community, rally your workplace, hospitals, and schools to install water fountains and encourage your family to use re-usable, washable bottles for water consumption on the go. New Dream's *Unbottle Water Campaign* is full of inspiring stories and practical tips to help eliminate bottled water in your community.

Recycling is another small step that we can take on an individual basis to help the environment by reducing the amount of household waste that ends up in landfill sites, where it produces the second most important greenhouse gas, methane. Compost, compost, compost; all your organic matter—the food waste, the grass clippings, the wood chips, the brown leaves—can be composted. The finished product can be utilized to feed our soil, which is in desperate need. Neighborhoods must begin to take responsibility on a local scale for the food waste they're producing.

In addition, every ton of waste that is recycled helps to minimize the huge environmental impacts of mining and processing resources. Recycling aluminum cans, for instance, saves the tropical rainforests from further devastation because these areas are often mined for bauxite (the ore used to make aluminum). So you can be confident that any recycling you initiate will play a vital role in preserving the Earth's natural resources.

Many items should never arrive to landfills in the first place. Before throwing out an item, think creatively in finding new uses for pre-loved objects (Pinterest is a great resources for ideas, www.pinterest.com). Or, if you do not have a use for an old item, maybe someone else could. In your community, set up a scheme similar to the German *Sperrmüll* days (literally, miscellaneous items), where people leave any unwanted furniture—such as an old sofa or chair, or carpet or building materials—on the curb outside their house. Neighbors take a look, particularly students, and second hand dealers often pass by to pick up anything they fancy and give it a new lease of life. The remainder (although there's often not much left) is taken away by municipal trucks, thus reducing the amount that would ordinarily go to the dump.

Alternatively, why not encourage a city-wide garage sale. For example, El Cerrito, California had its first citywide garage sale—to clear unwanted items from garages and to benefit the environment by promoting reuse—in 1990, and the event was such a success that the city has since made it an annual tradition. Now in its 23nd year, the garage sale is as popular as ever, expanding from one Saturday in October to two events per year: "[The citywide garage sale] helps people clear the clutter out of their homes and encourages reuse, putting unwanted items back into circulation. People look forward to the event; it gives them a chance to meet their neighbors and brings a sense of community," said Garth Schultz, environmental analyst for the city of El Cerrito.

Unlike the traditional take-make-consume-dispose linear economy of the past, the circular economy restores so-called "old" parts and products back to their original state using methods that consume fewer resources, encouraging the reuse of materials to the furthest extent possible. Remanufacturing takes an end-of-life part or product in order to return it to like-new, and focuses on the return and reuse of valuable materials, making them last for as long as possible. Some may be surprised to know that the United States is the undisputed leader in terms of producing and exporting remanufactured goods. In 2011, production of remanufactured goods in the United States totaled $43 billion and accounted for 2% of all sales of manufactured goods. Industries employing remanufacturing include the aerospace and automotive sectors predominantly, in addition to motor vehicle parts, IT products, consumer products, electrical apparatus, and office furniture.[53]

Hundreds of thousands of tons of office furniture is thrown away every year from businesses, the majority of which is in perfect working order and replaced simply for aesthetic reasons. An estimated 50% of office furniture sent to landfills each year is reusable,[54] and is a huge waste of resources of money. A remanufactured desk has 30% the carbon footprint and 35% the water footprint of that of a new desk, and remanufacturing office furniture can save up to 90% of the original energy input.[55] Urge your employers, before throwing out old office furniture, to ask around the local community—an NGO, church-based group, or other local initiative might be pleased to receive the "old" furniture.

Swapping is a great way to put your unwanted things back into circulation, preventing them from arriving at landfills, and you can receive something "new" in return. Many websites offer platforms to swap books (www.paperbackswap.com), movies (swapadvd.com), and music (swapacd.com) with people all across the world. Swap.com and gumtree.com offer the free swap of items, trade, and exchange goods. Cloths swap events among students are becoming increasingly popular, where quality clothing and accessories are simply traded. And food swaps are a fantastic outlet for sharing homemade, homegrown, or foraged foods, and offer an alternative to store-bought items, helping swappers eat locally, sustainably, and affordably (see www.foodswapnetwork.com for local events). You can even swap your house for a free holiday if you find a like-minded family (www.lovehomeswap.com).

Sharing resources is such a simple—yet effective—idea and can be as easy as sharing tools with neighbors, such as a ladder, power tools, or a pick-up truck; Seattle has gone a step further and set up a tool lending library. Alternatively, share skills by collaborating with neighbors to work on home projects as a neighborhood work group. Find like-minded people in your area to swap things and get things done for free. (Find local groups in your area www.localskillswap.com.) Why not look in your local area for swapping schemes, or set one up within your community? Toys, clothing, food, seeds, arts and crafts, books and media, even skills can be swapped—swap piano lessons for having your car serviced, babysitting for sessions with a personal trainer, hairdressing for math tuition for your kids—the possibilities are endless. The Shareable and New Dream website offer lots of helpful hints on how you can get started with swap and share schemes in your local community (http://www.newdream.org/ and http://www.shareable.net/).

To address climate change, we need a radically different ethic, one based on the values of caring, sharing, and mutual responsibility—the core values of almost all human societies and religions.

Urban gardens constitute a huge step towards the ultimate goal of creating cities that function more like cyclical ecosystems, where we're growing more food within city limits, and very importantly, processing our waste as well. They also help teach people about to sustainable consumption and production. But even more so, they offer a great opportunity for groups to get started with their first community project. The ethics of working together on community-based projects are being increasingly extended to co-operatives, which offer real community ownerships possibilities. Co-ops are an idea that has been around for centuries, but they are currently being described as the wave of the future. You may not know that 2012 was The United Nation's International Year of Co-ops, and co-ops are being strongly promoted by the UN's Food and Agriculture Organization (FAO) as a way to build food security for producers and consumers alike.

Co-operatives are formed to meet the goals and aspirations of their members, and members control all the decisions; they are not driven by the need to accumulate profit for investors. As such, their values and principles—including equality, democracy, self-help, and concern for community—reinforce a very different, more sustainable approach to business. Housing co-ops, energy co-ops, farming co-ops, bank co-ops, etc., offer a powerful tool for addressing challenges of economic instability and global climate change and present a real opportunity for social change.

"I'd much rather live in a world where there's community and people have joy in their lives and they work together, and they build and grow and live together and share skills and share resources," notes Matthew Stein, author, engineer, designer, and green builder.

There are many steps we can take as individuals and as small communities to wean ourselves off the current imperial set of living arrangements, and they all have in common that they require more thought than conventional practices. We need to optimize land use and make choices on an individual, family, and community level to develop more environmentally friendly lifestyles and build resilience for the future. A sustainable future is heading towards a more co-operative world:

> "The solution to both our social and ecological solutions is the same: community. Restore the community of caring and sharing, understand that community means the interconnection of people with the environment and natural communities that sustain us, restore power and resources to communities, and trust in the resilience of the community of life." Starhawk[56]

Have You Had Enough?

Now that we've had a look at the many possibilities that exist for engagement in green living, we've come to the point in the book where we need to reflect on the question: have we had enough? It seems the meat and dairy, as well as the chemical industries, including pharmaceutical companies, have an uncanny way of assaulting nature on both sides. The fishing industry is a perfect example of this as well. It raises fish in enclosed tanks, where they are more susceptible to disease due to cramped conditions and increased levels of toxins; all the while, it has been stripping the oceans of fish to use as feed for their caged fish farm swimmers.

Another example of this double-edged assault (two issues covered independently in previous sections) are the pesticides used on plants being raised for animal feed, that very often are leaching into and poisoning our soil and our waterways that are supplying our drinking water. As I showed much earlier in the discussion, beef cattle production, in particular, uses vast amounts of water and land. Grain and grasses occupying huge tracts of land require large amounts of water to simply feed a single cow during its lifetime. And this is one primary reason why water resources are rapidly dwindling. In the US alone, the large Ogallala fossil aquifer which lies under the Great Plains and supports much of the grain production in the American heartland is receding rapidly. Once a fossil aquifer goes dry, there's no restoring it—it's dead.

And they will not stop until consumer demand shifts the tide. In reality, nothing much happens to change any one situation until there is enough momentum (typically pain) for that change for a person or group to do something about it. In this case, and as related to what we've been discussing throughout the book, all that really is required is for a large enough group of people to become committed to thriving on the plant-based diet. Or, as an alternative, if that reality is too difficult, is for a large enough group of people to stop buying meat of any kind or dairy (including organic) from a grocery store, and only purchase from local farmers. That's it. If enough people did this, before long the meat and dairy industries would be forced to make significant changes, which would be beneficial for everyone, animals included.

At the time of this writing, California has become the first state in the nation to restrict water usage, calling for a full 25% reduction in nine months.[57] The 31-point plan, approved by Governor Jerry Brown, affects landscaping uses and the complex system of agricultural water rights and even establishes programs to replace old appliances. According to the US Drought Monitor, 99.85% of California has been suffering drought conditions for more than four years: more than 66% of the state is in "extreme drought" and 41% of the state is suffering from "exceptional" drought, the most severe.[58]

More dire predictions of the earth's future suggest that environmental destruction has been so great under our civilization that a complete collapse of nature is now unstoppable, and our children have nothing to look forward to but a diseased life on a devastated planet. I don't believe that this trajectory towards self-destruction has to continue. If enough of us stand our ground and work to turn the tide, we have the possibility of turning this planet into a heaven on earth. Green eating is one huge play in our struggle to introduce sanity as well as sustainability to the world, and make our peace with nature. Truly creative out-of-the-box thinking is the other.

The Message of the New Millennium

Let's begin our examination at how the good news about vegetarianism is getting out to a wider public by first looking at publications targeting those who are working in the trenches to keep Americans healthy: your family physicians.

These family doctors often subscribe to the *Journal American Family Physician,* and in November 1994 they would have seen a positively oriented piece on the health effects of vegetarian diets. According to the piece, people eating vegetarian diets often have lower weight and blood pressure than the population at large. It continues, "The lower intakes of cholesterol and saturated fat decrease cholesterol and low-density lipoprotein fractions in vegetarians. They have lower mortality rates attributable primarily to lower death rates from ischemic heart disease and certain cancers. High fiber intake also may reduce risk of other diseases such as bowel cancers, gallstones and diabetes." You could hardly mount a better defense for green eating than that. Even better, the report concludes that "considering the improvement in health that may be derived from vegetarianism, patients (especially those at risk for cardiovascular disease and cancer) should be encouraged to consume increasingly vegetarian diets."

This article suggests family doctors consider recommending vegetarian eating to some of their patients, which is a welcome change in that American doctors have often lagged in their ideas of the relation between diet and disease. Even more welcome is a similarly laudatory piece appearing in the November 1993 *Journal of the American Dietetic Association.* Recall this was the same journal that back in 1949 was happy to run an ad by Amour extolling the complete protein found in meat. Now, the group is holding positions that would make Amour pull any ad they might have been tempted to place. The magazine now notes, "It is the position of The American Dietetic Association that vegetarian diets are healthful and nutritionally adequate when appropriately planned." But that's hardly all.

The essay goes on to discuss the benefits of this way of green eating noting, for instance, that studies of vegetarians indicate that they often have lower mortality rates from several chronic degenerative diseases than non-vegetarians—a fact that may be attributed to diet as well as to other lifestyle characteristics.

Among the chronic illnesses noted in the piece is coronary heart disease where, it is said, mortality is lower in vegetarians than in non-vegetarians. It adds that vegetarians have low rates of hypertension and non-insulin dependent diabetes mellitus than do non-vegetarians.

In other words, the American Dietetic Association is now not only conceding that vegetarianism is an acceptable dietary choice, but also that it offers concrete health benefits superior to a meat eating diet.

The Future of Health & Nutrition

While the information I just shared about the impacts of green eating on chronic diseases is vital, it's not new; it's all been reported before in studies published in a vast variety of journals. What's particularly noteworthy here, though, is that the influential American Dietetic Association has now assimilated all of this information into its own world view and policy.

As said previously, this is the group that's instrumental in molding the way America's dietitians are trained. We saw in our small glance at the history of nutrition education, a previous generation of dietitians pronounced the gospel that a vegetarian diet was inadequate or, at best, difficult to practice. The story then was that if you weren't eating meat, you had to consciously combine vegetable and sometimes dairy sources of protein in a complicated mesh so that you were getting the "complete" protein that your body needs.

Now, as we've seen, with the growing evidence of the health benefits of green eating along with the mounting problems of animal-centered diet, the ADA is singing a different, more pleasing and truthful tune.

I just alluded to "growing problems," one of which is directly related to dieticians since they are concerned with advising the general public on what to eat. The problem that I am referring to is obesity, a major public health problem in the United States that is provoked by poor eating choices. It has become an epidemic in our country. As dieticians are now acknowledging, vegetarians, especially vegans, generally have closer to desirable weights than do non-vegetarians.

And while in years gone by, as we've established, the ADA warned that vegetarians were in dire danger of not receiving enough protein, now they realize that although most vegetarian diets meet or exceed the Recommended Dietary Allowances for protein, they often provide less protein than non-vegetarian diets, and this is a good thing! This lower protein intake seems to be associated with better calcium retention in vegetarians and improved kidney function in individuals with prior kidney damage. Furthermore, lower protein intakes may result in lower fat intake with the inherent advantages of this lessening, especially in relation to weight gain, because foods high in protein are frequently high in fat also.

The ADA article doesn't stop at saying vegetarian diets contain a beneficial amount of protein, but goes on to fill in this thought by noting that plant sources of protein alone can provide adequate amounts of the essential and nonessential amino acids, assuming that dietary protein sources from plants are reasonably varied and that caloric intake is sufficient to meet energy needs. Whole grains, legumes, vegetables, seeds, and nuts all contain essential and nonessential amino acids. Conscious combining of these foods within a given meal, as the complementary protein dictum suggests, is unnecessary.

Frankly, I wouldn't be surprised to see this article from the ADA in a book on the wonders of vegetarianism! That's how much the group has shifted its position on plant-based diets. To their credit, this important and far reaching group has acknowledged studies showing that vegetable foods provide everything that humans need for a healthy life.

So here is a second professional group, the first being family physicians, who are getting the message on the health value of going green.

Have We Reached a Tipping Point?

Let's open the pages of a few more journals directed at health professionals, particularly physicians, where the changes are rung on one of the major themes of this book: how green eating empowers health.

An article in a publication aimed at alternative practitioners, the *New Life Journal*, which appeared in February/March 2004 and was penned by Bill Najger, begins with these words directed toward other clinicians:

> According to research from Dr. Colin Campbell at Cornell University, diets that are rich in fruit, vegetables and grains, reduce the risk of various cancers and heart disease. Specifically, vegetarian diets are linked in his medical research to a reduced risk of obesity, diabetes, high blood pressure, dementia, high cholesterol, bowel disorders, gallstones, osteoporosis … and rheumatoid arthritis. Anyone suffering from these ailments may benefit from a vegetarian diet, and anyone who wishes to avoid such health problems may find a vegetarian diet is a strong preventative tool.

The self-evident thesis is that medical professionals should be looking into moving patients onto a green path, especially if they are suffering from a host of common ailments, or if wanting to avoid these diseases altogether.

Najger buttresses his argument by glancing at the physiologic effects of a vegetarian diet. One is that green eaters have lower total serum cholesterol levels, and lower blood pressure as well. Also, vegetarians have lower mortality rates than the population at large, because heart-disease and certain cancers occur less frequently in this group.

The article mentions the vital, health-promoting role fiber plays, something already brought up in this text. This particular author stresses that dietary fibers—especially soluble fibers such as guar gum, pectin, and oat gum—have been shown to lower total cholesterol levels. He notes that because vegetarians (especially vegans) may have fiber intakes two to three times those of omnivores, fiber intake may contribute to vegetarians' favorable lipid profiles. Higher fiber intake may also help reduce risks of other diseases such as bowel cancers, gallstones, and diabetes.

A second article directed at health workers appeared in *The Mayo Clinic Health Letter*. Its title tells the story: "Vegetarian Diets: They're No Longer Radical, Just Good for You," and that about sums up the change in attitude that's come about of late, as officialdom comes to accept the mountain of evidence showing that vegetarianism is the sensible dietary choice.

This particular essay looks to China for evidence, pinpointing a study of 6,500 families in China that showed those who ate the least meat were the healthiest. But it could have gone west instead of east, and examined people living in the Mediterranean, who have traditionally enjoyed health benefits stemming largely from their plant-centered diet.

This was the focus of another article in a health professionals' magazine, *The American Journal of Clinical Nutrition.* A piece on "the Mediterranean diet," labels it a dietary pattern that deserves to be preserved and promoted.

The piece focuses on the researcher Ancel Keys, who, beginning in the 1950s, examined the Mediterranean diet and helped establish it as the original prototype for the way people should be eating. Here are some of Keys's reflections on the diet and public health today:

> My concern about diet as a public health problem began in the early 1950s in Naples, where we observed very low incidences of coronary heart disease associated with what we later came to call the good Mediterranean diet. The heart of this diet is mainly vegetarian, and differs from American and northern European diets in that it is much lower in meat and dairy products and uses fruit for dessert. These observations led to our subsequent research in the Seven Countries Study, in which we demonstrated that saturated fat is the major dietary villain. Today, the healthy Mediterranean diet is changing and coronary heart disease is no longer confined to medical textbooks. Our challenge is to persuade children to tell their parents to eat as Mediterranean's do.

As I am trying to stress here, it is not only that these writers are emphasizing the value of green eating, but that they are doing it outside of scientific journals and in magazines read by health professionals. This means the message is becoming more widely distributed, and therefore accepted.

Practical Solutions for America's Medical Problems

Another place where the interest in vegetarianism is surfacing is in several university publications. I find this heartening, but not for the same reason I found the aforementioned publications exciting. These university journals are not for the educated general reader, but are scientific studies. I single them out, though, because of the historical heritage of the schools from which they come.

Howard University was founded shortly after the Civil War to be a place for newly freed African-Americans. While it is now open to all races, its history is that of being particularly a place for Black students and studies. So when researchers from Howard University Medical Center published a review article on the dietary management of blood pressure, they properly gave particular attention to the health difficulties of African-Americans. Here's some of what they had to say:

> Hypertension is a major cause of morbidity and mortality in the United States, particularly in the African-American population. Although there have been indications since the beginning of this century that blood pressure might be influenced by dietary factors, this has been generally ignored, and the mainstay of hypertension treatment has been the use of pharmacologic antihypertensives.

The literature is replete with evidence that vegetarian and low-sodium dietary patterns are associated with lower blood pressure levels. This implies that if many people could adopt vegetarian and low-salt dietary habits, the prevalence of hypertension would be significantly reduced.

The article goes on to discuss the importance of developing palatable and socio-culturally acceptable vegetarian menus for African-Americans in particular. So, as you see, scientists of a higher learning center for African-American scholarship are looking at the beneficial effects of a plant-based diet on African-Americans.

A second university that has a rich history related to promoting plant-based diets is Harvard. Along with Yale and a few other schools, Harvard has been seen as among the very best that the US has to offer. The fact that articles such as "Vegetable and Fruit Lowers Stroke Risk" are appearing in the *Harvard Heart Letter* is proof that the value of plant-oriented diets is gaining a hearing and acceptance at the highest levels of American society.

This particular article cites a study published in the April 12, 1995, issue of the *Journal of the American Medical Association*, which demonstrated a correlation between a vegetable- and fruit-rich diet and a reduced risk of stroke. Specifically, "men who ate the most vegetables and fruits had a 59% lower stroke rate than those who ate the least."

The *Harvard* article speculates that the protective factors present in these foods could be the potassium content of the fruits and vegetables, their folate, and their antioxidant vitamins.

The article concludes, "Even though the mechanisms responsible for this protective effect are not definitely known, this study reinforces the belief that eating large amounts of fruits and vegetables may be a fundamental step in reducing the risk of vascular disease-in this case, stroke."

Of course, each university in the US has its own unique virtues. I simply wanted to highlight a couple here that are delving into the positive effects of vegetarian-oriented diets, and to note that the values of such diets are being extolled across the spectrum of top schools.

What Exactly Is Happening Here?

My point in these last few sections is to demonstrate that voices in favor of vegetarian diets as a way to bolster one's health and steer clear of illness are reaching all venues and audiences. Scientists, health professionals and general readers who are concerned with a better understanding of the diet/disease link need not look far these days for evidence of this reality.

Before concluding this part of the discussion, I feel almost compelled, because I have been coming across so much new information in the course of writing this book, to share a bit more encouraging information about the health value of green eating. However, let me follow up on the last thing we read from the *Harvard* article, which concerned the attempt to assess what component of a vegetable or fruit is responsible for the food's helpful effects.

While the article mentioned some vitamin and mineral possibilities that might account for plant foods lowering stroke risk, the difficulty in locating the benefactors stems from the fact that plants are composed of hundreds, and perhaps thousands, of naturally occurring chemicals. That's why you could take the most sophisticated "nutritionally complete" regimen of vitamin and mineral pills and still not be as well-nourished as you would be if you ate the actual plant food that the regimen was trying to duplicate.

The chemical compounds in plant foods that provide such value are known as phytochemicals. Their nutritional value, though, is both understood in some aspects and not yet understood in others. We know the different phytochemicals in a single plant work in combination to create what we know as a health-promoting plant food, and one leading edge of scientific research now is set on uncovering these synergies, and the results are already very heartening. They assert that by substituting a synthetic or natural supplement that you could gain equal value.

One result of this ongoing research on phytochemicals was a June 1994 *Medical Update* article entitled "Would You Eat Food Containing Saponins, Indoles, or Phytic Acid? (Phytochemicals)." The article concluded that you would be wise to dine on all these substances because "at least 150 studies around the world have shown that people who eat the most fruits and vegetables are half as likely to have cancer as those who eat the least." While the piece noted that much work has to be done to assess whether phytochemicals are really involved in preventing this disease, it ended, "Nonetheless, the evidence strongly suggests the importance of these chemicals and the possible mechanisms involved."

The Journal of the American Medical Association published a study showing the effectiveness of fasting followed by one year of vegetarian eating in healing rheumatoid arthritis. A follow-up study in *Clinical Rheumatology* indicates that improvements resulting from this approach can be sustained through a two-year period.[59]

Whatever the mechanisms involved, plant foods are health-promoting and the documentation to this effect is virtually endless. Let me reach into my grab bag for a few final items testifying to the virtues of plants.

Revolution at the Dinner Table and Beyond

I've worked to dispel the numerous myths connected to the value of the vegetarian diet from a nutritional perspective, especially related to protein. My hope is that you are left with an exuberant sense of possibility related to the world of plant-based foods. There are literally hundreds of fruits and vegetables in the US alone—thousands when you count varietals. The world of plant-based eating is a wondrous and thrilling adventure that happens also to be linked to health and vitality, for us and the planet.

In his book *The Food Revolution: How Your Diet Can Help Save Your Life And Our World*, author, practicing vegan, and Founder and Board Chair Emeritus of EarthSave International John Robbins says:

> "Like blades of grass bursting through a crack in a thick slab of concrete, something is seeking to break through the walls we have put between us and our kinship with the Earth. It is the awesome power of Creation itself. It is the same force that turns the tides, brings rain to parched earth, entices the bee to the flower, and ignites new life in countless species.
>
> Maybe we aren't on a one-way road to oblivion. Maybe we're standing at a crossroad, facing what may be the most important choice human beings have ever faced, a choice between two directions. In one direction is what we will have if we do nothing to alter our present course. By doing nothing, we are choosing a world of pollution and extinctions, of widening chasms and deepening despair, a world where humanity moves ever farther from achieving its highest aspirations and ever nearer to living its darkest fears."[60]

In ending, I gave myself the task of noting how vegetarianism as a dietary and lifestyle choice is becoming more accepted, using as evidence how journals addressing health professionals, from family physicians to dieticians, and now the USDA, are now recommending the vegetarian diet that many of them 20 years ago would have condemned. They have been prompted to make this reversal especially because of the large body of medical evidence testifying to the dangers of meat- and milk-based diets and the corresponding benefits of green eating. So this is where vegetarianism has its first foothold in beginning to overturn America's meat and dairy fixation.

I dare say that this is just a first step and far from the only one needed to get more people to adopt a vegetarian world view. As I've insisted, if green eating and green living goes no further than this in its rationale, no further than being adopted for health reasons, it will remain stalled and we will die on the vine, so to speak.

Approaching this change as an essential aspect of an *environmental* movement, which I spoke of earlier, is not likely to entice many either. A 2013 Gallup poll[61] noted many things of interest, including increasing ire regarding the movement—the percentage of people saying they were "unsympathetic" to environmental causes doubled from 5% in the early 2000s, to its current level of 10%. Some attribute this increase to industry sponsored public relations campaigns made to discredit environmentalists. Still, only about half of Americans are generally concerned about climate change and approximately 65% about the quality of their environment.[62] Another Gallup poll, this one taken in 2014, shows concern about climate change near the bottom of a 15 point list, with only 24% admitting they worry a "great deal" about it. On a positive note, a Pew Research study noted that support for the increased use of fracking has declined, and there is broad public support for stricter limits on power plant emissions.[63]

A New Movement Founded in Vegetarian Living

NPR ran a story titled "Millennials: We Help The Earth But Don't Call Us Environmentalists,"[64] in which they highlighted the results of a 2014 Pew Research Center poll noting that 42% of both boomers and GenXers considered themselves an "environmentalist." Only 32% of millennials agreed. Pew said that while that may not seem substantial, it's statistically significant.[65] But even though young people in America are dissociating from the term "environmentalist," they still are involved in helping humans and the planet.

In fact, it appears that millennials are more aware than any of us of the dangers we face.[66] A study in *Statista* in March of 2014 looked at the different attitudes on climate change by generation (Millennials (18-36), GenX (37-48), Baby Boomers (49-67) and Matures (68+)). In answer to the question if they believed that climate change was real and that humans were to blame for most of it, 50% of millennials answered yes, whereas only 37% of Matures agreed. Baby Boomers and Gen Xers came in at 43% and 47%, respectively. This may be somewhat comforting, recognizing that future social, health, and environmental policies have a greater possibility of being shaped by a group aware of the issues at hand.

The NPR article featured a story about Lisa Curtis, Founder & CEO of Kuli Kuli, a company that helps West African villages economically and environmentally, a staunch environmentalist who *re*named herself a "social entrepreneur" to avoid the derogatory commentary associated with the word environmentalist. Titles aside, the article goes on to note that previous polls find millennials more likely than older Americans to favor developing alternative energy sources, and more likely than other generations to believe that humans are responsible for climate change.[67]

I'm not the only one holding this position. The Intergovernmental Panel on Climate Change's (IPCC) Fifth Assessment Report concluded by saying they had a "95 per cent certainty that the human influence on the climate system is clear and is evident from the increasing greenhouse gas concentrations in the atmosphere, positive radiative forcing, observed warming, and understanding of the climate system."[68] A 2010 report from the United Nations Environment Program's (UNEP) International Panel of Sustainable Resource Management echoed these sentiments stating that a global shift towards a vegan diet is critical for mitigating issues of hunger, fuel poverty and the worst impacts of climate change worldwide. The panel declared:

> Impacts from agriculture are expected to increase substantially due to population growth and increasing consumption of animal products. Unlike fossil fuels, it is difficult to look for alternatives: people have to eat. A substantial reduction of impacts would only be possible with a substantial worldwide diet change, away from animal products.[69]

As Robbins notes, "You see people who are environmentalists trying to conserve water washing their cars less often, installing low flow sinks and toilets, drought resistant landscaping, and legislation passing requiring low flow shower heads and so forth. These are all prudent and helpful measures, but all combined they don't even compare to what you save by eating one less hamburger."[70]

Help Wanted: Vegan Social Entrepreneurs

As my book has shown, a true vegetarian spirit goes way beyond concern with your personal health to a concern with the health of the planet and all its denizens. What I've tried to establish is the *multifaceted nature of the full vegetarian commitment.*

We have learned that green eating entails far more than simply doing something to improve your health, although that is a big part of it. Without health, it is very difficult to contribute to social change. It means taking a stand against the environmental destruction of the planet, which is an unwanted but unavoidable product of large scale livestock raising, among numerous other forms of unnecessary consumerism. It also means challenging ourselves to create sustainable solutions in every aspect of our lives.

Here at home, it means "getting off the grid as much as possible," the essence of which is articulated by author Gerry Ellen as possible but not so easy to do in America:

> Living off the grid is an ultimate change in consciousness. It is the desire to only have what you need, not take from the land [more than what is essential to live], and thrive in conditions that are about as raw as eating straight from your garden. And, you have to tend a garden. This whole idea of self-sufficiency in alignment with Mother Earth could have significant benefits besides saving you a great deal of money. It requires a willingness and compassion for plants, animals and all of life... Eco-conscious organic living is a good place to start. Being a minimalist is truly the essence of living off the grid.[71]

In general, living off the grid means making a commitment to converting from fossil fuels to renewable energy like solar power and wind energy; hydro-power can also be harnessed naturally; there are no harmful by-products and you can continually use these energies without harming or polluting the environment. It also means living simply: since there is no electricity, people who live off the grid use solar power and other forms of fuel for lighting or to fuel things like kerosene lamps, but occasionally cell phones and TVs, not microwaves.

In an article by John Platt appearing at Mother Nature Network, author Nick Rosen (*Off the Grid: Inside the Movement for More Space, Less Government, and True Independence in Modern America)* is quoted as saying: "Going off the grid is not a game; it is real life and a real choice for real people." He also notes that people go off the grid for a variety of reasons, and to various degrees. "You can't get off all of the grids all the time," he says. "It's a question of which grids you choose to get off of and in what way and for how long."[72] Some people live off the grid part of the year for leisure purposes and others get themselves off the public electrical or water systems but still participate in what Rosen calls the "car grid" or the "supermarket grid" or "bank grid." Even though most people choosing to live off the grid don't do it for environmental reasons, Platt notes that it, indeed, is a very green option, since the choice is automatically tied in to less consumerism. Still, Rosen acknowledged that it can be still be a lot of work, even on a small plot of land:

> Rosen says most families could go off the grid with as little as a half an acre, "as long as it's the right half-acre." Ideal locations would have some woodland, an area for agriculture, enough light for solar power and a good source of water, either a well or a stream. "The era of 40 acres and a mule has been replaced by the era of a half an acre and a laptop and a solar panel … But even a half an acre can be a lot of work—too much for most people. You're giving yourself a lot to do if you're running your own power plant, dealing with your own water supply, disposing of your own waste and pulling your own food."[73]

Even still… it's here to stay. A 2014 article in the *Guardian* said: "It's official. Off-grid energy is moving from the eco-fringe to mainstream. Last month US investment bank Morgan Stanley announced that the off-grid era had arrived: falling prices for renewable energy equipment and rising prices for energy supplied by power companies are fundamentally altering the business model of the trillion-dollar electricity industry."[74]

It might sound farfetched to be totally independent from fossil fuels but, in truth, it not only can be done, it is being done right now by a growing number of individuals. The *Guardian* article noted that over a million homes in the US are now currently off the grid, with the UK at around 100,000. Rosen estimates that this number is increasing by 10% a year according to an article that appeared in USA Today.[75] His website off-grid.net, along with a host of others (see resources section for more), provides information, forums, and community for those wanting to make this transition. In an interview with CNBC, James Wrathall, an attorney in the energy finance group at Sullivan & Worcester in Washington, D.C. stated, "I think consumers are gaining power in the equation and they are seeing these availabilities of this technology and they are seeing the benefit economically and they are going to demand it and they are going to get it... In the end, greater power of control is going to flow towards consumers."[76]

At first, employing these energy savings strategies can costs more, but the investment is worth it as you become more independent from local authorities and other purveyors to provide what you need to survive. Plus, you would be contributing to and influencing others. There is still a lot of fear and misconception about living off the grid; so by learning from experts and putting these practices into place, you can speak first-hand about its benefits and the good that you are doing in the world by putting them in place.

Living off the grid—at least in some way—might be something you've never considered, but you might want to pause and reflect on what you would do if you turned on the faucet and no water came out, as is happening in some towns in southern California, could not put fuel in your car because the gas pumps wouldn't work (no electricity), or had to bicycle or walk a couple of miles to get what you needed. While the scenarios I presented above might sound implausible, they are not. Global population and natural disasters are expected to increase, and as the strain on natural resources continues, systems will fail. That our government continues to be controlled by corporate factions means one thing: we must rely 100% on ourselves for what we need to live and survive.

Being a social entrepreneur also means raising the possibility of staving off world hunger in the only way that is possible, by shifting the well-off populations toward plant-heavy diets, and growing foods in ways that provide far greater economy and efficiency. But it is not enough to just switch to plant-based agriculture. Given the numbers of people on this earth, and our strain when it comes to water supply and mineral- depleted soils, we must become hyper-efficient in utilizing the resources that we do have toward the best outcomes. For certain, though, it means ending the suffering of penned and denatured animals with which we have broken the pact that once governed our ties between humans and other inhabitants of this earth.

Conclusion: The Healthy Vegetarian

The time for embracing real health is now. Yes, it requires change, but that's the nature of life. In reality, waiting longer is not an option: there is too much at stake, and there is no "Plan B." Our society is rife with disease, mostly attributed to our lifestyle, and the planet is nearing the end of its ability to sustain human life. The problems are vast, deep, political, and social, and very, very complicated. We are in the midst of a crisis—epidemics of obesity and diabetes, global warming water shortages and desertification, extreme environmental degradation and chemical pollution, and increasing rates of hunger, both at home and abroad. The solution is simple: *healthy vegetarianism*.

What I hope to have accomplished with this book is to paint a complete picture of the implications of both omnivorism and healthy vegetarianism, from the deeply political to the deeply personal. I wanted to show you that omnivorism is harming and killing us all in so many ways, on so many levels, and that most people in our world are not even cognizant of this fact. Its practice is deeply detrimental, and we simply cannot consider ourselves a healthy society until we completely let go of the unconscious, inhumane, health-depleting and resource-devastating ways of animal-based food industry.

In the preceding pages, I have carefully traced the harms of omnivorism and corresponding benefits of vegetarianism on multiple levels. I talked about why we're omnivores in the first place and what causes us to mistakenly believe that meat or dairy is a good source of nutrition. As you now know, this all emerged from the joining of a few very powerful forces—namely corporate agenda—through advertising and propaganda—along with government collusion and a cultural perception that eating animals indicates superior status, which is only true in the minds of those who subscribe to the doctrine of domination over nature, promoted by Judeo-Christianity at the beginning of the Common Era (C.E.), nearly two millennia ago. This, in turn, has invoked an incredibly powerful social current of omnivorism that can be extremely difficult to counter.

It's not our fault, really—but, for certain, the responsibility for changing it lies with each of us, solely and completely. We learn primarily from others and we've been taught by the authorities we have adhered to that eating meat is good for you and even necessary for good health, which is plainly untrue. Most of us don't want to believe that we live in a world where the objectives of private industry trump public health, yet this is what we've created. The forces of corporate dominance and greed are too difficult for any one individual to overcome alone, but through the collective actions of a growing number of aware and healthful people, I remain steadfast in my opinion that we can reach a tipping point, whereby the positive changes we all want to see will occur readily and automatically.

Over time, many individuals have fought this powerful social tide of omnivorism, and chosen vegetarianism. These vegetarian dissidents of the Western world have been around since before the onset of Christianity, as written by Porphyry in 275 CE, but also before Common Era through the Greek physician Hippocrates, for example—who is well-known as the father of modern medicine and coined the phrase "Let thy food be thy medicine; and thy medicine be thy food." Their ranks have included some incredibly prominent thinkers and social leaders, whose words and deeds have extended well beyond their time on the planet.

Some religious sects, particularly of Eastern traditions, have also practiced vegetarianism for thousands of years because they eschew the killing of God's creatures. They recognize that killing is murderous and, therefore, harmful. It is also important to remember that millions of people in our world are vegetarians, in part out of economic necessity or geographic considerations. But many wealthy people are now entirely plant-based, including not only famous politicians, actors and entertainers, physicians, artists, writers and philosophers, and international athletes, as well. While our vegetarian numbers may represent a small minority of the general population, they represent a growing enlightened group of human beings who have purposely chosen a healthier way for themselves and the world in which they live. We are the torch bearers and our flame is spreading.

As I've demonstrated, it's really quite easy to eliminate all animal products from your diet—the world offers so many creative possibilities, if we are but willing to venture there. Fruits and vegetables, legumes and tubers, grains, nuts, and seeds, when used properly, will provide you with all of the nutrients you need, including sufficient and superior protein. These foods will also return you to a normal body weight, improve your skin, hair, nails, and your sleep, increase your energy, heal your digestive tract, enhance your libido, and fortify your immune system.

Just from this perspective of physical health alone, which is only a small focus of the healthy vegetarian lifestyle, healthy vegetarians realize that by not eating animals they are reducing their risk for disease, and substantially. First, they are avoiding the myriad of noxious chemicals that they had been eating along with those hamburgers and steaks that will, over time, have adverse effects in your body. Then, there's the excess of saturated fat and protein that will tax a body's systems to the point of overload and eventual shutdown. The healthy vegetarian will avoid all of these complications.

Healthy vegetarianism also involves choosing natural foods, which have not been genetically modified. Genetic modifications by definition alter the DNA of the food organism, changing it to something unnatural. These "foods" are essentially created in a lab, hence the popular and well deserved name "Frankenfoods," and primarily by the largest poison producer in the land, Monsanto. Genetically modified organisms (GMOs) are not altered to improve nutritional value, but to increase profits—directly at the expense of all who consume them, and irrespective of any health and harm that may come to consumers. Organics are non-GMO; they are food as nature made it and intended it. Organic organisms also re-seed themselves, as organisms are supposed to. They are natural, and they're also treated with less harmful insect repellents. Don't fret about the slightly higher price; rejoice in the fact that you can still buy healthy, more nutritious food for yourself and your family and that there are options for reducing your expenses through home gardening, cooperative buying, and a growing number of farmer's markets.

Physical health is only one component of the healthy vegetarian lifestyle, however. Healthy vegetarianism is more than just a diet. It's a *consciousness*. It's an awareness of what you're contributing to and supporting when you choose this product over that one—vegan items over products from animals or that use animals in their processing. Healthy vegetarianism also involves a consciousness of the greater good as well as one of ecological and spiritual interdependence: This brings about actions based on the understanding that whatever they do affects the whole.

Healthy vegetarians are aware of the devastating repercussions of human behavior on our planet's ecosystems and that the planet upon which we rely for our very existence is deeply wounded, and choose ecological clothing and wears, recyclable over disposable products, and energy-saving devices whenever possible; they are aware that harming another human through words or act creates suffering and hatred, so they practice patience, kindness, and compassion in their interactions and relations, and they are aware that all living creatures are sensitive to pain, and participate in initiatives to end violence against all living beings.

Healthy vegetarianism is sustainable, because it includes the perspective and charge of living with "enough," so that all may have their basic needs met. It embraces a mindset that sustainable living is something to do perpetually, rather than sporadically, and that many more of us will be in a world of hurt very soon, if we do not change our ways now. The healthy vegetarian gets this, and participates joyfully in the solutions, regardless of the concern, sadness, and discouragement that might arise in them from time to time.

This brings me to a few words about healing. At the beginning of Part I, I shared a quote by author Haruki Murakami: "What happens when people open their hearts? They get better." If we want to get better, meaning healthy, as a person, as a nation, we need first open our hearts to what is occurring; then, we must connect with our feelings and let these feelings guide us to our *Why*; it is crucial at this very precarious time in human history that we become crystal clear about our *Why*. This way we really can find the strength and conviction to make the changes that will create our "better"—which is the healing for us and, therefore, the world.

For the healthy vegetarian, the peace and comfort that health brings to them and all inhabitants of this fundamentally glorious planet Earth is one of the most compelling *Why's*. As such, they are someone who chooses to live a healthy life despite the endless obstacles to doing so: she practices meditation and mindfulness over fret and worry; and he chooses a good night's rest over partying and late-night gorging. They frequent co-ops and health food stores, where they bring their own bags, and stay far away from the major box stores and conglomerates, especially those who do the greatest social harm. They host parties, movie screenings about important issues, and vegan potlucks, and gladly invite their omnivorous friends. They also take the time for themselves that they need in order to feel centered and balanced. They gently remove themselves from no-win situations and say no when they need to, preserving their own integrity and self-respect. They take care of their emotional, psychological, and intellectual health in addition to their physical health.

The healthy vegetarian wouldn't knowingly participate in anything that brings harm to anyone or anything. She understands the horrors endured by slaughterhouse workers and empathizes with the hurting, terrified creature being led to its death; she refuses to support this. He knows that eating meat contributes not only to global warming and the depletion of, well, *all* of our natural resources, but it also means that millions of people suffer from needless starvation; so he willingly speaks about his choice. It is impossible for the healthy vegetarian to indulge in a practice that means others starve to death; this is unequivocally opposite of where the moral compass of a healthy vegetarian points.

Healthy vegetarians are more evolved beings. They are meticulously aware of where food comes from and do everything they can to ensure no one or the planet suffers in bringing it to their table. They promote a lifestyle that is responsible, compassionate, and healthy not only for themselves, but for all of humankind *and* the wellbeing of the planet. They live sustainably; and they also know that by doing so they are creating healing in the world, which brings them happiness. It is the closest that they get to heaven on Earth, which is why they stay in action.

In a world where our population is growing rapidly and exponentially, we must live sustainably. We have no choice. In the late chapters of this book, I have given any number of healthful activities that you can personally undertake to create greater health and well-being in your life, in your community, and in the world at large. There are also plenty of exciting green initiatives in which you can become involved, as a hobby or, even, as a career. One thing is certain: refusing to live sustainably is akin to self-inflicted genocide. So the question to ask yourself, then, is, "How will I feel if I do not do everything that I can to make a difference right now—to shift my activities away from destruction to health?"

In reality, we can make a difference and turn the tide. You can make a difference: it's as simple as first choosing a plant-based diet over an animal-based one. Make this one small change at home, and you will be contributing to a huge change in the world. If you haven't already done this, just begin now and see what happens; you will likely be amazed and probably even pleasantly surprised—about how the choice of a healthy vegetarian lifestyle will change you and those around you. It may even help resolve some of the biggest problems that you currently face. And if enough of us do just this, it may even resolve some of the biggest problems that the world is facing, and that is something to feel great about.

If you are already enjoying the vegetarian diet and lifestyle and its benefits, I would ask you to consider where you might give more energy in support of the healthy vegetarian diet and sustainable lifestyle becoming more commonplace in our nation, or to a cause that you already know about or have identified through reading this book. Every bit of loving energy and effort that any of us can give to raising consciousness and helping to eliminate the suffering of our fellow humans and all living creatures on this planet makes a significant contribution to all life.

I need to end with a strong statement of the truth that we are facing as a population and species. Unless this path of healthy vegetarianism becomes a crowded one, there is little hope for us, and possibly for many of the species occupying this planet. But if you and your family members, neighbors and community—virtual and actual—would begin hiking along this metaphorical mountain trail, taking more steps together each day in support of the ideas and actions presented in this book, you cannot only expect better health, but you can expect a world and planet experiencing more love, more kindness, and more peace—a place where humans and other species have a better than fighting chance.

Appendices

Appendix A: Aging Gracefully Research Study

As suggested, participants in the study had problems with their hair, skin or both, and were all willing to make changes in their lifestyles in order to see what improvements might occur. At the first assessment point in the study, many subjects reported measurable benefits, such as the improvement of inflammatory conditions, better sleep, more energy, better digestion and less pain. Still, hair and teeth remained the same.

We then added two to ten times the normal dietary intake of phytonutrients, in the form of fresh fruit and vegetable juices or concentrated fruit and vegetable powders. We theorized that since processes that cause aging include damage to DNA from oxidative stress, the body must be saturated with phytonutrients to have an effect on long-term damage. We speculated that increasing phytonutrients would not only hold back further damage but roll back effects already present. Still, it was an open question whether this radical attempt to pour on the juices and powders could reduce system damage and reverse the DNA damage causing loss of hair or graying.

Let me make clear the components of the program.

The nutritional protocols called for a low-fat, high-complex-carbohydrate, primarily vegetarian diet, paired with eliminating foods and beverages with documented negative health effects.

Subjects adhered to the following regimen:

i) Exercise

Exercise included both aerobic and resistance training. The aerobics entailed sustaining 70% of optimal heart rate for at least 45 minutes of cardiac conditioning a day. Resistance training consisted of working on 8-10 various large muscle group machines a day, at 3-5 repetitions per circuit, times 5 circuits. This was done six days a week.

ii) Stress management techniques

The relaxation/meditation component consisted of participants setting aside at least two half-hour sessions a day in which to engage in such calming, centering activities as prayer, meditation, journaling, listening to tranquil music, walking, and/or yoga.

iii) Self-actualization leading to self-empowerment

For the study groups, emotional and physical support (in the form of talk therapy, hands-on exercise demonstration, and other personalized attention) were offered weekly in order to help participants shake their counterproductive habits, such as keeping to their exercise plan or avoiding junk food. Coaching also included dietary counseling on the benefits of a vegetarian diet for those suffering from circulatory, blood sugar, joint, and weight problems. There were group counseling sessions, small group discussions and one-on-one talk therapy sessions by licensed nutritional counselors.

Part of the reason for affording counseling was that we (planning the study) felt it was not enough to have participants change their activities and eating for the length of the program. Through education and consultation, we wanted to help our participants see their formerly unhealthy attitudes toward diet, exercise, and even personal relationships through new, more health-conscious eyes. Those who developed favorable attitudes in all three areas were better able to make the lifestyle changes which provided measurable results in both the short and long run.

iv) Nutrition: A live-foods diet

The dietary portion of the protocol was a complete sweep, eliminating all foods that can have adverse health effects. This amounted to eliminating all animal protein (beef, fish, poultry, and shellfish) as well as dropping dairy products, wheat, alcohol and caffeine, simple sugars and artificial sweeteners, soft drinks and carbonated

beverages, fried, barbecued, and processed foods, food additives, canned and salted foods, dried fruits, preservatives, coloring agents, flavorings, MSG, and yeast.
In place of so many objectionable foods, we substituted:

- Good-quality protein from vegetarian sources (such as beans, nuts, seeds, legumes, and starchy vegetables). Protein intake was approximately 0.9 g/kg of body weight (40–60g high quality protein for women and 60-80g for men).
- Nine servings of nutrient-dense fruits and vegetables (preferably organic) per day. Fiber intake was at least 35-50 grams.
- Four servings of beans and grains (such as brown rice, spelt, quinoa and millet).

Sprouts, sea vegetables, soy products, onions and garlic, olive oil, coconut oil, flaxseed oil, spring or filtered water, decaffeinated green and herbal teas as well as grain beverages were among the other included foods and beverages.

I mentioned that we came to the conclusion that only by saturating the body with phytochemicals and phytonutrients could we hope to reverse DNA damage. So for the "repair" portion of the program—we made juices from fresh vegetables and fruits and their natural powdered concentrates. Our active participants consumed them at a ratio of five vegetable juices to each fruit juice. Subjects began by drinking one 16-ounce glass of juice a day in week one and built up to eight glasses a day in week eight.

v) Supplementation

Aside from all the participants eating such a robust diet and drinking such vitality-infused juices, we recommended a broad-based intake of vitamin and mineral supplementation, among which were the following:

Omega 3 EPA & DHA, 1,500mg from flaxseed oil
Coenzyme Q 10, 100mg 3 x per day
Milk Thistle, 200mg
Linoleic Acid, 50mg
N Acetyl Cysteine, 500mg 2x per day

Grape Seed Extract, 200mg
Alpha Lipoic Acid, 500mg 3x per day
Quercitin, 100mg 3x per day
St. John's Wort, 300mg
Vitamin E 400 IU 2x per day
Selenium Methionine, 200mcg
Linoleic Acid, 100mg
Ascorbic Acid, 1000mg-8000mg (or up to bowel tolerance)
L-Carnosine, 500mg 3x per day
Acetyl-L-Carnotine, 200mg 3x per day
Acidophilus, 1 teaspoon per day
Superoxide Dismutase, 100mg 3x per day
Dimethyl Glysine, 150mg/per day
B Complex, 50mg once a day
Beta Carotene, 333IU/mg 5000IU
Niacinamide, 50mg
Di Calcium Pantothenate, 50mg
Vitamin B12, 800mcg

vi) Environmental hygiene

Lastly, in order to make sure that participants—who were now living and eating in a healthy way—weren't being sabotaged by a hostile environment, we asked them to reduce their exposure to air pollutants, allergens, toxins, and electromagnetic fields in their living and work environments. (Refer back to Chapter 7 where I spoke about what is required to create a sound, healthful environment.)

After our six-month study, we found statistically significant improvements for those who could adhere to such a rigorous program. These improvements were not solely in the target areas of skin and hair but in many aspects of mental and physical functioning. Participants rated each outcome measure as "worse," "unchanged," "slightly improved," "improved," or "much improved." The majority of the ratings fell into the "slightly improved" and "improved" categories. We broke down the participants' answers by sex and age, and were happy to find both men and women had similar positive outcomes as did participants below and above age 55.

To be a bit more specific:

- Hair and skin results: there were documented improvements in measures of hair, facial skin, body skin and nails. Hair measures most improved were thinning (good results in 69.8% of participants), texture (66.9%), luster (65.4%), balding (61.0%), graying (58.3%), hair loss per day/week (57.3%), and darkening (52.6%). Skin measures most improved were texture (86.7%) and tone (81.2%), followed by wrinkles (63.0%), blemishes (61.4%), and eyelids (37.4%).
- Physical, mental, and energy results: there was a high frequency of improvement in mental capabilities and energy. Energy function improved for 91.5% of participants, while overall mental function improved for 82.9%.

Appendix B: Sprouting Guide

They are so easy to cultivate that I can give you two methods to do so. I will follow this with a sprouting chart that fills you in on the amounts of dry seed, grain, or bean to use and their individual sprouting times. There are numerous books on the subject matter, if you have further interest in what I am presenting here. Note that whatever container you use, make sure there is room for an increase in size of from five to eight times the original material.

The simplest method is with a jar. Here's what you need to get started: (a) a wide mouth jar, (b) a rubber band, (c) a wire screen, cheesecloth or an old clean nylon stocking, and (d) a whole seed, bean, or grain.

- First, soak the seeds (or other plants you are using) in plenty of water overnight. Use approximately twice the volume of water as the volume you have of dry seed.
- Second, drain the water through the screen or cloth, and rinse the seeds well.
- Third, turn the jar upside down at an angle; place in a bowl, pot, or wire stand; and put in a dark, temperate place.
- Rinse the seeds through the screen twice daily in cool-to-mild water and three times daily in the summer. During this time, when the rising is finished, keep the jar inverted and gently shake the seeds to distribute them evenly around the walls of the jar.

Another easy method relies on using a pan rather than a jar. Soak the seeds overnight in the pan, again using twice as much water as dry material. After the second day, spread the seeds thinly and evenly on the bottom of a glass or screen tray, a colander or even in a straw basket. Sprinkle generously with water two to three times daily. Cover with a wet cheesecloth or paper towel.

Most sprouts are ready to eat when they've grown to ½ or whole inch long, except for alfalfa, buckwheat, and sunflower seed sprouts, which should be left a little longer. After the third day, place alfalfa sprouts in the sun to enhance the development of their chlorophyll.

When the sprouts have reached their desired length, put them in a closed jar or plastic container and store in the refrigerator. If properly covered, they will keep a few days, as long as any fresh vegetable.

The following chart will give you more details on the more popular sprouts.

SPROUTING CHART

Once you've grown any of these varieties of sprouts, you'll be able to add to your meals something that is nutrient rich, low in calories, easily digested, and a good source of B-complex vitamins. And sprouts are good neighbors, complementing other foods as they are added to main dishes, casseroles, soups, and salads.

Type	Soaking Time	Rinse/Drain (Times per Day)	Sprouting Time	Amt. in Qt. Jar
Alfalfa Seeds	12 hrs. (overnight)	2	3-6 days	3 tbs.
Buckwheat	12 hrs.	1	4-6 days	5 tbs.
Fenugreek Seeds	12 hrs.	1	4-6 days	3 tbs.
Garbanzo Beans	12 hrs.	2	3-5 days	1 cup
Lentils	12 hrs.	2	4-6 days	10 tbs.
Mung Beans	12 hrs.	2	4-6 days	6 tbs.
Mustard Seeds	None	1	5-7 days	3 tbs.

Radish Seeds	12 hrs.	1	5-7 days	3 tbs.
Red Clover Seeds	12 hrs.	2	5 days	3 tbs.
Rye	12 hrs.	1	4 days	5 tbs.
Soybeans	24 hrs.	2	6 days	1 cup
Sunflower Seeds	12 hrs.	1	8 days	8 tbs.
Wheat	12 hrs.	1	5 days	5 tbs.

Appendix C: Protein Content of Legumes, Grains, Grain Flours, Nuts, and Seeds

Protein is shown in grams per 100 grams, which is approximately 3.5oz or ½ cup

Legumes	g protein per 100 g (approx. 3.5 oz)
Tempeh (raw)	18.54
Soybeans	16.64
Kidney beans	15.35
Miso	11.69
Lentils	9.02
Pinto beans	9.01
Black beans	8.86
Chick-peas	8.86
Split peas	8.34
Navy beans	8.23
Tofu (raw)	8.08
Black-eyed peas	7.73
Broad beans	7.60
Adzuki beans	7.52
Mung beans	7.06

Grains (raw)	
Oat bran	17.30
Whole wheat	13.68
Buckwheat	13.25
Millet	11.02
Whole rye	10.34
Whole barley	9.91
Corn	9.42
Quinoa	4.40
Wild Rice	3.99
Amaranth	2.11
White Rice	2.02

Grains (flour)	
Wheat	13.21
Triticale	13.18
Buckwheat	12.62
Rye	10.88
Millet	10.75
Barley	10.50
Corn	6.93
Rice	5.95

Nuts and Seeds	
Pumpkin/squash seeds	30.23
Mustard seeds (ground)	26.08
Peanuts (raw)	25.80
Fenugreek seeds	23.00
Almonds	21.15
Sunflower seeds	20.78

Pistachio	20.27
Flaxseeds	18.29
Cashews	18.22
Chia seeds	16.54
Walnuts	15.23
Filberts	14.95
Brazil nuts	14.32
Pignolias	13.69
Sesame seeds	11.73
Pecans	9.17
Alfalfa seeds	3.99
Radish seeds (sprouted)	3.81

Source: National Nutrient Database for Standard Reference (Release 27), USDA Agricultural Research Service.

Appendix D: Average Weights for Men & Women

Ideal Body Weight Charts

For Men 25-59 years of age			
Height in Feet & Inches	Small Frame	Medium Frame	Large Frame
5’2”	128-134	131-141	138-150
5’3”	130-136	133-143	140-153
5’4”	132-138	135-145	142-156
5’5”	134-140	137-148	144-160
5’6”	136-142	139-151	146-164
5’7”	138-145	142-154	149-168
5’8”	140-148	145-157	152-172
5’9”	142-151	151-163	155-176
5’10”	144-154	151-163	158-180
5’11”	146-157	154-166	161-184
6’0”	149-160	157-170	164-188
6’1”	152-164	160-174	168-192
6’2”	155-168	165-178	172-197
6’3”	158-172	167-182	176-202
6’4”	162-176	171-187	181-207

For Women 25-59 years of age			
Height in Feet & Inches	Small Frame	Medium Frame	Large Frame
4'10"	102-111	109-121	118-131
4'11"	103-113	111-123	120-134
5'0"	104-115	113-126	122-137
5'1"	106-118	115-129	125-140
5'2"	108-121	118-132	128-143
5'3"	111-124	121-135	131-147
5'4"	114-127	124-138	134-151
5'5"	117-130	127-141	137-155
5'6"	120-133	130-144	140-159
5'7"	123-136	133-147	143-163
5'8"	126-139	136-150	146-167
5'9"	129-142	139-153	149-170
5'10"	132-145	142-156	152-173
5'11"	135-148	145-159	155-176
6'0"	138-151	148-162	158-179

FRAME SIZE

If you have always wondered what size frame you are, here is the method the insurance company used. This will be easier with the help of a friend.

1. Extend your arm in front of your body bending your elbow at a ninety degree angle to your body (your arm is parallel to your body).
2. Keep your fingers straight and turn the inside of your wrist to your body.
3. Place your thumb and index finger on the two prominent bones on either side of your elbow, and measure the distance between the bones with a tape measure or calipers.
4. Compare to the medium-framed chart below. Select your height based on what you are barefoot. If you are below the listed inches, your frame is small. If you are above, your frame is large.

ELBOW MEASUREMENTS FOR MEDIUM FRAME			
Height in 1" heels	Elbow	Height in 1" heels	Elbow
Men	**Breadth**	**Women**	Breadth
5'2"-5'3"	21/2"-27/8"	4'10"-4'11"	21/4"-21/2"
5'4"-5'7"	25/8"-27/8"	5'0"-5'3"	21/4"-21/2"
5'8"-5'11"	23/4"-3"	5'4"-5'7"	23/8"-25/8"
6'0"-6'3"	23/4"-31/8"	5'8"-5'11"	23/8"-25/8"
6'4"	27/8"-31/4"	6'0"	21/2"-23/4"

Source: http://www.healthdiscovery.net/links/calculators/ideal_bodyweight.htm

Appendix E: List of Organic Brands Owned by Major Food Corporations

(Note: list does not currently include private labels such as Walmart's Great Value or Target's Archer Farms brands.)

These companies are our favorite brands to support… they continue to operate independently, which enables them to uphold solid product integrity as well as freedom in educating about GMOs.

Brand	Company Owned By	Year
Alexia Foods	ConAgra	2007
Alta Dena	Dean	1999
Annie's Naturals	General Mills	2014
Arrowhead Mills	Hain Celestial	1998
Attune (Erewhon Cereals, etc.)	Post Foods	2013
Back To Nature	Kraft	2003
Barbara's	Wheatabix Food Co.	1986
Bearitos	Hain Celestial	1997
Bear Naked	Kellogg	2007
Ben & Jerry's Organic	Unilever	2003
Boca Foods	Kraft	2000
Bolthouse Farms	Campbell Soup	2012
Breadshop	Hain Celestial	1999
Breyer's Organic	Unilever	2006

Brand	Company Owned By	Year
Brown Cow	Dannon/Danone	2003
Campbell's Organic	Campbell Soup	2003
Casbah	Hain Celestial	1999
Cascadian Farm	General Mills	1999
Dagoba	Hershey Foods	2006
DeBole's	Hain Celestial	1998
DiGiorno Organic	Kraft	2006
Dole Organic	Dole	2001
Dove Organic	M&M Mars	2006
Earth's Best	Hain Celestial	1999
Ella's Kitchen	Hain Celestial	2013
Erewhon (see Attune)	Post Foods	2013
Food Should Taste Good	General Mills	2012
French Meadow	Rich Products Corp.	2007
Fruitti de Bosco	Walnut Acres	2001
Garden of Eatin	Hain Celestial	1998
Gerber Organic Baby Food	Nestle	2007
Gold Medal Organic	General Mills	2005
Golden Temple	Post / Hearthside	2011
Green & Black's	Cadbury Schweppes	2005
Happy Baby Organic Baby Food	Dannon/Danone	2013
Happy Family	Dannon/Danone	2013
Health Valley	Hain Celestial	1999
Heinz Organic	Heinz	2002
Hershey Organic	Hershey Foods	2007
Honest Tea	Coca Cola (40% stake)	2008
Horizon Organic	Dean	2004
Humboldt Creamery	Foster Farms	2009
Hunt's Organic	ConAgra	2005
Imagine	Hain Celestial	2002
Kashi	Kellogg	2000

Brand	Company Owned By	Year
Keebler Organic	Kellogg	2006
Kellogg's Organic	Kellogg	2006
Kettle (chips, etc.)	Diamond Foods	2010
Knudsen, R.W.	J.M. Smucker	1984
Kraft Organic	Kraft	2008
Larabar	General Mills	2008
Late July	Snyders (minority stake)	2007
Lightlife	ConAgra	2000
Maranatha	Hain Celestial	2008
Millina's Finest	Walnut Acres	2001
Millstone	J.M. Smucker	2008
Morningstar Farms	Kellogg	1999
Mott's Organic	Cadbury Schweppes	2004
Mountain Sun	Hain Celestial / Walnut Acres	2001
Muir Glen	Cascadian Farm	1998
Nabisco Organic	Kraft	2007
Naked Juice	Pepsi	2008
Nantucket Nectars Organic	Cadbury Schweppes	2004
Natural Touch	Kellogg	1999
Nile Spice	Hain Celestial	1998
Odwalla	Coca Cola	2001
Organic Cow of Vermont	Horizon	1999
Orville Redenbacher's Organic	ConAgra	2005
Pace Organic	Campbell's	2005
PAM Organic	ConAgra	2006
Peace Cereal	Post / Hearthside	2011
Peet's Coffee & Tea	Sara Lee / JAB / D.E. Master Blenders	2011
Planters Organic	Kraft	2007
Plum Organic Baby Food	Campbells	2013
PowerBar	Nestle	2006
Prego Organic	Campbell's	2005

Brand	Company Owned By	Year
Pria Grain Essentials	Nestle	2006
Ragu Organic	Unilever	2005
Rice Dream (Imagine)	Hain Celestial	2002
Santa Cruz Organic	J.M. Smucker Co.	1989
Seeds of Change	M&M Mars	1997
ShariAnn's	Walnut Acres	2001
Silk	White Wave Foods*	2013
Similac Organic Infant Formula	Abbott Nutrition	1950s
Soy Dream (Imagine)	Hain Celestial	2002
Spectrum Organics	Hain Celestial	2005
Stone Mill	Anheuser-Busch	2006
Stonyfield	Dannon/Danone	2001-2004
SunSpire	Hain Celestial	2008
Swanson's Organic	Campbell's	2005
Tostito's Organic	Pepsi	2003
Tropicana Organic	Pepsi	2007
V8 Organic	Campbell's	2005
Walnut Acres	Hain Celestial	2003
Westbrae	Hain Celestial	1997
Westsoy	Hain Celestial	1997
Wholesome & Hearty	Kellogg	2007
Wild Hop	Anheuser-Busch	2006
Willamette Valley Granola	Post / Hearthside	2011
Wolfgang Puck	Campbell Soup	2008

Source: http://gmo-awareness.com/shopping-list/family-organic-brands/

Resources

Vegetarian Lifestyle Magazines	
Vegetarian Times (print and online)	www.vegetariantimes.com
Natural Health Magazine (print and online)	www.naturalhealthmag.com
VegNews Magazine (print and online)	vegnews.com
Laika (print and online)	www.laikamagazine.com
Clean Eating Magazine (print and online)	www.cleaneatingmag.com
Vegan Lifestyle Magazine (print and online)	www.veganlifestylemagazine.com
Vegan Magazine (online only)	www.vegan-magazine.com
Vegan Food Magazine (online only)	www.veganfoodmagazine.com
Kiwi Magazine (print and online) – especially aimed at families	www.kiwimagonline.com
Vegetarian Restaurant Guides	
Veggie Heaven - reviews of vegetarian restaurants worldwide	veggieheaven.com
Book: The Artichoke Trail: A Guide to Vegetarian Restaurants, Organic Food Stores & Farmer's Markets in the US	Author: James A. Frost Hunter Travel Guides, Hunter Publishing (NJ)
Happy Cow, VegGuide, and Veg Dining offer comprehensives list of Vegetarian restaurants	www.happycow.net www.vegguide.org www.vegdining.com

Vegetarian Journal's Guide to Vegan and Vegetarian Restaurants in the U.S. and Canada	www.vrg.org/restaurant
Urbanspoon and Yelp also have sections on vegetarian restaurants	www.urbanspoon.com www.yelp.com
Healthy Consumer Products	
VeganEssentials	www.veganessentials.com
Alternative Outfitters	www.alternativeoutfitters.com
VeganKit	vegankit.com
The Vegan Store	www.veganstore.com
Green Harmony Living	greenharmonyliving.com
Organic Grace – non-toxic products	organicgrace.com
Basic Vegetarian and Nutrition information	
Vegetarian Resource Group (VRG)	www.vrg.org
Vegetarian Society	www.vegsoc.org
VeganKit	vegankit.com/eat
The Vegetarian Site	www.thevegetariansite.com
Vegetarian Nutrition	vegetariannutrition.net
North American Vegetarian Society (NAVS)	www.navs-online.org
Gary Null, Your Guide to Healthy Living	www.gnhealthyliving.com
Michael Gregor, M.D.	www.nutritionfacts.org
T. Colin Campbell Center for Nutrition Studies	nutritionstudies.org
Dr. McDougall's Health & Medical Center	www.drmcdougall.com
Dr. Fuhrman Smart Nutrition, Superior Health	www.drfuhrman.com
TreeHugger	www.treehugger.com
Real Goods	realgoods.com

Animal Rights Activism	
The Physicians Committee for Responsible Medicine (PCRM)	www.pcrm.org
People for the Ethical Treatment of Animals (PETA)	www.peta.org
Farm Sanctuary	www.farmsanctuary.org
The American Society for the Prevention of Cruelty to Animals (ASPCA)	www.aspca.org
Mercy for Animals (MFA)	www.mercyforanimals.org
Animal Liberation Front (ALF)	www.animalliberationfront.com
Action for Animals (AFA)	www.afa-online.org
Save Animals from Exploitation (SAFE)	safe.org.nz
Coalition to Abolish the Fur Trade (CAFT)	www.caft.org.uk
Organics Information	
Organic Consumers Association	www.organicconsumers.org
Sustainable Organic Resources Partnership (SORP)	www.sorp.org
Soil Science Society of America	www.soils.org
Permaculture Institute	www.permaculture.org
Ecological Farming Association	eco-farm.org
US Dietary Health Organizations	
The Academy of Nutrition and Dietetics (AND)— formerly the American Dietetic Association (ADA)	www.eatrightpro.org
American Society for Nutrition	www.nutrition.org
American Heart Association (AHA)	www.heart.org
American Diabetes Association	www.diabetes.org

U.S. Government organizations related to food and food safety	
US Department of Agriculture (USDA)	www.usda.gov
US Food and Drug Administration FDA	www.fda.gov
US Environmental Protection Agency (EPA)	www.epa.gov
Foodsafety.gov communicates food safety information provided by government agencies to the public.	Foodsafety.gov
Food and Agricultural Organization of the United Nations (FAO)	www.fao.org
Bureau for Food Security of the U.S. Agency for International Development (USAID)	www.usaid.gov
Department of Food Safety, World Health Organization (WHO)	www.who.int/foodsafety
USDA Handbook #8	http://www.scribd.com/doc/59945722/USDA-Handbook-8-Composition-of-Foods-Sausages-and-Luncheon-Meats#scribd
Food Politics resources/activism	
Food Democracy Now	www.fooddemocracynow.org
Slow Food	www.slowfoodusa.org
Slow Food Movement	www.slowfood.com
Slow Movement	www.slowmovement.com
The Institute for Agricultural and Trade Policy	www.iatp.org
Organic Trade Association	www.ota.com
Roots of Change	www.rootsofchange.org
The National Sustainable Agriculture Coalition (NSAC)	sustainableagriculture.net
Food First	foodfirst.org

John Robbins	johnrobbins.info
Organic Consumers Association	www.organicconsumers.org
The Land Institute	www.landinstitute.org
General Environmental Activism & Climate Change	
Greenpeace	www.greenpeace.org
Friends of the Earth	www.foe.org
EarthSave International	www.earthsave.org
Environment America	www.environmentamerica.org
International Tree Foundation	internationaltreefoundation.org
Sierra Club	www.sierraclub.org
Ecologic Institute	www.ecologic.eu
Conservation International	www.conservation.org
World Nature Organization (WNO)	www.wno.org
Climate Action Network	www.climatenetwork.org
The Environmental Working Group (EWG)	www.ewg.org
National Resources Defense Council (NRDC)	www.nrdc.org
General Social Activism	
Corporate Accountability International	www.stopcorporateabuse.org
Means of Exchange	www.meansofexchange.com
CATO Institute	www.cato.org
The Center for a New American Dream	www.newdream.org
Urban Institute	www.urban.org
Center for American Progress	www.americanprogress.org
Progressive News Sources	
Progressive Radio Network	prn.fm
Truthout	www.truth-out.org
Mother Jones	www.motherjones.com
The New Republic	www.newrepublic.com

YES! Magazine	www.yesmagazine.org
Mother Nature Network (MNN)	www.mnn.com
Moyers & Company	billmoyers.com
Fairness & Accuracy in Reporting (FAIR)	fair.org
Common Dreams	www.commondreams.org
AlterNet	www.alternet.org
The Progressive	www.progressive.org
The Nation	www.thenation.com
ThinkProgress	thinkprogress.org
Progressive Think Tank Organizations	
TED	www.ted.com
World Resources Institute (WRI)	www.wri.org
The Union of Concerned Scientists (UCS)	www.ucsusa.org
E3G	www.e3g.org
Ceres	www.ceres.org
Climate Institute	www.climate.org
Center for Community Change	www.communitychange.org
Ecotrust	www.ecotrust.org
The Environmental Law Institute (ELI)	www.eli.org
Environmental Defense Fund (EDF)	www.edf.org
Brighter Green	www.brightergreen.org
The Center for Climate and Energy Solutions (C2ES)	www.c2es.org
Spiritual Organizations Promoting Non-Violence	
Center for Nonviolent Communication (CNVC)	www.cnvc.org
Fellowship of Reconciliation (FOR)	forusa.org
Ahimsa Organization	ahimsazine.com

The Buddhist Association of the United States (BAUS)	www.baus.org
National Center for Complementary and Integrative Health (NCCIH), National Institutes of Health	nccih.nih.gov
US Yoga Federation	www.usayoga.org
American Yoga Association	www.americanyogaassociation.org
Community Focused Sites	
City Plants	www.cityplants.org
American Community Gardening Association (ACGA)	communitygarden.org
Co-operative Energy	www.cooperativeenergy.coop
Touchstone Energy	www.touchstoneenergy.com
Co-operative bank	www.ncb.coop
Shareable	www.shareable.net
National Association of Housing Cooperatives	coophousing.org
TimeBanks	timebanks.org
The National Farm to School Network	www.farmtoschool.org
Smart Growth	www.smartgrowth.org
Sustainable Agriculture Education Association	sustainableaged.org

Bibliography

Introduction

1. RL Phillips, "Role of lifestyle and dietary habits in risk of cancer among Seventh-day Adventists," *Cancer Res.*, 35(Suppl) (1975):3513-22.
2. DA Snowdon and RL Phillips, "Does a vegetarian diet reduce the occurrence of diabetes?" *Am J Public Health,* 75 (1985):507–12.
3. TJ Key et al., "Mortality in vegetarians and non-vegetarians: a collaborative analysis of 8300 deaths among 76,000 men and women in five prospective studies," *Public Health Nutr.*, 1 (1998):33–41.
4. T Huang et al., "Cardiovascular disease mortality and cancer incidence in vegetarians: a meta-analysis and systematic review," *Ann Nutr Metab.*, 60 (2012):233–40.
5. M de Lorgeril et al., "Mediterranean diet, traditional risk factors, and the rate of cardiovascular complications after myocardial infarction: final report of the Lyon Diet Heart Study," *Circulation,* 99 (1999):779–85.
6. SE Berkow and N Barnard, "Vegetarian diets and weight status," *Nutr Rev.,* 64 (2006):175–88.
7. M Malter, "Natural killer cells, vitamins, and other blood components of vegetarian and omnivorous men," *Nutr and Cancer,* 12 (1989):271-8.
8. Michael Bluejay, "Why going meatless saves the planet," *Vegetarianism and the Environment,* 2012.
9. "How Sustainable Agriculture Can Address the Environmental and Human Health Harms of Industrial Agriculture," *Environmental Health Perspectives,* 110(5), (May 2002). Accessed March 31, 2015 from http://wannaveg.com/
10. Kathy Freson, "The Startling Effects of Going Vegetarian for Just One Day," *Alternet.* (April 2, 2009) accessed on March 31, 2015 from http://www.chooseveg.com/environment. Unattributed statistics were calculated from scientific reports by Noam Mohr, a physicist with the New York University Polytechnic Institute.
11. NT Burkert et al., "Nutrition and Health – The Association between Eating Behavior and Various Health Parameters: A Matched Sample Study," *PLoS ONE,* 9(2014): e88278.

Part I

1. World Life Expectancy, "Dying of a broken heart," (LeDuc Media, 2011), Accessed March 3, 2015 from http://www.worldlifeexpectancy.com/news/broken-heart.

2. World Health Organization, 1948.
3. Jen Christensen, "A third of Americans use alternative medicine," (February 11, 2015), Accessed on March 31, 2015 from http://www.cnn.com/2015/02/11/health/feat-alternative-medicine-study/
4. Kathy Weiser, "Native American medicine - history and information," (Legends of America, 2012), Accessed March 3, 2015 from http://www.legendsofamerica.com/na-medicine.html.

Chapter 1

1. Lily Armstrong, "Carbon Monoxide Food Poisoning – what you need to know," *A Guide to Prevent Carbon Monoxide Poisoning* Accessed Mar 31, 2015 from http://www.carbon-monoxide-poisoning.com/article7-carbon-monoxide-food-poisoning.html
2. Martha Rosenberg, "We're Eating What? 9 Contaminants in US Meat," *OpEdNews.com*, (9/28/2013), Accessed Mar 31, 2015 from http://www.opednews.com/articles/2/We-re-Eating-What-9-Conta-by-Martha-Rosenberg-Animals_Animals_Beef_Cancer-130928-645.html.
3. "Carbon Monoxide: Masking the truth about meat?" *Food & Water Watch*, (2008), Accessed Mar 31, 2015 from http://documents.foodandwaterwatch.org/doc/CarbonMonoxide_web.pdf.
4. Kristen Michaelis, "Your apples are a year old," (foodrenegade.com, 2013), Accessed Mar 31, 2015 from http://www.foodrenegade.com/your-apples-year-old/.
5. James P Mattheis, "Keeping apples crunchy and flavorful after storage," *AgResearch Magazine*, (United States Department of Agriculture, October 2007), Accessed on April 12, 2015 from http://www.ars.usda.gov/is/AR/archive/oct07/apples1007.htm.
6. Valerie Liles, "List of chemicals used in food processing," (Demand Media Inc, 2011), Accessed March 31, 2015 from http://www.livestrong.com/article/419242-list-of-chemicals-used-in-food-processing/.
7. Joseph Mercola, "Aspartame: By far the most dangerous substance added to most foods today," (Joseph Mercola, 2011), Accessed March 3, 2015 from http://articles.mercola.com/sites/articles/archive/2011/11/06/aspartame-most-dangerous-substance-added-to-food.aspx
8. Samantha Olson, "Coca-Cola spreads lies about Aspartame and dangers of artificial sweetener," *Medical Daily* (IBT Media, Inc., 2014), Accessed March 3, 2015 from http://www.medicaldaily.com/coca-cola-spreads-lies-about-aspartame-and-dangers-artificial-sweetener-311300.
9. Coupon Sherpa, "Top 15 chemical additives in your food," (Phys.org, 2010), Accessed March 3, 2015 from http://phys.org/news183110037.html.
10. Barbara P Minton, "The Dangers of MSG," (Food Matters, 2010), Accessed April, 2015 from http://foodmatters.tv/articles-1/the-dangers-of-msg.
11. Kris Gunnars, "9 ways that processed foods are slowly killing people," (Authority Nutrition, 2014), Accessed March 3, 2015 from http://authoritynutrition.com/9-ways-that-processed-foods-are-killing-people/.
12. National Cancer Institute, "Acrylamide in food and cancer risk," (National Cancer Institute, 2008), Accessed March 3, 2015 from http://www.cancer.gov/cancertopics/causes-prevention/risk/diet/acrylamide-fact-sheet.

13. Acrylamide," International Agency for Research on Cancer, Accessed May 20, 2015 from http://monographs.iarc.fr/ENG/Monographs/vol60/mono60-16.pdf
14. K Svensson et al., "Dietary intake of acrylamide in Sweden," *Food and Chemical Toxicology*, 41 (2003):1581-1586.
15. Takashi Sugimura et al., "Heterocyclic amines: Mutagens/carcinogens produced during cooking of meat and fish," *Cancer Science,* 95 (2004):290-299.
16. "Heterocyclic Amines in cooked meats," (MedicineNet, Inc., 2005), Accessed March 3, 2015 from http://www.medicinenet.com/script/main/art.asp?articlekey=47818.
17. National Cancer Institute, "Chemicals in meat cooked at high temperatures and cancer risk," (National Cancer Institute, 2010), Accessed March 3, 2015 from http://www.cancer.gov/cancertopics/causes-prevention/risk/diet/cooked-meats-fact-sheet.
18. Alice G Walton, "How much sugar are Americans eating? [Infographic]," (Forbes.com LLC™, 2012), Accessed March 3, 2015 from http://www.forbes.com/sites/alicegwalton/2012/08/30/how-much-sugar-are-americans-eating-infographic/.
19. American Heart Association, "Frequently asked questions about sugar," (American Heart Association, Inc., 2014), Accessed March 3, 2015 from http://www.heart.org/HEARTORG/GettingHealthy/NutritionCenter/HealthyDietGoals/Frequently-Asked-Questions-About-Sugar_UCM_306725_Article.jsp.
20. Jacque Wilson, "WHO-proposed sugar recommendation comes to less than a soda per day," (Cable News Network, 2014), Accessed March 3, 2015 from http://www.cnn.com/2014/03/06/health/who-sugar-guidelines/.
21. American Liver Foundation, "NAFLD Non-Alcoholic Fatty Liver Disease," (American Liver Foundation, 2015), Accessed March 3, 2015 from http://www.liverfoundation.org/abouttheliver/info/nafld/.
22. R Jaffe and P Donovan, Your Health: A Professional User's Guide, (Sterling, VA: Health Studies Collegium, 1993).
23. P Belluck, "Children's Life Expectancy Being Cut Short by Obesity." The New York Times. Mar 17, 2005. Accessed 4/28/2012.
24. Stepaniak, J."The Name Game: Coming to Terms." Accessed Mar 17, 2015 from http://www.vegsource.com/jo/essays/namegame.htm.
25. Genesis 1:29.
26. G Mervyn et al., "Nonflesh Dietaries," *Journal of the American Dietetic Association,* 43 (1963):545.
27. George Parluski, "The History of the Vegetable Passion in the Orient," *Vegetarian Times* (March/April 1977): 17.
28. SS Altshuler, "The Historical and Biological Evolution of Human Diet," *American Journal of Digestive Disease,* 1 (1934):215.
29. "What's Wrong With Eating Meat?" *Amanda Marga Publications,* (1977): 5.
30. "Vegetarianism: A New Concept?" *National Health Journal* 2nd ed., 1 (Washington: Herald Pub. Assoc., 1973).
31. Colman McCarthy, "Meatless Meals: A Change in America's Menu," *Washington Post,* 13 Jan. 1976, 19.
32. Hardinge, "Nonflesh Dietaries."

33. Sarrat K Majunder, "Vegetarianism: Fad, Faith, or Fact?" *American Scientist,* 60 (March/April 1972).
34. Helen Zoe Veit, *Modern food, moral food: Self-control, science, and the rise of modern American eating in the early twentieth century* (Chapel Hill, North Carolina: The University of North Carolina Press, 2013)
35. S Lepkovsky, "The Bread Problem in War and Peace," *Physiological Review,* 24 (1944):239.
36. M Hindhede, "The Effect of Food Restriction During War on Mortality in Copenhagen," *Journal of the American Medical Association,* 74 (1920): 381.
37. A Strom and RA Jensen, "Mortality From Circulatory Diseases in Norway, 19401945," *Lancet,* 260 (1951):126.
38. "What's the current population of India?" (Yahoo, 2007) Accessed from https://answers.yahoo.com/question/index?qid=20080104100147AAtFgok
39. Accessed from http://en.wikipedia.org/wiki/Vegetarianism_in_specific_countries#India
40. "How many Vegetarians are there worldwide - or, What %tage of the world's population is vegetarian?" (Yahoo, 2007), Accessed from http://in.answers.yahoo.com/question/index?qid=20070221074745AARnMgh.
41. "The Connection between Psychological and Physical Health," Accessed from https://www.cqu.edu.au/__data/assets/pdf_file/0006/57282/The_Connection_between_Psychological_and_Physical_Health_slides_for_webinar_pdf.pdf
42. D Goldberg, "The detection and treatment of depression in the physically ill," *World Psychiatry*, 9 (2010):16-20.
43. "Review of Research Challenges Assumption that Success Makes People Happy: Happiness May Lead to Success via Positive Emotions," (American Psychological Association 2005), Accessed April, 2015 from http://www.apa.org/news/press/releases/2005/12/success.aspx.

Chapter 2

1. Remarks Bush made during a Social Security Conversation at the Athena Performing Arts Center in New York on May 24, 2005. Accessed March 31, 2015 from http://www.globalresearch.ca/may-i-quote-you-mr-president/3907
2. Robert F Kennedy, Jr., "CDC scientist still maintains agency forced researchers to lie about safety of mercury based vaccines," (Ring of Fire Radio, LLC., 2015), Accessed March 3, 2015 from http://www.ringoffireradio.com/2015/02/cdc-scientist-still-maintains-agency-forced-researchers-lie-safety-mercury-based-vaccines/
3. Ibid.
4. Marion Nestle, "Food Politics: How the Food Industry Influences Nutrition and Health" (University of California Press, 2002).
5. FDA News Release," (US Food and Drug Administration, 2008), Accessed April, 2015 from http://www.fda.gov/NewsEvents/Newsroom/PressAnnouncements/2008/ucm116836.htm.
6. About Cloned Animals," (Center for Food Safety), Accessed April, 2015 from http://www.centerforfoodsafety.org/issues/302/animal-cloning/about-cloned-animals
7. "Cloned animals," (RSPCA), Accessed April, 2015 from http://www.rspca.org.uk/adviceandwelfare/laboratory/biotechnology/clonedanimals.

8. "Factsheet on Animal Cloning," (The Humane Society of the United States, September 28, 2009) Accessed on March 15, 2015 from http://www.humanesociety.org/issues/cloning/qa/questions_answers.html.

9. Feng J He and Graham A MacGregor. "Effect of longer-term modest salt reduction on blood pressure." *Cochrane Database of Syst Rev.,* (2004). DOI: 10.1002/14651858.CD004937

10. Hillel W Cohen, et al., "Salt intake and cardiovascular mortality." *Am J Med.*, 120 (2007):e7.

11. World Health Organisation (2010). Creating an enabling environment for population-based salt reduction strategies: report of a joint technical meeting held by WHO and the Food Standards Agency, United Kingdom. Accessed on March 17, 2015 from http://whqlibdoc.who.int/publications/2010/9789241500777_eng.pdf

12. American Heart Association, "Frequently Asked Questions (FAQs) About Sodium" (May, 2014) Accessed on March 17, 2015 from http://www.heart.org/HEARTORG/GettingHealthy/NutritionCenter/HealthyEating/Frequently-Asked-Questions-FAQs-About-Sodium_UCM_306840_Article.jsp

13. Marion Nestle, "Food Politics: How the Food Industry Influences Nutrition and Health" (University of California Press, 2002).

14. Ibid.

15. Eric Schlosser, *Fast food nation: The dark side of the all-American meal* (Houghton Mifflin Company, 2001)

16. Helena Paul, "GM crops are driving genocide and ecocide - keep them out of the EU!" *The Ecologist*, (5 Feb 2014) Accessed on March 31, 2015 from http://www.theecologist.org/News/news_analysis/2267255/gm_crops_are_driving_genocide_and_ecocide_keep_them_out_of_the_eu.html

17. M Antoniou et al., "GMO Myths and Truths: An Evidence-Based Examination of the Claims Made for the Safety and Efficacy of Genetically Modified Crops," *Earth Open Source,* (June 2013):66.

18. "Roundup, An Herbicide, Could be Linked to Parkinson's, Cancer and Other Health Issues, Study Shows" (Reuters, April 25, 2013)

19. Gang Wang et al., "Parkinsonism after chronic occupational exposure to glyphosate," *Parkinsonism Relat Disord.*, 17 (2011):486-7.

20. Alejandra Paganelli et al., "Glyphosate-Based Herbicides Produce Teratogenic Effects on Vertebrates by Impairing Retinoic Acid Signaling," *Chem. Res. Toxicol.,* 23 (2010):1586-1595.

21. Sarath Gunatilake Channa Jayasumana and Priyantha Senanayake Glyphosate, "Hard Water and Nephrotoxic Metals: Are They the Culprits Behind the Epidemic of Chronic Kidney Disease of Unknown Etiology in Sri Lanka?" *Int. J. Environ. Res. Public Health,* 11 (2014):2125-2147.

22. Dario Aranda, "Cancer Danger in the GMO Fields" Pagina 12 (Argentina), June 23, 2014.

23. "Male Infertility," (American Pregnancy Association, 2014), Accessed April, 2015 from http://americanpregnancy.org/infertility/maleinfertility.html.

24. Amy Dean and Jennifer Armstrong, "Genetically Modified Foods," *American Academy of Environmental Medicine*, May 8, 2009. Accessed on April 3, 2015 from http://www.aaemonline.org/gmopost.html.

25. "GMO Dangers. Genetically Modified Foods: Are they Safe?" Institute for Responsible medicine. Accessed on April 3, 2015 from http://www.responsibletechnology.org/gmo-dangers

26. Claire Robinson, "Republication of the Seralini Study: Science Speaks for Itself." (GMOSeralini.org, June 24, 2014). Accessed on April 3, 2015 from http://www.gmoseralini.org/republication-seralini-study-science-speaks/.
27. Philip H Howard, "Organic Industry Structure: Acquisitions and Alliances, Top 100 Food Producers in America. 2013." Accessed on March 3, 2015 from https://www.msu.edu/~howardp/OrganicMay2013zoom.png
28. Beth Hoffman, "Who Owns Organic Brands And Why You Should Care," *Food & Drink* 5/25/2013. Accessed on March 3, 2015 from http://www.forbes.com/sites/bethhoffman/2013/05/25/who-owns-organic-brands-and-why-you-should-care/
29. Stephanie Ladwig Cooper, "Information and Funding Data from Cal" *Late and $5000+ Contributions Received* ONLY Accessed on Nov 13, 2012 from http://companiesopposegmofoodlabeling.blogspot.com/p/food-companies.html. See also http://cal-access.sos.ca.gov/Campaign/Committees/Detail.aspx?id=1344135&session=2011&view=late1
30. Andrew Dyke and Robert Whelan, "Memo to Consumers Union" (September 12, 2014), Accessed on March 3, 2015 from https://consumersunion.org/wp-content/uploads/2014/09/GMO_labeling_cost_findings_Exe_Summ.pdf.
31. "Electronic Code of Federal Regulations. e-CFR US Government Publishing Office." PART 205—NATIONAL ORGANIC PROGRAM. data is current as of May 1, 2015. Accessed on April 10, 2015 from http://www.ecfr.gov/cgi-bin/text-idx?rgn=div5&node=7:3.1.1.9.32
32. GMO-Awareness.com 2011–2014, Accessed on March 3, 2015 from http://gmo-awareness.com/shopping-list/family-organic-brands/.
33. "Family-Owned Organic GMO-Free Brands," (GMO-Awareness.com), Accessed April, 2015 from http://gmo-awareness.com/shopping-list/family-organic-brands/.
34. "Printable List of Monsanto Owned "Food" Producers," (REALfarmacy.com,) Accessed April, 2015 from http://www.realfarmacy.com/printable-list-of-monsanto-owned-food-producers/.
35. "Dietary Guidelines Advisory Committee Shows Plant-Based Diets Beat Animal Products for Health Promotion, Disease Prevention, Sustainability," (The Physicians Committee, 2015), Accessed April, 2015 from http://www.pcrm.org/media/news/dietary-guidelines-plant-based-promotion.
36. "Electronic Code of Federal Regulations".
37. Gary Null, *The New Vegetarian* (New York: Dell, 1978).
38. David Robinson Simon, *Meatonomics*, (Conari Press, 2013).
39. Harish, "Counting Animals: A Meat Industry Advertising," Blog post (May 7, 2012). Accessed on March 3, 2015 from http://www.countinganimals.com/meat-industry-advertising/
40. FJ Schlink and MC Phillips, *Meat Three Times a Day* (New York: Richard Smith, 1946), 54.
41. Ibid.
42. Boyce Rensberger, "Can Eating Less Meat Here Relieve Starvation in the World?" *New York Times,* (28 Nov. 1974), 44.
43. Ibid.
44. http://www.fas.usda.gov/dlp/circular/2006/06-03LP/bpppcc.pdf
45. "Per Capita Consumption of Poultry and Livestock, 1965 to Estimated 2015, in Pounds," National Chicken Council.(4/9/15), Accessed on March 3, 2015 from http://www.nationalchickencouncil.org/about-the-industry/statistics/per-capita-consumption-of-poultry-and-livestock-1965-to-estimated-2012-in-pounds/

46. "Seafood Choices: Overview of the US Seafood Supply," *Seafood Health Facts.* Accessed on March 3, 2015 from http://seafoodhealthfacts.org/pdf/seafood-choices-overview.pdf.
47. Jeanine Bentley, "Trends in US Per Capita Consumption of Dairy Products, 1970-2012," *USDA Economic Research Service.* (Jun 2, 2014).
48. "Egg Industry Fact Sheet Revised April 2015," United Egg Producers, *General US Stats.* Accessed on March 3, 2015 from http://www.unitedegg.org/GeneralStats/default.cfm.
49. Ibid.
50. Susan Levin, "Dairy Products and Bone Health, Letter to the Editor," *Journal of the American Dietetic Association,* (Jan 2007). Accessed on March 3, 2015 from http://www.pcrm.org/news/commentary070109.html
51. Oleg Sokolov, et al., "Autistic children display elevated urine levels of bovine casomorphin-7 immunoreactivity." *Peptides,* 56 (2014):68-71.
52. Jim Bartley and Susan Read McGlashan. "Does milk increase mucus production?" *Med Hypotheses,* 74 (2010):732-734.
53. MG Murray, et al., "Milk-induced wheezing in children with asthma." *Allergol Immunopathol (Madr).,* 41 (2013): 310-314.
54. Glenn Lorang, "We Raise Wheat for Feed," *Western Field* (September 1972): 25.
55. Rudolph Ballentine, *Diet and Nutrition* (Honesdale, Pa.: The Himalayan International Institute of Yoga Science and Philosophy, 1978).
56. Eric Barger, "A whopping 90 percent of Americans think they eat a healthy diet by January 4, 2001" Chrone.com Accessed on March 3, 2015 fromhttp://blog.chron.com/sciguy/2011/01/a-whopping-90-percent-of-americans-think-they-eat-a-healthy-diet/.
57. "Slow Food," (Slow Food, 2015), Accessed April, 2015 from http://www.slowfood.com/
58. Carle Honoré, "In Praise of Slow," Accessed April, 2015 from http://www.carlhonore.com/books/in-praise-of-slowness/
59. More information about the movement can be found on www.slowfood.com and www.slowmovement.com.
60. Pablo Monsivais, et al., "Time spent on home food preparation and indicators of healthy eating," *American Journal of Preventive Medicine,* 47 (2014):796-802.
61. Emily Caldwell, "Exercise or make dinner? Study finds adults trade one healthy act for another," (American Association for the Advancement of Science (AAAS), 2013), Accessed March 3, 2015 from http://www.eurekalert.org/pub_releases/2013-04/osu-eom040913.php
62. Ibid.
63. Mark Bittman, "The truth about home cooking," *Time* (Time Inc., 2014), Accessed March 3, 2015 from http://time.com/3483888/the-truth-about-home-cooking/
64. Centers for Disease Control and Prevention National Center for Health Statistics. Health, United States (2013). Accessed on March 3, 2015 from http://www.cdc.gov/nchs/fastats/obesity-overweight.htm.
65. "Food Security Status of US Households in 2013," US Department of Agriculture. Updated Jan 12, 2015. Accessed on March 3, 2015 from http://www.ers.usda.gov/topics/food-nutrition-assistance/food-security-in-the-us/key-statistics-graphics.aspx.
66. Carmen DeNavas-Walt and Bernadette D. Proctor, "Income and Poverty in the United States: 2013." *US Census Bureau, Current Population Reports,* (US Government Printing Office: Washington, DC, 2014): 60-249. Accessed on March 3, 2015 from http://www.census.gov/

content/dam/Census/library/publications/2014/demo/p60-249.pdf . See also http://www.worldhunger.org/articles/Learn/us_hunger_facts.htm

67. James B Mason, *Vegetarian Times* (January/February 1980): 40.

68. Economic Research Service, "Food availability (per capita) data system," (United States Department of Agriculture, 2014), Accessed March 3, 2015 from http://www.ers.usda.gov/data-products/food-availability-%28per-capita%29-data-system.aspx.

69. "US and international meat consumption chart," (ProCon.org, 2012), Accessed March 3, 2015 from http://vegetarian.procon.org/view.resource.php?resourceID=004716

70. Janet Larsen, "Meat consumption in China now double that in the United States," (Earth Policy Institute, 2012), Accessed March 3, 2015 from http://www.earth-policy.org/plan_b_updates/2012/update102

71. Karen Flynn, "Americans eating less meat, even as rest of world eats more," (Researchscape International, 2013), Accessed March 3, 2015 from http://www.researchscape.com/health/meat-consumption-trends

Chapter 3

1. Web Sites Plus, "Our food supply, environment, etc," Accessed March 3, 2015 from http://www.websites-host.com/toxic-food.html

2. Ker Than, "Organophosphates: A common but deadly pesticide," *National Geographic* (National Geographic Society, 2013), Accessed March 3, 2015 from http://news.nationalgeographic.com/news/2013/07/130718-organophosphates-pesticides-indian-food-poisoning/

3. R Blaylock (ed). "The Great Cancer Lie: It is Preventable and Beatable," *Blaylock Wellness Report.* (October, 2008).

4. K Pommer, "New Proteoloytic enzymes for the production of savory ingredients," *Cereal Foods World,* 40 (1995):745-748.

5. John L Gittleman, "Adaptation," *Encyclopædia Britannica* (Encyclopædia Britannica, Inc., 2014), Accessed March 3, 2015 from http://www.britannica.com/EBchecked/topic/5263/adaptation

6. Scott Holmberg, "Hidden Danger In Our Food," Channel 7 News (ABC), 7 November 1984.

7. Jo Robinson, "Grass-Fed Products are Clean and Safe," Accessed from http://www.eatwild.com/foodsafety.html.

8. Centers for Disease Control October 16, 2007. CDC estimates 94,000 invasive drug-resistant staph infections occurred in the US in 2005; Study establishes baseline for MRSA infection estimates. Accessed on March 3, 2015 from http://www.cdc.gov/media/pressrel/2007/r071016.htm.

9. Neal Barnard, "Meat Too Tough to Eat," *The Hartford Courant*, 28 Aug. 2006.

10. "Antibiotics Can Lead to Tainted Meat," *USA Today,* 6 Sept. 1984, Dl

11. "Chloramphenicol Use by Cattlemen Said to Be Dangerous," *Vegetarian Times* (September 1984): 6.

12. Ibid.

13. John Robbins, "The Truth About GrassFed Beef," blog entry (Dec. 19, 2012). Accessed on March 3, 2015 from http://foodrevolution.org/blog/the-truth-about-grassfed-beef/.

14. From Field to Feeder: Beef Cattle," (Homestead Organics, 2003), Accessed April, 2015 from http://www.homesteadorganics.ca/beef.aspx.

15. "Pesticide Environmental Fate One Line Summary: DDT," (Washington, DC.: US Environmental Protection Agency,1989); Augustijn-Beckers et al., "SCS/ARS/CES Pesticide Properties Database for Environmental Decisionmaking II," *Additional Properties Reviews of Environmental Contamination and Toxicology*, Vol. 137(1994). Accessed on March 3, 2015 http://pmep.cce.cornell.edu/profiles/extoxnet/carbaryl-dicrotophos/ddt-ext.html.

16. "Persistent Bioaccumulative and Toxic (PBT) Chemical Program: DDT," (US Environmental Protection Agency), Accessed from http://www.epa.gov/pbt/pubs/ddt.htm.

17. "Dangerous Chemicals in Meat," *Natural Living Newsletter* 40.

18. Robert Ballentine, "Dietary Suggestions for Chronic Pain," Accessed on March 3, 2015 from http://www.holistichealthservices.com/research/chronic_pain.html.

19. Paul Goettlich, "RoundupÒ: A Product of el Diablo," Mindfully.org, (25 May 2003). Accessed on March 3, 2015 from http://www.mindfully.org/Pesticide/2003/Roundup-El-Diablo25may03.htm.

20. AM Liebstein and Neil L Ehmki, "The Case for Vegetarianism," *American Mercury* (April 1950): 27.

21. Ibid.

22. Angela Fraser, et al., "What you can't see, can't hurt. Your kids and you! Preventing food-borne illness in your child care center or day care home," (Michigan State University, 1995), Accessed from http://web2.msue.msu.edu/bulletins/Bulletin/PDF/E2568.pdf.

23. Al B Wagner, "Bacterial Food Poisoning," (Texas A&M University), Accessed from http://aggie-horticulture.tamu.edu/extension/poison.html.

24. University of Pennsylvania School of Medicine, "Bacterial Toxin Closes Gate On Immune Response, Researchers Discover," (Science Daily, 2008), Accessed February 19, from http://www.sciencedaily.com/releases/2008/02/080213140826.htm.

25. Accessed from http://www.consumerreports.org/cro/consumer-protection/recalls-and-safety-alerts-3-08/rise-in-beef-contamination/recalls-beef-contamination.htm

26. David Migoya, "USDA Condones Use of Recalled Meat in Processed Food," *The Denver Post* (2 Aug 2002); Accessed on March 3, 2015 from http://archives.foodsafety.ksu.edu/fsnet/2002/8-2002/fsnet_august_3.htm.

27. Accessed from http://www.fsis.usda.gov/Fact_Sheets/Fighting_BAC_by_Chilling_Out/index.asp

28. Vince Patton, "Tillamook, Milk and GMO Hormones," (18 Feb 2005); Accessed on March 3, 2015 from http://www.mindfully.org/GE/2005/Monsanto-Posilac-rBGH18feb05.htm.

29. Samuel Epstein, "Monsanto's rBGH Genetically Modified Milk Ruled Unsafe by the United Nations;" Accessed on March 3, 2015 from www.mindfully.org/GE/Monsanto-rBGH-BGH-Unsafe-UN18aug99.htm.

30. Brian Tokar, "Monsanto: A Checkered History," reprinted from *The Ecologist,* Sep/Oct 1998, www.mindfully.org; http://www.mindfully.org/Industry/Monsanto-Checkered-HistoryOct98.htm

31. Samuel Epstein, "Monsanto's rBGH Genetically Modified Milk Ruled Unsafe by the United Nations," Accessed on March 3, 2015 from www.mindfully.org/GE/Monsanto-rBGH-BGH-Unsafe-UN18aug99.htm.

32. See *Hormone Research* 53 (2000):53-67, and "The devil in the milk," (Mercola, 2009), Accessed from http://www.mercola.com/2000/sep/10/milk_cancer.htm.

33. Samuel S Epstein, "What's In Your Milk?" Cancer Prevention Coalition, (2006); Accessed on March 3, 2015 from http://www.preventcancer.com/publications/WhatsInYourMilkRelease.htm.

34. Robert E Fontaine, et al., "Epidemic Salmonellosis From Cheddar Cheese: Surveillance and Prevention," *American Journal of Epidemiology,* 3 (1980):247251; "Officials Recall Cheeses After Link to 28 Deaths," *New York Times,* 14 June 1985, A12.

35. Cow's Milk: "A Natural Choice?" *Toronto Vegetarian Association*, (15 Mar 2005); Accessed on March 3, 2015 from http://veg.ca/content/view/139/110/.

36. "Human Health/Diet," *Delaware Action for Animals;* Accessed on March 3, 2015 from http://www.da4a.org/health.htm.

37. Robert Cohen, "Behold the Power of Antibiotics," *Dairy Education Board*, sponsor of notmilk.com; Accessed on February 2, 2008 from http://www.notmilk.com/forum/777.html

38. "Deadly Poisons From the Deep," *FishingHurts.com Webpage*, PETA, 2006; Accessed January 14, 2008.

39. Richard H Schwartz, "Troubled Waters: The Case Against Eating Fish," *Vegetarian Voice*, (2004).

40. Ibid.

41. Ibid.

42. Christine Stencel, "Consumers need better guidance to fully weigh possible benefits and risks when making seafood choices," *The National Academies*, press release,(17 Oct 2006); Accessed January 17, 2008 from http://www8.nationalacademies.org/onpinews/newsitem.aspx?RecordID=11762.

43. Ibid.

44. Hope Ferdowsian and Susan Levin, "Fish Still Not a Healthy Choice," *The Providence Journal*, 24 Oct. 2006; Accessed on March 3, 2015 from http://www.pcrm.org/news/commentary061024.html .

45. Amy Joy Lanou and Patrick Sullivan, "Something's Fishy on Federal Dietary Committee," *Physicians Committee for Responsible Medicine,* (13 Apr2004); Accessed on March 3, 2015 from http://www.pcrm.org/news/commentary0404.html.

46. Ibid.

47. X Hugan et al., "Consumption advisories for salmon based on risk of cancer and noncancer health effects." *Environmental Research,* 101 (2006):263-274.

48. "World fish stocks facing grim future" UN Food and Agriculture Organization. 19 May 2006.

49. J Alder, et al., "Forage Fish: From Ecosystems to Markets," *Annual Review of Environment and Resources*, 33 (2008):153-166.

50. Ibid.

51. "Big-Fish Stocks Fall 90 Percent Since 1950, Study Says," *National Geographic News* (National Geographic, 2003), Accessed April, 2015 from http://news.nationalgeographic.com/news/2003/05/0515_030515_fishdecline.html.

52. Ken Stier, "Fish Farming's Growing Dangers," *Time* (19 Sept 2007).

53. Wai Lang Chu, "Study warns excess fish farming drug use promotes resistance" *Drug Researcher.com,* (21 Jun 2006); Accessed on March 3, 2015 from http://www.drugresearcher.com/content/35563.

54. See "Pure Salmon Campaign," Accessed on March 3, 2015 from www.puresalmon.org.

55. "Opinion of the Scientific Committee on Animal Nutrition on the Use of Canthaxanthin in Feed for Salmon and Trout, Laying Hens and Other Poultry," (Brussels: European Commission, Health and Consumer Protection, 2002); Accessed on March 17, 2015 from http://ec.europa.eu/food/fs/sc/scan/out81_en.pdf

56. JG Dorea, "Fish meal in animal feed and human exposure to persistent bioaccumulative and toxic substances," *Journal of Food Protection,* 69 (2006):2777-2785.
57. "Farm Raised Fish Not So Safe." Environmental Working Group Report. (20 Mar 2008); http://nutrionresearchcenter.org/healthnews/farm-raised -fish-not-so-safe
58. D Hayward et al., "Polybrominated dipheylethers and polychlorinated biphenyls in commercially wild caught and farm-raised fish fillets in the United States." *Environmental Research,* 103 (2007):46-54.
59. "Agribusiness: Sector profile, 2015," (The Center for Responsive Politics, 2015), Accessed April, 2015 from https://www.opensecrets.org/lobby/indus.php?id=A.
60. Ibid.
61. Paul A Lauto, "Meat Company Exposed For Illegal Slaughter And Sale To Schools Of Downer Cattle," (2013), Accessed April, 2015 from http://www.liattorney.com/scales-of-justice/meat-company-exposed-for-illegal-slaughter-and-sale-to-schools-of-downer-cattle.
62. "Requirements for the Disposition of Non-Ambulatory Disabled Veal Calves," (USDA, Spring 2014). (9 CFR 309.13(b)) Accessed on March 3, 2015 from http://www.reginfo.gov/public/do/eAgendaViewRule?pubId=201404&RIN=0583-AD54
63. Michael Markarian, "Make a PACT to Stop Animal Cruelty," (Humane Society Legislative Fund, 2015), Accessed April, 2015 from http://blog.hslf.org/political_animal/.
64. Sam Zuckerman, "Food Ad Rogues' Gallery," *Nutrition Action* (September 1984):5.
65. "CDC estimates of foodborne illness in the United States: Contribution of different food commodities (categories) to estimated domestically-acquired illnesses and deaths, 1998-2008," (Centers for Disease Control and Prevention, 2013), Accessed March 3, 2015 from http://www.cdc.gov/foodborneburden/attribution-image.html#foodborne-illnesses
66. http://www.umm.edu/altmed/articles/food-poisoning-000064.htm
67. Lauren Neergaard, "Food poisoning can be long-term health problem," Pantagram.com, (22 Jan. 2008); Accessed on March 3, 2015 from http://www.pantagraph.com/articles/2008/01/22/news/doc4794de83d9002067069057.txt.
68. "Raw milk/cheese (Listeria, salmonella, e.coli, etc.) contamination reports," *Pritzker-Ruohonen Law;* Accessed on March 3, 2015 from http://www.pritzkerlaw.com.
69. Accessed from http://www.consumerreports.org/cro/consumer-protection/recalls-and-safety-alerts-3-08/rise-in-beef-contamination/recalls-beef-contamination.htm
70. Victoria Kim, "Undercover tape of abused cattle being slaughtered at a Chino plant raises questions about inspection process." *Los Angeles Times,* (7 Feb. 2008).
71. Lydia Zuraw, "2.5 Million Pounds of Meat, Poultry Recalled for Pathogen Contamination in 2014," (Food Safety News, 2015), Accessed April, 2015 from http://www.foodsafetynews.com/2015/01/fsis-releases-summary-of-2014-recalls/#.VV2oUIvleFJ.
72. "California Slaughterhouse Shuts Down After Massive Beef Recall," *Huffington Post* (02/11/2014) Updated: 04/13/2014.
73. Accessed from http://www.farmedanimal.net/faw/faw8-5.htm
74. Ibid.
75. Institute of Medicine, "Cattle Inspection," (The National Academies Press, 1990), Accessed from http://books.nap.edu/openbook.php?record_id=1588&page=11.

76. "Food Safety As It Relates to the North American Free Trade Agreement," Testimony of William Lehman before the House Energy and Commerce Committee (18 February 1993).
77. Ibid.
78. Peter M Schantz, "Trichinosis in the United States, 1975: Increase in Cases Attributed to Numerous CommonSource Outbreaks," *The Journal of Infectious Diseases,* 136 (1977):712715.
79. Ibid.
80. "Listeria (Listeriosis)," Centers for Disease Control and Prevention (December 4, 2013), Accessed April 4, 2015 from http://www.cdc.gov/listeria/risk.html
81. Scott Holmberg, "Hidden Danger In Our Food," Channel 7 News (ABC), 7 November 1984.
82. Harold E Sours and Owan G Smith, "Outbreaks of Foodborne Disease in the United States, 19721978," *The Journal of Infectious Diseases,* 142 (1980):122125.
83. Senate Select Committee on Nutrition and Human Needs, *Dietary Goals for the United States* (Washington, D.C., 1977).
84. "Paleo Leap," (Paleo Leap, LLC, 2015), Accessed March 3, 2015 from http://paleoleap.com/.
85. Smith et al., "Unrestricted Paleolithic diet is associated with unfavorable changes to blood lipids in healthy subjects," Int J Exerc Sci., 7 (2014):128-139.
86. Indre Viskontas and Kishore Hari "Interview with Michael Pollan: 17 Michael Pollan - The Science of Eating Well (And Not Falling For Diet Fads)" (Jan 16, 2014)
87. Rob Dunn, "Human Ancestors Were Nearly All Vegetarians," *Scientific American,* (Jul 23, 2012).
88. Karen Hardy et al., "Neanderthal medics? Evidence for food, cooking, and medicinal plants entrapped in dental calculus," *Naturwissenschaften,* 99 (2012):617-626.
89. Erica Eelson, "Can Seven Billion Humans Go Paleo?" *Earth Island Journal.* (Feb 2, 2015). Accessed on March 3, 2015 from http://www.earthisland.org/journal/index.php/elist/eListRead/can_seven_billion_humans_go_paleo/.
90. DL Katz and S Meller, "Can We Say What Diet Is Best for Health?" *Annual Review of Public Health,* 35 (2014):83-103.
91. A Akesson, "Low-risk diet and lifestyle habits in the primary prevention of myocardial infarction in men: a population-based prospective cohort study," *J Am Coll Cardiol.*, 64 (2014):1299-1306.
92. H Du et al., "Fresh fruit consumption, blood pressure and cardiovascular disease risk: a prospective cohort study of 0.5 million adults in the China Kadoorie Biobank," Report presented at: European Society of Cardiology Congress 2014 Barcelona, Spain(Sept 1, 2014).
93. S Li et al., "Low carbohydrate diet from plant or animal sources and mortality among myocardial infarction survivors," *J Am Heart Assoc.* , 3 (2014): e001169.
94. Centers for Disease Control and Prevention. CDC Features. (Feb 12, 2014). http://www.cdc.gov/features/heartmonth/. Accessed on January 9, 2015 from http://www.pcrm.org/health/diets/ffl/employee/animal-protein-linked-to-early-death.
95. Ibid.
96. MS Farvid, et al., "Dietary protein sources in early adulthood and breast cancer incidence: prospective cohort study," *BMJ, 348* (2014):g3437.
97. Physicians Committee for Responsible Medicine, "Five protein myths," (The Physicians Committee, 2015), Accessed March 3, 2015 from http://www.pcrm.org/health/reports/five-protein-myths.
98. United States Department of Agriculture, "Steak," Accessed April, 2015 from http://www.google.com/search?q=how+much+fat+in+sirloin+steak&ie=utf-8&oe=utf-8&gws_rd=ssl.

99. KN Sourbeer et al., "Metabolic syndrome components and prostate cancer risk: results from the Reduce study," Presented at: American Urological Association 2014 Annual Meeting; (Orlando, Fla. May 20, 2014).

100. S Li et al., "Low carbohydrate diet from plant or animal sources and mortality among myocardial infarction survivors." *J Am Heart Assoc.*, 3 (2014):e001169.

Chapter 4

1. "Scientific Report of the 2015 Dietary Guidelines Advisory Committee," USDA, 2015.

2. Kathleen M Zelman, "Dietary fiber: Insoluble vs. soluble," (WebMD, LLC., 2010), Accessed March 3, 2015 from http://www.webmd.com/diet/insoluble-soluble-fiber.

3. Ibid.

4. DP Burkitt and NS Painter, "Dietary Fiber and Disease," *Journal of the American Medical Association,* 229 (1974):10681074.

5. Burkitt and Painter, 1974.

6. Ibid.

7. Ibid.

8. "Meat and Potatoes Still Number One," *USA Today,* (4 Dec 1984).

9. Pape MaWhinney, et al., "Human Prion Disease and Relative Risk Associated with Chronic Wasting Disease," *Emerging Infectious Diseases,* 12 (2006):1527-35.

10. Kate Marsh et al., "Health Implications of a Vegetarian Diet: A Review," *American Journal of Lifestyle Medicine,* 6 (2012):250-267.

11. Baungartner RN et al, "Predictors of skeletal muscle mass in elderly men and women," *Mech aging development,* 107 (1999):123-36.

12. "Vegetarian Diets Can Help Prevent Chronic Diseases, American Dietetic Association Says," *Science Daily*. (Jul 3, 2009). Accessed on March 14, 2013 from: http://www.sciencedaily.com/releases/2009/07/090701103002.htm

13. VR Young and PL Pellet, "Plant proteins in relation to human protein and amino acid nutrition. *Am J Clin Nutr*. 59 (1994):1203S-1212S.

14. Ioan Drăgan et al., "Studies regarding the efficiency of Supro isolated soy protein in Olympic athletes. *Rev Roum Physiol.*, 29 (1992):63-70.

15. "54 million Americans affected by Osteoporosis and low bone mass," (National Osteoporosis Foundation, 2014), Accessed March 3, 2015 from http://nof.org/news/2948

16. Robert G Cumming and Robin J Klineberg. "Case-control study of risk factors for hip fractures in the elderly." *Am J Epidemiol.,* 139 (1994):493-503.

17. Jacqueline Hoare, et al., "The National Diet and Nutrition Survey – Adults aged 19-64 years," Summary Report. *Food Standards Agency*, 5, (2004). HMSO: London.

18. Justine Butler, "Boning up on Calcium!," (Vegetarian and Vegan Foundation, 2005), Accessed March 3, 2015 from http://www.vegetarian.org.uk/factsheets/calciumfactsheet.html

19. "Food and your bones," (National Osteoporosis Foundation), Accessed March 3, 2015 from http://nof.org/foods

20. LJ Beilin and BM Margetts, "Vegetarian Diet and Blood Pressure," *Biblthca Cardiology,* 41(1987):85105.

21. LJ Beilin, et al., "Vegetarian Diet and Blood Pressure Levels: Incidental or Causal Association?" *The American Journal of Clinical Nutrition,* 48 (1988):806810.

22. GBD 2013 Mortality and Causes of Death Collaborators. "Global, regional, and national age-sex specific all-cause and cause-specific mortality for 240 causes of death, 1990-2013: a systematic analysis for the Global Burden of Disease Study 2013.".*Lancet* 385 (2015):117–171.
23. Caldwell B Esselstyn, "Prevent and Reverse Heart Disease." Avery (February 1, 2007).
24. Caldwell B Esselstyn, Jr, et al., "A way to reverse CAD?" *Journal of Family Practice,* 63 (2014):356-364.
25. IL Rouse et al., "Vegetarian Diet, Blood Pressure and Cardiovascular Risk," *Australian & New Zealand Journal of Medicine,* 14 (1984):439443.
26. B Armstrong et al, "Blood Pressure in SeventhDay Adventist Vegetarians," *American Journal of Epidemiology,* 105 (1977): 444449.
27. [216] R0 West and 0B Hayes, "Diet and Serum Cholesterol Levels," *The American Journal of Clinical Nutrition,* 21 (1968):853862.
28. J Ruys and JG Hickie, "Serum Cholesterol and Triglyceride Levels in Australian Adolescent Vegetarians," *British Medical Journal,* (1976): 87.
29. LA Simons et al., "The Influence of a Wide Range of Absorbed Cholesterol on Plasma Cholesterol Levels in Man," *The American Journal of Clinical Nutrition,* 31 (1978):13341339.
30. L Phillips, et al., "Coronary Heart Disease Mortality Among SeventhDay Adventists with Differing Dietary Habits: A Preliminary Report," *The American Journal of Clinical Nutrition,* 31 (October 1978):S191S198.
31. Francesca L Crowe, et al., "Risk of hospitalization or death from ischemic heart disease among British vegetarians and nonvegetarians: results from the EPIC-Oxford cohort study," *American Journal of Clinical Nutrition,* (2013).ajcn.112.044073.
32. "Introduction," (EPIC-Oxford), Accessed March 3, 2015 from http://www.epic-oxford.org/introduction/
33. Robert A Koeth et al. "Intestinal microbiota metabolism of L-carnitine, a nutrient in red meat, promotes atherosclerosis." *Nature Medicine,* 19 (2013):576–585.
34. "Vegetarian diets," (American Heart Association, 2014), Accessed March 16, 2015 from http://www.heart.org/HEARTORG/GettingHealthy/NutritionCenter/Vegetarian-Diets_UCM_306032_Article.jsp
35. Manish J Parswani, et al., "Mindfulness-based stress reduction program in coronary heart disease: A randomized control trial," *International Journal of Yoga,* 6 (2013):111–117.
36. Jon Kabat-Zinn, "An outpatient program in behavioural medicine for chronic pain patients based on the practice of mindfulness meditation: Theoretical consideration and preliminary results." *Gen Hosp Psychiatry,* 4 (1982):33–47.
37. John J Miller et al., "Three-year follow-up and clinical implications of a mindfulness meditation-based stress reduction intervention in the treatment of anxiety disorders." *Gen Hosp Psychiatry,* 17 (1995):192–200.
38. Wolfgang Linden et al. "Psychosocial interventions for patients with coronary artery disease: a meta-analysis," *Arch Intern Med.,* 156 (1996):745–752.
39. JW Zamarra, et al., "Usefulness of the TM program in the treatment of patients with coronary artery disease." *Am. J. Cardiol.,* 78 (1996):77-80.
40. Ibid.
41. Dean Ornish et al., "Effects of stress management training and dietary changes in treating ischemic heart disease." *JAMA,* 249 (1983):54-59.

42. TJ Key et al., "Mortality in Vegetarians and Nonvegetarians: Detailed Findings From a Collaborative Analysis of 5 Prospective Studies," *American Journal of Clinical Nutrition,* 70 (1999):516S-524S
43. Gary Fraser et al., "Vegetarian diets and cardiovascular risk factors in black members of the Adventist Health Study-2." *Public Health Nutrition,* 18 (2015):537-545.
44. "Leading causes of death." FastStats. Centers for Disease Control and Prevention. 2013. http://www.cdc.gov/nchs/fastats/leading-causes-of-death.htm
45. FJ He et al., "Fruit and Vegetable Consumption and Stroke: Meta-Analysis of Cohort Studies," *The Lancet,* 367 (2006):320-326.
46. PN Appleby et al., "Hypertension and Blood Pressure Among Meat Eaters, Fish Eaters, Vegetarians and Vegans in EPIC-Oxford," *Public Health Nutrition,* 5 (2002):645-654.
47. "Welcome to Adventist Health Studies," (Loma Linda University), Accessed March 16, 2015 from http://www.llu.edu/public-health/health/index.page?
48. FR Ellis FR and P Mumlord, "The nutritional status of vegans and vegetarians" *Proc Nutr Soc.,* 26 (1967):205-12.
49. Neal Barnard, "Witness statement," (Mc spotlight), Accessed from http://www.mcspotlight.org/people/witnesses/nutrition/barnard_neal.html.
50. Ibid.
51. B Armstrong and R Doll, "Environmental Factors and Cancer Incidence and Mortality in Different Countries with Special Reference to Dietary Practices," *International Journal of Cancer,* 15 (1975):617631.
52. RL Phillips et al., "Cancer Mortality among Comparable Members Versus Nonmembers of the SeventhDay Adventist Church," *Banbury Report 4: Cancer Incidence in Defined Populations*, New York: (Cold Spring Harbor Laboratory, 1980), 93107.
53. Michael J Orlich et al., "Vegetarian Dietary Patterns and the Risk of Colorectal Cancers." *JAMA Intern Med.,* 175 (2015):767-776.
54. Loma Linda University Adventist Health Sciences Center. "Vegetarians may be at lower risk of heart disease, diabetes and stroke." *ScienceDaily*. (17 Apr 2011). Accessed on March 3, 2015 from www.sciencedaily.com/releases/2011/04/110413133026.htm.
55. RL Phillips, "Cancer Among SeventhDay Adventists," *Journal of Environmental Pathology and Toxicology,* 3 (1980):157169.
56. Atif B Awad and Carol S Fink, "Phytosterols as Anticancer Dietary Components: Evidence and Mechanism of Action," *Journal of Nutrition,* 130 (2000):2127-2130.
57. Eduardo De Stefani, et al., "Plant Sterols and Risk of Stomach Cancer: A Case-Control Study in Uruguay," *Nutrition and Cancer,* 37 (2000):140-144.
58. AL Normén et al., "Plant Sterol Intakes and Colorectal Cancer Risk in the Netherlands Cohort Study on Diet and Cancer," *The American Journal of Clinical Nutrition,* 74 (2001):141-148.
59. MJ Goldberg et al., "Comparison of the Fecal Microflora of SeventhDay Adventists with Individuals Consuming a General Diet: Implications Concerning Colonic Carcinoma," *Annals of Surgery,* (1977): 97100.
60. N Turjman, et al., "Faecal BileAcids and Neutral Sterols in SeventhDay Adventists and the General Population in California," in Kasper and Golbel (eds.), *Colon and Cancer,* Falk Symposium 32, (Lancaster, England: MTP Press, Ltd., 1982): 291297.

61. BM Calkins, et al., "Diet, Nutrition, Intake, and Metabolism in Populations at High and Low Risk for Colon Cancer," *The American Journal of Clinical Nutrition,* 40 (1984):887895.
62. SM Finegold and VL Sutter, "Fecal Flora in Different Populations, with Special Reference to Diet," *The American Journal of Clinical Nutrition,* 31 (1978):S116S122.
63. PP Nair, et al., "Diet, Nutrition Intake, and Metabolism in Populations at High and Low Risk for Colon Cancer," *The American Journal of Clinical Nutrition,* 40 (1984):931936.
64. PK Mills, et al., "Cohort Study of Diet, Lifestyle, and Prostate Cancer in Adventist Men," *Cancer,* 64 (1989):598604.
65. BJ Howie and TD Shultz, "Dietary and Hormonal Interrelationships Among Vegetarian SeventhDay Adventists and Nonvegetarian Men," *The American Journal of Clinical Nutrition,* 42 (1985):127134.
66. PK Mills et al., "Cancer Incidence Among California SeventhDay Adventists, 19761982," *The American Journal of Clinical Nutrition,* 59 (1994):1136S-1142S.
67. American Cancer Society, "What's new in prostate cancer research and treatment?" (American Cancer Society 2015), Accessed March 16, 2015 from http://www.cancer.org/cancer/prostatecancer/detailedguide/prostate-cancer-new-research.
68. Dennis Thompson, Jr., "Eat vegetarian, prevent prostate cancer?" (Everyday Health Media, LLC, 2011), Accessed March 16, 2015 from http://www.everydayhealth.com/prostate-cancer/eat-vegetarian-prevent-prostate-cancer.aspx.
69. WW Bassett et al., "Impact of obesity on prostate cancer recurrence after radical prostatectomy: data from CaPSURE," *Urology*, 66 (2005):1060-1065.
70. [256] PK Mills et al., "Dietary Habits and Past Medical History as Related to Fatal Pancreas Cancer Risk Among Adventists," *Cancer,* 61 (1988):25782585.
71. PK Mills et al., "Risk Factors for Tumors of the Brain and Cranial Meninges in SeventhDay Adventists," *Neuroepidemiology,* 8 (1989):266275.
72. BK Armstrong et al., "Diet and Reproductive Hormones: A Study of Vegetarian and Nonvegetarian Postmenopausal Women," *Journal of the National Cancer Institute,* 67 (1981):761767.
73. Kathleen O'Grady, "Early puberty for girls: The new "normal" and why we need to be concerned," *Women's Health Activist Newsletter* (National Women's Health Network, 2009), Accessed March 16, 2015 from https://nwhn.org/early-puberty-girls-new-%E2%80%9Cnormal%E2%80%9D-and-why-we-need-be-concerned.
74. A Sanchez et al., "A Hypothesis on the Etiological Role of Diet on Age of Menarche," *Medical Hypotheses,* 7 (1981):13391345.
75. J Sabate et al., "Lower Height of LactoOvovegetarian Girls at Preadolescence: An Indicator of Physical Maturation Delay," *Journal of the American Dietetic Association,* 92 (1992):12631264.
76. FA Tylavsky and JB Anderson, "Dietary Factors in Bone Health of Elderly Lactoovovegetarian and Omnivorous Women," *The American Journal of Clinical Nutrition,* 48 (1988):842849.
77. AG Marsh, et al., "Cortical Bone Density of Adult Lactoovovegetarian and Omnivorous Women," *Journal of the American Dietetic Association,* 76 (1980):148151.
78. D Feskanich et al., "Dietary calcium, and bone fractures in women: a 12-year prospective study," *American Journal of Public Health,* 876 (1997):992-7.

79. Vivian Goldschmidt, "Debunking the milk myth: Why milk is bad for you and your bones," (Save Institute, 2010), Accessed March 16, 2015 from http://saveourbones.com/osteoporosis-milk-myth/.

80. Robert G Cumming and Robin J Klineberg. "Case-control study of risk factors for hip fractures in the elderly." *Am J Epidemiol.,* 139 (1994):493-503.

81. Lan T Ho-Pham et al. "Effect of vegetarian diets on bone mineral density: a Bayesian meta-analysis." *American Society for Nutrition,* 90 (2009): 43-950.

82. Lan T Ho-Pham et al. "Vegetarianism, bone loss, fracture and vitamin D: a longitudinal study in Asian vegans and non-vegans." *Eur J Clin Nutr.,* 66 (2012):75-82.

83. The Nutrition Source, "Calcium and milk: What's best for your bones and health?" (Harvard T.H. Chan School of Public Health, 2008), Accessed March 16, 2015 from http://www.hsph.harvard.edu/nutritionsource/calcium-full-story/

84. E Linkosalo, "Dietary Habits and Dental Health in Finnish SeventhDay Adventists," *Proceedings of the Finnish Dental Society,* 84 (1988):109115.

85. DC Nieman et al., "Hematological, Anthropometic, and Metabolic Comparisons Between Vegetarian and Nonvegetarian Elderly Women," *International Journal of Sports Medicine,* 10 (1989):243250.

86. J Sabate et al., "Anthropometric Parameters of Schoolchildren with Different Lifestyles," *American Journal of Diseases of Children,* 144 (1990):11591163.

87. DA Snowdon and RL Phillips, "Does a Vegetarian Diet Reduce the Occurrence of Diabetes?" *American Journal of Public Health,* 75 (1985):507512.

88. HA Kahn, et al., "Association between Reported Diet and AllCause Mortality: TwentyOne Year FollowUp on 27,530 Adult SeventhDay Adventists," *American Journal of Epidemiology,* 119 (1984):775787.

89. IW Webster and 0K Rawson, "Health Status of SeventhDay Adventists," *The Medical Journal of Australia,* (1979):417420.

90. N Nnakwe et al., "Calcium and Phosphorus Nutritional Status of Lactoovovegetarian and Omnivore Students Consuming Meals in a Lactoovovegetarian Food Service," *Nutrition Reports International,* 29 (1984):365369.

91. DC Nieman et al., "Dietary Status of SeventhDay Adventist Vegetarian and NonVegetarian Elderly Women," *Journal of the American Dietetic Association,* 89 (1989):17631769.

92. IF Hunt et al., "Food and Nutrient Intake of SeventhDay Adventist Women," *The American Journal of Clinical Nutrition,* 48 (1988):850851.

93. KA Lombard and DM Mock, "Biotin Nutritional Status of Vegans, Lacto-ovo-vegetarians, and Nonvegetarians," *The American Journal of Clinical Nutrition,* 50 (1989):486490.

94. BM Calkins, "Consumption of Fiber in Vegetarians and Nonvegetarians," in 0A Spiller and D Chern, *CRC Handbook of Dietary Fiber in Human Nutrition* (Boca Raton, Fl.: CRC Press, 1986): 407414.

95. TD Shultz and JE Leklem, "Vitamin B6 Status and Bioavailability in Vegetarian Women," *The American Journal of Clinical Nutrition,* 46 (1987):647651.

96. RL Phillips and DA Snowdon, "Mortality Among SeventhDay Adventists in Relation to Dietary Habits and Lifestyle," in R.L. Ory (ed.), *Plant Proteins: Applications, Biological Effects, and Chemistry,* (Washington, D.C.: American Chemical Society, 1986).

97. UD Register, "The SeventhDay Adventist Diet and LifeStyle and the Risk of Major Degenerative Disease," in *Frontiers in Longevity Research*:7482.

98. Francesca L Crowe, et al., "Risk of hospitalization or death from ischemic heart disease among British vegetarians and nonvegetarians: results from the EPIC-Oxford cohort study," *American Journal of Clinical Nutritio,n* (2013).ajcn.112.044073.

99. "Vegetarianism Can Reduce the Risk of Heart Disease by Up to a Third," *ScienceDaily*. (Jan 30, 2013). Accessed on March 3, 2015 from http://www.sciencedaily.com/releases/2013/01/130130121637.htm. Accessed March 21, 2013.

100. SF Knutsen, "Lifestyle and the Use of Health Services," *The American Journal of Clinical Nutrition*, 59 (1994):1171S1 175S.

Chapter 5

1. WS Collens and GB Dobkin, "Phylogenetic Aspects of the Cause of Human Atherosclerotic Disease," *Circulation*, 32 (1965):7.

2. Philip L White and Nancy Selvey, *Let's Talk About Foods* (Acton, Mass.: Publishing Sciences Group, 1974).

3. Alex Hershaft and Lori Sonken, "Mark Hegsted: A Closeup of the Federal Government's Chief Nutritionist," *Vegetarian Times*, 41 (May 1983).

4. DM Hegsted, et al., "Lysine and Methionine Supplementation of AllVegetable Diets for Human Adults," *Journal of Nutrition*, 56 (1955):555-576.

5. "Meatless Diet Urged by Mexican Government," *Vegetarian Times* (June 1982): 7.

6. "AMA Attacks Vegetarian Diet," *Vegetarian Times* (May/June 1979):810.

7. Ibid.

8. FR Ellis, "The Nutritional Status of Vegans and Vegetarians," *Proceedings of the Nutrition Society*, 26 (1967):205211.

9. Lignans for Life, "Lignans health benefits," (Products Development, LLC.), Accessed March 16, 2015 from http://www.lignans.net/health-benefits.html.

10. Igho J Onakpoya et al., "The effect of chlorogenic acid on blood pressure: a systematic review and meta-analysis of randomized clinical trials." *Journal of Human Hypertension*, 29 (2014):77-81.

11. Adrian J Parr et al., "Dihydrocaffeoyl polyamines (kukoamine and allies) in potato (Solanum tuberosum) tubers detected during metabolite profiling." *J. Agric. Food Chem.*, 53 (2005):5461-6.

12. Mitsuyoshi Kano et al., "Antioxidative activity of anthocyanins from purple sweet potato, Ipomoera batatas cultivar Ayamurasaki." *Biosci Biotechnol Biochem.*, 69 (2005):979-88.

13. Priya Ramnani et al., "Prebiotic effect of fruit and vegetable shots containing Jerusalem artichoke inulin: a human intervention study." *British Journal of Nutrition*, 104 (2010):233-240.

14. Anne L Coleman et al., "Glaucoma risk and the consumption of fruits and vegetables among older women in the study of osteoporotic fractures." *Am J Ophthalmol.*, 145 (2008):1081-9.

15. Stip Purup et al. "Differential Effects of Falcarinol and Related Aliphatic C17-Polyacetylenes on Intestinal Cell Proliferation." *J Agric Food Chem.*, 57 (2009):8290-8296.

16. Alhaji U. N'jai et al. "Spanish black radish (Raphanus sativus L. Var. niger) diet enhances clearance of DMBA and diminishes toxic effects on bone marrow progenitor cells." *Nutr Cancer*, 64 (2012):1038-48.

17. Francesco Forastiere et al., "Consumption of fresh fruit rich in vitamin C and wheezing symptoms in children." *Thorax* 55, (2000):283-288.

18. Xiang Wu et al. "Are isothiocyanates potential anti-cancer drugs?" *Acta Pharmacologica Sinica,* 30 (2009):501–512.

19. Masataka Shiraki et al, "Vitamin K2 (menatetrenone) effectively prevents fractures and sustains lumbar bone mineral density inosteoporosis." *J Bone Miner Res.,* 15 (2000):515-21.

20. Stip Purup et al., "Differential Effects of Falcarinol and Related Aliphatic C17-Polyacetylenes on Intestinal Cell Proliferation." *J Agric Food Chem.,* 57 (2009):8290-8296.

21. Pamela J Mink et al., "Flavonoid intake and cardiovascular disease mortality: a prospective study in postmenopausal women." *Am J Clin Nutr.,* 85 (2007):895-909.

22. Carlotta Galeone et al., "Onion and garlic use and human cancer." *Am J Clin Nutr.* 84 (2006):1027-32.

23. Garlic and Cancer Prevention Factsheet," (National Cancer Institute. 2008). Accessed on March 15, 2015 from http://www.cancer.gov/cancertopics/causes-prevention/risk/diet/garlic-fact-sheet

24. Martha L Slattery et al., "Carotenoids and colon cancer." *American Society for Clinical Nutrition,* 71 (2000):575-582.

25. Vasil G. Georgiev et al. "Antioxidant activity and phenolic content of betalain extracts from intact plants and hairy root cultures of the red beetroot Beta vulgaris cv. Detroit dark red." *Plant Foods Hum Nutr.,* 65 (2010):105-11.

26. Seung-Hee Kim and Kyung-Chul Choi. "Anti-cancer Effect and Underlying Mechanism(s) of Kaempferol, a Phytoestrogen, on the Regulation of Apoptosis in Diverse Cancer Cell Models." *Toxicol Res.,* 29 (2013):229–234.

27. Priya Ramnani et al., "Prebiotic effect of fruit and vegetable shots containing Jerusalem artichoke inulin: a human intervention study." *British Journal of Nutrition,* 104 (2010):233-240.

28. Prebiotic Canada, "Inulin," (Prebiotic Canada), Accessed March 16, 2015 from http://www.prebiotic.ca/inulin.html.

29. André Dejam and Mark T. Gladwin, "Effects of Dietary Nitrate on Blood Pressure." *N Engl J Med.,* 356 (2007):1590.

30. Igho J Onakpoya et al., "The effect of chlorogenic acid on blood pressure: a systematic review and meta-analysis of randomized clinical trials." *Journal of Human Hypertension,* 29 (2014):77-81.

31. Srinibas Das et al., "Cancer modulation by glucosinolates: A review." *Current Science,* 79 (2000):1665-1670.

32. Teresita Guardia et al., "Anti-inflammatory properties of plant flavonoids. Effects of rutin, quercetin, and hesperidin on adjuvant arthritis in rat." *Farmaco,* 56 (2001):683-687.

33. Sarah Egert et al., "Quercetin reduces systolic blood pressure and plasma oxidised low-density lipoprotein concentrations in overweight subjects with a high-cardiovascular disease risk phenotype: a double-blinded, placebo-controlled cross-over study." *Br J Nutr.,* 102 (2009):1065-74.

34. Dorothy R Pathak et al., "Joint association of high cabbage/sauerkraut intake at 12-13 years of age and adulthood with reduced breast cancer risk in polish migrant women: results from the US component of the Polish women's health study." Presented at the 4th annual American Association for Cancer Research Conference on Frontiers in Cancer Prevention Research conference. (Baltimore, Maryland, October 2005).

35. JP San Giovanni et al., "The relationship of dietary carotenoid and vitamin A, E, and C intake with age-related macular degeneration in a case-control study: AREDS Report No. 22," *Arch. Ophthalmol.,* 125 (2007):1225–32.

36. Stuart Richer et al., "Double-masked, placebo-controlled, randomized trial of lutein and antioxidant supplementation in the intervention of atrophic age-related macular degeneration: the Veterans LAST study (Lutein Antioxidant Supplementation Trial)."*Optometry,* 75 (2004):216–30.

37. Kiminori Matsubara et al., "Inhibitory effect of glycolipids from spinach on in vitro and ex vivo angiogenesis." *Oncol Rep.,* 14 (2005):157-60.

38. Jennifer Di Noia, "Defining Powerhouse Fruits and Vegetables: A Nutrient Density Approach: A Nutrient Density Approach." *Prev Chronic Dis.,* 11 (2014):130390.

39. Talwinder Singh Kahlon et al., "Steam cooking significantly improves in vitro bile acid binding of collard greens, kale, mustard greens, broccoli, green bell pepper, and cabbage." *Nutrition Research,* 28 (2008):351-7.

40. Jennifer Di Noia, "Defining Powerhouse Fruits and Vegetables: A Nutrient Density Approach: A Nutrient Density Approach." *Prev Chronic Dis.,* 11 (2014):130390.

41. Rose K. Davidson et al., "Sulforaphane Represses Matrix-Degrading Proteases and Protects Cartilage From Destruction In Vitro and In Vivo." *Arthritis & Rheumatism,* 65 (2013):3130–3140.

42. Stuart Richer et al., "Double-masked, placebo-controlled, randomized trial of lutein and antioxidant supplementation in the intervention of atrophic age-related macular degeneration: the Veterans LAST study (Lutein Antioxidant Supplementation Trial)." *Optometry, 75* (2004):216–30.

43. María-Isabel Covas et al,. "EUROLIVE Study Group. The effect of polyphenols in olive oil on heart disease risk factors: a randomized trial." *Ann Intern Med.,* 145 (2006):333-41.

44. Francesco Visioli and Elena Bernardini, "Extra Virgin Olive Oil's Polyphenols: Biological Activities." *Curr Pharm Des.,* 17 (2011):786-804.

45. Silvia Terés et al., "Oleic acid content is responsible for the reduction in blood pressure induced by olive oil." *Proc Natl Acad Sci U S A.,* 105 (2008):13811-13816.

46. Ulrike Peters et al., "Serum Lycopene, Other Carotenoids, and Prostate Cancer Risk: a Nested Case-Control Study in the Prostate, Lung, Colorectal, and Ovarian Cancer Screening Trial. "*Cancer Epidemiol Biomarkers Prev.,* 16 (2007): 962-968.

47. American Cancer Society. Accessed April 2015 from http://www.cancer.org/treatment/treatmentsandsideeffects/complementaryandalternativemedicine/dietandnutrition/lycopene

48. Mahyar Etminan et al., "The role of tomato products and lycopene in the prevention of prostate cancer: a meta-analysis of observational studies." *Cancer Epidemiol Biomarkers Prev.,* 13 (2004):340-345.

49. John Shi and Marc Le Maguer, "Lycopene in tomatoes: chemical and physical properties affected by food processing." *Crit Rev Biotechnol.,* 20 (2000):293-334.

50. Muneeza Rizwan et al., "Tomato paste rich in lycopene protects against cutaneous photodamage in humans in vivo: a randomized controlled trial," *British Journal of Dermatology,* 164 (2011):154-162.

51. Cristina Ribeiro Barros Cardoso et al., "Influence of topical administration of n-3 and n-6 essential and n-9 nonessential fatty acids on the healing of cutaneous wounds." *Wound Repair Regen.,* 12 (2004):235-243.

52. Paulo AR Jorge et al., "Effect of eggplant on plasma lipid levels, lipidic peroxidation and reversion of endothelial dysfunction in experimental hypercholesterolemia." *Arq. Bras. Cardiol.,* 70 (1998):87-91.

53. Pu Jing et al., "Effect of glycosylation patterns of Chinese eggplant anthocyanins and other derivatives on antioxidant effectiveness in human colon cell lines." *Food Chem.*, 172 (2015):183-9.
54. Pamela Maher, "Modulation of multiple pathways involved in the maintenance of neuronal function during aging by fisetin," *Genes Nutr.*, 4 (2009):297–307.
55. Arpad Szallasi and Peter M Blumberg, "Vanilloid receptors: new insights enhance potential as a therapeutic target." *Pain,* 68 (1996):195-208.
56. Raúl U Hernández-Ramírez et al., "Dietary intake of polyphenols, nitrate and nitrite and gastric cancer risk in Mexico City." *Int J Cancer,* 125 (2009):1424–1430.
57. "Nutritional Information," (Maine Coast Sea Vegetables), Accessed March 16, 2015 from http://www.seaveg.com/shop/index.php?main_page=page&id=3&chapter=1.
58. Emily DeLacey, "Trace minerals: What they are and their importance," (FitDay), Accessed March 16, 2015 from http://www.fitday.com/fitness-articles/nutrition/vitamins-minerals/trace-minerals-what-they-are-and-their-importance.html.
59. Nutrient data for this listing was provided by USDA SR-21. "Nutrition Facts: Seaweed, agar, raw," (Nutrition Data), Accessed April, 2015 from http://nutritiondata.self.com/facts/vegetables-and-vegetable-products/2615/2#ixzz3YNUsOvRA.
60. Kanten (Agar Agar) World. "Facts about Kanten".Blog post. (July 19, 2007). http://kanten-Accessed on March 3, 2015 from world.blogspot.com/2007/07/facts-about-kanten.html.
61. Christine Dawczynski et al., "Amino acids, fatty acids, and dietary fibre in edible seaweed products." *Food Chem.*, 103 (2007):891–899.
62. Paul MacArtain et al., "Nutritional value of edible seaweeds." *Nutr Rev.,* 65 (2007):535–543.
63. Albana Cumashi et al., "A comparative study of the anti-inflammatory, anticoagulant, antiangiogenic, and antiadhesive activities of nine different fucoidans from brown seaweeds." *Glycobiology,* 17 (2007):541-552.
64. Matthew D Wilcox et al., "The modulation of pancreatic lipase activity by alginates." *Food Chemistry*, 146 (2014):479-484.
65. Tae-Wook Chung et al., "Marine Algal Fucoxanthin Inhibits the Metastatic Potential of Cancer Cells." *Biochemical and Biophysical Research Communications,* 439 (2013):580-85.
66. Pamela Maher, "Modulation of multiple pathways involved in the maintenance of neuronal function during aging by fisetin." *Genes Nutr.* , 4 (2009):297–307.
67. Adrian R Whyte and Claire M Williams. "Effects of a single dose of a flavonoid-rich blueberry drink on memory in 8 to 10 y old children." *Nutrition,* 31 (2015):531-4.
68. Robert Krikorian et al., "Blueberry Supplementation Improves Memory in Older Adults." *J Agric Food Chem.,* 58 (2010):3996–4000.
69. Ruth Jepson et al., Cranberries for preventing urinary tract infections. *Cochrane Database Syst Rev.*, 1 (2004):CD001321.
70. Ora Burger et al., "Inhibition of Helicobacter pylori adhesion to human gastric mucus by a high-molecular-weight constituent of cranberry juice." *Crit Rev Food Sci Nutr.,* 42 (2002):279-84.
71. Khushwant S Bhullar and Basil P Hubbard. "Lifespan and healthspan extension by resveratrol." *Biochim Biophys Acta.,* 1852 (2015):1209-1218.
72. "Ellagic acid," (Memorial Sloan Kettering Cancer Center, 2012), Accessed April, 2015 from https://www.mskcc.org/cancer-care/integrative-medicine/herbs/ellagic-acid.
73. Robert Krikorian et al., "Concord grape juice supplementation improves memory function in older adults with mild cognitive impairment." *Br J Nutr.,* 103 (2010):730-4.

74. Bente L Halvorsen et al., "Content of redox-active compounds (ie, antioxidants) in foods consumed in the United States." *Am J Clin Nutr.,* 84 (2006):95-135.
75. "Ellagic acid," (Memorial Sloan Kettering Cancer Center, 2012), Accessed April, 2015 from https://www.mskcc.org/cancer-care/integrative-medicine/herbs/ellagic-acid.
76. Liisa J Nohynek et al., "Berry phenolics: antimicrobial properties and mechanisms of action against severe human pathogens." *Nutr Cancer,* 54 (2006):18-32.
77. Tadashi Nakanishi et al., "Catechins inhibit vascular endothelial growth factor production and cyclooxygenase-2 expression in human dental pulp cells." *International Endodontic Journal,* 48 (2015):277–282.
78. Lisa Brown et al., "Cholesterol-lowering effects of dietary fiber: a meta-analysis." *Am J Clin Nutr.,* 69 (1999):30-42.
79. Basharat Yousuf et al., "Health Benefits of Anthocyanins and Their Encapsulation for Potential Use in Food Systems: A Review." *Crit Rev Food Sci Nutr.,* 6 (2015):0.
80. Susanne Burkhardt et al., "Detection and quantification of the antioxidant melatonin in Montmorency and Balaton tart cherries (Prunus cerasus)." *J Agric Food Chem.,* 49 (2001):4898-902.
81. Barbara K Butland et al., "Diet, lung function, and lung function decline in a cohort of 2512 middle aged men." *Thorax,* 55 (2000):102-8.
82. Loïc Le Marchand et al., "Intake of Flavonoids and Lung Cancer." *JNCI J Natl Cancer Inst.,* 92 (2000):154-160.
83. Paul Knekt et al., "Quercetin intake and the incidence of cerebrovascular disease." *Eur J Clin Nutr.,* 54 (2000):415-7.
84. Lydia A Bazzano, "Effects of soluble dietary fiber on low-density lipoprotein cholesterol and coronary heart disease risk." *Curr Atheroscler Rep.,* 10 (2008):473-7.
85. Nicole M Wedick et al., "Dietary flavonoid intakes and risk of type 2 diabetes in US men and women." *Am J Clin Nutr.,* 95 (2012):925-33.
86. Neal D. Freedman et al., "Fruit and vegetable intake and esophageal cancer in a large prospective cohort study." *Int J Cancer,* 121 (2007):2753-60.
87. "Health Benefits Of Citrus Limonoids Explored," Science News, USDA / Agricultural Research Service, (Apr 9, 2005)
88. "Diet, nutrition and the prevention of chronic diseases," Report of the joint WHO/FAO expert consultation. WHO Technical Report Series, No. 916 (TRS 916).
89. "*Food, Nutrition, Physical Activity, and the Prevention of Cancer: a Global Perspective,*" World Cancer Research Fund, American Institute for Cancer Research, (Washington, DC: American Institute for Cancer Research; 2007).
90. Ken Fujioka et al., "The effects of grapefruit on weight and insulin resistance: relationship to the metabolic syndrome." *J Med Food,* 9 (2006):49-54.
91. Abdul Waheed et al., "Naringenin inhibits the growth of *Dictyostelium* and MDCK-derived cysts in a TRPP2 (polycystin-2)-dependent manner." *British Journal of Pharmacology,* 171 (2014):2659–2670.
92. Marcia Wood, "Citrus Compound: Ready To Help Your Body!" *Agricultural Research Magazine,* 53 (Feb. 2005):16-17.
93. Martha P Tarazona-Díaz et al., "Watermelon Juice: Potential Functional Drink for Sore Muscle Relief in Athletes." *J. Agric. Food Chem.,*61 (2013):7522–7528.

94. Douglas S Kalman, et al., "Comparison of coconut water and a carbohydrate-electrolyte sport drink on measures of hydration and physical performance in exercise-trained men." *Journal of the International Society of Sports Nutrition,* 9 (2012):1.
95. Alberto Ascherio et al., "Intake of Potassium, Magnesium, Calcium, and Fiber and Risk of Stroke Among US Men." *Circulation,* 98 (1998):1198-1204.
96. Helena Gylling et al., "Plant sterols and plant stanols in the management of dyslipidaemia and prevention of cardiovascular disease." *Atherosclerosis,* 232 (2014):346-60.
97. Eudokia K Mitsou et al., "Effect of banana consumption on faecal microbiota: a randomized, controlled trial." *Anaerobe,* 17 (2011):384-7.
98. Michael B Sporn and Karen T Liby, "Is lycopene an effective agent for preventing prostate cancer?" *Cancer Prev Res.,* 6 (2013):384-6.
99. Jhoti Somanah et al., "Effects of a short term supplementation of a fermented papaya preparation on biomarkers of diabetes mellitus in a randomized Mauritian population." *Prev Med.,* 54 (2012):S90-7.
100. Sarah Brien et al., "Bromelain as a Treatment for Osteoarthritis: a Review of Clinical Studies." *Evid Based Complement Alternat Med.,* 1 (2004):251–257.
101. Michael Aviram and Leslie Dornfield, "Pomegranate juice consumption inhibits serum angiotensin converting enzyme activity and reduces systolic blood pressure." *Atherosclerosis,* 158 (2001):195–198.
102. Michael Aviram et al., "Pomegranate juice consumption for 3 years by patients with carotid artery stenosis reduces common carotid intima-media thickness, blood pressure and LDL oxidation."*Clin Nutr.,* 23 (2004):423-33.
103. Juma M Alkaabi et al., "Glycemic indices of five varieties of dates in healthy and diabetic subjects." *Nutr J.,* 10 (2011):59.
104. Wasseem Rock et al., "Effects of date (Phoenix dactylifera L., Medjool or Hallawi Variety) consumption by healthy subjects on serum glucose and lipid levels and on serum oxidative status: a pilot study." *J Agric Food Chem.,* 57 (2009):8010-7.
105. Pauline Koh-Banerjee et al., "Changes in whole-grain, bran, and cereal fiber consumption in relation to 8-y weight gain among men." *American Journal of Clinical Nutrition,* 80 (2004):1237-45.
106. Lydia A Bazzano et al., "Dietary Fiber Intake and Reduced Risk of Coronary Heart Disease in US Men and Women. The National Health and Nutrition Examination Survey I Epidemiologic Follow-up Study." *Arch Intern Med.,* 163 (2003):1897-1904.
107. Michael McIntosh and Carla Miller, "A diet containing food rich in soluble and insoluble fiber improves glycemic control and reduces hyperlipidemia among patients with type 2 diabetes mellitus." *Nutr Rev.,* 59 (2001):52-5.
108. Danik M Martirosyan et al., "Amaranth oil application for coronary heart disease and hypertension." *Lipids in Health and Disease,* 6 (2007):1.
109. Massimo F Marcone et al., "Amaranth as a rich dietary source of beta-sitosterol and other phytosterols. " *Plant Foods for Human Nutrition, 58 (2003):207-11.*
110. Kay M Behall et al., "Diets containing barley significantly reduce lipids in mildly hypercholesterolemic men and women." *Am J Clin Nutr.*, 80 (2004):1185-93.
111. Vida Skrabanja et al., "Nutritional Properties of Starch in Buckwheat Products: Studies in Vitro and in Vivo." *J. Agric. Food Chem.*, 49 (2001):490–496.

112. Romina P Pedreschi, "Fractionation of phenolic compounds from a purple corn extract and evaluation of antioxidant and antimutagenic activities." Master's thesis, Texas A&M University. Texas A&M University. Available electronically from http : //hdl .handle . net /1969 .1 /2343.

113. Chun-Ho Bae et al.,"Effects of phosphorylated cross-linked resistant corn starch on the intestinal microflora and short chain fatty acid formation during *in vitro* human fecal batch culture. " *Food Science and Biotechnology,* 22 (2013):1649-1654.

114. Andrew L Carvalho-Wells et al., "Determination of the in vivo prebiotic potential of a maize-based whole grain breakfast cereal: a human feeding study." *British Journal of Nutrition,* 21 (2010):1-4.

115. Anoma Chandrasekara and Fereidoon Shahidi. "Content of insoluble bound phenolics in millets and their contribution to antioxidant capacity. " *Journal of Agricultural and Food Chemistry, 58 (2919): 6706-14.*

116. Candida J Rebello et al., "Acute effect of oatmeal on subjective measures of appetite and satiety compared to a ready-to-eat breakfast cereal: a randomized crossover trial." *J Am Coll Nutr.,* 32 (2013):272–9.

117. Anne R Lee et al., "The effect of substituting alternative grains in the diet on the nutritional profile of the gluten-free diet." *J Hum Nutr Diet,* 22 (2009):359-63.

118. Lena Galvez Ranilla et al., "Evaluation of indigenous grains from the Peruvian Andean region for antidiabetes and antihypertension potential using in vitro methods." *J Med Food,* 12 (2009):704-13.

119. Elisa Pojer et al., "The Case for Anthocyanin Consumption to Promote Human Health: A Review." *Comprehensive Reviews in Food Science and Food Safety* 12 (2913):483-508.

120. Ola K. Magnusdottir et al., "Whole Grain Rye Intake, Reflected by a Biomarker, Is Associated with Favorable Blood Lipid Outcomes in Subjects with the Metabolic Syndrome – A Randomized Study." *PLoS One* 9 (2014):e110827.

121. Constance Kies and Hazel M Fox, "Protein nutritive value of wheat and triticale grain for humans, studied at two levels of protein intake." *Cer. Chem.*, 47 (1970):671-678.

122. David P Rose et al., "High-fiber diet reduces serum estrogen concentrations in premenopausal women." *Am J Clin Nutr.,* 54 (1991):520-5.

123. Carol J Haggans et al., "The effect of flaxseed and wheat bran consumption on urinary estrogen metabolites in premenopausal women." *Cancer Epidemiol Biomarkers Prev.,* 9 (2000):719-25.

124. Michael Greger, "Increased Lifespan From Beans," (2013), Accessed April, 2015 from http://nutritionfacts.org/video/increased-lifespan-from-beans/.

125. Chizuko Maruyama et al., "Azuki Bean Juice Lowers Serum Triglyceride Concentrations in Healthy Young Women." *J Clin Biochem Nutr.,* 43 (2008):19–25.

126. Jian He and M Monica Giusti, "Anthocyanins: natural colorants with health-promoting properties." *Annu Rev Food Sci Technol.,* 1 (2010):163-87.

127. Marcelo Hernández-Salaza et al., "*In vitro* fermentability and antioxidant capacity of the indigestible fraction of cooked black beans (*Phaseolus vulgaris* L.), lentils (*Lens culinaris* L.) and chickpeas (*Cicer arietinum* L.)" *Journal of the Science of Food and Agriculture,* 90 (2010):1417-1422.

128. Elaine Lanza et al., "High dry bean intake and reduced risk of advanced colorectal adenoma recurrence among participants in the Polyp Prevention Trial." *J Nutr.*, 136 (2006):1896–1903.

129. FAO/WHO, Expert consultation on protein quality evaluation. Food and Agriculture Organization of the United Nations, Rome, (1990).

130. Jane K Pittaway et al., "Dietary supplementation with chickpeas for at least 5 weeks results in small but significant reductions in serum total and low-density lipoprotein cholesterols in adult women and men." *Ann Nutr Metab.*. 50 (2006):512-8.

131. Siegfried W Souci et al., *Food Composition and Nutrition Tables*, (Stuttgart, Germany: Medpharm Scientific Publishers, 2008).

132. Thomas H Crook et al., "Effects of Phosphatidylserine in Age-Associated Memory Impairment." *Neurology,* 41(1991):644-649.

133. David Benton et al., "The Influence of phosphatidylserine supplementation on mood and heart rate when faced with an acute stressor," *Nutritional Neuroscience,* 4 (2001):169–78.

134. KV Rajagopalan, "Molybdenum: an essential trace element in human nutrition," *Annu Rev Nutr.,* 8 (1988):401-427.

135. Alessandro Menotti et al., "Food intake patterns and 25-year mortality from coronary heart disease: cross-cultural correlations in the Seven Countries Study. The Seven Countries Study Research Group," *Eur J Epidemiol,* 15 (1999):507-15.

136. Saman Abeysekara et al., "A pulse-based diet is effective for reducing total and LDL-cholesterol in older adults." *Br J Nutr.,* 108 Suppl 1 (2012):S103-10.

137. Helen M Hermsdorff et al., "A legume-based hypocaloric diet reduces proinflammatory status and improves metabolic features in overweight/obese subjects," *Eur J Nutr.,* 50 (2011):61-9.

138. David JA Jenkins et al., "Exceptionally low blood glucose response to dried beans: comparison with other carbohydrate foods," *Br Med J.*, 281(1980):578-80.

139. Sharon Thompson et al., "Bean and rice meals reduce postprandial glycemic response in adults with type 2 diabetes," *Nutr J.*, 11(2012):23.

140. Stephen T Talcott et al., "Polyphenolic content and sensory properties of normal and high oleic acid peanuts," *Food Chemistry,* 90 (2005):379-388.

141. Leonard Stoloff, "Aflatoxin as a cause of primary liver-cell cancer in the United States: A probability study." *Nutrition and Cancer* 5 (1983):165-186.

142. SH Sicherer et al., "US prevalence of self-reported peanut, tree nut, and sesame allergy: 11-year follow-up," *J Allergy Clin Immunol.,* 125 (2010):1322-6.

143. Donna M Winham et al., "Pinto bean consumption reduces biomarkers for heart disease risk," *J Am Coll Nutr.,* 26 (2007):243-9.

144. James W Anderson et al., "Meta-analysis of the effects of soy protein intake on serum lipids." *N Engl J Med.,* 333 (1995):276-282.

145. Paraskevi Detopoulou et al., "Dietary choline and betaine intakes in relation to concentrations of inflammatory markers in healthy adults: the ATTICA study," *American Journal of Clinical Nutrition,* 87 (2008):424-430.

146. Armin Zittermann et al., "Short-term effects of high soy supplementation on sex hormones, bone markers, and lipid parameters in young female adults," *Eur J Nutr.,* 43 (2004):100-8.

147. Yu-Ming Chen et al., "Soy isoflavones have a favorable effect on bone loss in Chinese postmenopausal women with lower bone mass: a double-blind, randomized, controlled trial." *J Clin Endocrinol Metab.,* 88 (2003):4740-7.

148. "Adoption of Genetically Engineered Crops in the US" USDA Economic Research Service. August 2014 [using data from USDA, National Agricultural Statistics Service, June Agricultural Survey].
149. Hasnah Haron et al., "Absorption of calcium from milk and tempeh consumed by postmenopausal Malay women using the dual stable isotope technique," *Int J Food Sci Nutr.,* 61 (2010):125-37.
150. Xing Tong et al., "Meta-analysis of the relationship between soybean product consumption and gastric cancer."*Zhonghua Yu Fang Yi Xue Za Zhi,* 44 (2010):215-20.
151. "Edamame," (National Soybean Research Laboratory), Accessed March 16, 2015 from http://nsrl.illinois.edu/content/edamame.
152. Sylvie Tremblay, "What are the health benefits of eating nuts & seeds?" *SFGate* (Demand Media, Inc.), Accessed March 16, 2015 from http://healthyeating.sfgate.com/health-benefits-eating-nuts-seeds-6701.html.
153. Ying Bao et al., "Association of Nut Consumption with Total and Cause-Specific Mortality." *N Engl J Med,.* 369 (2013):2001-2011.
154. Meathead, "Why Raw Sprouts May be the Riskiest Food in Your Grocery Store," *Huffington Post,* (06/11/201; Updated: 08/11/2011).
155. Pera R Jambazian et al., "Almonds in the diet simultaneously improve plasma alpha tocopherol concentrations and reduce plasma lipids," *Journal of the American Dietetic Associatio,n* 105 (2005):449-454.
156. Paul A Davis and Christine K Iwahashi, "Whole almonds and almond fractions reduce aberrant crypt foci in a rat model of colon carcinogenesis," *Cancer Letters,* 165 (2001):27–33.
157. André F Amaral et al., "Pancreatic cancer risk and levels of trace elements," *Gut,* 61 (2012):1583-8.
158. Leonard Tedong et al., "Hydro-ethanolic extract of cashew tree (Anacardium occidentale) nut and its principal compound, anacardic acid, stimulate glucose uptake in C2C12 muscle cells," *Molecular Nutrition & Food Research,* 54 (2010):1753-62.
159. Vladimiar Vuksan et al., "Supplementation of conventional therapy with the novel grain Salba (Salvia hispanica L.) improves major and emerging cardiovascular risk factors in type 2 diabetes: results of a randomized controlled trial," *Diabetes Care,* 30 (2007):2804–2810.
160. Malak A Al-Yawer et al., "Garden Cress Seed Could be A Factual Galactagogue." *The Iraqi Postgraduate Medical Journal,* 5 (2006):62-67.
161. Marina S Touillaud et al., "Dietary Lignan Intake and Postmenopausal Breast Cancer Risk by Estrogen and Progesterone Receptor Status," *JNCI J Natl Cancer Inst.,* 99 (2007):475-486.
162. Wendy Demark-Wahnefried et al., "Pilot study of dietary fat restriction and flaxseed supplementation in men with prostate cancer before surgery: exploring the effects on hormonal levels, prostate-specific antigen, and histopathologic features," *Urology,* 58 (2001):47-52.
163. An Pan et al., "Effects of a Flaxseed-Derived Lignan Supplement in Type 2 Diabetic Patients: A Randomized, Double-Blind, Cross-Over Trial." *PLoS ONE,* 2 (2007):e1148.
164. Umesh Rudrappa, "Pecans nutrition facts," (www.nutrition-and-you.com, 2014), Accessed March 16, 2015 from http://www.nutrition-and-you.com/pecans.html.
165. Craig S Patch et al., "Plant Sterols as Dietary Adjuvants in the Reduction of Cardiovascular Risk: Theory and Evidence." *Vasc Health Risk Manag.,* 2 (2006):157–162.

166. Georgina M Hughes et al., "The effect of Korean pine nut oil (PinnoThin™) on food intake, feeding behaviour and appetite: A double-blind placebo-controlled trial." *Lipids Health Dis.,* 7 (2008):6.

167. Gemma Brufau et al., "Nuts: source of energy and macronutrients." *Br J Nutr.,* 96 (2006):S24-8.

168. Colin D Kay et al., "Pistachios increase serum antioxidants and lower serum oxidized-LDL in hypercholesterolemic adults," *Journal of Nutrition,* 140 (2010):1093-8.

169. Heeok Hong et al., "Effects of pumpkin seed oil and saw palmetto oil in Korean men with symptomatic benign prostatic hyperplasia," *Nutr Res Pract.,* 3 (2009):323–327.

170. Rajesh Naithani et al., "Antiviral activity of phytochemicals: a comprehensive review." *Mini Rev Med Chem.,* 8 (2008):1106-33.

171. Satomi Kita et al., "Antihypertensive effect of sesamin. I. Protection against deoxycorticosterone acetate-salt-induced hypertension and cardiovascular hypertrophy," *Biol Pharm Bull,* 18 (1995):1016-9.

172. Wen-Huey Wu et al., "Sesame Ingestion Affects Sex Hormones, Antioxidant Status, and Blood Lipids in Postmenopausal Women," *J. Nutr.,* 136 (2006):1270-1275.

173. George A Eby and Karen L Eby, "Rapid recovery from major depression using magnesium treatment." *Medical Hypotheses*, 67 (2006):362–370.

174. Kelly A Shaw et al., "Tryptophan and 5-hydroxytryptophan for depression," *Cochrane Database Syst Rev.,* (2001):CD003198.

175. Margareta Öhrvall et al., "Gamma, but not alpha, tocopherol levels in serum are reduced in coronary heart disease patients." *J Intern Med.,* 239 (1996):111–7.

176. Margareta Kristenson et al., "Antioxidant state and mortality from coronary heart disease in Lithuanian and Swedish men: concomitant cross sectional study of men aged 50," *BMJ,* 314 (1997):629–33.

177. Yoshihiro Kokubo et al., "Association of dietary intake of soy, beans, and isoflavones with risk of cerebral and myocardial infarctions in Japanese populations: the Japan Public Health Center-based (JPHC) study cohort I," *Circulation,* 116 (2007):2553-62.

178. Makio Kobayashi, "Immunological functions of soy sauce: hypoallergenicity and antiallergic activity of soy sauce," *Journal of Bioscience and Bioengineering,* 100 (2005):144-151.

179. Stephenie L Darke and MaryAnne Drake, "Comparison of salty taste and time intensity of sea and land salts from around the world," *Journal of Sensory Studies*, 26 (2010):25–34.

180. Ibid.

181. Mamdouh Abou-Zaid et al., "High-performance liquid chromatography characterization and identification of antioxidant polyphenols in maple syrup," *Pharmaceutical Biology,* 46 (2008):117-125.

182. JW White, Jr. and Landis W Doner, "Honey Composition and Properties." Beekeeping in the United States. Agriculture Handbook Number 335 (1980).

183. *Methicillin-resistant Staphylococcus aureus* (MRSA) Infections, CDC, Last updated 28 May 2014, Accessed 11 June 2014.

184. NS Al-Waili and KY Saloom, "Effects of topical honey on post-operative wound infections due to gram positive and gram negative bacteria following caesarean sections and hysterectomies." *Eur J Med Res.,* 4 (1999):126-30.

185. "Links Medical Receives Both FDA & EU Market Clearance for Advance Wound Care Products with Medical-Grade Manuka Honey" (Business Wire, July 2012), Accessed April 15, 2015 from

http://www.businesswire.com/news/home/20120710006966/en/Links-Medical-Receives-FDA-EU-Market-Clearance#.VVelp7mqqko

186. "Manuka Honey Information" (Honey Centre, 2007), Accessed April 15, 2015 from http://honeycentre.com/Manuka_Honey_Info.php

187. Wenfu Mao et al., "Honey constituents up-regulate detoxification and immunity genes in the western honey bee Apis mellifera." *Proc Natl Acad Sci U S A,* 110 (2012):8842-8846.

188. M Sanford and R Hoopingarner. The Hive and the honey bee. (1992). J Graham (ed). Hamilton, IL: Dadant. From "Why honey is not vegan," (Vegetus.org) Accessed April 16, 2015 from http://vegetus.org/honey/kill.htm

189. "Tests Show Most Store Honey Isn't Honey," (Food Safety News, November 7, 2011). Accessed April 16, 2015 from http://www.foodsafetynews.com/2011/11/tests-show-most-store-honey-isnt-honey/#.VVeFcUaVyM9

190. Hans-Joachim F Zunft et al., "Carob pulp preparation rich in insoluble fibre lowers total and LDL cholesterol in hypercholesterolemic patients," *Eur J Nutr.*, 42 (2003):235-42.

191. Shigenori Kumazawa et al., "Antioxidant activity of polyphenols in carob pods," *J Agric Food Chem.,* 16 (2002):373-7.

192. "Inulin" (Prebiotic Canada), Accessed April 21, 2015 from http://www.prebiotic.ca/inulin.html

193. Bahram Pourghassem Gargari et al., "Effects of High Performance Inulin Supplementation on Glycemic Control and Antioxidant Status in Women with Type 2 Diabetes." *Diabetes Metab J.,* 37 (2013):140–148.

194. "What Are the Benefits of Coconut Sugar?" (Livestrong.com, April 16, 2015), Accessed 2 May, 2015 from http://www.livestrong.com/article/367337-what-are-the-benefits-of-coconut-sugar/

195. Katherine M Phillips et al., "Total antioxidant content of alternatives to refined sugar," *J Am Diet Assoc.,* 109 (2009):64-71.

196. Silvia Terés et al., "Oleic acid content is responsible for the reduction in blood pressure induced by olive oil," *Proc Natl Acad Sci U S A,* 105 (2008):13811-13816.

197. María-Isabel Covas, "Olive oil and the cardiovascular system," *Pharmacological Research,* 55 (2007):175–186.

198. Cécilia Samieri et al,, "Olive oil consumption, plasma oleic acid, and stroke incidence. The Three-City Study," *Neurology,* 77 (2011):418-25.

199. Matthew J Killeen et al., "Hydroxytyrosol: An examination of its potential role in cardiovascular disease, inflammation, and longevity," *AgroFood Industry Hi-Tech.*, 22 (2011):16-9.

200. Christa Meisinger et al., "Plasma oxidized low-density lipoprotein, a strong predictor for acute coronary heart disease events in apparently healthy, middle-aged men from the general population," *Circulation,* 112 (2005):651-7.

201. Concepción Romero et al., "In Vitro Activity of Olive Oil Polyphenols against Helicobacter pylori," *J Agric Food Chem.*, 55 (2007):680-686.

202. Claudio Pelucchi et al., "Olive Oil and Cancer Risk: An Update of Epidemiological Findings through 2010," *Curr Pharm Des.*, 17 (2011):805-12.

203. Alaa H Abuznait et al., "Olive-oil-derived oleocanthal enhances β-amyloid clearance as a potential neuroprotective mechanism against Alzheimer's disease: in vitro and in vivo studies," *ACS Chem Neurosci.*, 4 (2013):973-82.

204. Marie-Pierre St-Onge and Peter JH Jones, "Greater rise in fat oxidation with medium-chain triglyceride consumption relative to long-chain triglyceride is associated with lower initial body

weight and greater loss of subcutaneous adipose tissue," *International Journal of Obesity,* 27 (2003):1565–1571.

205. Hans Kaunitz and Conrado S Dayrit, "Coconut oil consumption and coronary heart disease," *Philippine Journal of Internal Medicine,* 30 (1992):165-171.

206. Joseph Mercola, "Coconut oil: This cooking oil is a powerful virus-destroyer and antibiotic…," (Joseph Mercola, 2010), Accessed March 16, 2015 from http://articles.mercola.com/sites/articles/archive/2010/10/22/coconut-oil-and-saturated-fats-can-make-you-healthy.aspx.

207. Etienne Guillot et al., "Intestinal absorption and liver uptake of mediumchain fatty acids in non-anaesthetized pigs," *Br.J Nutr.,* 69 (1993):2.

208. Phienvit Tantibhedhyangkul and Sami A Hashim, "Medium-chain triglyceride feeding in premature infants: effects on calcium and magnesium absorption," *Pediatric,s* 61 (1978):537-45.

209. David L Hachey et al., "Human lactation II: endogenous fatty acid synthesis by the mammary gland," *Pediatr Res.,* 25 (1989):63–8.

210. Yeou-mei Christiana Liu, "Medium-chain triglyceride (MCT) ketogenic therapy". *Epilepsia,* 49 (2008):33-36.

211. Moutairou A Egounlety and Ogugua C Aworh, "Effect of soaking, dehulling, cooking and fermentation with Rhizopus oligosporus on the oligosaccharides, trypsin inhibitor, phytic acid and tannins of soybean (Glycine max Merr.), cowpea (Vinga unguiculata L. Walp) and groundbean (Macrotyloma geocarpa Harms*)," J. Food Eng,* 56 (2003):249-254.

212. Laila A Shekib, "Nutritional improvement of lentils, chick pea, rice and wheat by natural fermentation," *Plant Foods Hum Nutr.,* 46 (1994):201-5.

213. Irene TH Liem et al., "Production of vitamin B-12 in tempeh, a fermented soybean food," *Appl Environ Microbiol.*, 34 (1977):773–776.

214. Marja Tolonen et al., "Plant-derived biomolecules in fermented cabbage," *Journal of Agricultural and Food Chemistry,* 50 (2002):6798–6803.

215. NM Ali et al., "Antioxidant and Hepatoprotective Effect of Aqueous Extract of Germinated and Fermented Mung Bean on Ethanol-Mediated Liver Damage" *BioMed Research International,* 2013 (2013), Article ID 693613.

216. Jose M Saavedra et al., "Feeding of Bifidobacterium bifidum and Streptococcus thermophilus to infants in hospital for prevention of diarrhoea and shedding of rotavirus," *Lancet,* 344 (1994):1046-1049.

217. Georges M Halpern et al., "Treatment of irritable bowel syndrome with Lacteol Fort: a randomized, double-blind, cross-over trial," *Am J Gastroenterol.,* 91 (1996):1579 – 85.

218. Krzysztof Niedzielin et al., "A controlled, double-blind, randomized study on the efficacy of Lactobacillus plantarum299V in patients with irritable bowel syndrome," *Eur J Gastroenterol Hepatol.*, 13 (2001):1143 – 7.

219. Jerome Boudeau et al., "Inhibitory effect of probiotic Escherichia coli strain Nissle 1917 on adhesion to and invasion of intestinal epithelial cells by adherent-invasive E. coli strains isolated from patients with Crohn's disease," *Aliment Pharmacol Ther.,* 18 (2003):45 – 56.

220. Stjepan Kosalec et al., "Antifungal activity of fluid extract and essential oil from anise fruits (Pimpinella anisum L., Apiaceae)," *Acta Pharm.*, 55 (2005):377-85.

221. SH Park, and I Seong, "Antifungal Effects of the Extracts and Essential Oils from Foeniculum vulgare and Illicium verum against Candida albicans," *Korean J Med Mycol.,* 15 (2010):157-164.

222. Jyh-Ferng Yang, et al., "Chemical Composition and Antibacterial Activities of *Illicium verum* Against Antibiotic-Resistant Pathogens," *Journal of Medicinal Food,* 13 (2010):1254-1262.
223. Lei Zhang and Bal L Lokeshwar, "Medicinal properties of the Jamaican pepper plant Pimenta dioica and Allspice," *Curr Drug Targets,* 13 (2012):1900-6.
224. Trevor Daly et al., "Carotenoid content of commonly consumed herbs and assessment of their bioaccessibility using an in vitro digestion model," *Plant Foods Hum Nutr.,* 65 (2010):164-9.
225. Alam Khan et al., "Bay Leaves Improve Glucose and Lipid Profile of People with Type 2 Diabetes," *J Clin Biochem Nutr.*, 44 (2009):52–56.
226. Ila Das et al., "Antioxidative effects of the spice cardamom against non-melanoma skin cancer by modulating nuclear factor erythroid-2-related factor 2 and NF-κB signalling pathways" *Br J Nutr.,* 108 (2012):984-97.
227. GM McCarthy and DJ McCarty, "Effect of topical capsaicin in the therapy of painful osteoarthritis of the hands," *J Rheumatol.,* 19 (1992):604-7.
228. Mehmet Boga et al., "Antioxidant and anticholinesterase activities of eleven edible plants," *Pharm Biol.*, 49 (2011):290-295.
229. Alam Khan et al., "Cinnamon Improves Glucose and Lipids of People With Type 2 Diabetes," *Diabetes Care, 26 (2003)*:3215-3218.
230. Manuel Viuda-Martos et al., "Antioxidant activity of essential oils of five spice plants widely used in a Mediterranean diet," *Flavour Fragr J.,* 25(2010):13-19.
231. H Wangenstee et al., "Antioxidant activity in extracts from coriander," *Food Chemistry,* 88 (2004):293-297.
232. CI Wright et al., "Herbal medicines as diuretics: a review of the scientific evidence," *J Ethnopharmacol,* 114 (2007):1-31.
233. Venkateswarlu Korthikunta et al., "In vitro anti-hyperglycemic activity of 4-hydroxyisoleucine derivatives," *Phytomedicine,* 22 (2015):66-70.
234. Nithya Neelakantan et al., "Effect of fenugreek (Trigonella foenum-graecum L.) intake on glycemia: a meta-analysis of clinical trials," *Nutr J.* 13 (2014):7.
235. Rita de Cássia da Silveira e Sá et al., "A Review on Anti-Inflammatory Activity of Monoterpenes," *Molecules,* 18 (2013):1227-1254.
236. HG Grigoleit and P Grigoleit, "Peppermint oil in irritable bowel syndrome," *Phytomedicine,* 12 (2005):601-6.
237. S Das et al., "Cancer modulation by glucosinolates: A review," *Current Science* 79 (2000):1665-1670.
238. N Brenner et al., "Chronic Nutmeg Psychosis," *Journal of the Royal Society of Medicine,* 86 (1993):179–180.
239. X Wu et al., "Lipophilic and Hydrophilic Antioxidant Capacities of Common Foods in the United States," *J. Agric. Food Chem.*, 52 (2004) :4026–4037.
240. SM Henning et al., "Antioxidant capacity and phytochemical content of herbs and spices in dry, fresh and blended herb paste form," *Int J Food Sci Nutr.,* 62 (2011):219-225..
241. Benford Mafuvadze et al., "Apigenin Induces Apoptosis and Blocks Growth of Medroxyprogesterone Acetate-Dependent BT-474 Xenograft Tumors," *Hormones and Cancer* 3 (2012):160-171.
242. Margriet Westerterp-Plantenga et al., "Metabolic effects of spices, teas, and caffeine," *Physiol Behav.*, 89 (2006):85-91.

243. UH Park et al., "Piperine, a component of black pepper, inhibits adipogenesis by antagonizing PPARγ activity in 3T3-L1 cells," *J Agric Food Chem.*, 60 (2012):3853-60.

244. PB Yaffe et al., "Piperine impairs cell cycle progression and causes reactive oxygen species-dependent apoptosis in rectal cancer cells," *Exp Mol Pathol.*, 94 (2013):109-14.

245. Seenivasan Prabuseenivasan, "*In vitro* antibacterial activity of some plant essential oils" *BMC Complement Altern Med.,* 6 (2006):39.

246. J Tai et al., "Antiproliferation effect of Rosemary (Rosmarinus officinalis) on human ovarian cancer cells in vitro," *Phytomedicine,* 19 (2012):436-43.

247. Heather A. Hausenblas et al., "Saffron (Crocus sativus L.) and major depressive disorder: a meta-analysis of randomized clinical trials," *Journal of Integrative Medicine,* 11 (2013): 377–83.

248. NT Tildesley, "Salvia lavandulaefolia (Spanish sage) enhances memory in healthy young volunteers," *Pharmacol Biochem Behav.,* 75 (2003):669-74.

249. Benford Mafuvadze et al., "Apigenin Induces Apoptosis and Blocks Growth of Medroxyprogesterone Acetate-Dependent BT-474 Xenograft Tumors," *Hormones and Cancer,* 3 (2012):160-171.

250. CF Bagamboula et al., "Inhibitory effect of thyme and basil essential oils, carvacrol, thymol, estragol, linalool and p-cymene towards *Shigella sonnei* and *S. flexneri*," *Food Microbio,.* 21 (2004):33-42.

251. H Mith, "Antimicrobial activities of commercial essential oils and their components against food-borne pathogens and food spoilage bacteria," *Food Sci Nutr.,* 2 (2014):403-16.

252. "Can turmeric prevent or treat cancer?" (Cancer Research UK, January 30, 2013), Accessed 8 April, 2015 from http://www.cancerresearchuk.org/about-cancer/cancers-in-general/cancer-questions/can-turmeric-prevent-bowel-cancer

253. "Cruciferous vegetables," (Wikipedia), Accessed from http://en.wikipedia.org/wiki/Cruciferous_vegetables.

254. Jon Michnovicz et al., "Altered estrogen metabolism and excretion in humans following consumption of indole-3-carbinol," *Nutr Cancer,* 16 (1991):59-66.

255. GY Wong et al., "Dose ranging study of indole-3-carbinol for breast cancer prevention," *J Cell Biochem.,* 28 (1997):111-16.

256. S Das et al., "Cancer modulation by glucosinolates: A review," *Current Science,* 79 (2000):1665-1670.

257. CX Cohen et al., "Fruit and vegetable intakes and prostate cancer risk," *J Natl Cancer Inst.,* 92 (2000):61-68.

258. CX Zhang et al., "Greater vegetable and fruit intake is associated with a lower risk of breast cancer among Chinese women," *Int J Cancer,* 125 (2009):181-188.

259. Sarah J Nechuta et al., "Cruciferous Vegetable Intake After Diagnosis of Breast Cancer and Survival: a Report From the Shanghai Breast Cancer Survival Study, "Abstract #LB-322. In *Annual Meeting of the American Association for Cancer Research, 2012 Mar 31-Apr 4.* (Chicago, Il; 2012).

260. Joel Fuhrman, "Dr. Fuhrman's Anti-Cancer Solution," (Dr Fuhrman Disease Proof, 2006), Accessed from http://www.diseaseproof.com/archives/healthy-food-dr-fuhrmans-anticancer-solution.html.

261. Lester Packer and Enrique Cadenas, "Lipoic acid: energy metabolism and redox regulation of transcription and cell signaling," *J Clin Biochem Nutr.,* 48 (2011):26–32.

262. Gerritje S Mijnhout et al., "Alpha lipoic Acid for symptomatic peripheral neuropathy in patients with diabetes: a meta-analysis of randomized controlled trials," *Int J Endocrinol.,* (2012): 456279.

263. Nate Matusheski, et al., "Epithiospecifier Protein from Broccoli (Brassica oleraceaL. Ssp.italica) Inhibits Formation of the Anticancer Agent Sulforaphane," *Journal of Agricultural and Food Chemistry,* 54 (2006):2069–76.

264. Gerry K Schwalfenberg, "The Alkaline Diet: Is There Evidence That an Alkaline pH Diet Benefits Health?" *J Environ Public Health,* 2012 (2012):727630.

265. World Cancer Research Fund/American Institute for Cancer Research, "Food, Nutrition, Physical Activity, and the Prevention of Cancer: a Global Perspective," Washington DC: AICR, 2007.

266. Olaf Sommerburg et al., "Fruits and vegetables that are sources for lutein and zeaxanthin: the macular pigment in human eyes," *Br J Ophthalmol.,* 82 (1998):907-910

267. World Cancer Research Fund/American Institute for Cancer Research, "Food, Nutrition, Physical Activity, and the Prevention of Colorectal Cancer," Continuous Update Project Report. (2011).

268. "Eating Green Leafy Vegetables Keeps Mental Abilities Sharp," (Newswise, 2015), Accessed April, 2015 from http://www.newswise.com/articles/eating-green-leafy-vegetables-keeps-mental-abilities-sharp.

269. William Faloon, "How many Americans are magnesium deficient?" *Life Extension,* 11 (2005):7 http://www.lef.org/magazine/2005/9/awsi/Page-01.

270. Emmett Hughes, "Magnesium: A best-kept secret," (American Chiropractic Association), Accessed March 16, 2015 from http://www.acatoday.org/content_css.cfm?CID=3956.

271. D King et al., "Dietary magnesium and C-reactive protein levels," *J Am Coll Nut.,* 24 (2005):166-71.

272. Nancy Piccone, "The silent epidemic of iodine deficiency," *Life Extension,* 17 (2011): 42-51 http://www.lef.org/magazine/2011/10/The-Silent-Epidemic-of-Iodine-Deficiency/Page-01.

273. Ida Calado Junio and Lourdes Partible Bisco, "Formulation and standardization of seaweeds flakes," *E–International Scientific Research Journal,* V (2013):183-194.

274. "Nutritional Information," (Maine Coast Sea Vegetables), Accessed March 16, 2015 from http://www.seaveg.com/shop/index.php?main_page=page&id=3&chapter=1.

275. S Dugasani et al., "Comparative antioxidant and anti-inflammatory effects of [6]-gingerol, [8]-gingerol, [10]-gingerol and [6]-shogaol" *J Ethnopharmacol.,* 127 (2010):515–20.

276. RD Altman and KC Marcussen, "Effects of a ginger extract on knee pain in patients with osteoarthritis," *Arthritis Rheum.*, 44 (2001):2531–8.

277. Francesca Borrelli et al., "Effectiveness and safety of ginger in the treatment of pregnancy-induced nausea and vomiting," *Obstet Gynecol.,* 105 (2005):849-56.

278. Julie Jurenka, "Anti-inflammatory properties of curcumin, a major constituent of Curcuma longa: a review of preclinical and clinical research," *Altern Med Rev.,* 14 (2009):141-53.

279. PR Holt et al., "Curcumin therapy in inflammatory bowel disease: a pilot study," *Dig Dis Sci.,* 50 (2005):2191-3.

280. V Kuptniratsaikul et al., "Efficacy and safety of Curcuma domestica extracts in patients with knee osteoarthritis," *J Altern Complement Med.,* 15 (2009):891-7.

281. Ann-Lii Cheng et al., "Phase I Clinical Trial of Curcumin, a Chemopreventive Agent, in Patients with High-risk or Pre-malignant Lesions." *Anticancer Research,* 21 (2001):2895-2900.

282. Hee Jin Kim et al., "A comprehensive review of the therapeutic and pharmacological effects of ginseng and ginsenosides in central nervous system," *J Ginseng Res.,* 37 (2013): 8–29.

283. SJ Fulder, "Ginseng and the hypothalamic-pituitary control of stress," *Am J Chin Med.,* 9 (1981):112–8.

284. J Liu et al., "Stimulatory effect of saponin from *Panax ginseng* on immune function of lymphocytes in the elderly," *Mech Ageing Dev.,* 83 (1995):43–53.

285. R Luke Bucci. "Selected herbals and human exercise performance," *Am J Clin Nutr.*, 72 (2000):624-636.

286. Morton Walker, "Adaptogens: nature's answer to stress," *Townsend Lett Doctors* (1994):751–5.

287. P Chatterjee et al., "Evaluation of anti-inflammatory effects of green tea and black tea: A comparative *in vitro* study," *J Adv Pharm Technol Res.*, 3 (2012): 136–138.

288. Igho Onakpoya et al,. "The effect of green tea on blood pressure and lipid profile: a systematic review and meta-analysis of randomized clinical trials," *Nutr Metab Cardiovasc Dis.,* 24 (2014):823-36.

289. G Sibi, "Inhibition of lipase and inflammatory mediators by *Chlorella* lipid extracts for antiacne treatment," *J Adv Pharm Technol Res.,* 6 (2015):7–12.

290. RE Merchant and CA Andre, "A review of recent clinical trials of the nutritional supplement Chlorella pyrenoidosa in the treatment of fibromyalgia, hypertension, and ulcerative colitis." *Altern Ther Health Med.*, 7 (2001):79-91.

291. Suzana Makpol et al., "*Chlorella Vulgaris* Modulates Hydrogen Peroxide-Induced DNA Damage and Telomere Shortening of Human Fibroblasts Derived from Different Aged Individuals," *Afr J Tradit Complement Altern Med.*, 6 (2009): 560–572.

292. Judy Foreman, "More Evidence For 'Stinking Rose' Garlic's Cancer-Fighting Potential," (wbur's Common Health, August 16, 2013), Accessed 18 April, 2015 from http://commonhealth.wbur.org/2013/08/more-evidence-for-stinking-rose-garlics-cancer-fighting-potential

293. DY Lee et al., "Anti-Inflammatory Activity of Sulfur-Containing Compounds from Garlic," *J Med Food,* 15 (2012):992–999.

294. Aaron T Fleischauer and Lenore Arab, "Garlic and Cancer: A critical review of the epidemiologic literature," *J. Nutr.,* 131 (2001):1032S–1040S.

295. Hiroyuki Nakagawa et al., "Growth inhibitory effects of diallyl disulfide on human breast cancer cell lines." *Carcinogenesis,* 22 (2001):891-897.

296. Bolan Yu et al., "Spirulina is an effective dietary source of zeaxanthin to humans," *British Journal of Nutrition,* 108 (2012):611–619.

297. Dorothy Pattison et al., "Dietary β-cryptoxanthin and inflammatory polyarthritis: results from a population-based prospective study," *Am J Clin Nutr.*, 82 (2005):451-455.

298. Khushwant S Bhullar and Basil P Hubbard, "Lifespan and healthspan extension by resveratrol," *Biochim Biophys Acta,* 1852 (2015): 209-1218.

299. Jay K Udani et al., "Effects of Açai (Euterpe oleracea Mart.) berry preparation on metabolic parameters in a healthy overweight population: a pilot study." *Nutr J.*, 10 (2011):45.

300. "Goji have an ORAC of 3173," Oxygen Radical Absorbance Capacity (ORAC) of Selected Foods, Release 2. Nutrient Data Laboratory, (US Department of Agriculture, Agricultural Research Service. 2010).

301. Peter Bucheli et al., "Goji Berry Effects on Macular Characteristics and Plasma Antioxidant Levels," *Optometry & Vision Science,* 88 (2011):257-262.

302. Harunobu Amagase and Dwight M Nance, "A randomized, double-blind, placebo-controlled, clinical study of the general effects of a standardized Lycium barbarum (Goji) Juice, GoChi," *J Altern Complement Med.,* 14 (2008):403-12.

303. M Aviram and L Dornfield, "Pomegranate juice consumption inhibits serum angiotensin converting enzyme activity and reduces systolic blood pressure," *Atherosclerosis,* (2001) 158:195–198.

304. M Aviram et al., "Pomegranate juice consumption for 3 years by patients with carotid artery stenosis reduces common carotid intima-media thickness, blood pressure and LDL oxidation," *Clin Nutr* 23 (2004):423-33.

305. Robin Goldwyn Blumenthal, "Drink Up! America is finally eating its vegetables -- from a bottle. How fresh juice is becoming big business for Starbucks and your local juice bar," *Barron's* (July 23, 2012) Accessed on March 3, 2015 from http://online.barrons.com/articles/SB50001424053111904346504577531063244598398.

306. Gary Null, *Reverse Arthritis and Pain Naturally: A Proven Approach to a Pain-Free Life* (Essential Publishing, 2013). Nutrition Intervention Reverses Arthritis Symptoms.

307. Damian Carrington and George Arnett, "Clear differences between organic and non-organic food, study finds," *The Guardian* (2014), Accessed March 16, 2015 from http://www.theguardian.com/environment/2014/jul/11/organic-food-more-antioxidants-study.

308. Deborah Kotz, "Time in the Sun: How Much Is Needed for Vitamin D?" *US News & World Report*, (June 23, 2008) Accessed on March 3, 2015 from http://health.usnews.com/health-news/family-health/heart/articles/2008/06/23/time-in-the-sun-how-much-is-needed-for-vitamin-d

309. Jennifer Daniels, "A silent killer - The war on constipation!" (rense.com), Accessed March 16, 2015 from http://rense.com/general65/constipation.htm.

310. Erin Coleman, "The best fiber foods for vegetarians," *SFGate* (Demand Media, Inc.), Accessed March 16, 2015 from http://healthyeating.sfgate.com/fiber-foods-vegetarians-8591.html.

311. Terri Coles, "14 high-fibre foods you should be eating every day," *The Huffington Post Canada* (The Huffington Post Canada, 2013), Accessed Mach 16, 2015 from http://www.huffingtonpost.ca/2013/10/31/high-fibre-foods_n_4178239.html.

312. Theodore M Brasky et al., "Plasma Phospholipid Fatty Acids and Prostate Cancer Risk in the SELECT Trial." *J Natl Cancer Inst.*, (2013) doi:10.1093/jnci/djt174

313. Dr. Mark Hyman, "Can fish oil cause prostate cancer?" (November 21, 2014) Accessed 17 April, 2015 from http://drhyman.com/blog/2013/07/26/can-fish-oil-cause-prostate-cancer/

314. Alexandra J Richardson and Paul Montgomery, "The Oxford-Durham Study: A Randomized Controlled Trial of Dietary Supplementation with Fatty Acids in Children with Developmental Coordination Disorder," *Pediatrics,* 115 (May 2005):1360-1366.

315. M Johnson et al., "Omega-3/Omega-6 Fatty Acids for Attention Deficit Hyperactivity Disorder: A Randomized Placebo-Controlled Trial in Children and Adolescents," *Journal of Attention Disorders,* (30 April 2008): Epub ahead of print, PMID 18448859.

316. M Tully et al., "Low Serum Cholesteryl Ester-Docosahexaenoic Acid Levels in Alzheimer's Disease: A Case-Control Study," *British Journal of Nutrition* 89 (2003):483-489.

317. Fredrik Jernerén et al., "Brain atrophy in cognitively impaired elderly: the importance of long-chain ω-3 fatty acids and B vitamin status in a randomized controlled trial," *Am J Clin Nutr.,* ajcn103283 (2015).

318. Ze Liu et al., "Omega-3 Fatty Acids and Other FFA4 Agonists Inhibit Growth Factor Signaling in Human Prostate Cancer Cells," *JPET,* 352 (2015):380-394.

319. "Study shows how omega-3 inhibits cancer cell growth," (Life Extension, 2015), Accessed April, 2015 from http://www.lifeextension.com/WhatsHot/2015/3/March-Whats-Hot-Articles/Page-01#Study-shows-how-omega-3-inhibits-cancer-cell-growth.

320. Raymond W Kwong et al., "Effect of Purified Omega-3 Fatty Acids on Reducing Left Ventricular Remodeling after Acute Myocardial Infarction (OMEGA-REMODEL Study: A Double-Blind Randomized Clinical Trial)," Paper presented at the American College of Cardiology's 64th Annual Scientific Session in San Diego, USA, (March 2015).

321. "Omega-3 helps heart attack survivors," (Life Extension, 2015), Accessed April, 2015 from http://www.lifeextension.com/WhatsHot/2015/3/March-Whats-Hot-Articles/Page-01#Omega-3-helps-heart-attack-survivors.

322. Accessed from http://www.vegsoc.org/info/omega3.htm

323. Elizabeth Brown, "Foods high in Linoleic acid," *SFGate* (Demand Media, Inc.), Accessed March 16, 2015 from http://healthyeating.sfgate.com/foods-high-linoleic-acid-9573.html.

324. WJ Rayment, "Prostaglandins," (InDepthInfo), Accessed March 16, 2015 from http://www.indepthinfo.com/biology/prostaglandins.htm.

325. Accessed from Holistichealthservices.com

326. Ray Sahelian, "Prostaglandin influence on health, role of food and diet," (2014), Accessed from http://www.raysahelian.com/prostaglandin.html.

327. BC Davis and PM Kris-Etherton, "Achieving Optimal Essential Fatty Acid Status in Vegetarians: Current Knowledge and Practical Implications," *American Journal of Clinical Nutrition,* 78 (2003):640S-646S.

328. Accessed from http://borntoexplore.org/omega.htm

329. Accessed from http://www.lef.org/magazine/mag2003/dec2003_report_omega_01.htm

330. Robert R Ballentine, "Dietary suggestions for chronic pain," (Holistic Health Services), Accessed from http://www.holistichealthservices.com/research/chronic_pain.html.

331. Accessed from http://borntoexplore.org/omega.htm

332. Accessed from http://www.lef.org/magazine/mag2003/dec2003_report_omega_01.htm

333. A Pan et al., "A-linolenic acid and risk of cardiovascular disease: a systematic review and meta-analysis," *Am J Clin Nutr.*, 96 (2012):1262-1273.

334. Kevin Gianni, "Dr. Gabriel Cousens on the importance of supplementing with vitamin B12," *Natural News* (Natural News Network, 2008), Accessed March 16, 2015 from http://www.naturalnews.com/023075_food_kids_Gabriel_Cousens.html.

335. Jack Norris, "B12 in plant foods," (VeganHealth.org, 2003), Accessed March 16, 2015 from http://www.veganhealth.org/b12/plant#seaweeds.

336. "Is tempeh a reliable source vitamin B12?" (Tempeh.info), Accessed March 16, 2015 from http://www.tempeh.info/health/vitaminB12.php.

337. "Nutritional Information," (Maine Coast Sea Vegetables), Accessed March 16, 2015 from http://www.seaveg.com/shop/index.php?main_page=page&id=3&chapter=1.

338. Jack Norris, "B12 in plant foods," (VeganHealth.org, 2003), Accessed March 16, 2015 from http://www.veganhealth.org/b12/plant#seaweeds.

339. Lief Hallberg, et al., "The role of vitamin C in iron absorption," *International Journal for Vitamin and Nutrition Research,* 30 (1989):103-108.

340. FR Ellis, "The Nutritional Status of Vegans and Vegetarians," *Proceedings of the Nutrition Society* 26 (1967):205211.
341. Mervyn G Hardinge and FJ Stare, "Do Human Beings Need Meat?" *Journal of Clinical Nutrition,* 2 (1954):73.
342. James G Bergan and Phyllis T Brown, "Nutritional Status of 'New' Vegetarians," *Journal of the American Dietetic Association,* 76 (1980):151154.
343. DS Miller and P Mumford, *Getting the Most Out of Food* (London: Van den Bergh, 1966), 9.
344. Eleanor Williams, "Making Vegetarian Diets Nutritious," *American Journal of Nursing* (1975):21682173.
345. Daisy Whitebread, "Top 10 vegetables highest in Calcium," (HealthAliciousNess, 2010), Accessed March 16, 2015 from http://www.healthaliciousness.com/articles/high-calcium-vegetables.php.
346. "Phytoestrogens," (Wikipedia,) Accessed from http://en.wikipedia.org/wiki/Phytoestrogens.
347. MJ McCann et al., "Role of Mammalian Lignans in the Prevention and Treatment of Prostate Cancer," *Nutrition and Cancer,* 52 (2005):1-14.
348. MS Morton et al., "Measurement and Metabolism of Isoflavonoids and Lignans in the Human Male," *Cancer Letters,* 114 (1997):145-51.
349. W Zhang et al., "Dietary Flaxseed Lignan Extract Lowers Plasma Cholesterol and Glucose Concentrations in Hypercholesterolaemic Subjects," *British Journal of Nutrition,* 99 (2008):1301-1309.
350. K Yamashita, "Enhancing Effects on Vitamin E Activity of Sesame Lignans," *Journal of Clinical Biochemistry and Nutrition,* 35 (2004):17-28.
351. Y Naito, "Tasty Seeds Have Hidden Health Benefits," *The Japan Times Online* (16 Oct 2000), Accessed on February 16, 2015 from http://search.japantimes.co.jp/cgi-bin/fl20001016a1.html
352. M Vanharanta et al., "Risk of Cardiovascular Disease–Related and All-Cause Death According to Serum Concentrations of Enterolactone," *Archives of Internal Medicine,* 163 (2003):1099-1104.
353. Johanna Dwyer, "Health Implications of Vegetarian Diets," *Comprehensive Therapy,* 9 (1983):2328.
354. JA Scharffenberg, "Vegetarian Diets," *American Journal of the Disabled Child,* 133 (1979):1204.
355. Ben Best, "The 2014 Cardiovascular Disease Prevention Symposium," (Life Extension, 2014), Accessed April, 2015 from http://www.lef.org//Magazine/2014/7/The-2014-Cardiovascular-Disease-Prevention-Symposium/Page-01.
356. Ibid.
357. D Donald Kasarda, "Can an increase in Celiac Disease be attributed to an increase in the gluten content of wheat as a consequence of wheat breeding?" *Journal of Agricultural and Food Chemistry,* 61 (2013): 1155 1159.
358. Mark Hyman, "Three hidden ways wheat makes you fat," (Dr. Mark Hyman, 2014), Accessed March 16, 2015 from http://drhyman.com/blog/2012/02/13/three-hidden-ways-wheat-makes-you-fat/#close.
359. "Dr Mark Hyman," (Dr. Mark Hyman), Accessed March 16, 2015 from http://drhyman.com/blog/author/admin/#close.
360. Arthur Agatston, "Gluten: 5 things you need to know," *Cable News Network (CNN)* (Turner Broadcasting System, Inc 2013), Accessed March 16, 2015 from http://edition.cnn.com/2013/04/05/health/gluten-5-things/.

361. Ibid.
362. Colby Vorland, "Distraction during eating reduces fullness & increases subsequent consumption," *Nutsci.org* (Nutsci.org, 2011), Accessed March 16, 2015 from http://nutsci.org/2011/01/31/distraction-during-eating-reduces-fullness-increases-subsequent-consumption/.
363. Mollie Bloudoff-Indelicato, "Beaver Butts Emit Goo Used for Vanilla Flavoring." (*National Geographic*, October 1, 2013). Accessed on March 16, 2015 from http://voices.nationalgeographic.com/2013/10/01/beaver-butts-emit-goo-used-for-vanilla-flavoring/
364. National List of Allowed and Prohibited Substances. National Organic Program. Accessed from http://www.ams.usda.gov/AMSv1.0/NOPPetitionedSubstancesDatabase
365. Food Biotechnology in the United States: Science, Regulation, and Issues. Congressional Research Service Report, U.S. Department of State. June 1999. Accessed from http://fpc.state.gov/6176.htm
366. EPA Memorandum from William Burnham, Health Effects Division: Office of Pesticide Programs' List of Chemicals Evaluated for Carcinogenic Potential, February 19, 1997. Accessed from http://www.nrdc.org/health/kids/ocar/chap5.asp
367. Pesticides in the Diets of Infants and Children. National Research Council, p. 13. Accessed from http://www.ncbi.nlm.nih.gov/books/NBK236275/
368. Pesticide Data Program: Annual Summary Calendar Year 1995. Agricultural Marketing Service. U.S. Department of Agriculture, May 1997. Accessed from http://cfpub.epa.gov/eroe/index.cfm?fuseaction=detail.viewReference&ch=48&lShowInd=0&subtop=312&lv=list.listByChapter&r=201566
369. Shelby, M.D. NTP-CERHR monograph on the potential human reproductive and developmental effects of bisphenol A. NTP CERHR MON. 2008 Sep;(22):v, vii-ix, 1-64 passim.
370. Markey E. Ban Poisonous Additives Act of 2009. HR 1523. Accessed from https://www.govtrack.us/congress/bills/111/hr1523
371. Bisphenol A (BPA): Use in Food Contact Application. Update on Bisphenol A (BPA) for Use in Food Contact Applications. January 2010; March 30, 2012; Updated March 2013; July 2014; November 2014.
372. Bisphenol A - Toxic Plastics Chemical in Canned Food. Environmental Working Group. March 2007. Accessed from http://www.ewg.org/research/bisphenol
373. "Bisphenol A (BPA): Use in Food Contact Application Update on Bisphenol A (BPA) for Use in Food Contact Applications" (Food and Drug Administration 01/06/2015).
374. "FDA Regulations No Longer Authorize the Use of BPA in Infant Formula Packaging Based on Abandonment; Decision Not Based on Safety" (CFSAN Constituent Update July 11, 2013; Food and Drug Administration updated 6/9/2014) Accessed on March 3, 2015 from http://www.fda.gov/Food/NewsEvents/ConstituentUpdates/ucm360147.htm.
375. "Behind the Bean: the heroes and Charlatans of the natural and organic soy foods industry." The Social, Environmental, and Health Impacts of Soy. The Cornucopia Institute. 2009.
376. Ibid.
377. SJ Towns and CM Mellis, "Role of acetyl salicylic acid and sodium metabisulfite in chronic childhood asthma. *Pediatrics* 73 (1984):631-637.
378. "'Inactive' Ingredients in Pharmaceutical Products: Update (Subject Review). Committee on Drugs." *Pediatrics, 99 (1997):*268-278.

379. "Committee on Toxicity of Chemicals in Food, Consumer Products and the Environment: Statement on Research Project (T07040) Investigating the Effect of Mixtures of Certain Food Colours and a Preservative on Behaviour in Children." COT statement 2007/04.
380. "Healthy Home Tips: Tip 6 - Skip the Non-stick to Avoid the Dangers of Teflon." Environmental Working Group. Accessed from http://www.ewg.org/research/healthy-home-tips/tip-6-skip-non-stick-avoid-dangers-teflon
381. Ibid.
382. Eleanor Williams, "Making Vegetarian Diets Nutritious," *American Journal of Nursing* (1975):21682173.
383. Ibid.
384. Ibid.
385. "Nutritional Facts," (Potatoes Goodness Unearthed, 2012), Accessed March 16, 2015 from http://www.potatogoodness.com/nutrition/nutritional-facts/.
386. Daiva Gorczyca et al., "Impact of Vegetarian Diet on Serum Immunoglobulin Levels in Children," *Clinical Pediatrics,* (2013) 10.1177/0009922812472250
387. Rosalind S Gibson et al., "Is iron and zinc nutrition a concern for vegetarian infants and young children in industrialized countries?" *The American Journal of Clinical Nutrition,* 100 (2014):459S-468S.
388. Markus Keller, "Vegetarische Ernährung bei Kindern und Jugendlichen," (Vegetarierbund Deutschland, 2013), Accessed March 16, 2015 from https://vebu.de/themen/gesundheit/kinderjugendliche.
389. D. Gorczyca et al., "An impact of the diet on serum fatty acid and lipid profiles in Polish vegetarian children and children with allergy," *Eur J Clin Nutr.,* 65 (2011):191-195.
390. Leslen Newman, "Natural Wonder," *Vegetarian Times* (March/April 1979):80.
391. Michael F Roizen and Mehmet C Oz, *You: on a Diet* (New York: Free Press, 2006).
392. Ron Pikarski, "Bringing Vegetarianism into the Gourmet Limelight," *Vegetarian Times* (January/February 1980): 3132.
393. Ibid.
394. Frank J Hurd and Rosalie Hurd, *Ten Talents* (Collegedale, Tenn.: The College Press, 1968), 5.
395. Abhay Kumar Pati, "Ayurveda for Health," *International Journal of Holistic Health & Medicine,* 1 (1982): 5.
396. Ibid.
397. Rudolph Ballentine, *Diet and Nutrition* (Honesdale, Pa.: Himalayan International Institute of Yoga Science and Philosophy, 1978), 317.
398. Yoni Freedhoff, "A review of David Kessler's The End of Overeating," *Weighty Matters* (Weighty Matters, 2010), Accessed March 16, 2015 from http://www.weightymatters.ca/2010/03/review-of-david-kesslers-end-of.html.
399. Abhay Kumar Pati, "Ayurveda for Health," *International Journal of Holistic Health & Medicine* 1 (1982):5.

Chapter 6

1. *Journal of the American Dietetic Association*, 25 (1949):202.
2. Ibid. 17, no. 6 (June/July 1941).
3. Ibid. (September 1948).

4. Ibid. 31 (1955).
5. Ibid. (September 1964).
6. Ibid. 17, no. 1 (January 1941).
7. Centers for Disease Control and Prevention, "Multistate Outbreak of Listeriosis Linked to Blue Bell Creameries Products" (April 21, 2015) Accessed on April 28, 2015 from http://www.cdc.gov/listeria/outbreaks/ice-cream-03-15/.
8. Robert Goodhart and Maurice Shils, *Modern Nutrition in Health and Disease* (Philadelphia: Lea and Febiger, 1980), 91.
9. Elle Paula, "What roles does protein play in the body?" *SFGate* (Demand Media, Inc.), Accessed March 16, 2015 from http://healthyeating.sfgate.com/roles-protein-play-body-3918.html.
10. P Evenepoel et al., "Digestibility of cooked and raw egg protein in humans as assessed by stable isotope techniques," *J. Nutr.* (1998) 128:1716-22
11. Mervyn G Hardinge, "Do Human Beings Need Meat?" *Review and Herald* (27 February 1969).
12. Ibid.
13. Ibid.
14. Editorial, *Lancet* 2 (1959): 956.
15. Hardinge.
16. Arturi I Virtanen, *Federation Proceedings 27,* no. 6 (1968): 1374.
17. Hardinge.
18. Physicians Committee for Responsible Medicine, "Vegetarian diets for children: Right from the start," (The Physicians Committee, 2002), Accessed March 16, 2015 from http://pcrm.org/health/diets/vegdiets/vegetarian-diets-for-children-right-from-the-start.
19. John McDougall, M.D., radio interview with author on "Natural Living," WBAI, New York, (26 March 1987).
20. Hara Marano, "The Problem with Protein," *New York* (5 March 1979): 51.
21. Ibid.
22. Ibid.
23. Physicians Committee for Responsible Medicine, "Doctors tell Arby's to retract 'Protein is better in meat form' tweet," (The Physicians Committee, 2014), Accessed March 16, 2015 from http://www.pcrm.org/media/news/doctors-tell-arbys-to-retract-protein-tweet.
24. USDA Dietary Guidelines Advisory Committee, "Food groups—Current intakes and trends," Dietary Guidelines Advisory Committee 2015) Accessed March 16, 2015, from http://www.health.gov/dietaryguidelines/2015-scientific-report/06-chapter-1/d1-3.asp.
25. Michael Greger, "protein," (NutritionFacts.org, 2015), Accessed March 16, 2015 from http://nutritionfacts.org/topics/protein/.
26. K Marsh et al., "Health implications of a vegetarian diet; a review," *Am J Lifestyle Med.,* 6 (2012):250-267.
27. Hara Marano, "The Problem with Protein," *New York* (5 March 1979): 51.
28. Physicians Committee for Responsible Medicine, "Five protein myths," (The Physicians Committee, 2015), Accessed March 3, 2015 from http://www.pcrm.org/health/reports/five-protein-myths.
29. N Barnard et al., "Meat consumption as a risk factor for type 2 diabetes," *Nutrients,* 6 (2014):897-910.

30. THT Chiu et al., "Taiwanese vegetarians and omnivores: dietary composition, prevalence of diabetes and IFG," *PLOS One,* (2014) DOI: 10.1371/journal.pone.0088547
31. M Van Nielen et al,. "Dietary protein intake and incidence of type 2 diabetes in Europe: the EPIC-INTERACT case-cohort study," *Diabetes Care,* 37 (2014):1854-62.
32. AJ Gaskins et al., "Dietary patterns and semen quality in young men," *Hum Reprod.*, 27 (2012):2899-2907.
33. EF Schisterman et al., "Lipid concentrations and semen quality: the LIFE study," *Andrology*, 2 (2014):408-415.
34. JE Chavarro et al., "Protein intake and ovulatory infertility," *Am J Obstet Gynecol.,* 198 (2008):210.e1-7.
35. Karen and Michael Iacobbo, *Vegetarian America: A History.* (Praeger, 2014).
36. T Osborne and LB Mendel, "Amino Acids in Nutrition and Growth," *Journal of Biological Chemistry,* 17 (1914):324.
37. John McDougall, M.D., radio interview with author on "Natural Living," WBAI, New York, 26 March 1987.
38. William Rose, "The Amino Acid Requirements of Adult Man, XVI, the Role of the Nitrogen Intake," *Journal of Biological Chemistry,* 217 (1955):997.
39. McDougall, radio interview.
40. John McDougall, M.D., radio interview with author on "Natural Living," WBAI, New York, 26 March 1987.
41. J McDougall, "Building the high performance athletic body," (September 2003) Accessed on March 30, 2013 from. http://www.drmcdougall.com.
42. The National Research Council, "Dietary reference intakes for energy, carbohydrate, fiber, fat, fatty acids, cholesterol, protein, and amino acids *(Macronutrients),*" Institute of Medicine of the National Academies (Washington, D.C., 2005) Accessed March 16, 2015, from http://books.nap.edu/openbook.php?record_id=10490.
43. National Agricultural Library, "Food search," Accessed March 16, 2015 from http://ndb.nal.usda.gov/ndb/foods?fgcd=Vegetables+and+Vegetable+Products&manu=&lfacet=&count=&max=35&sort=&qlookup=&offset=&format=Abridged&new=&measureby=.
44. Keith Akers, *A Vegetarian Sourcebook* (New York: Putnam, 1983).
45. William Rose, "The Amino Acid Requirements of Adult Man, XVI, the Role of the Nitrogen Intake," *Journal of Biological Chemistry,* 217 (1955): 997.
46. John A McDougall and Mary A McDougall, *The McDougall Plan for Super Health and LifeLong Weight Loss* (New Jersey: New Century Publishers, 1983).
47. McDougall, *The McDougall Plan,* 99.

Chapter 7

1. "A sample entry from the encyclopedia of religion and nature," *Encyclopedia of Religion and Nature* (Continuum, 2005), Accessed March 16, 2015 from http://www.religionandnature.com/ern/sample/Kalland--ReligiousEnvtlParadigm.pdf.
2. Suzanne Sutton, "Ellen White, SeventhDay Adventists and Vegetarianism," *Vegetarian Times* (November/December 1977): 37.

3. Seventh Day Adventist Church. Office of Archives, Statistics and Research. North American Division (1913-2014), Accessed March 15, 2015 from http://www.adventiststatistics.org/view_Summary.asp?FieldID=D_NAD.
4. Accessed from http://www.llu.edu/llu/health/mortality.html
5. JC McKenzie, "Social and Economic Implications of Minority Food Habits," *Proceedings of the Nutrition Society,* 26 (1967): 198.
6. Louis A Berman, "Why is Jewish Vegetarianism Different from All Others?" *Vegetarian Times* (April 1980): 4445.
7. "A sample entry from the encyclopedia of religion and nature," *Encyclopedia of Religion and Nature* (Continuum, 2005), Accessed March 16, 2015 from http://www.religionandnature.com/ern/sample/Kalland--ReligiousEnvtlParadigm.pdf.
8. Swami BV Tripurari, *Ancient Wisdom for Modern Ignorance*, (1995).
9. "A tribute to Hinduism: the book," Accessed from http://www.hinduwisdom.info/Nature_Worship.htm.
10. Hardinge.
11. Nathaniel Altman, "The Spiritual Side of Vegetarianism," *Vegetarian Times* (November/December 1977): 36.
12. Abantika Ghosh and Vijaita Singh, "Census: Hindu share dips below 80%, Muslim share grows but slower," *The Nation* New Delhi, Updated: January 24, 2015, Accessed on March 3, 2015 from http://indianexpress.com/article/india/india-others/census-hindu-share-dips-below-80-muslim-share-grows-but-slower/.
13. Jane Srivastava, "Vegetarianism and Meat-Eating in 8 Religions," *Hinduism Magazine* (June 2007). Accessed on March 3, 2015 from http://www.hinduismtoday.com/modules/smartsection/item.php?itemid=1541.
14. Nirmala George, "India's diehard Hindus push to ban beef in blow to poor," (Dawn, 2015), Accessed April, 2015 from http://www.dawn.com/news/1176364/indias-diehard-hindus-push-to-ban-beef-in-blow-to-poor.
15. Billy HC Kwok, "Horrifying Photos of China's Dog-Eating Festival—and the Activists Who Are Trying to Stop It," *New Republic* (August 27, 2014). Accessed on March 3, 2015 from http://www.newrepublic.com/article/119223/photos-yulin-chinas-dog-meat-eating-festival-2014.
16. Chris Wright, "International" Forbes Magazine (2/11/2014). Accessed March 31, 2015 from http://www.forbes.com/sites/chriswright/2014/02/11/when-chinas-food-runs-out/
17. Maki, "Just Hungry. Japan: A Survival Guide For Vegans" Blog entry, posted on 5 Mar 2009. Accessed on March 3, 2015 from http://justhungry.com/japan-survival-guide-vegans
18. Karen Atwood, "Japanese vegetarians campaign for Tokyo's 50,000 restaurants to offer meat free dishes," *The Independent* (December 28, 2014). Accessed on March 3, 2015 from http://www.independent.co.uk/life-style/food-and-drink/news/japanese-vegetarians-campaign-for-tokyos-50000-restaurants-to-offer-meat-free-dishes-9946598.html
19. Ibid.
20. Darla Erhard, "Nutrition Education for the Now Generation," *Journal of Nutrition Education,* (1971): 135.
21. Darla Erhard, "The New Vegetarians," *Nutrition Today* (January/February 1974): 20.
22. Erhard, "Nutrition Education."

23. Ibid.
24. Bhagwan Shree Rajneesh, "The Spiritual Side of Vegetarianism," *Vegetarian Times* (March 1980): 62.
25. Erhard, "Nutrition Education."
26. Ibid.
27. *Lancet* 285 (1963): 43.
28. William Adolph, "Vegetarian China," *Scientific American* (September 1938): 133
29. Ibid.
30. "Insomnia," (Life Extension). Accessed March 31, 2015 from http://www.lef.org/Protocols/Lifestyle-Longevity/Insomnia/Page-03.
31. Terry Lyles, *Cracking the stress code: Eliminate harmful stress and achieve life mastery in 4 simple steps* (Essential Publishing, Inc, 2015)
32. Gary Null, *Get healthy now!: A complete guide to prevention, treatment, and healthy living* (Seven Stories Press, 2011)
33. Mayo Clinic, "Red wine and resveratrol: Good for your heart?" (Mayo Foundation for Medical Education and Research, 2014). Accessed March 31, 2015 from http://www.mayoclinic.org/diseases-conditions/heart-disease/in-depth/red-wine/art-20048281.
34. Michael V Holmes et al., "Association between alcohol and cardiovascular disease: Mendelian randomisation analysis based on individual participant data," *BMJ,* 349 (2014):g4164.
35. T Blake, Some Surprising Benefits of Meditation. *Kajama.* Accessed on November 20, 2012 from http://www.kajama.com/index.php?file=articledetail&id=936FD18C-EB29-4BA7-B83E-1FE277B39305&PageNum=1
36. J. Littman, "Finally—Scientific Proof that Our Thoughts Affect Our Health. (We Already Knew That!)," *Empower Network* (Oct 15, 2012).
37. Manish J Parswani, et al., "Mindfulness-based stress reduction program in coronary heart disease: A randomized control trial," *International Journal of Yoga,* 6 (2013):111-117.
38. Kristen Domonell, "5 surprising health benefits of yoga," *The Huffington Post* (The Huffington Post, 2014), Accessed March 31, 2015 from http://www.huffingtonpost.com/2014/02/12/yoga-health-benefits_n_4768746.html.
39. Yoga Health Foundation, "Health Benefits of Yoga explained," (Yoga Health Foundation, 2012), Accessed March 31, 2015 from http://www.yogahealthfoundation.org/health_benefits_of_yoga_explained.
40. Associated Press, "Out of Keystone debate's glare, pipelines going in nationwide," *Associated Press* (Fuelfix.com, 2015), Accessed March 31, 2015 from http://fuelfix.com/blog/2015/03/16/out-of-keystone-debates-glare-pipelines-going-in-nationwide/.
41. GaiaTheory.org, "Overview," (Entrepreneurial Earth LLC). Accessed March 31, 2015 from http://www.gaiatheory.org/overview/.
42. Bec Crew, "New study reveals 84% of vegetarians return to meat," *ScienceAlert* (ScienceAlert Pty Ltd., 2014), Accessed March 31, 2015 from http://www.sciencealert.com/new-study-reveals-84-of-vegetarians-return-to-meat.
43. "The Roseto Effect," (University of Illinois, 1999), Accessed April, 2015 from http://www.uic.edu/classes/osci/osci590/14_2%20The%20Roseto%20Effect.htm
44. Gary Null, *Reverse arthritis & pain naturally: A proven approach to a pain-free life* (Essential Publishing, Inc, 2013)

45. FJ Dalal, "Nonviolence and health," (Jain Study Circular), Accessed March 31, 2015 from http://www.jainstudy.org/Vegetarianism.htm#4.
46. Cassadaga Spiritualist Camp, "What is Spiritualism..." (Cassadaga Spiritualist Camp), Accessed March 31, 2015, 2015 from http://www.cassadaga.org/whatitis.htm.
47. Katie Byron, *Do The Work,* (Byron Katie International), Accessed from http://thework.com/do-work.
48. John Clark Smith, "Vegetarian As Art," *Vegetarian Times* (September/October 1979):21.
49. Colman McCarthy, "Meatless Meals: A Change in America's Menu," *Washington Post,* (13 Jan. 1976), 19.
50. F James Garrett, "George Bernard Shaw," *Vegetarian Times* (July/August 1977).
51. "Classics: The Vegetarian Diet According to Shaw," *Vegetarian Times* (March/April 1979):5051.
52. Barbara Sarkesian, "Thoreau," *Vegetarian Times* (December 1976/January 1977):20.
53. Daniel Wesolowski, "Henry Thoreau," *Vegetarian Times* (November/December 1977):39.
54. Sarkesian, "Thoreau."
55. Helen and Scott Nearing, "Living the Good Life at 95," *Vegetarian Times* (no. 23, 1978):3839.
56. Rynn Berry, Jr., "Cloris!" *Vegetarian Times* (May/June 1979): 15.
57. Judy Klemesrud, "Vegetarianism: Growing Way of Life, Especially Among the Young," *New York Times,* (10 March 1976), 47; Suzanne Sutton, "Superstars," *Vegetarian Times* (March/April 1977):3637.
58. Ann Johnson and Torney Smith, "Susan Smith Jones: More than Just a Pretty Face," *Vegetarian Times* (November/December 1979):2023.
59. Bob Lewanski, "Vegetarians Who Pump Iron," *Vegetarian Times* (March/April 1979):1922.
60. Robyn M. Grasing, "John Marino: A World Record Holder on Nutrition," *Vegetarian Times* (January/February 1979): 3031.
61. "Still Skiing at Eighty Four," *Life and HealthNational Health Journal* (1973) 1.
62. "Great Vegan Athletes," *Cyclist* (Great Vegan Athletes), Accessed March 31, 2015 from http://www.greatveganathletes.com/cyclists.

Chapter 8

1. Ricardo Lopez, "Most workers hate their jobs or have 'checked out,' Gallup says," *Los Angeles Times* (Los Angeles Times, 2013), Accessed March 31, 2015 from http://www.latimes.com/business/la-fi-mo-employee-engagement-gallup-poll-20130617-story.html.
2. Susan W Butterworth, "Influencing patient adherence to treatment guidelines," *Journal of Managed Care Pharmacy* (2008) 14(6 (suppl S-b)), S21-S25
3. "Friedrich Nietzsche," (Goodreads, Inc.), Accessed March 31, 2015 from http://www.goodreads.com/author/show/1938.Friedrich_Nietzsche.
4. Viktor E Frankl, *Man's search for meaning* (Beacon Press, 2006)
5. Ibid.

Part II

1. Jonny Citizen, "Top 10 environmental issues facing our planet," *Planet Earth Herald* (Planet Earth Herald), Accessed March 31, 2015 from http://planetearthherald.com/top-10-environmental-issues/

2. Derek Markham, "Global warming effects and causes: A top 10 list," (PlanetSave, 2009), Accessed March 31, 2015 from http://planetsave.com/2009/06/07/global-warming-effects-and-causes-a-top-10-list/
3. Center for Biological Diversity, "The extinction crisis," (Center for Biological Diversity), Accessed March 31, 2015 from http://www.biologicaldiversity.org/programs/biodiversity/elements_of_biodiversity/extinction_crWoSs/
4. Ibid.
5. Jonny Citizen, "Top 10 environmental issues facing our planet," *Planet Earth Herald* (Planet Earth Herald), Accessed March 31, 2015 from http://planetearthherald.com/top-10-environmental-issues/
6. "What is ozone and where is it in the atmosphere?" (The Ozone Hole, Inc.), Accessed March 31, 2015 from http://www.theozonehole.com/twenty.htm.
7. Jonny Citizen, "No fish left in in the oceans 50 years from now?" (Planet Earth Herald, 2012), Accessed March 31, 2015 from http://planetearthherald.com/no-fish-left-in-50-years-from-now/
8. Alexander Haro, "The oceans could be dead by the year 2048," *The Inertia* (The Inertia, 2014), Accessed March 31, 2015 from http://www.theinertia.com/environment/the-oceans-could-be-dead-by-the-year-2048/
9. Ryan Grenoble, "World's oldest trees dying at alarming rate: Study (VIDEO)," *The Huffington Post* (2012), Accessed March 31, 2015 from http://www.huffingtonpost.com/2012/12/10/oldest-trees-dying_n_2272775.html.

Chapter 9

1. Peter Singer and Jim Mason, *The way we eat: Why our food choices matter* (Rodale, 2006)
2. Eric Schlosser, *Fast food nation: The dark side of the all-American meal* (Houghton Mifflin Company, 2001)
3. Ibid.
4. "Cow's Milk: A Cruel and Unhealthy Product", Accessed on March 3, 2015 from http://www.peta.org/issues/animals-used-for-food/animals-used-food-factsheets/cows-milk-cruel-unhealthy-product/
5. Oxford Vegetarians; Accessed on March 3, 2015 from http://www.ivu.org/oxveg/.
6. www.sfvegan.org/Worldwide_Animal_Slaughter_Statistics.pdf
7. "Food," (Animal Equality United Kingdom, Accessed March 31, 2015 from http://www.animalequality.net/food.
8. James B Mason, "Animals," *Vegetarian Times* (March 1980): 52. Accessed on March 3, 2015 from http://www.da.gov.ph/wps/portal/bai. Select Features, then Chicken, then Production Management.
9. Ibid.
10. Ross Flume Hall, *Food for Naught* (New York: Vintage, 1974), 91.
11. Mason, "Animals."
12. Ibid., 53.
13. CD Van Houweling, "Drugs In Animal Feeds? A Question Without An Answer," FDA *Papers* (September 1967): 1115.
14. Hall, 100.
15. Ibid.

16. W Anderson, "Porcine Stress Syndrome Problem Updated by Vet," *Feedstuffs* (May 1972): 21.
17. Michael W Fox, "Philosophy, Ecology, Animal Welfare, and the 'Rights Question,'" in *Ethics and Animals* (Clifton, NJ: Humana Press, Inc., 1983), 308.
18. "Cut Stress and You'll Control Dark Cutters," *Feedlot Management* 14(1972): 5051.
19. Mo, "Feeling the pain of others," (ScienceBlogs, 2009), Accessed March 31, 2005 from http://scienceblogs.com/neurophilosophy/2009/12/17/feeling-the-pain-of-others/.
20. "Cut Stress."
21. Hall.
22. William K. Stevens, "For Steaks, A Gilded Age is Fading," *New York* Times, (7 Jan. 1981), p.C6.
23. Clark Smith, "Vegetarianism As Art," *Vegetarian Times* (September/October 1979):2021.
24. Michael W. Fox, "The Hidden Costs of Modern Farming," A *Special Awareness Report* (The Humane Society of the United States, 1981).
25. Richard Rhodes, "Watching the Animals," 9192.
26. Louis A. Berman, "Why Is Jewish Vegetarianism Different From All Others?" *Vegetarian Times* (April 1980): 43.
27. DeDee Benrey, "The World According to Isaac Singer," *Vegetarian Times* (March 1983):14.
28. Michael W Fox, "The Question of Animal Rights," *The Veterinary Record* (11 July 1981):3739.
29. Tamara Ross, "Animal, Vegetable, Mineral," *Nursing Mirror* (July 1980).
30. Mark Braunstein, "On Being Radically Vegetarian," *Vegetarian Times* (March 1980):7273.
31. R Brooks and JR Kernm, "Vegan Diet and Lifestyle: A Preliminary Study by Postal Questionnaire," *Proceedings of the Nutrition Society,* 38 (1979):15A.
32. Nathaniel Altman, "The Spiritual Side of Vegetarianism," *Vegetarian Times* (November/December 1977):3638.
33. James B. Mason, "Vegetarianism is a Human Rights Struggle," *Vegetarian Times* (June 1980):4849.
34. Ibid.
35. Fox, *Ethics and Animals.*
36. Ibid.
37. Charles Wilson and Eric Schlosser, *Chew on this: everything you don't want to know about fast food* (Houghton Mifflin, 2007)
38. *World Health Organization: visit: http://www.who.int/violence_injury_prevention (2002).*
39. The Peace Alliance, "Statistics on violence & peace," (The Peace Alliance, 2013), Accessed April 5, 2015 from http://peacealliance.org/tools-education/statistics-on-violence/.
40. EG Krug et al., eds, "World report on violence and health," (Geneva, World Health Organization, 2002). Via CDC.
41. The Economic Dimensions of Interpersonal Violence, (World Health Organization, 2004.)
42. Global Peace Index, (2014) Accessed in April 2015 from http://www.visionofhumanity.org/#page/indexes/global-peace-index/2014/USA/OVER]
43. UN Report on violence against women worldwide, (2015).
44. "Global and Regional Estimates of Violence against Women," (World Health Organization, 2013).
45. *2012 US Peace Index*, (Institute for Economics and Peace)
46. Ibid.
47. *World Report on Violence and Health,* (World Health Organization 2002).

48. Centers for Disease Control, "Web-based Injury Statistics Query and Reporting System (WISQARS)" (Atlanta, GA: US Department of Health and Human Services, CDC, 2013). Accessed on March 3, 2015 from http://www.cdc.gov/injury/wisqars/index.html.]

49. Return on investment: Evidence-based options to improve statewide outcomes. October 2013 (Printed on 3-20-14). Olympia: Washington State Institute for Public Policy.

50. The Juvenile Justice System in Washington State: Recommendations to Improve Cost-Effectiveness, 2002.

51. National Research Center's Analysis of the Longmont Community Justice Partnership 2007-2009 http://www.lcjp.org/images/stories/pdf/LCJP_2007-2009_Report_Final.pdf

52. "Improving School Climate; Findings from Schools Implementing Restorative Practices" a report from the International Institute for Restorative Practices, 2009.

53. Preventing youth violence and delinquency through a universal school-based prevention approach. Prevention Science, (2006).

54. NBC Nightly News, January 2015.

55. Adapted with permission from "Simple Changes, Big Rewards: A Practical, Easy Guide for Healthy, Happy Living," a special health report (Harvard Health Publications). Accessed on March 3, 2015 from http://www.helpguide.org/articles/work-career/volunteering-and-its-surprising-benefits.htm.

56. Anthony Rivas, "People who volunteer may be happier, healthier, and live longer," *Medical Daily* (IBT Media, Inc., 2013), Accessed April 5, 2015 from http://www.medicaldaily.com/people-who-volunteer-may-be-happier-healthier-and-live-longer-254147

57. United Health Group, "Volunteering linked to better physical, mental health," (UnitedHealth Group, 2013), Accessed April 5, 2015 from http://www.unitedhealthgroup.com/newsroom/articles/feed/unitedhealth%20group/2013/0619healthvolunteering.aspx.

58. Bert N Uchino, *Social Support and Physical Health: Understanding the Health Consequences of Relationships*, (New Haven, CT: Yale University Press; 2004).

59. BH Brummett et al., *Psychosom Med.* 63 (2001):267-72.

60. JK Kiecolt-Glaser et al., *Annu Rev Psychol.* 53 (2002):83-107; PA Thoit, *J Health Soc Behav.*, (1995):53-79.

61. United States Environmental Protection Agency, *Municipal Solid Waste Generation, Recycling, and Disposal in the United States: Facts and Figures for 2011.* (Washington, DC: , 2013). Accessed on February 9, 2015 from <http://www.epa.gov/osw/nonhaz/municipal/pubs/MSWcharacterization_508_053113_fs.pdf>.

62. Heeral Bhalala, "Will the US ever learn to recycle?" (Center for Leadership in Global Sustainability, 2013), Accessed April 5, 2015 from http://cligs.vt.edu/recycle/.

63. Clarissa A León, "These top 10 food companies control nearly everything we eat: A new map puts our food system in a whole new light." (AlterNet, 2014), Accessed April 5, 2015 from http://www.alternet.org/food/food-brands-climate-change.

64. Damian Carrington and George Arnett, "Clear differences between organic and non-organic food, study finds," *The Guardian* (2014), Accessed March 16, 2015 from http://www.theguardian.com/environment/2014/jul/11/organic-food-more-antioxidants-study.

65. Tony Henderson, "Newcastle University study proves organic food is better for you," *The Journal* (Trinity Mirror North East, 2014), Accessed April 5, 2015 from http://www.thejournal.co.uk/news/newcastle-university-study-proves-organic-7411542.

66. Eat Local Grown, "Top 10 most common GMO foods," Accessed April 5, 2015 from http://eatlocalgrown.com/article/12060-top-gmo-foods.html.
67. Margaret Floyd, "Why do many processed foods contain soy?" (ShareCare, Inc.), Accessed April 5, 2015 from http://www.sharecare.com/health/soy-supplements/why-processed-foods-contain-soy.
68. Lawrence Robinson, et al., "Are organic foods right for you? Understanding the benefits of organic food and the risks of GMOs and pesticides," (Helpguide.org, 2015), Accessed April 5, 2015 from http://www.helpguide.org/articles/healthy-eating/organic-foods.htm.
69. Jennifer Morris, et al., "School-based gardens can teach kids healthier eating habits," *California Agriculture,* 54 (2000):40-46.

Chapter 10

1. RN Lubowski et al, "How the Land Is Used," *Major Uses of Land in the United States, 2002/EIB-14* (Economic Research Service/USDA). Accessed on March 3, 2015 from http://www.ers.usda.gov/Publications/EIB14/.
2. Frances Moore Lappé, *Diet for a Small Planet* (New York: Ballantine, 1971).
3. Frances Moore Lappé and Joseph Collins, *Food First: Beyond the Myth of Scarcity* (New York: Ballantine, 1977)
4. Ibid.
5. United Nations, Department of Economic and Social Affairs, Population Division, "World Population Prospects: The 2012 Revision, Highlights and Advance Tables," Working Paper No. ESA/P/WP.228. (2013) Accessed on March 3, 2015 fromhttp://www.worldometers.info/world-population/
6. Alex Hershaft, *Solving the Population/Food Crisis by Eating for Life* (Washington, D.C.: Vegetarian Information Service, 1985).
7. "FAQ & Answers," (Save The Amazon Rainforest), Accessed April, 2015 from http://savetheamazonrainforest.com/web_folders/faq_answers/.
8. NE Stork, "Measuring Global Biodiversity and Its Decline," in ML Reaka-Kudla et al, (eds) *Biodiversity II: Understanding and Protecting our Natural Resources.* (Washington, DC: Joseph Henry Press 1997). Accessed on March 3, 2015 from http://www.rain-tree.com/facts.htm
9. DH Boucher, *Brazil's success in reducing deforestation. UCS Tropical Forest and Climate Briefing #8.* (Cambridge, MA: Union of Concerned Scientists, 2011). Accessed on March 3, 2015 from http://www.newsweek.com/brazils-deforestation-rates-are-rise-again-315648
10. K Morales and T Vinicius, "Amazon rainforest: biodiversity and biopiracy," *STUDENT BMJ,* 13 (2003):386-7.
11. Rainforest Facts, Raintree (December 2012) Accessed on March 3, 2015 from http://www.raitree.com/facts.htm.
12. "Honey Bee Health and Colony Collapse Disorder" Agricultural Research Service, US Department of Agriculture. (March 2015) Accessed on March 3, 2015 from https://www.organicconsumers.org/essays/gmos-are-killing-bees-butterflies-birds-and
13. "Protecting the Pollinators: Spotlight" Agriculture and Consumer Protection Department. (UN Food and Agriculture Organisation, 2005). Accessed on March 3, 2015 from http://www.bbc.com/future/story/20140502-what-if-bees-went-extinct
14. S Suchail et al, "Characteristics of imidacloprid toxicity in two Apis mellifera subspecies," *Environmental Toxicology and Chemistry,* 19 (2000):1901–1905.

15. George Monbiot, "Neonicotinoids are the new DDT killing the natural world," (5th August 2013) Accessed on March 3, 2015 from http://www.monbiot.com/2013/08/13/ddt-2-0/
16. TC Van Dijk et al, "Macro-Invertebrate Decline in Surface Water Polluted with Imidacloprid," *PLoS ONE* 8 (2013):e62374.
17. George Monbiot, "Another Silent Spring?" (July 15, 2014). Accessed March 31, 2015 from http://www.monbiot.com/2014/07/15/another-silent-spring/.
18. Lappé, *Food First.*
19. Lester R Brown and Edward C Wolf, *Soil Erosion: Quiet Crisis in the World Economy,* World Watch Paper No. 60 (New York: 1984).
20. EA Scholin, et al. "Mortality of sea lions along the central California coast linked to a toxic diatom bloom," *Nature,* 403 (2000):80-84.
21. RJ Diaz and R Rosenberg, "Spreading Dead Zones and Consequences for Marine Ecosystems." *Science* 321 (2008):926–9.
22. J Barfroff, "How the food we feed farm animals is destroying the environment," *One Green Planet,* (September 18, 2014).
23. A Gallo, "Algae Blooms Making Toledo Water Undrinkable Are Thriving," *The Wall Street Journal,* (August 3, 2014).
24. RB Alexander et al, "Differences in Phosphorus and Nitrogen Delivery to the Gulf of Mexico from the Mississippi River Basin," *Environ. Sci. Technol.,* 42 (2008):822–830.
25. US Department of Agriculture, "Pastured poultry in Alabama," Natural Resources Conservation Service, USDA (2010).
26. David Pimental, "Soil Erosion: A Food and Environmental Threat" *Journal of the Environment.* 8 (2006):119-137.
27. H Eswaran, et al., "Land degradation: an overview." In: Bridges, EM., ID. Hannam, LR. Oldeman, FWT. Pening de Vries, SJ. Scherr, and S Sompatpanit (eds.). Responses to Land Degradation. Proc. 2nd. International Conference on Land Degradation and Desertification, Khon Kaen, Thailand. Oxford Press, New Delhi, India (2001).
28. "What If the World's Soil Runs Out?" World Economic Forum. *Time Magazine.* Dec. 14, 2012.
29. United Nations Convention to Combat Desertification (UNCCD), United Nations Environment Programme, Accessed April 15, 2015 from http://www.unep.org/ecosystemmanagement/News/PressRelease/tabid/426/language/en-US/Default.aspx?DocumentID=664&ArticleID=6918&Lang=en
30. Lappé, *Diet for a Small Planet.*
31. Seth King, "Iowa Rain and Wind Deplete Farmlands," *New York Times,* 5 Dec. 1976, 61.
32. Curtis Harnack, "In Plymouth County, Iowa, the Rich Topsoil's Going Fast. Alas," *New York Times, 11* July 1980.
33. Lappé, *Diet for a Small Planet.*
34. Ibid.
35. Ibid.
36. US Department of Agriculture, *Soil and Water Resources Conservations ActSummary of Appraisal,* Review Draft, 1980, 18.
37. Lappé, *Diet for a Small Planet*
38. "Study Says Soil Erosion Could Cause Famine," *New York Times, 30* Sept. 1984, 20.
39. Brown, *Soil Erosion.*

40. "Study Says Soil Erosion Could Cause Famine," *New York Times.*
41. Ibid.
42. Brown, Soil *Erosion.*
43. General Comment No. 15. "The right to water," (UN Committee on Economic, Social and Cultural Rights, November 2002).
44. IPCC Fourth Assessment Report: Climate Change 2007 (AR4).
45. Ibid.
46. UNDP. Habitat II, Dialogue III: Water for thirsty cities, Report of the Dialogue. United Nations Development Programme, United Nations Conference on Human Settlements, June 1996, Istanbul.
47. IPCC Fourth Assessment Report: Climate Change 2007 (AR4).
48. Jesse McKinley, "Drought Adds to Hardships in California," *The New York Times*, February 21, 2009.
49. "Livestock impacts on the environment," Agriculture and Consumer Protection Department. UN Food and Agriculture Organisation (2006). Accessed on March 3, 2015 from http://www.eateco.org/Environment/Water.htm.
50. "Livestock's long shadow: Environmental issues and options," UN Food and Agriculture Organisation (2006). Accessed on March 3, 2015 from ftp://ftp.fao.org/docrep/fao/010/a0701e/a0701e04.pdf
51. Ibid.
52. George Bargstrom, paper presented at the annual meeting of the American Association for the Advancement of Science, (1981); radio interview with author 5 October 1979.
53. "The Browning of America," *Newsweek* (22 February 1981): 26.
54. Ibid.
55. K Caldeira and ME Wickett, "Anthropogenic carbon and ocean pH." *Nature* 425 (2003): 365–365.
56. Frank J Millero, "Thermodynamics of the carbon dioxide system in the oceans." *Geochimica et Cosmochimica Acta,* 59 (1995):661–677.
57. Robert E Service, "Rising Acidity Brings an Ocean Of Trouble." *Science,* 337 (2012):146–148.
58. Burden of disease from Household Air Pollution for 2012. WHO Report.
59. Hazrije Mustafić, et al. "Main Air Pollutants and Myocardial Infarction: A Systematic Review and Meta-analysis." *JAMA,* 307 (2012):713-721.
60. EPA, *Endangerment Finding,* 74 FR 66498.
61. Hong Chen, et al., "A Systematic Review of the Relation Between Long-term Exposure to Ambient Air Pollution and Chronic Diseases," *Reviews on Environmental Health,* 23 (2011):243–298.
62. Confalonieri, U., et al. B. Human health. In: *Climate Change 2007: Impacts, Adaptation and Vulnerability. Contribution of Working Group II to the Fourth Assessment Report of the Intergovernmental Panel on Climate Change* Parry, M.L., O.F. Canziani, J.P. Palutikof, P.J. van der Linden and C.E. Hanson, (eds.), (2007). Cambridge University Press, Cambridge, United Kingdom.
63. "7 million premature deaths annually linked to air pollution," News release. (World Health Organization, March 25, 2010). Accessed on April 5, 2015 from http://www.who.int/mediacentre/news/releases/2014/air-pollution/en/
64. "Gebrselassie opts out of marathon." (BBC Sport, March 10, 2008), Accessed April 15, 2015 from http://news.bbc.co.uk/sport2/hi/olympics/athletics/7287578.stm.

65. "Henin trying to manage asthma, might skip Olympics." (ESPN, August, 4 2008), Accessed April 15, 2015 from http://sports.espn.go.com/sports/tennis/news/story?id=3095205

66. "The Benefits and Costs of the Clean Air Act from 1990 to 2020." Summary Report. EPA. March 2011.

67. "Maintaining Air Quality in a Transboundary Air Basin: Georgia Basin-Puget Sound." 2005 Report. Canada-United States Air Quality Agreement.

68. US Geological Survey, "The Quality of Our Nation's Waters— Nutrients and Pesticides" *U.S. Geological Survey Circular* 1225, (1999).

69. CD Cook, "The spraying of America," *Earth Island Journal.* Article adapted from Cook, *C.D. Diet for a Dead Planet: How the Food Industry Is Killing Us.* (The New Press, May 29, 2006). Accessed on March 3, 2015 from http://www.earthisland.org/journal/index.php/eij/article/the_spraying_of_america/

70. "Beijing Olympics Experiment Reveals Biological Link between Air Pollution Exposure and Cardiovascular Disease," *HealthCanal.* (June 5, 2012). Accessed on March 3, 2015 from http://www.healthcanal.com/blood-heart-circulation/29872-beijing-olympics-experiment-reveals-biological-link-between-air-pollution-exposure-and-cardiovascular-disease.html

71. DQ Rich et al., "Association Between Changes in Air Pollution Levels During the Beijing Olympics and Biomarkers of Inflammation and Thrombosis in Healthy Young Adults," *JAMA,* 307 (2012):2068-2078.

72. "Beijing Olympics Experiment Reveals Biological Link between Air Pollution Exposure and Cardiovascular Disease," *HealthCanal.* (June 5, 2012). Accessed on March 3, 2015 from http://www.healthcanal.com/blood-heart-circulation/29872-beijing-olympics-experiment-reveals-biological-link-between-air-pollution-exposure-and-cardiovascular-disease.html.

73. D Pimental and CW Hall, *Food and Energy Resources: Food Science and Technology* (Academic Press, 1984).

74. Lappé, *Diet for a Small Planet.*

75. "Livestock's long shadow: Environmental issues and options," (UN Food and Agriculture Organisation, 2006). Accessed on March 3, 2015 from http://www.fao.org/docrep/010/a0701e/a0701e00.HTM

76. E Hertwich et al. "UNEP Assessing the Environmental Impacts of Consumption and Production: Priority Products and Materials," A Report of the Working Group on the Environmental Impacts of Products and Materials to the International Panel for Sustainable Resource Management (2010) Accessed on March 3, 2015 from http://www.unep.org/resourcepanel/Portals/24102/PDFs/PriorityProductsAndMaterials_Report.pdf

77. K Senior, "When Will Fossil Fuels Run Out?" *CarbonCounted,* (April 22, 2015). Accessed on May 3, 2015 from http://www.carboncounted.co.uk/when-will-fossil-fuels-run-out.html

78. *Monthly Energy Review.* U.S. Energy Information Administration, (March 2015). DOE/EIA-0035(2015/03), Accessed on May 3, 2015 from http://www.eia.doe.gov/emeu/mer/pdf/pages/sec1_7.pdf

79. "U.S. Energy Facts," U.S. Energy Information Administration, (March 2015). Accessed on May 3, 2015 from http://www.eia.gov/energyexplained/index.cfm?page=us_energy_home

80. "Climate Change milestone demands shift to renewable energy," *WWF,* (May 3, 2015). Accessed on May 6, 2015 from http://wwf.panda.org/wwf_news/?208477/Climate-Change-milestone-demands-shift-to-renewable-energy

81. *US Greenhouse Gas Inventory Report: 1990-2013,* (EPA, April 2015). Accessed on March 3, 2015 from http://epa.gov/climatechange/ghgemissions/gases/ch4.html.

82. *Methane and Nitrous Oxide Emissions from Natural Sources,* EPA Report, (Washington D.C., US Environmental Protection Agency, April 2010).

83. "Overview of Greenhouse Gases: Methane Emissions," U.S. Environmental Protection Agency, April 2015. Accessed on May 3, 2015 from http://epa.gov/climatechange/ghgemissions/gases/ch4.html.

84. "Livestock impacts on the environment," Spotlight 2006. Agriculture and Consumer Protection Department. (UN Food and Agriculture Organisation, 2006). Accessed on March 3, 2015 from http://www.fao.org/ag/magazine/0612sp1.htm.

85. H Steinfeld et al., "FAO. 2006. Livestock's long shadow – Environmental issues and options," in C Nellemann et al (eds) *The Environmental Food Crisis – The Environment's Role in Averting Future Food Crises.*

86. United Nations Environment Programme, GRID-Arendal, Arendal. (Rome: UNEP, 2009).

87. N Fiala, "Meeting the demand: an estimation of potential future greenhouse gas emissions from meat production," *Ecological Economics,* 67 (2008):412–419.

88. Steinfeld et al.

89. Ibid.

90. Fiala 2008.

91. UNEP (2009). (eds. Nellemann, C, MacDevette, M, Manders, T, Eickhout, B, Svihus, B, Prins, AG and Kaltenborn, BP). "The Environmental Food Crisis – The Environment's Role in Averting Future Food Crises." United Nations Environment Programme, GRID-Arendal, Arendal.

92. M Gill et al., "Mitigating climate change: the role of domestic livestock," *Animal* 4 (2010):323–333.

93. JMG Barclay, "Meat, a damaging extravagence: a response to Grumett and Gorringe," *The Expository Times.* 123 (2012):70-73.

94. D Tilman and M Clark, "Global diets link environmental sustainability and human health," *Nature,* 515 (2014):518–522.

95. "Irrigation and Water Use," U.S. Department of Agriculture, Economic Research Service. (June 2013). Accessed on March 3, 2015 from http://www.ers.usda.gov/topics/farm-practices-management/irrigation-water-use/background.aspx.

96. MI Jacobson, "Six Arguments for a Greener Diet Argument #4: More and Cleaner Water," (Center for Science in the Public Interest. 2006). Accessed on March 3, 2015 from http://www.cspinet.org/EatingGreen/pdf/arguments4.pdf

97. "Meat Production Wastes Natural Resources," (PETA), Accessed April 2015 from http://www.peta.org/issues/animals-used-for-food/meat-wastes-natural-resources/

98. CJ Peters, et al., "Testing a complete-diet model for estimating the land resource requirements of food consumption and agricultural carrying capacity: The New York State example," *Renewable Agriculture and Food Systems*, 22 (2007):145-153.

99. C McGlade and P Ekins, "The geographical distribution of fossil fuels unused when limiting global warming to 2 °C," *Nature*, 517 (2015):187–190.

100. Brown, ibid., quoted in Matthew Wald, "Corn Farmers Smile as Ethanol Prices Rise, but Experts on Food Supplies Worry," *New York Times* (Jan 16, 2006).

101. Ibid.

102. Ibid.

103. "Stop The Rush To Corn Biofuel," Editorial, *Christian Science Monitor* (Aug. 12, 2008), Accessed on March 5, 2010 from http://www.csmonitor.com/2008/0812/p08s01-comv.html

104. Ibid.

105. Ibid.

106. "Guardian Newspaper Report Admits Widespread Failure of GM Btbrinjal," *GMWatch* (June 5, 2014).

107. Deirdre Fulton, "GMO Corn No Longer Resistant to Bugs," *Common Dreams* (July 30, 2014).

108. Pushpa M Bhargava, "US is trying to control our food production," *Hindustan Times*, (August 7, 2014), Accessed on March 3, 2015 from http://www.hindustantimes.com/comment/analysis/us-is-trying-to-control-our-food-production/article1-1249456.aspx.

109. "Karnataka bans Mahyco's Cotton Seeds" *Business Standard* (India) (March 28, 2014).

110. "Ten Years of Failure, Farmers Deceived by GM Corn" *MASIPAG* (Philippines (October 16, 2013).

111. "In Historic Ruling, Brazilian Court Prevents the Release of Transgenic Corn from Bayer" *Terra de Direitos* (Brazil) (March 13, 2014).

112. "UN Report Says Small Scale Organic Farming Only Way to Feed the World." *Technology Water*. (December 14, 2013). Accessed on March 3, 2015 from http://www.technologywater.com/post/69995394390/un-report-says-small-scale-organic-farming-only-way-to

113. "New Wave of Herbicide-Tolerant Crops Awaiting Likely U.S. Approval," *eNews Park Forest* (August 8, 2014), Accessed on March 3, 2015 from http://www.enewspf.com/latest-news/science/science-a-environmental/54647-new-wave-of-herbicide-tolerant-crops-awaiting-likely-u-s-approval.html.

114. US Greenhouse Gas Inventory Report: 1990-2013. EPA. (April 2015).

115. Energy Explained. US Energy Information Administration, US Department of Energy (August 2014).

116. Ibid.

117. "Fukushima Nuclear Radiation Spikes 7,000% as Contaminated Water Pours into the Ocean," *Global Research News* (March 1, 2015). Accessed on May 3, 2015 from http://www.globalresearch.ca/fukushima-radiation-spikes-7000-as-contaminated-water-pours-into-the-ocean/5434258.

118. US Greenhouse Gas Inventory Report: 1990-2013. EPA. (April 2015).

119. *Advancing the Science of Climate Change*. National Research Council Report (2010). The National Academies Press, Washington, DC, USA.

120. *Methane and Nitrous Oxide Emissions from Natural Sources*. EPA Report (April 2010). US Environmental Protection Agency, Washington, DC, USA.

121. Summary Report: Global Anthropogenic Non-CO2 Greenhouse Gas Emissions: 1990 – 2030. US Environmental Protection Agency, Washington, DC, USA. (December 2012).

122. Summary Report: Global Anthropogenic Non-CO2 Greenhouse Gas Emissions: 1990 – 2030. US Environmental Protection Agency, Washington, DC, USA. (December 2012).

123. Summary Report: Global Anthropogenic Non-CO2 Greenhouse Gas Emissions: 1990 – 2030. US Environmental Protection Agency, Washington, DC, USA. (December 2012).

124. *Methane and Nitrous Oxide Emissions from Natural Sources*. EPA Report (April 2010). U.S. Environmental Protection Agency, Washington, DC, USA.

125. "Nitrous Oxide Emissions: Overview of Greenhouse Gases," US Environmental Protection Agency, (April 2015), Accessed on May 1, 2015 from http://www.epa.gov/climatechange/ghgemissions/gases/n2o.html
126. Jan-Martin Rhiemeier and Jochen Harnisch, *Sectoral Emission Reduction Potentials and Economic Costs for Climate Change: F-gases (HFCs, PFCs and SF6)*. Kanaalweg, Netherlands: Ecofys, 2009.
127. "The Inside Story: A Guide to Indoor Air Quality" (1995), by the US EPA Office of Air and Radiation and U.S. Consumer Product Safety Commission, (EPA 402-K-93-007).
128. Anne C Steinemann, et al., "Chemical emissions from residential dryer vents during use of fragranced laundry products." *Air Quality, Atmosphere and Health,* 6 (2013):151-156.
129. "Indoor Air Chemistry: Cleaning Agents, Ozone and Toxic Air Contaminants." California Air Resources Board. May 2006. Accessed from http://www.arb.ca.gov/research/apr/past/01-336.pdf
130. "Clean Air Act Amendments 1990." U.S. Environmental Protection Agency. Accessed from http://www2.epa.gov/laws-regulations/summary-clean-air-act
131. PW Harvey and P Darbre, "Endocrine disruptors and human health: Could estrogenic chemicals in body care cosmetics adversely affect breast cancer incidence in women? A review of evidence and call for further research." *Journal of Applied Toxicology* 24 (2004):167–76.
132. JE Nagel, et al., "Paraben allergy." *J Am Med Assoc.,* 237 (1977):1594–5.
133. Rolf U Halden, "On the Need and Speed of Regulating Triclosan and Tricolocarban in the United States." *Environmental Science & Technology* 48 (2014):3603-3611.
134. "Triclosan: What Consumers Should Know." FDA Consumer Health Information. FDA 2010. Accessed from http://www.fda.gov/ForConsumers/ConsumerUpdates/ucm205999.htm
135. O Albert and B Jegou, "A critical assessment of the endocrine susceptibility of the human testis to phthalates from fetal life to adulthood." *Human Reproduction Update* 20 (2013):231-249.
136. EU Phthalates Directive 2005/84/EC. Accessed from http://eur-lex.europa.eu/legal-content/EN/ALL/?uri=CELEX:32005L0084
137. "PVC Policies Across the World." PVC Factsheet. Center for Health, Environment & Justice. Accessed from http://chej.org/wp-content/uploads/Documents/PVC/2009/Fact-Sheets/110909%20PVC%20Policies%20Across%20the%20World.pdf
138. "Detox my Fashion," (Greenpeace, 2014), Accessed 14 April, 2015 from http://www.greenpeace.org/international/en/campaigns/detox/fashion/
139. Kevin Brigden, et al., "Hazardous chemicals in branded textile products on sale in 25 countries/regions during 2013." Greenpeace Research Laboratories Technical Report 06/201. December 2013.

Chapter 11

1. Food and Agricultural Organization of the United Nations (FAO), Food Security Indicators, 2013. Accessed on March 3, 2015 from http://kff.org/global-indicator/population-undernourished/
2. Alex Hershaft, *Solving the Population/Food Crisis by Eating for Life* (Washington, D.C.: Vegetarian Information Service, 1985).
3. "Food Wastage Footprint: Impacts on Natural Resources," Food and Agriculture Organization of the United Nations (FAO). (2013), Accessed on February 27, 2015 from http://news.nationalgeographic.com/news/2014/10/141013-food-waste-national-security-environment-science-ngfood/

4. "Meat, CashCrop Exports, Contribute to Starvation in Brazil," *Vegetarian Times* (August 1984): 810.
5. Sarrat K Malunder, "Vegetarianism: Fad, Faith or Fact?" *American Scientist*, 60 (1972):177179.
6. James Bonner, "The Population Dilemma," Bulletin no. 95 (January 21, 1965).
7. Frances Moore Lappé and Joseph Collins, *Food First: Beyond the Myth of Scarcity* (New York: Ballantine, 1977).
8. EA Spencer et al., "Diet and body mass index in 38000 EPIC-Oxford meat-eaters, fish-eaters, vegetarians and vegans," *International Journal of Obesity*, 27 (2003):728–734.
9. D Pimental et al., "Will limits of the earth's resources control human numbers?" (Feb 1999). Accessed May 2015 from http://www.jayhanson.us/page174.pdf.
10. Frances Moore Lappé, *Diet for a Small Planet* (New York: Ballantine, 1971).
11. *By-Product Feedstuffs in Dairy Cattle Diets in the Upper Midwest,* (College of Agricultural and Life Sciences: University of Wisconsin at Madison, 2008).
12. *"Crop Production," USDA. National Agricultural Statistics Service. (March 8, 2013). Accessed on February 15, 2015 from* http://www.epa.gov/agriculture/ag101/cropmajor.html
13. Lappé, *Diet for a Small Planet.*
14. R S Harris, "Influence of Culture on Man's Diet," *Arch Environmental Health,* 5 (1962):144152.
15. Ross Hume Hall, *Food for Naught* (New York: Vintage, 1974).
16. Lappé, *Diet for a Small Planet.*
17. Hershaft, *Solving the Population/Food Crisis.*
18. Lappé, *Diet for a Small Planet.*
19. Ibid.
20. "Bill Clinton's Heavy Hand on Haiti's Vulnerable Agricultural Economy: The American Rice Scandal," *Council on Hemispheric Affairs* (April 13, 2010) Accessed on March 3, 2015 from http://www.coha.org/haiti-research-file-neoliberalism%E2%80%99s-heavy-hand-on-haiti%E2%80%99s-vulnerable-agricultural-economy-the-american-rice-scandal/
21. Lappé, *Food First.*
22. Alan Benz, *The Nutrition Factor: Its Role in National Development* (Washington, D.C.: The Brookings Institution, 1973), 65.
23. Lappé, *Food First.*
24. Alan Riding, "Malnutrition Taking Bigger Toll Among Mexican Children," *New York Times,* (6 March 1978), 2.
25. Lappé, *Food First.*
26. Ibid.
27. Ibid.
28. Rensberger, "Starvation in the World."
29. Physicians Committee for Responsible Medicine, "Taxing America's Health: Subsidies for Meat and Dairy Products," (May 2011). Accessed March 20, 2015 from http://www.pcrm.org/search/?cid=2586
30. *National Retail Report – Beef. Advertised Prices for Beef at Major Retail Supermarket Outlets ending during the period of 04/17 thru 04/23.* USDA Agricultural Marketing Service, Livestock, Poultry, and Grain Market News. (April 2015). Accessed April 15, 2015 from http://www.ams.usda.gov/mnreports/lswbfrtl.pdf

31. "Average Retail Food and Energy Prices, U.S. and Midwest Region," U.S. Bureau of Labor Statistics, Mid-Atlantic Information Office. Accessed April 3, 2015 from http://www.bls.gov/regions/mid-atlantic/data/AverageRetailFoodAndEnergyPrices_USandMidwest_Table.htm.

32. C Brown and M Sperow, "Examining the Cost of an All-Organic Diet," *Journal of Food Distribution Research*, 36 (2005):20-26.

33. "Organic poultry profile," Agricultural Marketing Resource Center. (January 2013). Accessed March 31, 2015 from Accessed on March 3, 2015 from http://www.agmrc.org/commodities__products/livestock/poultry/organic-poultry-profile-625/

34. M Lipka, "Is organic chicken worth the price?" *Reuters*, (July 14, 2014). Accessed April 15, 2015 from Accessed on March 3, 2015 from http://www.reuters.com/article/2014/07/17/us-money-chicken-organic-idUSKBN0FM24Q20140717

35. J Bunge and A Chen, "Tyson Expects U.S. Chicken Demand to Outpace Beef, Pork." *The Wall Street Journal*, (November 17, 2014). Accessed April 3, 2015 from http://www.wsj.com/articles/tyson-sales-rise-on-higher-beef-pork-prices-1416229004

36. *National Retail Report - Fruits and Vegetables. Advertised Prices for Fruits & Vegetables at Major Retail Supermarket Outlets ending during the period of 04/11 to 04/23.* (USDA, Agricultural Marketing Service, April 17, 2015). Accessed April 20, 2015 from http://www.ams.usda.gov/mnreports/fvwretail.pdf.

37. Amazon.com, Results for "organic brown rice, Accessed April 11, 2015 from http://www.amazon.com/s/ref=nb_sb_noss_1?url=search-alias%3Daps&field-keywords=organic%20brown%20rice&sprefix=organic+br%2Caps.

38. National Retail Report - Fruits and Vegetables. Advertised Prices for Fruits & Vegetables at Major Retail Supermarket Outlets ending during the period of 04/11 to 04/23. USDA, Agricultural Marketing Service. (April 17, 2015). Accessed April 20, 2015 from http://www.ams.usda.gov/mnreports/fvwretail.pdf.

39. C Jones-Shoeman, "Know the true cost of your beef," *Natural News*, (July 16, 2011). Accessed April 20, 2015 from http://www.naturalnews.com/033011_beef_cost.html.

40. Ingredients weight chart, King Arthur Flour. (2015). Accessed April 20, 2015 from http://www.kingarthurflour.com/recipe/master-weight-chart.html.

41. Nuts and Seeds: Natural Weight-Loss Foods. HowStuffWorks (April 18, 2006). Accessed April 20, 2015 from http://health.howstuffworks.com/wellness/food-nutrition/natural-foods/natural-weight-loss-food-nuts-and-grains-ga.htm.

42. C Jones-Shoeman, "Know the true cost of your beef." *Natural News* (July 16, 2011), Accessed April 15, 2015 from http://www.naturalnews.com/033011_beef_cost.html

43. Sonya Lunder, "FDA Clears BPA In Cans, Again," (Environmental Working Group, 2015), Accessed April, 2015 from http://www.ewg.org/enviroblog/2015/01/fda-clears-bpa-cans-again.

44. S Bae and Y-C Hong, "Exposure to Bisphenol A From Drinking Canned Beverage Increases Blood Pressure," *Hypertension,* 65 (2015):313-319.

45. "Bisphenol A (BPA): Use in Food Contact Application," U.S. Food and Drug Administration. Accessed March 31, 2015 from http://www.fda.gov/food/ingredientspackaginglabeling/foodadditivesingredients/ucm064437.htm#summary; S. Lunder, "FDA Clears BPA In Cans, Again," *EWG*, (January 8, 2015). Accessed on March 3, 2015 from http://www.ewg.org/enviroblog/2015/01/fda-clears-bpa-cans-again.

46. Megan Gannon, "We're In Serious Denial About Our Weight," *Huffington Post*, (June 11, 2014). Accessed on March 3, 2015 from http://www.huffingtonpost.com/2014/06/11/overweight-denial-obesity-weight-americans_n_5484154.html.

Chapter 12

1. Bill Mollison, *Permaculture: A Designers' Manual,* (Tagari Publications 1988).
2. Accessed from http://permacultureprinciples.com/principles
3. Accessed from http://starhawk.org/permaculture-solutions-for-climate-change/
4. RJ Stoner and JM Clawson. *A High Performance, Gravity Insensitive, Enclosed Aeroponic System for Food Production in Space (1997-1998).* Principal Investigator, NASA SBIR NAS10-98030.
5. Accessed from http://www.greenroofs.com/projects/pview.php?id=1461
6. B Ong, "Green plot ratio: an ecological measure for architecture and urban planning," *Landscape and Urban Planning,* 63 (2003):197-211.
7. Y Dreizin et al., "Integrating large scale seawater desalination plants within Israel's water supply system," *Desalination* 220 (2008):132-139.
8. Menachem Elimelech and William A Phillip, "The Future of Seawater Desalination: Energy, Technology, and the Environment," *Science,* (2011). 333:712-717
9. Simon Gottelier, "A desalination boom in California could help it deal with 'exceptional' drought," *The Guardian,* (30 June 2014)
10. *2012 Annual Consumer Report on the Quality of Tap Water.* (City of Cape Coral).
11. Gottelier.
12. Ibid.
13. "Running Pure: The importance of forest protected areas to drinking water." A research report for the World Bank/WWF Alliance for Forest Conservation and Sustainable Use. August 2003.
14. *Convenient Solutions to an Inconvenient Truth: Ecosystem-based Approaches to Climate Change.* (Environment Department, The *World Bank,* June 2009).
15. Matthew Tallis et al.,"Estimating the removal of atmospheric particulate pollution by the urban tree canopy of London, under current and future environments," *Landscape and Urban Planning.* 103 (2011):129-138.
16. "Thirty-five Water Conservation Methods for Agriculture, Farming, and Gardening. Part 4," *Big Picture Agriculture.* http://www.bigpictureagriculture.com/2013/02/more-crop-per-drop-water-agriculture-325.html
17. Michael Amaranthus, "Mycorrhizal fungi awareness emerging in new soil health paradigm," *Australian Farm Journal,* (February 2011).
18. M Malesu, et al., "Rainwater Harvesting for Agricultural Production and Ecological Sustainability," *Green Water Management Handbook.* (Nairobi: The World Agroforesty Centre, 2007).
19. Albert Bates, *The Biochar Solution:* Carbon Farming and Climate Change. New Society Publishers
20. Michael Mortimore et al., "Sustainable Growth in Machakos," *ILEIA Newsletter* 9(4). (December 1993).
21. "What you need to know about energy," National Academy of Sciences,(2008), Accessed on March 3, 2015 from http://www.nap.edu/reports/energy/supply.html.
22. US Senate Committee on Environment & Public Works Hearing Statements 07, August 2003.
23. Accessed from www.walkingschoolbus.org/

24. Marcio Santilli, "Tropical deforestation and the Kyoto Protocol: An editorial essay," *Climatic Change* 71 (2005):267–276.

25. Bradley Rowe, D. "Green roofs as a means of pollution abatement," *Environmental Pollution,* 159 (2011):2100-2110.

26. Accessed from www.london.gov.uk

27. Matthew Tallis et al., "Estimating the removal of atmospheric particulate pollution by the urban tree canopy of London, under current and future environments," *Landscape and Urban Planning.* 103 (2011:129-138.

28. "SA Urban Forests: Million Trees Program. Over six years of achievement 2003-2009," *Government of South Australia.*

29. Accessed from www.denverwater.org/Conservation/Xeriscape/XeriscapePlans/

30. Accessed from http://www.sdcc.ie/services/planning/strategic-development-zones/clonburris

31. Simon Joss, et al., *Eco-Cities — A Global Survey 2011,* (University of Westminster).

32. Accessed from http://www.2030districts.org/seattle/case-studies

33. William D Solecki et al., "Mitigation of the heat island effect in urban New Jersey," *Global Environmental Change Part B: Environmental Hazards,* 6 (2005):39-49.

34. Accessed from www.cubaagriculture.com/agriculture-today.htm

35. John Paull, "Incredible Edible Todmorden: Eating the Street," *Farming Matters* 27 (2011):28-29.

36. W Passchier-Vermeer and W. Passchier, "Noise exposure and public health," *Environmental Health Perspectives,* 108 (2000):123–131.

37. S Wakefield et al., "Growing urban health: Community gardening in South-East Toronto," *Health Promotion International,* 22 (2007):92-101.

38. General Comment No. 15. "The right to water," (UN Committee on Economic, Social and Cultural Rights, November 2002).

39. Ibid.

40. "Poor sanitation threatens public health," Joint News Release WHO/UNICEF.

41. *WRI. World resources, 1992-1993.* New York, Oxford University Press, 1992.

42. A Prüss-Üstün et al, *Safer water, better health: costs, benefits and sustainability of interventions to protect and promote health,* (World Health Organization, 2008).

43. World Health Organization. *Creating healthy cities in the 21st century.* (Geneva: World Health Organization, 1996).

44. Uno Winblad, "Towards an ecological approach to sanitation," *Sanitation Promotion.* SIDA - SDC - WSSCC – WHO (1998), 292.

45. Yoloquetzatl. Ceballos, "Urine as fertilizer in Mexico City. Sanitation Promotion. SIDA - SDC – WSSCC," (WHO. 1998), 292.

46. FH King, *Farmers of Forty Centuries: permanent agriculture in China, Korea and Japan.* (Pennsylvania: Rodale Press, 1973, originally published in 1909).

47. S Matsui, "Nightsoil collection and treatment in Japan (1997)," In: *Ecological Alternatives in Sanitation.* Proceedings from Sida Sanitation Workshop. Stockholm, Sweden.

48. *Ecological alternatives in sanitation.* Publications on Water Resources No. 9, Sida. Stockholm, Sweden.

49. Surendra K Pradhan. et al., "Use of Human Urine Fertilizer in Cultivation of Cabbage (*Brassica oleracea*)—Impacts on Chemical, Microbial, and Flavor Quality," *J. Agric. Food Chem.,* 55 (2007):8657–8663.

50. Joseph Jenkins, *The Humanure Handbook: A Guide to Composting Human Manure* (Chelsea Green Publishing, 2005).
51. PH Gleick and HS Cooley, "Energy implications of bottled water," *Environmental Research Letters*, 4 (2009):014009.
52. Accessed from http://www.bundyontap.com.au/
53. Remanufactured Goods: An Overview of the United States and Global Industries, Markets, and Trade. USITC, (2012).
54. "Reuse of Office Furniture – Incorporation into the 'Quick Wins' Criteria. A study of the market potential for reused and remanufactured office furniture in the UK," *CRR*, (2009).
55. "Alternative Business Model Caste Study: Remanufacturing Office Furniture," *WRAP*, (2014).
56. Accessed from http://starhawk.org/permaculture-solutions-for-climate-change/
57. Executive Order B-29-15. Executive Department, State of California. (April 2015). Accessed on March 3, 2015 from http://gov.ca.gov/docs/4.1.15_Executive_Order.pdf; ."California water restrictions should cover oil companies, activists say," *RT*, (April 3, 2015). Accessed April 15, 2015 from http://rt.com/usa/246429-california-water-mandate-oil-companies/
58. US Drought Monitor: California. The National Drought Mitigation Center, USDA. Accessed March 31, 2015 from http://www.theguardian.com/us-news/2015/apr/05/california-water-restrictions-have-not-stopped-the-sprinklers-from-flowing
59. M Haugen et al., "The influence of fast and vegetarian diet on parameters of nutritional status in patients with rheumatoid arthritis," *Clin Rheumatol.,* 12 (1993):62–9.
60. J Robbins, *The Food Revolution: How Your Diet Can Help Save Your Life And Our World.* (Conari Press, 2010). Accessed on March 3, 2015 from http://johnrobbins.info/other-books-by-john/the-food-revolution/
61. M Tobin, "Gallup finds rising hostility toward environmentalists," *EcoWest*, (May 30, 2013). Accessed on March 3, 2015 from http://ecowest.org/2013/05/30/gallup-finds-rising-hostility-toward-environmentalists/
62. "Environment," (Gallup, 2015), Accessed April, 2015 from http://www.gallup.com/poll/1615/environment.aspx
63. "How Americans view the top energy and environmental issues," (Pew Research Center, January 15, 2015). Accessed on March 3, 2015 from http://www.pewresearch.org/key-data-points/environment-energy-2/
64. "Millennials: We Help The Earth But Don't Call Us Environmentalists," *NPR*, (October 11, 2014). Accessed on March 3, 2015 from http://www.npr.org/2014/10/11/355163205/millennials-well-help-the-planet-but-dont-call-us-environmentalists
65. "Millennials in Adulthood: Pew Research Survey," *Pew Research Center* (Feb. 14-23, 2014).
66. United States Survey: How do you feel about global climate change? (by generation), *Statista*, (March 2014). Accessed on March 3, 2015 from http://www.statista.com/statistics/297260/united-states-global-climate-change-public-opinion-generation/
67. "Millennials: We Help The Earth But Don't Call Us Environmentalists." NPR.
68. *Climate Change 2014: Synthesis Report*. Contribution of Working Groups I, II and III to the Fifth Assessment Report of the Intergovernmental Panel on Climate Change [Core Writing Team, RK Pachauri and LA Meyer (eds.)].(Geneva, Switzerland:IPCC, 2014).

69. E Hertwich et al., *UNEP Assessing the Environmental Impacts of Consumption and Production: Priority Products and Materials,* A Report of the Working Group on the Environmental Impacts of Products and Materials to the International Panel for Sustainable Resource Management (2010).
70. John Robbins, "Eating for the Environment" (all-creatures.org) Environmental Articles Archive. Accessed on March 3, 2015 from http://www.all-creatures.org/articles/env-eatingfor.html.
71. G Ellen, "What Does it Mean to "Live Off the Grid?" " *Elephant Journal.* (September 24, 2013). Accessed on March 3, 2015 from http://www.elephantjournal.com/2013/09/what-does-it-mean-to-live-off-the-grid/
72. J Platt, "Going off the grid: Why more people are choosing to live life unplugged," *Mother Nature Network*, (November 14, 2012), Accessed on March 3, 2015 from http://www.mnn.com/lifestyle/responsible-living/stories/going-off-the-grid-why-more-people-are-choosing-to-live-life-un
73. N Rosen, "Off-grid living: it's time to take back the power from the energy companies," *The Guardian*, (April 11, 2014). Accessed on March 3, 2015 from http://www.theguardian.com/lifeandstyle/2014/apr/11/power-energy-companies
74. Rosen, *The Guardian.*
75. W Koch, "Could you live off-grid? More Americans give it a try," *USA TODAY*, (August 9, 2010), Accessed March 31, 2015 from http://content.usatoday.com/communities/greenhouse/post/2010/08/americans-living-off-grid/1.
76. C Thompson, "Why living off the grid will get a lot easier in 25 years," *CNBC*, (November 27, 2014). Accessed on March 3, 2015 from http://www.cnbc.com/id/102170511.

INDEX

B

C

D

G

H

M

N

O

P